TEXTBOOK *of* CLINICAL ECHOCARDIOGRAPHY

FOURTH EDITION

TEXTBOOK *of* CLINICAL ECHOCARDIOGRAPHY

CATHERINE M. OTTO, MD

J. Ward Kennedy-Hamilton Endowed Professor of Cardiology
Director, Training Programs in Cardiovascular Disease
University of Washington School of Medicine
Associate Director, Echocardiography Laboratory
Co-Director, Adult Congenital Heart Disease Clinic
University of Washington Medical Center
Seattle, Washington

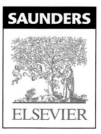

SAUNDERS

ELSEVIER

SAUNDERS
ELSEVIER

1600 John F. Kennedy Boulevard
Suite 1800
Philadelphia, PA 19103-2899

TEXTBOOK OF CLINICAL ECHOCARDIOGRAPHY, FOURTH EDITION ISBN: 978-1-4160-5559-4
Copyright © 2009 by Saunders, an imprint of Elsevier, Inc.

Notice

Knowledge and best practice in this field are constantly changing. As new research and experience broaden our knowledge, changes in practice, treatment and drug therapy may become necessary or appropriate. Readers are advised to check the most current information provided (i) on procedures featured or (ii) by the manufacturer of each product to be administered, to verify the recommended dose or formula, the method and duration of administration, and contraindications. It is the responsibility of the practitioner, relying on their own experience and knowledge of the patient, to make diagnoses, to determine dosages and the best treatment for each individual patient, and to take all appropriate safety precautions. To the fullest extent of the law, neither the Publisher nor the Author assumes any liability for any injury and/or damage to persons or property arising out of or related to any use of the material contained in this book.

The Publisher

Previous editions copyrighted 2004, 2000, 1995.

Library of Congress Cataloging-in-Publication Data
Otto, Catherine M.
  Textbook of clinical echocardiography / Catherine M. Otto. – 4th ed.
    p.; cm.
  Includes bibliographical references and index.
  ISBN 978-1-4160-5559-4
1. Echocardiography. I. Title.
[DNLM: 1. Echocardiography. 2. Heart Diseases–ultrasonography.   WG 141.5.E2 O91t 2009]
RC683.5.U5O87 2009
616.1'207543–dc22

                                        2009007994

Executive Publisher: Natasha Andjelkovic
Developmental Editor: Anne Snyder
Design Direction: Lou Forgione

ISBN: 978-1-4160-5559-4

Printed in China.

Last digit is the print number: 9 8 7 6 5 4 3 2

PREFACE

Echocardiography is an integral part of clinical cardiology with important applications in the initial diagnosis, clinical management, and decision making for patients with a wide range of cardiovascular diseases. In addition to examinations performed in the echocardiography laboratory, echocardiographic techniques are now used in a variety of other clinical settings, including the coronary care unit, intensive care unit, operating room, emergency department, catheterization laboratory, and electrophysiology laboratory, both for diagnosis and for monitoring the effects of therapeutic interventions. There continues to be expansion of echocardiographic applications given the detailed and precise anatomic and physiologic information that can be obtained with this technique at a relatively low cost and with minimal risk to the patient.

This textbook on general clinical echocardiography is intended to be read by individuals new to echocardiography and by those interested in updating their knowledge in this area. The text is aimed primarily at cardiology fellows on their basic echocardiography rotation but also will be of value to residents and fellows in general internal medicine, radiology, anesthesiology, and emergency medicine, as well as to cardiac sonography students. For physicians in practice, this textbook provides a concise and practical update. For additional clinical examples, practical tips for data acquisition, and self-assessment questions, the *Echocardiography Review Guide*, by Schwaegler and Otto (Elsevier/Saunders 2007) parallels the information provided in this textbook. A more advanced discussion of the impact of echocardiographic data in clinical medicine is available in a larger reference book, *The Practice of Clinical Echocardiography*, *3rd edition* (CM Otto [ed], 2007), also published by Elsevier/Saunders. The DVD that accompanies that book includes cases with cine images and interactive multiple choice questions for each chapter.

This book is structured around a clinical approach to echocardiographic diagnosis. First, a framework of basic principles is provided with chapters on ultrasound physics, normal tomographic transthoracic and transesophageal views, intracardiac flow patterns, indications for echocardiography, and evaluation of left ventricular systolic and diastolic function. A chapter on advanced echocardiographic modalities introduces the concepts of 3D echocardiography, myocardial mechanics, contrast echocardiography, and intracardiac echocardiography. Clinical use of these modalities is integrated into subsequent chapters as appropriate. Some of these modalities, such as intracardiac and intravascular echocardiography, typically are utilized by cardiologists with training in interventional procedures. Physicians and sonographers who plan to utilize these modalities in their clinical practices are referred to chapters in *The Practice of Clinical Echocardiography* and other suggested reading.

This framework of basic principles then is built upon in subsequent chapters, organized by disease category (for example, cardiomyopathy or valvular stenosis), corresponding to the typical indications for echocardiography in clinical practice. In each chapter, basic principles for echocardiographic evaluation of that disease category are reviewed, the echocardiographic approach and differential diagnosis are discussed in detail, limitations and technical considerations are emphasized, and alternate diagnostic approaches are delineated. Schematic diagrams are used to illustrate basic concepts; echocardiographic images and Doppler data show typical and unusual findings in patients with each disease process. Transthoracic and transesophageal images, Doppler data, and advanced imaging modalities are used throughout the text, reflecting their use in clinical practice. Tables are used frequently to summarize studies validating quantitative echocardiographic methods.

A selected list of annotated references is included at the end of each chapter. These references are suggestions for the individual who is interested in reading more about a particular subject. Additional relevant articles can be found in the suggested readings or in *The Clinical Practice of Echocardiography*. An online medical reference database is the best way to obtain more recent publications and to obtain a comprehensive list of all journal articles on a specific topic.

A special feature of this book that grew out of my experience teaching fellows and sonographers is The Echo Exam section at the end of the book. This section serves as a summary of the important concepts in each chapter and provides examples of the quantitative calculations used in the day-to-day clinical practice of echocardiography. The information in The Echo Exam is arranged as lists, tables, and figures for clarity. My hope is that The Echo Exam will also serve as a quick reference guide when a review is needed and in daily practice in the echocardiography laboratory.

In the fourth edition, the text of all the chapters has been revised to reflect recent advances in the field, the suggested readings have been updated, and the majority of the figures have been replaced with recent examples that more clearly illustrate the disease process. In the first chapter, the sections on ultrasound physics have been expanded to provide the knowledge base needed for certification examinations in echocardiography. Many sections in other chapters have been extensively revised, including diastolic dysfunction, advanced echocardiographic modalities, cardiomyopathies, and adult congenial heart disease. The use of transesophageal imaging is explicitly integrated into each chapter. Updated guidelines for echocardiography have been included in each chapter when available. A new chapter on "Intraoperative Transesophageal Echocardiography" has been added to provide an introduction to this clinical application and to highlight some of the unique aspects of echocardiographic evaluation of patients undergoing surgical or percutaneous intervention. This chapter includes details of echocardiographic evaluation of patients undergoing mitral valve repair, acute and chronic aortic disease, and management of intracardiac instrumentation, such as left ventricular assist devices.

It should be emphasized that this textbook is only a starting point or frame of reference for learning echocardiography. Appropriate training in echocardiography includes competency in the acquisition and interpretation of echocardiographic and Doppler data in real time. Additional training is needed for performance of stress and transesophageal examinations. Further, echocardiography continues to evolve so that as new techniques, such as 3D echocardiography, become practical and widely available, practitioners will need to update their knowledge. Obviously, a textbook cannot replace the experience gained in performing studies on patients with a range of disease processes, and still photographs do not replace the need for acquisition and review of real-time data. Clearly defined guidelines for training in echocardiography have been published, as referenced in Chapter 5, that serve as guidelines for determining clinical competency in this technique. Although this textbook is not a substitute for appropriate training and experience, I hope it will enhance the learning experience of those new to the field and provide a review for those currently engaged in the acquisition and interpretation of echocardiography. Every patient deserves a clinically appropriate and diagnostically accurate echocardiographic examination; each of us needs to continuously strive toward that goal.

Catherine M. Otto, MD

ACKNOWLEDGMENTS

Many people have provided input to each edition of the *Textbook of Clinical Echocardiography* and the book is immeasurably enhanced by their contributions—not all can be individually thanked here. My appreciation extends to the many readers who provided suggestions for improvement; comments from readers are always welcome. The cardiac sonographers at the University of Washington deserve special thanks for the outstanding quality of their echocardiographic examinations and for our frequent discussions of the details of image acquisition and the optimal echocardiography examination. Their skill in obtaining superb images provides the basis of many of the figures in this book. My thanks to David Diedrick, RDCS; Pam Clark, RDCS; Sarah Curtis, RDCS; Caryn D'Jang, RDCS; Merrit Foley, RDCS; Michelle Fujioka, RDCS; Carol Kraft, RDCS; Yelena Kovolenko, RDCS; Amy Loscher, RDCS; Chris McKenzie, RDCS; Joanna Sangco; Becky Schwaegler, RDCS; Erin Trent, RDCS; and Todd Zwink, RDCS.

My gratitude extends to my colleagues at the University of Washington who shared their expertise and helped identify images for the book, with special thanks to Kelley Branch, MD; Peter Cawley, MD; Michael Chen, MD; Rosario Freeman, MD; Jorg Dziersk, MD; and Karen Stout, MD. The University of Washington Cardiology Fellows also provided thoughtful (and sometimes humbling) insights with particular recognition to Joshua Buckler, MD; Kier Huehnergarth, MD; Eric Krieger, MD; David Owens, MD; Jordan Prutkin, MD; Bipin Ravindran, MD; and Justin Strote, MD. My thanks to Lester C. Permut, MD, for taking the time to help update the tables summarizing congenital heart surgery. Several of my colleagues generously provided illustrations for this edition: Michael Laflamme, MD, provided coronary histology examples; Donald C. Oxorn, MD, provided several intraoperative transesophageal images; Douglas K. Stewart, MD, provided the coronary angiograms, ventriculograms, and intravascular ultrasound images; James H. Caldwell contributed examples of radionuclide studies; and Florence H. Sheehan provided 3D echocardiographic examples for this book. In addition, my gratitude includes my colleagues from around the world who generously provided images, including Harry Acquatella, MD, Centro Medico, San Bernardino, Caracas; Judy W. Hung, MD, Massachusetts General Hospital, Boston, MA; and Nozomi Watanabe, MD, Kawasaki University, Okayama, Japan. Appreciation is also extended to those individuals who kindly gave permission for reproduction of previously published figures. Starr Kaplan is to be commended for her skills as a medical illustrator and for providing such clear and detailed anatomic drawings.

Finally, many thanks to my editor, Natasha Andjelkovic, at Elsevier for providing the support needed to write this edition, and to Anne Snyder and the production team for all the detail-oriented hard work that went into making this book a reality.

CONTENTS

GLOSSARY Abbreviations Used in Figures, Tables, and Equations

2D = two-dimensional
3D = three-dimensional
A-long = apical long-axis
A-mode = amplitude mode (amplitude versus depth)
A = late diastolic ventricular filling velocity with atrial contraction
A' = diastolic tissue Doppler velocity with atrial contraction
A2C = apical two-chamber
A4C = apical four-chamber
AcT = acceleration time
AF = atrial fibrillation
AMVL = anterior mitral valve leaflet
ant = anterior
Ao = aortic or aorta
AR = aortic regurgitation
AS = aortic stenosis
ASD = atrial septal defect
ATVL = anterior tricuspid valve leaflet
AV = atrioventricular
AVA = aortic valve area
AVR = aortic valve replacement

BAV = bicuspid aortic valve
BP = blood pressure
BSA = body surface area

c = propagation velocity of sound in tissue
CAD = coronary artery disease
cath = cardiac catheterization
C_m = specific heat of tissue
cm/s = centimeters per second
cm = centimeters
CMR = cardiac magnetic resonance imaging
CO = cardiac output
cos = cosine
CS = coronary sinus
CSA = cross-sectional area
CT = computed tomography
CW = continuous-wave
Cx = circumflex coronary artery

D = diameter
DA = descending aorta
dB = decibels
dP/dt = rate of change in pressure over time
dT/dt = rate of increase in temperature over time
dyne $\cdot$ s $\cdot$ cm^{-5} = units of resistance

E = early-diastolic peak velocity
E' = early-diastolic tissue Doppler velocity

ECG = electrocardiogram
echo = echocardiography
ED = end-diastole
EDD = end-diastolic dimension
EDV = end-diastolic volume
EF = ejection fraction
endo = endocardium
epi = epicardium
EPSS = E-point septal separation
EROA = effective regurgitant orifice area
ES = end-systole
ESD = end-systolic dimension
ESV = end-systolic volume
ETT = exercise treadmill test

Δf = frequency shift
f = frequency
FL = false lumen
F_n = near field
F_o = resonance frequency
F_s = scattered frequency
FSV = forward stroke volume
F_T = transmitted frequency

HCM = hypertrophic cardiomyopathy
HOCM = hypertrophic obstructive cardiomyopathy
HPRF = high pulse repetition frequency
HR = heart rate
HV = hepatic vein
Hz = Hertz (cycles per second)

I = intensity of ultrasound exposure
IAS = interatrial septum
ID = indicator dilution
inf = inferior
IV = intravenous
IVC = inferior vena cava
IVCT = isovolumic contraction time
IVRT = isovolumic relaxation time

kHz = kilohertz

l = length
LA = left atrium
LAA = left atrial appendage
LAD = left anterior descending coronary artery
LAE = left atrial enlargement
lat = lateral
LCC = left coronary cusp
LMCA = left main coronary artery
LPA = left pulmonary artery

LSPV = left superior pulmonary vein
L-TGA = corrected transposition of the great arteries
LV = left ventricle
LV-EDP = left ventricular end-diastolic pressure
LVH = left ventricular hypertrophy
LVID = left ventricular internal dimension
LVOT = left ventricular outflow tract

M-mode = motion display (depth versus time)
MAC = mitral annular calcification
MI = myocardial infarction
MR = mitral regurgitation
MS = mitral stenosis
MV = mitral valve
MVA = mitral valve area
MVL = mitral valve leaflet
MVR = mitral valve replacement

n = number of subjects
NBTE = nonbacterial thrombotic endocarditis
NCC = noncoronary cusp

ΔP = pressure gradient
P = pressure
PA = pulmonary artery
PAP = pulmonary artery pressure
PCI = percutaneous coronary intervention
PDA = patent ductus arteriosus or posterior descending artery (depends on context)
PE = pericardial effusion
PEP = preejection period
PET = positron-emission tomography
PISA = proximal isovelocity surface area
PLAX = parasternal long-axis
PM = papillary muscle
PMVL = posterior mitral valve leaflet
post = posterior (or inferior-lateral) ventricular wall
PR = pulmonic regurgitation
PRF = pulse repetition frequency
PRFR = peak rapid filling rate
PS = pulmonic stenosis
PSAX = parasternal short-axis
PV = pulmonary vein
PVC = premature ventricular contraction
PVR = pulmonary vascular resistance
PWT = posterior wall thickness

Q = volume flow rate
Q_{p} = pulmonic volume flow rate
Q_{s} = systemic volume flow rate

r = correlation coefficient
R = ventricular radius
R_{FR} = regurgitant instantaneous flow rate
RA = right atrium
RAE = right atrial enlargement
RAO = right anterior oblique
RAP = right atrial pressure

RCA = right coronary artery
RCC = right coronary cusp
R_{e} = Reynolds number
RF = regurgitant fraction
RJ = regurgitant jet
R_{o} = radius of microbubble
ROA = regurgitant orifice area
RPA = right pulmonary artery
RSPV = right superior pulmonary vein
RSV = regurgitant stroke volume
RV = right ventricle
RVE = right ventricular enlargement
RVH = right ventricular hypertrophy
RVOT = right ventricular outflow tract

s = second
SAM = systolic anterior motion
SC = subcostal
SEE = standard error of the estimate
SPPA = spatial peak pulse average
SPTA = spatial peak temporal average
SSN = suprasternal notch
ST = septal thickness
STJ = sinotubular junction
STVL = septal tricuspid valve leaflet
SV = stroke volume or sample volume (depends on context)
SVC = superior vena cava

$T^{1}/_{2}$ = pressure half-time
TD = thermodilution
TEE = transesophageal echocardiography
TGA = transposition of the great arteries
TGC = time gain compensation
Th = wall thickness
TL = true lumen
TN = true negatives
TOF = tetralogy of Fallot
TP = true positives
TPV = time to peak velocity
TR = tricuspid regurgitation
TS = tricuspid stenosis
TSV = total stroke volume
TTE = transthoracic echocardiography
TV = tricuspid valve

v = velocity
V = volume or velocity (depends on context)
VAS = ventriculo-atrial septum
Veg = vegetation
$V_{\max}$ = maximum velocity
VSD = ventricular septal defect
VTI = velocity-time integral

WPW = Wolff-Parkinson-White syndrome

$\mathcal{Z}$ = acoustic impedance

Symbols	Greek Name	Used for
α	alpha	Frequency
γ	gamma	Viscosity
Δ	Delta	Difference
θ	theta	Angle
λ	lambda	Wavelength
μ	mu	Micro-
π	pi	Mathematical constant (approx. 3.14)
ρ	rho	Tissue density
σ	sigma	Wall stress
τ	tau	Time constant of ventricular relaxation

UNITS OF MEASURE

Variable	Unit	Definition
Amplitude	dB	Decibels = a logarithmic scale describing the amplitude ("loudness") of the sound wave
Angle	degrees	Degree = $(\pi/180)$rad. Example: intercept angle
Area	cm^2	Square centimeters. A two-dimensional measurement (e.g., end-systolic area) or a calculated value (e.g., continuity equation valve area)
Frequency (f)	Hz kHz MHz	Hertz (cycles per second) Kilohertz = 1000 Hz Megahertz = 1,000,000 Hz
Length	cm mm	Centimeter (1/100 m) Millimeter (1/1000 m or 1/10 cm)
Mass	g	Grams. Example: LV mass

Variable	Unit	Definition
Pressure	mmHg	Millimeters of mercury, 1 mmHg = 1333.2 dyne/cm^2, where dyne measures force in $cm \cdot g \cdot s^{-2}$
Resistance	dyne $\cdot$ s $\cdot$ cm^{-5}	Measure of vascular resistance
Time	s ms μs	Second Millisecond (1/1000 s) Microsecond
Ultrasound intensity	W/cm^2 mW/cm^2	Where watt (W) = joule per second and joule = $m^2 \cdot kg \cdot s^{-2}$ (unit of energy)
Velocity (v)	m/s cm/s	Meters per second Centimeters per second
Velocity-time integral (VTI)	cm	Integral of the Doppler velocity curve (cm/s) over time (s), in units of cm
Volume	cm^3 mL L	Cubic centimeters Milliliter, 1 mL = 1 cm^3 Liter = 1000 mL
Volume flow rate (Q)	 L/min mL/s	Rate of volume flow across a valve or in cardiac output L/min = liters per minute mL/s = milliliters per second
Wall stress	dyne/cm^2 kdyn/cm^2 kPa	Units of meridional or circumferential wall stress Kilodynes per cm^2 Kilopascals where 1 kPa = 10 kdyn/cm^2

KEY EQUATIONS

Ultrasound Physics

Frequency $\quad f = \text{cycles/s} = \text{Hz}$

Wavelength $\quad \lambda = c/f = 1.54/f(\text{MHz})$

Doppler equation $\quad v = c \times \Delta f/[2F_T(\cos\theta)]$

Bernoulli equation $\quad \Delta P = 4V^2$

LV Imaging

Stroke volume $\quad \text{SV} = \text{EDV} - \text{ESV}$

Ejection fraction $\quad \text{EF}(\%) = (\text{SV/EDV}) \times 100\%$

Wall stress $\quad \sigma = \text{PR}/2\text{Th}$

Doppler Ventricular Function

Stroke volume $\quad \text{SV} = \text{CSA} \times \text{VTI}$

Rate of pressure rise $\quad dP/dt = 32 \text{ mm Hg/time from 1 to 3 m/s of MR CW jet(sec)}$

Pulmonary Pressures and Resistance

Pulmonary systolic pressure $\quad \text{PAP}_{\text{systolic}} = 4(V_{\text{TR}})2 + \text{RAP}$

PAP (when PS is present) $\quad \text{PAP}_{\text{systolic}} = 4(V_{\text{TR}})2 + \text{RAP}] - \Delta P_{\text{RV-PA}}$

Pulmonary vascular resistance $\quad \text{PVR} \cong 10\,(V_{\text{TR}})/\text{VTI}_{\text{RVOT}}$

Aortic Stenosis

Maximum pressure gradient (integrate over ejection period for mean gradient) $\quad \Delta P_{\max} = 4\,(V_{\max})^2$

Continuity equation valve area $\quad \text{AVA}(\text{cm}^2) = [\pi(\text{LVOT}_D/2)^2 \times \text{VTI}_{\text{LVOT}}]/\text{VTI}_{\text{AS-Jet}}$

Simplified continuity equation $\quad \text{AVA}(\text{cm}^2) = [\pi(\text{LVOT}_D/2)^2 \times V_{\text{LVOT}}]/V_{\text{AS-Jet}}$

Velocity ratio $\quad \text{Velocity ratio} = V_{\text{LVOT}}/V_{\text{AS-Jet}}$

Mitral Stenosis

Pressure half time valve area $\quad \text{MVA}_{\text{Doppler}} = 220/\text{T}^1/_2$

Aortic Regurgitation

Total stroke volume $\quad \text{TSV} = \text{SV}_{\text{LVOT}} = \text{CSA}_{\text{LVOT}} \times \text{VTI}_{\text{LVOT}})$

Forward stroke volume $\quad \text{FSV} = \text{SV}_{\text{MA}} = (\text{CSA}_{\text{MA}} \times \text{VTI}_{\text{MA}})$

Regurgitant volume $\quad \text{RV} = \text{TSV} - \text{FSV}$

Regurgitant orifice area $\quad \text{ROA} = \text{RSV}/\text{VTI}_{\text{AR}}$

Mitral Regurgitation

Total stroke volume OR 2D LV stroke volume $\quad \text{TSV} = \text{SV}_{\text{MA}} = (\text{CSA}_{\text{MA}} \times \text{VTI}_{\text{MA}})$

Forward stroke volume $\quad \text{FSV} = \text{SV}_{\text{LVOT}} = (\text{CSA}_{\text{LVOT}} \times \text{VTI}_{\text{LVOT}})$

Regurgitant volume $\quad \text{RV} = \text{TSV} - \text{FSV}$

Regurgitant orifice area $\quad \text{ROA} = \text{RSV}/\text{VTI}_{\text{AR}}$

PISA method

Regurgitant flow rate $\quad R_{\text{FR}} = 2\pi r^2 \times V_{\text{aliasing}}$

Orifice area (maximum) $\quad \text{ROA}_{\max} = R_{\text{FR}}/V_{\text{MR}}$

Regurgitant volume $\quad \text{RV} = \text{ROA} \times \text{VTI}_{\text{MR}}$

Aortic Dilation

Predicted sinus diameter

Children (<18 years): Predicted sinus dimension = 1.02 + (0.98 BSA)

Adults (age 18–40 years): Predicted sinus dimension = 0.97 + (1.12 BSA)

Adults (>40 years): Predicted sinus dimension = 1.92 + (0.74 BSA)

Ratio = Measured maximum diameter/Predicted maximum diameter

Pulmonary (Q_p) to Systemic (Q_s) Shunt Ratio

$Q_p : Q_s = [\text{CSA}_{\text{PA}} \times \text{VTI}_{\text{PA}}]/[\text{CSA}_{\text{LVOT}} \times \text{VTI}_{\text{LVOT}}]$

1

Principles of Echocardiographic Image Acquisition and Doppler Analysis

A n understanding of the basic principles of ultrasound imaging and Doppler echocardiography is essential both during data acquisition and for correct interpretation of the ultrasound information. Although at times current instruments provide instantaneous images so clear and detailed that it seems as if we can "see" the heart and blood flow directly, in actuality, we always are looking at images and flow data generated by complex analyses of ultrasound waves reflected and backscattered from the patient's body. Knowledge of the strengths of this technique and, more important, its limitations is critical for correct clinical diagnosis and patient management. On the one hand, echocardiography can be used for decision making with a high degree of accuracy in a variety of clinical settings. On the other hand, if an ultrasound artifact is mistaken for an anatomic abnormality, a patient might undergo needless, expensive, and potentially risky other diagnostic tests or therapeutic interventions.

In this chapter, a brief (and necessarily simplified) overview of the basic principles of cardiac ultrasound imaging and flow analysis is presented. The reader is referred to the Suggested Reading at the end of the chapter for more information on these subjects. Since the details of image processing, artifact formation, and Doppler physics become more meaningful with experience, some readers may choose to return to this chapter after reading other sections of this book and after participating in some echocardiographic examinations.

ULTRASOUND WAVES

Sound waves are mechanical vibrations that induce alternate refractions and compressions of any physical medium through which they pass (Fig. 1–1). Like other waves, sound waves are described in terms of (Table 1–1):

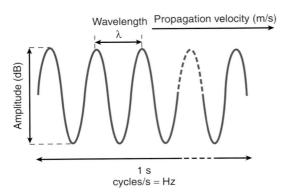

Figure 1–1 Schematic diagram of an ultrasound wave.

❏ Frequency: cycles per second (cycles/s), or hertz (Hz)
❏ Velocity of propagation
❏ Wavelength: millimeters (mm)
❏ Amplitude: decibels (dB)

Frequency (*f*) is the number of ultrasound waves in a 1-second interval. The units of measurement are hertz, abbreviated Hz, which simply means cycles per second. A frequency of 1000 cycles/s is 1 kilohertz (kHz), and 1 million cycles/s is 1 megahertz (MHz). Humans can hear sound waves with frequen-cies between 20 Hz and 20 kHz; frequencies higher than this range are termed *ultrasound*. Diagnostic medical ultrasound typically uses transducers with a frequency between 1 and 20 MHz.

The speed that a sound wave moves through the body, called the *velocity of propagation* (*c*), is different for each type of tissue. For example, the velocity of propagation in bone is much faster (about 3000 m/s) than in lung tissue (about 700 m/s). However, the velocity of propagation in soft tissues, including myocardium, valves, blood vessels, and blood is relatively uniform, averaging about 1540 m/s.

Wavelength is the distance from peak to peak of an ultrasound wave. Wavelength can be calculated by dividing the frequency (*f* in Hz) by the propagation velocity (*c* in m/s).

$$\lambda = c/f \qquad (1-1)$$

Since the propagation velocity in the heart is constant at 1540 m/s, using units of MHz for transducer frequency and dividing by 1000 to convert m to mm, the wavelength for any transducer frequency can be calculated as

$$\lambda(\text{mm}) = 1.54/f$$

TABLE 1–1 Ultrasound Waves			
	Definition	**Examples**	**Clinical Implications**
Frequency (*f*)	The number of cycles per second in an ultrasound wave. *f* = cycles/s = Hz	Transducer frequencies are measured in MHz (1,000,000 cycles/s). Doppler signal frequencies are measured in kHz (1000 cycles/s).	Different transducer frequencies are used for specific clinical applications, because the transmitted frequency affects ultrasound tissue penetration, image resolution, and the Doppler signal.
Velocity of Propagation (*c*)	The speed that ultrasound travels through tissue	The average velocity of ultrasound in soft tissue is about 1540 m/s.	The velocity of propagation is similar in various soft tissues (blood, myocardium, liver, fat, etc.) but is much lower in lung and much higher in bone.
Wavelength (λ)	The distance between ultrasound waves: λ = c/f = 1.54/f (in MHz)	Wavelength is shorter with a higher frequency transducer and longer with a lower frequency transducer.	Image resolution is greatest (~1 mm) with a shorter wavelength (higher frequency). Depth of tissue penetration is greatest with a longer wavelength (lower frequency).
Amplitude (dB)	Height of the ultrasound wave or "loudness" measured in decibels (dB)	A log scale is used for decibels. On the decibel scale, 80 dB represents a 10,000-fold and 40 dB indicates a 100-fold increase in amplitude.	A very wide range of amplitudes can be displayed using a gray-scale display for both imaging and spectral Doppler.

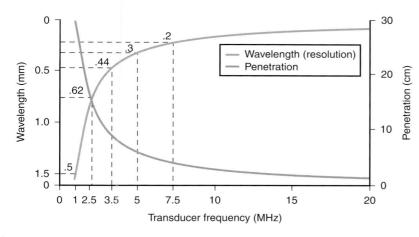

Figure 1–2 Graph of transducer frequency (*horizontal axis*) versus wavelength and penetration of the ultrasound signal in soft tissue. Wavelength has been plotted inversely to show that resolution increases with increasing transducer frequency while penetration decreases. The specific wavelengths for transducer frequencies of 1, 2.5, 3.5, 5, and 7.5 MHz are shown.

as shown in Figure 1–2. For example, the wavelength emitted by a 5-MHz transducer can be calculated as

$$\lambda = 1540 \text{ m/s}/5,000,000 \text{ cycles/s} = 0.000308 \text{ m}$$
$$= 0.308 \text{ mm}$$

or as:

$$\lambda = 1.54/s = 0.308 \text{ mm}$$

Wavelength is important in diagnostic applications for at least two reasons:

❏ Image resolution is no greater than 1 to 2 wavelengths (typically about 1 mm).
❏ The depth of penetration of the ultrasound wave into the body is directly related to wavelength; shorter wavelengths penetrate a shorter distance than longer wavelengths.

Thus, there is an obvious tradeoff between image resolution (shorter wavelength or higher frequency preferable) and depth penetration (longer wavelength or lower frequency preferable).

The acoustic pressure or *amplitude* of an ultrasound wave indicates the energy of the ultrasound signal. Power is the amount of energy per unit time. Intensity (I) is the amount of power per unit area:

$$\text{Intensity } (I) = \text{power}^2 \qquad (1\text{–}2)$$

This relationship shows that if ultrasound power is doubled, intensity is quadrupled. Instead of using direct measures of pressure energy, ultrasound amplitude is described relative to a reference value using the decibel scale. Decibels are familiar to all of us as the standard description of the loudness of a sound. Decibels (dB) are logarithmic units based on a ratio of the measured amplitude (A_2) to a reference amplitude (A_1) such that

$$dB = 20 \log(A_2/A_1) \qquad (1\text{–}3)$$

Thus, a ratio of 1000 to 1 is

$$20 \times \log(1000) = 20 \times 3 = 60 \text{ dB}$$

a ratio of 100 to 1 is

$$20 \times \log(100) = 20 \times 2 = 40 \text{ dB}$$

and a ratio of 2 to 1 is

$$20 \times \log(2) = 20 \times 0.3 = 6 \text{ dB}$$

A simple rule to remember is that a 6-dB change represents a doubling or halving of the signal amplitude or that a 40-dB change represents a 100 times difference in amplitude (Fig. 1–3). If acoustic intensity is used instead of amplitude, the constant 10 replaces 20 in the equation so that a 3-dB change represents doubling and a 20-dB change indicates a 100-fold difference in amplitude. Either of these decibel scales may be used to refer to transmitted or received ultrasound waves or to describe attenuation effects. The advantages of the decibel scale are that a very large range can be compressed into a smaller number of values and that low-amplitude (weak) signals can be displayed alongside very high-amplitude (strong) signals. In an echocardiographic image, amplitudes typically range from 1 to 120 dB. The decibel scale is the standard format both for echocardiographic image display and for the Doppler spectral display, although other amplitude scales may be an option.

ULTRASOUND-TISSUE INTERACTION

Propagation of ultrasound waves in the body to generate ultrasound images and Doppler data depends on a tissue property called *acoustic impedance* (Table 1–2). Acoustic impedance (Z) depends on tissue density (ρ) and on the propagation velocity in that tissue (c):

$$Z = \rho c \qquad (1\text{–}4)$$

Although the velocity of propagation differs between tissues (e.g., bone has a propagation velocity about twice as fast as blood), tissue density is the primary determinant of acoustic impedance for diagnostic ultrasound. Lung tissue has a very low density as compared with bone, which has a very high density. Soft tissues such

Figure 1–3 Graph of the decibel scale (*horizontal axis*) showing the logarithmic relationship with the amplitude ratio (*vertical axis*). Note that a doubling or halving of the amplitude ratio corresponds to a 6-dB change, and a 100-fold difference in amplitude corresponds to a 20-dB change.

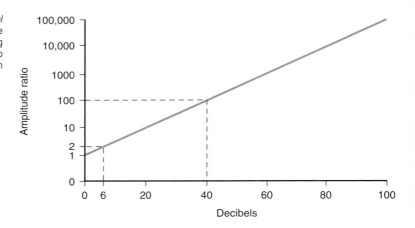

TABLE 1–2 Ultrasound-Tissue Interaction

	Definition	Examples	Clinical Implications
Acoustic impedance (Z)	A characteristic of each tissue defined by tissue density (ρ) and propagation of velocity (c) as: $Z = \rho \times c$	Lung has a low density and low propagation velocity, whereas bone has a high density and high propagation velocity. Soft tissues have smaller differences in tissue density and acoustic impedance.	Ultrasound is reflected from boundaries between tissues with differences in acoustic impedance (e.g., blood versus myocardium).
Reflection	Return of ultrasound signal to the transducer from a smooth tissue boundary	Reflection is used to generate 2D cardiac images.	Reflection is greatest when the ultrasound beam is perpendicular to the tissue interface.
Scattering	Radiation of ultrasound in multiple directions from small structures, such as blood cells.	The change in frequency of signals scattered from moving blood cells is the basis of Doppler ultrasound.	The amplitude of scattered signals is 100 to 1000 times less than reflected signals.
Refraction	Deflection of ultrasound waves from a straight path due to differences in acoustic impedance	Refraction is used in transducer design to focus the ultrasound beam.	Refraction in tissues results in double-image artifacts.
Attenuation	Loss in signal strength due to absorption of ultrasound energy by tissues	Attenuation is frequency dependent, with greater attenuation (less penetration) at higher frequencies.	A lower frequency transducer may be needed for apical views or in larger patients on transthoracic imaging.
Resolution	The smallest resolvable distance between two specular reflectors on an ultrasound image	Resolution has three dimensions—along the length of the beam (axial), lateral across the image (azimuthal), and in the elevational plane.	Axial resolution is most precise (as small as 1 mm), so imaging measurements are best made along the length of the ultrasound beam.

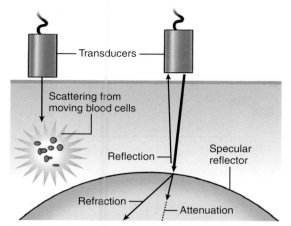

Figure 1–4 Diagram of the interaction between ultrasound and body tissues. Doppler analysis is based on the scattering of ultrasound in all directions from moving blood cells with a resulting change in frequency of the ultrasound received at the transducer. 2D imaging is based on reflection of ultrasound from tissue interfaces (specular reflectors). Attenuation limits the depth of ultrasound penetration. Refraction, a change in direction of the ultrasound wave, results in imaging artifacts.

as blood and myocardium have much smaller differences in acoustic impedance. Acoustic impedance determines the transmission of ultrasound waves through a tissue; differences in acoustic impedance result in reflection of ultrasound waves at tissue boundaries.

The interaction of ultrasound waves with the organs and tissues of the body can be described in terms of (Fig. 1–4):

◻ Reflection
◻ Scattering
◻ Refraction
◻ Attenuation

Reflection

The basis of ultrasound imaging is *reflection* of the transmitted ultrasound signal from internal structures. Ultrasound is reflected at tissue boundaries and interfaces, with the amount of ultrasound reflected dependent on (1) the relative change in acoustic impedance between the two tissues and (2) the angle of reflection. Smooth tissue boundaries with a lateral dimension greater than the wavelength of the ultrasound beam act as specular, or "mirror-like," reflectors. The amount of ultrasound reflected is constant for a given interface, although the amount received back at the transducer varies with angle because (like light reflected from a mirror) the angles of incidence and reflection are equal. Thus, optimal return of reflected ultrasound occurs at a perpendicular angle (90°). Remembering this fact is crucial for obtaining diagnostic ultrasound images. It also accounts for ultrasound "dropout" in a two-dimensional (2D) or three-dimensional (3D) images when too little or no reflected ultrasound reaches the transducer due to a parallel alignment between the ultrasound beam and tissue interface.

Scattering

Scattering of the ultrasound signal, instead of reflection, occurs with small structures, such as red blood cells suspended in fluid, because the radius of the cell (about 4 µm) is smaller than the wavelength of the ultrasound signal. Unlike a reflected beam, scattered ultrasound energy may be radiated in all directions. Only a small amount of the scattered signal reaches the receiving transducer, and the amplitude of a scattered signal is 100 to 1000 times (40–60 dB) less than the amplitude of the returned signal from a specular reflector. Scattering of ultrasound from moving blood cells is the basis of Doppler echocardiography.

The *extent* of scattering depends on:

◻ Particle size (red blood cells)
◻ Number of particles (hematocrit)
◻ Ultrasound transducer frequency
◻ Compressibility of blood cells and plasma

Although experimental studies show differences in backscattering with changes in hematocrit, variation over the clinical range has little effect on the Doppler signal. Similarly, the size of red blood cells and the compressibility of blood cells and plasma do not change significantly. Thus, the primary determinant of scattering is transducer frequency.

Scattering also occurs within tissues, such as the myocardium, from interference of backscattered signals from tissue interfaces smaller than the ultrasound wavelength. Tissue scattering results in a pattern of *speckles* that can be used to measure tissue motion by tracking these speckles from frame to frame, as discussed in Chapter 4.

Refraction

Ultrasound waves can be *refracted*—deflected from a straight path—as they pass through a medium with a different acoustic impedance. Refraction of an ultrasound beam is analogous to refraction of light waves as they pass through a curved glass lens (e.g., prescription eyeglasses). Refraction allows enhanced image quality by using acoustic "lenses" to focus the ultrasound beam. However, refraction also occurs in unplanned ways during image formation, resulting in ultrasound artifacts, most notably a double-image artifact.

Attenuation

Attenuation is the loss of signal strength as ultrasound interacts with tissue. As ultrasound penetrates into the body, signal strength is progressively *attenuated* due to absorption of the ultrasound energy by conversion to heat, as well as by reflection and scattering. The degree of attenuation is related to several factors including the:

◻ Attenuation coefficient of the tissue
◻ Transducer frequency
◻ Distance from the transducer
◻ Ultrasound intensity (or power)

The attenuation coefficient (α) for each tissue is related to the decrease in ultrasound intensity (measured in $-$dB) from one point (I_1) to a second point (I_2) separated by a distance (l) as described by the equation:

$$I_2 = I_1 \cdot e^{-2\alpha l} \qquad (1-5)$$

The attenuation coefficient for air is very high (about $1000\times$) compared with soft tissue, so that any air between the transducer and the cardiac structures of interest causes substantial signal attenuation. This is avoided on transthoracic examinations by use of a water-soluble gel to form an airless contact between the transducer and the skin; on transesophageal echocardiography (TEE) attenuation is avoided by maintaining close contact between the transducer and the esophageal wall. The air-filled lungs are avoided by careful patient positioning and the use of acoustic "windows" that allow access of the ultrasound beam to the cardiac structures without intervening lung tissue. Other intrathoracic air (e.g., pneumomediastinum, residual air after cardiac surgery) also results in poor ultrasound tissue penetration due to attenuation, resulting in suboptimal image quality.

The power output of the transducer is directly related to the overall degree of attenuation. However, an increase in power output may cause thermal and mechanical bioeffects as discussed in "Bioeffects and Safety" below.

Overall attenuation is also frequency dependent such that lower ultrasound frequencies penetrate deeper into the body than higher frequencies. The depth of penetration for adequate imaging tends to be limited to approximately 200 wavelengths. This translates roughly into a penetration depth of 30 cm for a 1-MHz transducer, 6 cm for a 5-MHz transducer, and 1.5 cm for a 20-MHz transducer, although diagnostic images at depths greater than these postulated limits can be obtained with state-of-the-art equipment. Thus, attenuation, as much as resolution, dictates the need for a particular transducer frequency in a specific clinical setting. For example, visualization of distal structures from the apical approach in a large adult patient often requires a low-frequency transducer. From a TEE approach, the same structures can be imaged (at better resolution) with a higher-frequency transducer. The effects of attenuation are minimized on displayed images by using different gain settings at each depth, an instrument control called time-gain (or depth-gain) compensation.

TRANSDUCERS

Piezoelectric Crystal

Ultrasound transducers use a piezoelectric crystal both to generate and to receive ultrasound waves (Fig. 1–5). A piezoelectric crystal is a material (such

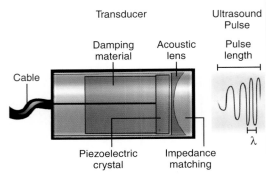

Figure 1–5 Schematic diagram of an ultrasound transducer. The piezoelectric crystal both produces and receives ultrasound signals, with the electric input/output transmitted to the instrument via the cable. Damping material allows a short pulse length (improved resolution). The shape of the piezoelectric crystal, an acoustic lens, or electronic focusing (with a phased-array transducer) are used to modify the beam geometry. The material of the transducer surface provides impedance matching with the skin. The ultrasound pulse length for 2D imaging is short (1–6 ms), typically consisting of two wavelengths (λ). "Ring down"—the decrease in frequency and amplitude in the pulse—depends on damping and determines bandwidth (the range of frequencies in the signal).

as quartz or a titanate ceramic) with the property that an applied electric current results in alignment of polarized particles perpendicular to the face of the crystal with consequent expansion of crystal size. When an alternating electric current is applied, the crystal alternately compresses and expands, generating an ultrasound wave. The frequency that a transducer emits depends on the nature and thickness of the piezoelectric material.

Conversely, when an ultrasound wave strikes the piezoelectric crystal, an electric current is generated. Thus, the crystal can serve both as a "receiver" and as a "transmitter." Basically, the ultrasound transducer transmits a brief burst of ultrasound and then switches to the "receive mode" to await the reflected ultrasound signals from the intracardiac acoustic interfaces. This cycle is repeated temporally and spatially to generate ultrasound images. Image formation is based on the *time delay* between ultrasound transmission and return of the reflected signal. Deeper structures have a longer time of flight than shallower structures, with the exact depth calculated based on the speed of sound in blood and the time interval between the transmitted burst of ultrasound and return of the reflected signal.

The burst, or pulse, of ultrasound generated by the piezoelectric crystal is very brief, typically 1 to 6 μs, since a short pulse length results in improved axial (along the length of the beam) resolution. Damping material is used to control the ring-down time of the crystal and, hence, the pulse length. Pulse length also is determined by frequency, since a shorter time is needed for the same number of cycles at higher frequencies.

The range of frequencies contained in the pulse is described as its *frequency bandwidth*. A wider bandwidth allows better axial resolution due to the ability of the system to produce a narrow pulse. Transducer bandwidth also affects the range of frequencies that can be detected by the system, with a wider bandwidth allowing better resolution of structures distant from the transducer. The stated frequency of a transducer represents the center frequency of the pulse.

Types of Transducers

The simplest type of ultrasound transducer is based on a single piezoelectric crystal (Table 1–3). Alternate pulsed transmission and reception periods allow repeated sampling along a single line, with the sampling rate limited only by the time delay needed for return of the reflected ultrasound wave from the depth of interest. An example

TABLE 1–3 Ultrasound Transducers

	Definition	Examples	Clinical Implications
Type	Transducer characteristics and configuration Most cardiac transducers use a phased array of piezoelectric crystals.	Transthoracic (adult and pediatric) Non-imaging CW Doppler 3D echocardiography TEE Intracardiac	Each transducer type is optimized for a specific clinical application. More than one transducer may be needed for a full examination.
Transmission frequency	The central frequency emitted by the transducer	Transducer frequencies vary from 2.5 MHz for TTE to 20 MHz for intravascular imaging.	A higher frequency transducer provides improved resolution but less penetration. Doppler signals are optimal at a lower transducer frequency than used for imaging.
Power output	The amount of ultrasound energy emitted by the transducer	An increase in transmitted power increases the amplitude of the reflected ultrasound signals.	Excessive power output may result in bioeffects measured by the mechanical and thermal indexes.
Bandwidth	The range of frequencies in the ultrasound pulse	Bandwidth is determined by transducer design.	A wider bandwidth allows improved axial resolution for structures distant from the transducer.
Pulse (or burst) length	The length of the transmitted ultrasound signal	A higher frequency signal can be transmitted in a shorter pulse length compared to a lower frequency signal.	A shorter pulse length improves axial resolution.
PRF	The number of transmission-receive cycles per second	The PRF decreases as imaging (or Doppler) depth increases because of the time needed for the signal to travel from and to the transducer.	PRF affects image resolution and frame rate (particularly with color Doppler).
Focal depth	Beam shape and focusing are used to optimize ultrasound resolutions at a specific distance from the transducer.	Structures close to the transducer are best visualized with a short focal depth, distant structures with a long focal depth.	The length and site of a transducer's focal zone are primarily determined by transducer design, but adjustment during the exam may be possible.
Aperture	The surface of the transducer face where ultrasound is transmitted and received	A small non-imaging CW Doppler transducer allows optimal positioning and angulation of the ultrasound beam.	A larger aperture allows a more focused beam. A smaller aperture allows improved transducer angulation on TTE imaging.

of using the transducer for simple transmission-reception along a single line is an A-mode (amplitude versus depth) or M-mode (depth versus time) cardiac recording when a high sampling rate is desirable.

Formation of a 2D or 3D cardiac ultrasound image uses an array of ultrasound crystals arranged in the transducer to provide a tomographic or volumetric dataset of signals. Each element in the transducer array can be controlled electronically both to direct the ultrasound beam across the region of interest and to focus the transmitted and received signals. Echocardiographic imaging uses a *sector scanning* format with the ultrasound signal originating from a single location (the narrow end of the sector), resulting in a fanlike shape of the image. Sector scanning is optimal for cardiac applications, because it allows a fast frame rate to show cardiac motion and a small transducer size (aperture or "footprint") to fit into the narrow acoustic windows used in echocardiography. A 3D ultrasound transducer may use a more complex array of crystals to generate a volume of image data, instead of a tomographic dataset (see Chapter 4).

Most transducers can provide simultaneous imaging and Doppler analysis; for example, 2D imaging and a superimposed color Doppler display. Quantitative Doppler velocity data are recorded with the image "frozen" or with only intermittent image updates, so that the ultrasound crystals can be used to optimize the Doppler signal. Although continuous-wave Doppler signals can be obtained using two elements of a combined transducer, use of a dedicated non-imaging transducer with two separate crystals (with one crystal continuously transmitting and the other continuously receiving the ultrasound waves) is recommended when accurate high-velocity recordings are needed. The final configuration of a transducer depends on transducer frequency (higher frequency transducers are smaller) and beam focusing, as well as the intended clinical use—for example, transthoracic versus TEE imaging.

Beam Shape and Focusing

An unfocused ultrasound beam is shaped like the light from a flashlight with a tubular beam for a short distance that then diverges into a broad cone of light (Fig. 1–6). Even with current focused transducers, ultrasound beams have a 3D shape that affects measurement accuracy and contributes to imaging artifacts. Beam shape and size depend on several factors, including:

❏ Transducer frequency
❏ Distance from the transducer
❏ Aperture size and shape
❏ Beam focusing

Aperture size and shape and beam focusing can be manipulated in the design of the transducer, but the effects of frequency and depth are inherent to ultrasound physics. For an unfocused beam, the initial segment of the beam is columnar in shape (near field F_n) with a length dependent on the diameter D of the transducer face and wavelength (λ):

$$F_n = D^2/4\lambda \qquad (1\text{--}6)$$

For a 3.5-MHz transducer with a 5-mm diameter aperture, this corresponds to a columnar length of 1.4 cm. Beyond this region the ultrasound beam diverges (far field), with the angle of divergence θ determined as:

$$\sin \theta = 1.22\lambda/D \qquad (1\text{--}7)$$

This equation indicates a divergence angle of 6° beyond the near field, resulting in an ultrasound beam width of about 4.4 cm at a depth of 20 cm for this 3.5-MHz transducer. With a 10-mm diameter aperture, F_n would be 5.7 cm and beam width at 20 cm would be about 2.5 cm (Fig. 1–7).

The shape and focal depth (narrowest point) of the primary beam can be altered by making the surface of the piezoelectric crystal concave or by adding an

Figure 1–6 Schematic diagram of beam geometry for an unfocused (*left*) and focused (*right*) transducer. The length of the near zone and the divergence angle in the far field depend on transducer frequency and aperture. The focal zone of a focused transducer can be adjusted, but beam width still depends on depth. Side lobes (and grating lobes with phased-array transducers) occur with both focused and unfocused transducers and, like the central beam, are three dimensional.

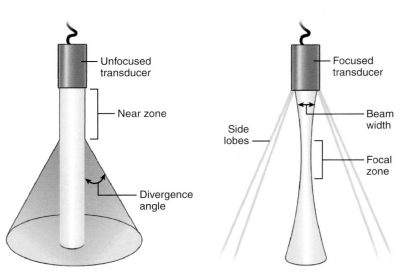

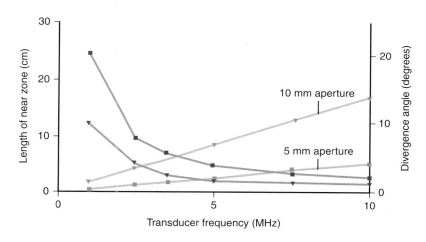

Figure 1–7 Graph of transducer frequency (*horizontal axis*) versus length of the near zone (*yellow lines*) and divergence angle (*blue lines*) for an unfocused 5- (*squares*) and 10-mm (*triangles*) diameter aperture transducer. Equations 1–6 and 1–7 were used to generate these curves.

acoustic lens. This allows generation of a beam with optimal characteristics at the depth of most cardiac structures, but again, divergence of the beam beyond the focal zone occurs. Some transducers allow manipulation of the focal zone during the examination. Even with focusing, the ultrasound beam generated by each transducer has a lateral and an elevational dimension that depends on the transducer aperture, frequency, and focusing. Beam geometry for phased-array transducers also depends on the size, spacing, and arrangement of the piezoelectric crystals in the array.

In addition to the main ultrasound beam, dispersion of ultrasound energy laterally from a single-crystal transducer results in formation of *side lobes* at an angle θ from the central beam where $\sin \theta = m\lambda/D$, and *m* is an integer describing sequential side lobes (i.e., 1, 2, 3, and so on) (Fig. 1–8). Reflected or backscattered signals from these side lobes may be received by the transducer, resulting in image or flow artifacts. With phased-array transducers additional accessory beams at an even greater angle from the primary beam, termed *grating lobes*, also occur as a result of constructive interference of ultrasound wave fronts (Fig. 1–9). Both the side lobes and the grating lobes affect the lateral and elevational resolution of the transducer.

Resolution

Image resolution occurs for each of three dimensions: (1) *axial resolution*, that is, along the length of the ultrasound beam, (2) *lateral resolution*, that is, the resolution side to side across the 2D image, and (3) *elevational resolution*, that is, the thickness of the tomographic "slice" (Fig. 1–10).

Of these three, axial resolution is most precise, so quantitative measurements are made most reliably using data derived from a perpendicular alignment between the ultrasound beam and the structure of interest. Axial resolution depends on the transducer frequency, bandwidth, and pulse length but is independent of depth (Table 1–4). Determination of the smallest resolvable distance between two specular reflectors with ultrasound is complex but is typically about twice the transmitted wavelength; higher frequency (shorter wavelength) transducers have greater axial resolution. For example, with a 3.5-MHz transducer axial resolution is about 1 mm, versus 0.5 mm with a 7.5-MHz transducer. A wider bandwidth also improves resolution by allowing a shorter pulse, thus avoiding overlap between the reflected ultrasound signals from two adjacent reflectors.

Lateral resolution varies with the depth of the specular reflector from the transducer, being most dependent on beam width at each depth. With a narrow beam width in the focal region, lateral resolution may approach axial resolution, and a point target will appear as a point on the 2D image. At greater depths, beam width diverges so a point target results in a reflected signal as wide as the beam width. The lack of lateral resolution at greater depths accounts for the "blurring" of the image in the far field. If the 2D image is examined carefully, progressive widening of the echo signals from similar targets along the ultrasound beam can be appreciated (Fig. 1–11). Erroneous interpretations occur when the effects of beam width are not recognized. For example, beam width artifact from a strong specular reflector in the tomographic plane may appear as a linear abnormal structure. Other factors that affect lateral resolution are transducer frequency, aperture, bandwidth, and side and grating lobe levels.

Resolution in the elevational plane is more difficult to recognize on the 2D image but is equally important in the echocardiographic examination. The thickness of the tomographic plane is variable over the 2D image, depending on transducer design and focusing, both of which affect beam width in the elevational plane at each depth. In general, cardiac ultrasound images have a "thickness" of approximately 3 to 10 mm depending on depth and the specific transducer used. The tomographic image

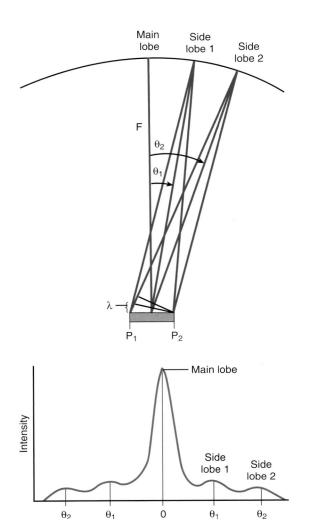

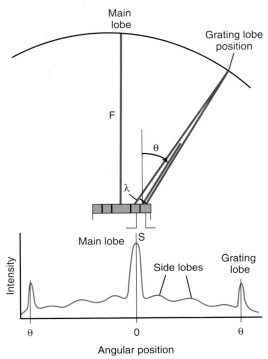

Figure 1–9 *Top,* Diagram showing the position of grating lobes in phased-array transducers. The position of grating lobes is determined by the spacing between the centers of independent crystal elements in the transducer. At any point where the path length between the two crystal elements differs by one wavelength, a grating lobe is formed. The grating lobe is formed at an angle θ that depends on the wavelength λ of the crystals and spacing S between the crystal elements. *Bottom,* The beam intensity plot formed at focal length F. *(From Geiser EA: Echocardiography: Physics and instrumentation. In Skorton DJ, Schelbert AR, Wolf GL, Brundage BH (eds): Marcus Cardiac Imaging, 2nd ed. Philadelphia: WB Saunders, 1996, p 283. Used with permission.)*

Figure 1–8 *Top,* Diagram showing the positions at which side lobes will form. Side lobes occur at the points where the distances traversed by the ultrasound pulse from each edge of the crystal face differ by exactly one wavelength. Note that the distance from the left edge of the crystal point at point P_1 to the position of side lobe 1 is exactly one wavelength longer than the distance from point P_2 at the extreme right edge of the crystal to the position of side lobe 1. *Bottom,* The beam intensity plot formed by sweeping along an arc at focal length F. *(From Geiser EA: Echocardioagraphy: Physics and instrumentation. In Skorton DJ, Schelbert AR, Wolf GL, Brundage BH (eds): Marcus Cardiac Imaging, 2nd ed. Philadelphia: WB Saunders, 1996, p 280. Used with permission.)*

generated by the instrument, in effect, includes reflected and backscattered signals from this entire thickness. Strong reflectors adjacent to the image plane may appear to be "in" the image plane due to elevational beam width. Even more distant strong reflectors may appear superimposed on the tomographic plane due to side lobes in the elevational plane. Examples include a calcified aortic valve appearing as a "mass" in the left atrium (LA) on apical views or a linear echo in the aortic lumen from an adjacent calcified atheroma appearing as a possible dissection flap. These principles of ultrasound imaging also apply to 3D echocardiography.

ULTRASOUND INSTRUMENTS AND IMAGING MODALITIES

M-Mode

Historically, cardiac ultrasound began with a single-crystal transducer display of the amplitude (A) of reflected ultrasound versus depth on an oscilloscope screen. An A-mode display may still be shown on the 2D image screen to aid the examiner in optimal adjustment of the instrument controls. Repeated pulse transmission-and-receive cycles allow rapid updating of the amplitude-versus-depth information so that rapidly moving structures, such as the aortic or mitral valve leaflets, can be identified by their characteristic timing and pattern of motion (Fig. 1–12).

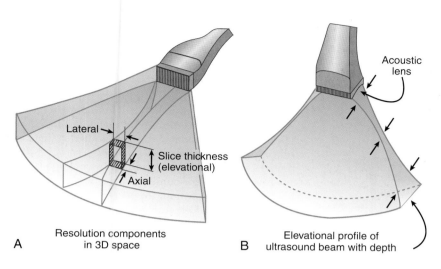

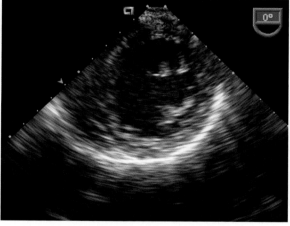

Figure 1–10 *Left,* The axial, lateral, and elevational slice thickness in three dimensions are shown for a phased-array transducer ultrasound beam. Axial resolution along the direction of the beam is independent of depth; lateral resolution and elevational resolution are strongly depth dependent. Lateral resolution is determined by transmit and receive focus electronics; elevational resolution is determined by the height of the transducer elements. At the focal distance, axial is better than lateral and is better than elevational resolution. *Right,* Elevational resolution profile with an acoustic lens across the transducer array produces a focal zone in the slice thickness direction. *(Redrawn from Bushberg JT, Seibert JA, Leidholdt EM, Boone JM: The Essential Physics of Medical Imaging. Philadelphia: Lippincott Williams & Wilkins, 2002, Fig. 6–21.)*

TABLE 1–4	Determinants of Resolution in Ultrasound Imaging

Axial Resolution

Transducer frequency
Transducer bandwidth
Pulse length

Lateral Resolution

Transducer frequency
Beam width (focusing) at each depth*
Aperture (width) of transducer
Bandwidth
Side and grating lobe levels

Elevational Resolution

Transducer frequency
Beam width in elevational plane

*Most important.

Figure 1–11 Two-dimensional echocardiographic view of the left ventricle (LV) from a TEE approach at end-diastole. Even with excellent image quality, as in this example, the effect of beam width can be appreciated by comparing the length of reflections from the endocardium near the transducer and more distal reflectors. Note the relative "dropout" of the epicardium and endocardium when parallel to the ultrasound beam.

With the time dimension shown explicitly on the horizontal axis and each amplitude signal along the length of the ultrasound beam converted to a corresponding gray-scale level, a *motion (M) mode display* is produced. M-mode data are shown on the video monitor either "scrolling" or "sweeping" across the screen at 50 to 100 mm/s. Two-dimensional imaging allows guidance of the M-mode beam to ensure an appropriate angle between the M-line and the structures of interest.

Because only a single "line of sight" is included in an M-mode tracing, the repetition frequency of the pulse transmission-and-receive phase of the transducer (the pulse repetition frequency, PRF) is limited only by the time needed for the ultrasound beam to travel to the maximum depth of interest and back to the transducer. Even a depth of 20 cm requires only 0.26 ms (given a speed of propagation of 1540 m/s), allowing a pulse frequency up to 3850 times per second. In actual practice, sampling rates of about 1800 times per second are used. This extremely high sampling rate is valuable for accurate evaluation of rapid normal intracardiac motion such as valve opening and closing. In addition, continuously moving structures, such as the ventricular endocardium, may be identified more accurately when motion versus time, as well as depth, is displayed clearly on the M-mode recording. Other examples of rapid intracardiac motion best demonstrated with M-mode imaging include the high-frequency fluttering of the anterior mitral leaflet in patients with aortic regurgitation and the rapid oscillating motion of valvular vegetations.

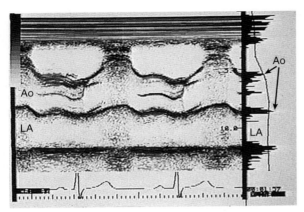

Figure 1–12 An A-mode (along right edge) and M-mode recording of aortic root (Ao), left atrium (LA), and aortic valve motion. On the A-mode recording, the anterior and posterior aortic root (with valve closure in the center) and posterior left atrial wall are clearly identified. The rapid sampling rate of M-mode recording allows visualization of aortic valve motion. The line representing the time-gain compensation curve is shown at the *right* of the image, superimposed on the A-mode signal.

Two-dimensional Echocardiography

Image Production

A 2D echocardiographic image is generated from the data obtained by electronically "sweeping" the ultrasound beam across the tomographic plane. For each scan line, short pulses (or bursts of ultrasound) are emitted at a frequency (PRF) determined by the time needed for ultrasound to travel to and from the maximum image depth. The pulse repetition period is the total time from pulse to pulse, including the length of the ultrasound signal and the time interval between signals.

Since a finite time is needed for each scan line of data (depending on the depth of interest), the time needed to acquire all the data for one image frame is directly related to the number of scan lines and the imaging depth. Thus, PRF is lower at greater imaging depths and higher at shallow depths. In addition, there is a tradeoff between scan line density and image frame rate—the number of images per second. For cardiac applications a high frame rate (≥30 frames per second) is desirable for accurate display of cardiac motion. This frame rate allows 33 ms per frame or 128 scan lines per 2D image at a displayed depth of 20 cm.

The reflected ultrasound signals for each scan line are received by the piezoelectric crystal and a small electric signal generated with (1) an amplitude proportional to incident angle and acoustic impedance and (2) timing proportional to distance from the transducer. This signal undergoes complex manipulation to form the final image displayed on the monitor. Typical processing includes signal amplification, time-gain compensation (TGC), filtering (to reduce noise), compression, and rectification. Envelope detection generates a bright spot for each signal along the scan line, which then undergoes analog-to-digital

scan conversion, since the original polar coordinate data must be fit to a rectangular matrix with appropriate interpolation for missing matrix elements. This image is subject to further "postprocessing" to enhance the visual appreciation of tomographic anatomy and is displayed in "real time" (nearly simultaneous with data acquisition) on the monitor screen.

Although standard ultrasound imaging is based on reflection of the fundamental transmitted frequency from tissue interfaces, *tissue harmonic imaging (THI)* instead is based on the harmonic frequency energy generated as the ultrasound signal propagates through the tissues. These harmonic frequencies result from the nonlinear effects of the interaction of ultrasound with tissue and have two properties key to generation of harmonic images. First, the strength of the harmonic signal increases with depth of propagation. Second, stronger fundamental frequencies produce stronger harmonics. Thus, harmonic imaging reduces near-field and side-lobe artifacts and improves endocardial definition, particularly in patients with poor fundamental frequency images (Fig. 1–13). THI improves visualization of the left ventricular endocardium, which allows border tracing for calculation of ejection fraction, reduces measurement variability, and results in visualization of more myocardial segments during stress echocardiography. However, although THI improves lateral resolution by 20% to 50%, it reduces axial resolution by 40% to 100%. Thus, valves and other planar objects may appear thicker with harmonic as compared with fundamental frequency imaging, so that caution is needed when diagnosing valve abnormalities or making measurements of chamber or vessel size.

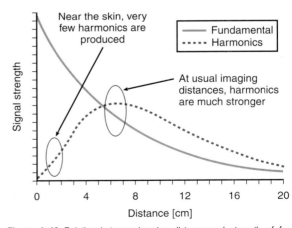

Figure 1–13 Relation between imaging distance and strength of fundamental and harmonic frequencies. As ultrasound pulse propagates, strength of fundamental frequency declines while strength of harmonic frequency increases. At usual imaging distances for cardiac structures, strength of harmonic frequency is maximized. In this schematic, harmonic frequency strength is exaggerated; harmonic frequency signal strength is much lower than fundamental frequency signal strength. *(From Thomas JD, Rubin DN: Tissue harmonic imaging: Why does it work? J Am Soc Echocardiogr 11:803–808, 1998.)*

Instrument Settings

Many of the elements in the process of image formation are features of a particular transducer and instrument that cannot be modified by the operator. However, for each patient and echocardiographic view, optimal image quality depends on selection of a specific transducer and careful adjustment of instrument settings. Standard imaging controls available in most ultrasound systems include:

❐ *Power output*: This control adjusts the total ultrasound energy delivered by the transducer in the transmitted bursts, thus resulting in higher amplitude reflected signals (see "Bioeffects and Safety").

❐ *Gain*: In contrast to power output, the gain control adjusts the displayed amplitude of the received signals, similar to the volume control in an audio system.

❐ *Time-gain compensation*: The TGC panel allows differential adjustment of gain along the length of the ultrasound beam to compensate for the effects of attenuation. Near-field gain can be set lower (since reflected signals are stronger), with a gradually increased gain over the midfield ("ramp" or "slope") and a higher gain in the far field (since reflected signals are weaker). A TGC curve is shown at the *right side* of Figure 1–12. On some instruments, near-field and far-field gains beyond the range of the TGC are adjusted separately.

❐ *Depth*: The displayed depth affects the PRF and frame rate of the image, as well as allowing maximal display of the area of interest on the screen. Standard depth settings show the entire plane (from the transducer down), while "resolution" or "magnification" modes focus on a specific depth range of interest.

❐ *Dynamic range/compression*: The amplitude range (in dB) of the reflected signal is greater than the display capacity of ultrasound systems, so the signal is compressed into a range of values from white to black, or gray scale. The number of levels of gray in the image, or *dynamic range*, can be adjusted to provide an image with marked contrast between light and dark areas or a gradation of gray levels between the lightest and darkest areas. A variation of standard gray scale is to use color intensity for each amplitude value.

Other typical instrument controls include preprocessing and postprocessing settings that change the appearance of the displayed image. Note that image quality and resolution depend on scan-line density (as well as the factors listed in Table 1–4). Scan-line density (or frame rate or both) can be increased by using a lower depth setting or by narrowing the sector to less than the standard 60° wide image.

Imaging Artifacts

Imaging artifacts include (1) extraneous ultrasound signals that result in the appearance of "structures" that are not actually present (at least at that location), (2) failure to visualize structures that are present, and (3) an image of a structure that differs in size and/or shape from its actual appearance. Obviously, recognition of image artifacts is important for both the individual performing the study and the individual interpreting the echocardiographic data (Table 1–5).

The most common image "artifact" is *suboptimal image quality* due to poor ultrasound tissue penetration related to the patient's body habitus with interposition of high attenuation tissues (e.g., lung or bone) or an increased distance (e.g., adipose tissue) between the transducer and cardiac structures. While, strictly speaking, poor image quality is not an "artifact," a low signal-to-noise ratio makes accurate diagnosis difficult and precludes quantitative measurements. In many patients with suboptimal ultrasound penetration, image quality often is improved by use of THI. In some cases TEE imaging may be needed to make an accurate diagnosis.

Acoustic shadowing (Fig. 1–14) occurs when a structure with a marked difference in acoustic impedance (e.g., prosthetic valve, calcium) blocks transmission of the ultrasound wave beyond that point. The image appears devoid of reflected signals distal to this structure, since no signal penetrates beyond the shadowing structure. The shape of the shadow (like a light shadow) follows the ultrasound path, so a small structure near the transducer casts a large shadow. When shadowing occurs, an alternate acoustic window is needed for evaluation of the area of interest. In some cases, a different transthoracic view will suffice. In other cases (e.g., prosthetic mitral valve), TEE imaging may be necessary.

Reverberations (Fig. 1–15) are multiple linear high-amplitude echo signals originating from two strong specular reflectors resulting in back-and-forth reflection of the ultrasound signal before it returns to the transducer. On the image, reverberations appear as relatively parallel, irregular, dense lines extending from the structure into the far field. Like acoustic shadowing, prominent reverberations limit evaluation of structures in the far field. In less dramatic cases, reverberations may appear to represent abnormal structures. For example, in the parasternal long-axis view, a linear echo in the aortic root may originate as a reverberation from anterior structures (e.g., ribs) rather than representing a dissection flap.

The term *beam width artifact* is applied to two separate sources of image artifacts. First, remember that all the structures within the 3D volume of the ultrasound beam are displayed in a single tomographic plane. In the focal zone of the beam, the 3D volume is quite small and the tomographic "slice" is narrow. In the far zone, however, strong reflectors at the edge of a larger beam will be superimposed on structures in the central zone of the beam even though signal intensity falls off at the edges of the beam. In addition, strong reflectors in side lobes of the beam will be displayed in the tomographic section

TABLE 1–5 Ultrasound Imaging Artifacts

Artifact	Mechanism	Example(s)
Suboptimal image quality	Poor ultrasound tissue penetration	Body habitus (obesity, lung disease) Past cardiac surgery
Acoustic shadowing	Reflection of all the ultrasound signal by a strong specular reflector	Prosthetic valve Calcification
Reverberations	Reverberation between two strong parallel reflectors	Prosthetic valve
Beam width	Superimposition of structures within the beam profile (including side lobes) into a single tomographic image	Aortic valve "in" left atrium Atheroma "in" aortic lumen
Lateral resolution	Displayed width of a point target varies with depth.	Excessive width of calcified mass or prosthetic valve
Refraction	Deviation of ultrasound signal from a straight path along the scan line	Double aortic valve or LV image in short-axis view
Range ambiguity	Echo from previous pulse reaches transducer on next cycle.	Second, deeper heart image
Electronic processing	Instrument specific	Variable

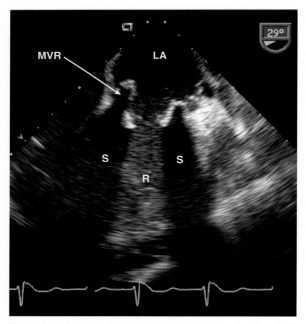

Figure 1–14 Example of acoustic shadowing and reverberations. TEE view of the LA and LV shows shadowing (S) by the sewing ring of a tissue mitral valve with reverberations (R) from the valve further obscuring the LV.

corresponding to the main beam. This type of beam width artifact can result in an image "showing" a calcified aortic valve in the middle of the LA in an apical four-chamber view (Fig. 1–16).

The second type of beam width artifact is a consequence of varying lateral resolution at different imaging depths. A point target appears as a line whose length depends on the beam characteristics at that depth and the amplitude of the reflected signal. For example, the struts on a prosthetic valve can appear much longer than their actual dimension due to poor lateral resolution. Sometimes beam width artifacts can be mistaken for abnormal structures such as a valvular vegetation, an intracardiac mass, or an aortic dissection flap.

The appearance of a side-by-side double image results from ultrasound *refraction* as it passes through a tissue proximal to the structure of interest. This artifact often is seen in parasternal short-axis views of the aortic valve or left ventricle (LV), where a second valve or LV is "seen" medial to and partly overlapping the actual valve or LV. The explanation for this appearance is that the transmitted ultrasound beam is deviated from a straight path (the scan line) by refraction as it passes through a tissue near the transducer. When this refracted beam is reflected back to the transducer by a tissue interface, the reflected signal is assumed to have originated from the scan line of the transmitted pulse (Fig. 1–17) and thus is displayed on the image in the wrong location.

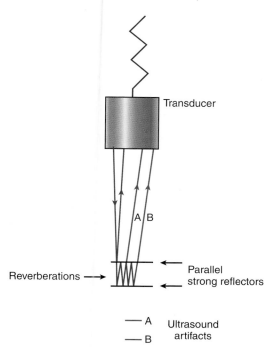

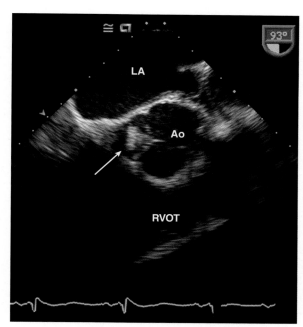

Figure 1–16 Example of beam width artifact. Apparent "mass" attached to the aortic valve on this off-axis TEE view is the noncoronary cusp of the aortic valve seen "en face." Imaging in other planes demonstrated a normal trileaflet aortic valve.

Figure 1–15 Reverberation artifacts result for the interaction of ultrasound with two parallel strong reflectors. The transmitted ultrasound beam (*red with down arrow*) is reflected from the first reflector and returns to the transducer (*red with up arrow*), resulting in an ultrasound signal that corresponds to the correct depth of the reflector. However, ultrasound signals also reflect back and forth between the two strong reflectors, with some signals returning to the transducer after two (A), three (B), or more reverberation cycles. The longer time from transmission to reception of these late-returning signals results in their display on the ultrasound image at points distal to the actual reflector. The exact distance is determined by the separation of the two reflectors and the number of back-and-forth reflections between them as shown for artifacts A and B. In clinical imaging, reverberation artifacts can either appear as a signal linear signal distal to the actual object or as a band of signals obscuring distal structures (see Fig. 1–14) due to multiple parallel reflectors.

Electronic processing artifacts can be difficult to identify and vary from instrument to instrument. In addition, types of artifacts other than those listed have been described.

Range ambiguity occurs when echo signals from an earlier pulse cycle reach the transducer on the next "listen cycle" for that scan line, resulting in deep structures appearing closer to the transducer than their actual location. The appearance of an anatomically unexpected echo within a cardiac chamber often is due to range ambiguity, as can be demonstrated by the disappearance or a change in position of this artifact when the depth setting (and PRF) is changed. Another type of range ambiguity is the appearance of an apparent second heart, deeper than the actual heart—a double image on the vertical axis. This type of range ambiguity results from echoes being re-reflected by a structure close to the transducer (such as a rib), being re-reflected by the cardiac structures and thus received at the transducer at a time *twice* normal. This artifact can be eliminated (or obscured) by decreasing the depth setting or adjusting the transducer position to a better acoustic window.

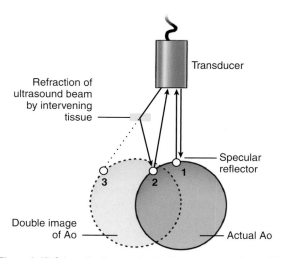

Figure 1–17 Schematic diagram showing the mechanism of a double-image artifact on 2D echocardiography. An ultrasound pulse reflected from point 1 of the LV endocardium returns to the transducer and is shown appropriately as a bright spot in the correct position on the 2D image. Later in the scan an ultrasound pulse is refracted by an intervening tissue so that the beam is reflected back to the transducer from point 2. However, this reflected signal is shown along the transmission scan line (point 3), because this is the presumed origin of the reflected signal. Ao, aorta in cross-section.

Echocardiographic Measurements

Echocardiographic measurements are most accurate using axial resolution, for example, along the length of the ultrasound beam. Measurements can be made using the *leading edge–to–leading edge* convention or at the white-black interface on the tissue. The rationale for measuring from the leading edge is that the first reflection detected from the tissue interface is the best measure of its actual location, with signals arriving slightly later due to reflections from within the tissue, reverberations, and ring-down artifact. The leading edge convention is used for M-mode studies, and much of the literature validating echocardiographic measurements and using these measurements for clinical decision making is based on this measurement approach.

On 2D images identification of the leading edge is challenging—for example, in a parasternal long axis view, separating the leading edge of the LV septal endocardium for signals originating within the septal myocardium. Instead, 2D measurements of cardiac chambers and great vessels are made using the white-black interface; LV internal dimensions are measured from the white-black interface of the septum to the white-black interface of the posterior wall. With current image quality, the white-black interface is a reasonable representation of the actual tissue-blood interface, because the leading edge of the endocardial echo and white-black interface are nearly identical. For measurements of great vessels, such as the aorta, the white-black interface convention is more reproducible than attempts to identify a leading edge on 2D images. Measurement of small solid or planar structures is problematic, although this approach is often used as an estimate of size or thickness.

DOPPLER ECHOCARDIOGRAPHY

Doppler Velocity Data

Doppler Equation

Doppler echocardiography is based on the change in frequency of the backscattered signal from small moving structures (red blood cells) intercepted by the ultrasound beam (Table 1–6). A visual analogy is that Doppler scattering from blood is similar to scattering of light in fog, while imaging is similar to reflections from a mirror. A stationary target, if much smaller than the wavelength, will scatter ultrasound in all directions, with the frequency of the scattered signal being the same as the transmitted frequency when observed from any direction. A moving target, however, will backscatter ultrasound to the transducer so that the frequency observed when the target is moving *toward* the transducer is higher and the frequency observed when the target is moving *away* from the transducer is lower than the original transmitted frequency (Fig. 1–18). This Doppler effect is known to all of us from audio examples

of the change in sound of a car horn, siren, or train whistle as it moves toward (higher pitch) and then away (lower pitch) from the observer.

The difference in frequency between the transmitted frequency (F_T) and the scattered signal received back at the transducer (F_S) is the Doppler shift:

$$\text{Doppler shift} = (F_S - F_T) \qquad (1\text{–}8)$$

Doppler shifts are in the audible range (0–20 kHz) for intracardiac velocities using diagnostic ultrasound transducer frequencies. The relationship between the Doppler shift and blood flow velocity (v, in m/s) is expressed in the Doppler equation:

$$v = c(F_S - F_T)/[2F_T(\cos\theta)] \qquad (1\text{–}9)$$

where c is the speed of sound in blood (1540 m/s), θ is the intercept angle between the ultrasound beam and the direction of blood flow, and 2 is a factor to correct for the transit time both *to* and *from* the scattering source (Fig. 1–19).

Note that intercept angle is critically important in calculation of blood flow velocity. The cosine of an angle of 0° or 180° (parallel toward or away from the transducer) is 1, allowing this term to be ignored when the ultrasound beam is aligned parallel to the direction of blood flow. In contrast, the cosine of 90° is *zero*, indicating that no Doppler shift will be recorded if the ultrasound beam is perpendicular to blood flow.

In cardiac Doppler applications the ultrasound beam is aligned as closely as possible to parallel with the direction of blood flow so that the cos θ can be assumed to be 1. Because the direction of intracardiac blood flow can be difficult to ascertain and is not predictable from the 2D image, especially with abnormal flow patterns, attempts to "correct" for intercept angle may result in significant errors in velocity calculations. Even when blood flow direction is apparent in a 2D plane, direction in the elevational plane remains unknown. Deviation from a parallel intercept angle up to 20° results in a calculated velocity only 6% less than the actual blood flow velocity. However, a 60° intercept angle results in a calculated velocity that is only half the actual velocity. Intercept angle is particularly important for high-velocity jets, such as in valvular stenosis. Although angle correction for the presumed direction of blood flow is used in some peripheral vascular applications, this approach is not acceptable for cardiac applications due to the likelihood that the "correction" will be erroneous.

Spectral Analysis and Doppler Instrument Controls

When the backscattered signal is received at the transducer, the difference between the transmitted and backscattered signals is determined by "comparing" the two waveforms. This is a complex process, since multiple frequencies are present in the backscattered signal. Typically, the frequency content of the signal

TABLE 1–6 Doppler Physics

	Definition	Examples	Clinical Implications
Doppler effect	The change in frequency of ultrasound scattered from a moving target: $v = c \times \Delta F / [2\, F_T (\cos \theta)]$	A higher velocity corresponds to a higher Doppler frequency shift, ranging from 1 to 20 kHz for intracardiac flow velocities.	Ultrasound systems display velocity, which is calculated using the Doppler equation, assuming cos θ equals 1.
Intercept angle	The angle (θ) between the direction of blood flow and the ultrasound beam.	When the ultrasound beam is parallel to the direction of blood flow (0° or 180°), cos θ is 1 and can be ignored in the Doppler equation.	Velocity is underestimated when the intercept angle is not parallel. This can lead to errors in hemodynamic measurements.
CW Doppler	Continuous ultrasound transmission with reception of Doppler signals from the entire length of the ultrasound beam.	CW Doppler allows measurements of high-velocity signals but does not localize the depth of origin of the signal.	CW Doppler is used to measure high velocities in valve stenosis and regurgitation.
Pulsed Doppler	Pulsed ultrasound transmission with timing of reception determining depth of the backscattered signal.	Pulsed Doppler samples velocities from a specific site but can only measure velocity over a limited range.	Pulsed Doppler is used to record low-velocity signals at a specific site, such as LV outflow velocity or LV inflow velocity.
PRF	The number of pulses transmitted per second.	The PRF is limited by the time needed for ultrasound to reach and return from the depth of interest. PRF determines the maximum velocity that can be unambiguously measured.	The maximum velocity measurable with pulsed Doppler is about 1 m/s at 6 cm depth.
Nyquist limit	The maximum frequency shift (or velocity) measurable with pulsed Doppler, equal to ½ PRF	The Nyquist limit is displayed as the top and bottom of the velocity range with the baseline centered.	The greater the depth, the lower the maximum velocity measurable with pulsed Doppler.
Signal aliasing	The phenomenon that the direction of flow for frequency shifts greater than the Nyquist limit cannot be determined.	With aliasing of the LV outflow signal, the peak of the velocity curve is "cut off" and appears as flow in the opposite direction.	Aliasing can result in inaccurate velocity measurements, if not recognized.
Sample volume	The intracardiac location where the pulsed Doppler signal originated.	Sample volume depth is determined by the time interval between transmission and reception. Sample volume length is determined by the duration of the receive cycle.	Sample volume depth and length are adjusted to record the flow of interest.
Spectral analysis	Method used to display Doppler velocity data versus time, with gray scale indicating amplitude.	Spectral analysis is used for both pulsed and CW Doppler.	The velocity scale, baseline position, and time scale of the spectral display are adjusted for each Doppler velocity signal.

CW, continuous-wave; PRF; pulse repetition frequency.

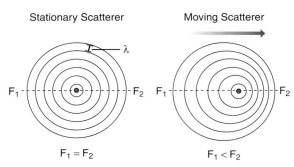

Stationary Scatterer   **Moving Scatterer**

$F_1 = F_2$ $F_1 < F_2$

Figure 1–18 The Doppler effect. A stationary scatterer (*left*) scatters ultrasound symmetrically in all directions with a wavelength identical to the transmitted wavelength and with the same frequency in all directions (no Doppler shift). A moving scatterer (*right*) also scatters ultrasound symmetrically in all directions. However, the frequency will be higher when the scatterer is moving toward the transducer (F_2) than when it is moving away from the transducer (F_1) due to the movement of the scatterer resulting in waves closer together in advance of and further apart behind the moving object.

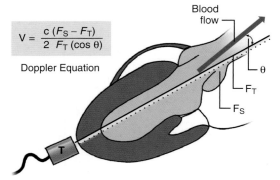

$$V = \frac{c\,(F_S - F_T)}{2\ F_T\,(\cos\theta)}$$

Doppler Equation

Figure 1–19 The Doppler equation. The velocity V of blood flow can be calculated from the speed of sound in blood c, transducer frequency F_T, backscattered frequency F_S, and the cosine of the angle θ between the ultrasound beam and direction of blood flow. T, transducer.

is analyzed by a process known as a *fast Fourier transform* that derives the component frequencies of a complex signal. Alternate methods of frequency analysis also may be used, such as the analog Chirp-Z method.

The display generated by this frequency analysis is termed *spectral analysis* (Fig. 1–20). By convention, this display shows time on the horizontal axis, the zero baseline in the center, and frequency shifts toward the transducer above and frequency shifts away from the baseline. Since multiple frequencies exist at any time point, each frequency signal is displayed as a pixel on the vertical axis, with the gray scale indicating the amplitude (or loudness) and the position on the vertical axis indicating the blood flow velocity (or frequency shift) component. Thus, at each time point the spectral display shows:

❐ Blood flow direction
❐ Velocity (or frequency shift)
❐ Signal amplitude

Each of these components is displayed at 4-ms intervals (or 250 times per second) simultaneous with data acquisition.

Continuous-wave Doppler Ultrasound

Continuous-wave Doppler uses two ultrasound crystals; one continuously transmits and one continuously receives the ultrasound signal. The major advantage of this Doppler modality is that very high-frequency shifts (velocities) can be measured accurately, since sampling is continuous. The potential disadvantage of continuous-wave Doppler is that signals from the entire length of the ultrasound beam are recorded simultaneously. However, even with overlap of flow data, a given signal often is characteristic in timing, shape, and direction, allowing correct identification of the origin of the signal. In some cases, other methods (2D echo, color, pulsed Doppler) must be used to determine the depth of origin of the Doppler signal.

Continuous-wave Doppler optimally is performed with a dedicated, non-imaging transducer with two crystals. This type of transducer has a high signal-to-noise ratio and a small footprint, allowing it to fit into small acoustic windows (e.g., between ribs) and to be angled to obtain a parallel intercept angle between the ultrasound beam and the direction of blood flow. Use of a simultaneous imaging transducer may be helpful in some cases, but signal quality may be poorer, angulation is more difficult, and the 2D image may distract the operator from optimizing the *flow* signal instead of the anatomic image (which may not coincide).

Careful technique yields a Doppler spectral signal that has a smooth contour with a well-defined edge and maximum velocity, as well as with clearly defined onset and end of flow. The audible signal is tonal and smooth. A continuous-wave Doppler velocity curve is "filled in," because lower velocity signals proximal and distal to the point of maximum velocity also are recorded. Note that while the maximum frequency shift depends on the intercept angle between the Doppler beam and the flow of interest, amplitude (gray-scale intensity), shape, and audible quality are less dependent on intercept angle. Thus, a "good quality" Doppler signal may be recorded at a non-parallel intercept angle, resulting in underestimation of flow velocity. The empirical method to ensure a parallel intercept angle is to examine the flow of interest from multiple windows with transducer angulation both in the plane of view and in the elevational plane to discover the highest-frequency shift. The highest value found is then assumed to represent a parallel intercept angle.

Pulsed Doppler Ultrasound

Pulsed Doppler echocardiography allows sampling of blood flow velocities from a specific intracardiac depth. A pulse of ultrasound is transmitted, and then, after a time interval determined by the depth of interest, the transducer briefly "samples" the backscattered signals. This transducer cycle of transmit-wait-receive is repeated at an interval termed the *pulse*

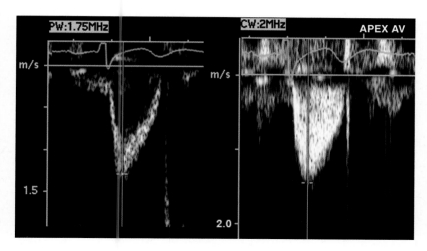

Figure 1–20 Examples of pulsed (*left*) and continuous-wave (CW, *right*) spectral Doppler displays. LV outflow recorded from an apical approach is shown in the standard format. The baseline has been moved from the middle of the vertical axis to display the antegrade flow signal. Velocities toward the transducer are shown above and velocities away from the transducer below the baseline. The velocity range is determined by the Nyquist limit (½ PRF) with pulsed Doppler echo. Velocities are shown in shades of gray corresponding to the amplitude (decibels) of the signal. Note the "envelope" of flow with pulsed Doppler because flow is sampled at a specific intracardiac location with relatively uniform blood flow velocities. With CW Doppler the curve is "filled in" due to multiple blood flow velocities along the entire length of the ultrasound beam.

repetition frequency (PRF) (Fig. 1–21). Since the "wait" interval is determined by the depth of interest—the time it takes ultrasound to travel to and from this depth—each transducer cycle is longer for increasing depths. Thus, the PRF also is depth dependent, being high at shallow depths and low for more distant sites.

The depth of interest in pulsed Doppler echo is called the *sample volume*, because signals from a small volume of blood are sampled, with the width and height of this volume dependent on beam geometry. The length of the sample volume can be varied by adjusting the length of the transducer "receive" interval. Typically, a sample volume length of 3 mm is used to balance range resolution and signal quality, but a longer (5–10 mm) or shorter (1–2 mm) sample volume may be useful in specific cases.

Because pulsed Doppler echo repeatedly samples the returning signal, there is a maximum limit to the frequency shift (or velocity) that can be measured unambiguously. A waveform must be sampled at least twice in each cycle for accurate determination of wavelength. A visual analogy is a motion picture film of a moving wagon wheel. If the frame rate is at least twice as fast as the rotation of the wheel, the forward rotation of the wheel is "seen." If the frame rate and rotation speed are the same, the wheel will appear to stay still. Even slower frame rates result in the appearance of the wheel going backward (Fig. 1–22). This phenomenon of ambiguity in the speed and/or direction of the sampled signal is known as *signal aliasing*. For the frequency of an ultrasound waveform to be correctly identified, it must be sampled at least twice per wavelength. Thus, the maximum detectable frequency shift (the *Nyquist limit*) is one half the PRF.

If the velocity of interest exceeds the Nyquist limit by a small degree, signal aliasing is seen with the signal cut off at the edge of the display and the "top" of the waveform appearing in the reverse channel (Fig. 1–23). In these cases baseline shift (in effect an electronic "cut and paste") restores the expected velocity curve and allows calculation of maximum velocity. When velocities further exceed the Nyquist limit, repeat "wraparound" of the signal occurs first into the reverse channel, then back to the forward channel, and so on. Occasionally, the shape of the

Pulsed Doppler Ultrasound

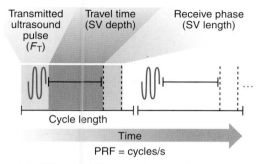

Figure 1–21 With pulsed Doppler ultrasound the transducer goes through a repetitive cycle of transmission of an ultrasound pulse at the transducer frequency (F_T), a waiting period determined by the time needed for the signal to travel to and from the depth of interest, and a receive phase when the backscattered signals are sampled. The travel-time duration determines sample volume depth. The duration of the receive phase determines sample volume length.

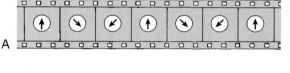
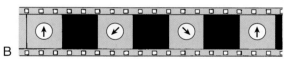

Figure 1–22 Visual analogy for aliasing. The filmstrip in (**A**) shows a wheel rotating clockwise. If the frame rate of the film (or sampling rate) is halved as in (**B**), the wheel will appear to move counterclockwise when the film is played. (*From Otto CM, Pearlman AS: Echocardiography 2:141, 1985.*)

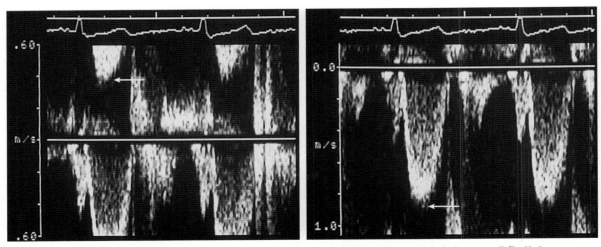

Figure 1–23 The velocity of LV outflow recorded from an apical approach exceeds the Nyquist limit so that aliasing occurs (*left*) with the appearance of the peak of the outflow curve in the reverse channel (*arrow*). This degree of aliasing can be resolved by shifting the baseline (*right*), in effect an electronic "cut and paste" of the spectral display.

waveform can be discerned (Fig. 1–24), but more often only an undifferentiated band of velocity signals can be appreciated (Fig. 1–25). Both nonlaminar disturbed flow and aliased laminar high-velocity flow will appear (and sound) similar on spectral analysis. Methods that can be used to resolve aliasing include:

☐ Using continuous-wave Doppler ultrasound
☐ Increasing the PRF to the maximum for that depth
☐ Increasing the number of sample volumes (high-PRF Doppler)
☐ Using a lower frequency transducer
☐ Shifting the baseline

Continuous-wave Doppler is the most reliable approach to resolving aliasing for very high velocities. The other approaches are useful when the aliased velocity exceeds the Nyquist limit by a modest degree (e.g., ≤ twice the Nyquist limit).

High-PRF Doppler is the deliberate use of range ambiguity to increase the maximum velocity that can be measured with pulsed Doppler echo (Fig. 1–26). When the transducer sends out a pulse, backscattered signals from the entire length of the ultrasound beam return to the transducer. Range resolution is achieved by sampling only those signals in the short time interval corresponding to the depth of interest. However, signals from exactly twice as far away as the sample volume will reach the transducer during the "receive" phase of the next cycle. Thus, signals from "harmonics" at $2\times$, $3\times$, $4\times$, and so on from the sample volume depth, have the potential of being analyzed. Usually signal strength is low and there are few moving scatterers at these depths, so that this range ambiguity can be ignored. If, instead, the sample volume is placed purposely at one-half the depth of interest, backscattered signals from this sample volume (SV_1) and a second sample volume (SV_2)

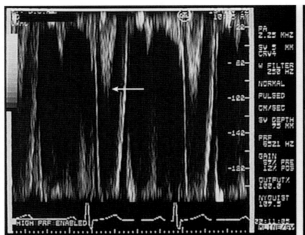
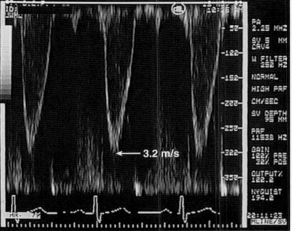

Figure 1–24 In this case LV outflow velocity exceeds twice the Nyquist limit, so that aliasing persists even after baseline shift (*left*). The "wrapped around" peak velocity is clearly seen (*arrow*). With high-PRF Doppler the maximum velocity is resolved in this patient with a subaortic membrane (*right*).

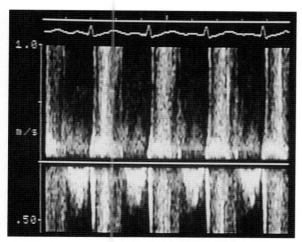

Figure 1–25 Severe aliasing results in a band of frequency shifts due to multiple "wraparounds" of the velocity signal. The maximum velocity cannot be reliably identified unless CW Doppler ultrasound is used.

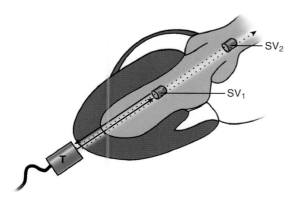

Figure 1–26 High-PRF Doppler ultrasound. High-PRF Doppler is based on the concept that with a given sample volume depth (SV_1) some ultrasound will penetrate beyond that depth. Backscattered signals from exactly twice the set depth (SV_2) will return to the transducer (T) during the receive phase of the next cycle. Thus, signals from both sample volume depths are recorded simultaneously.

twice as far away (i.e., the depth of interest) will return to the transducer during the "receive" phase (albeit one cycle later). This recording of the signal of interest at a higher PRF allows measurement of higher velocities without signal aliasing. An even higher PRF can be achieved by using additional (three or four) proximal sample volumes. Of course, the limitation of this approach is range ambiguity. The spectral analysis now includes signals from each of the sample volume depths. As with continuous-wave Doppler, the origin of the signal of interest must be determined based on ancillary data. However, high PRF Doppler is useful for evaluation of velocities that are just above the aliasing limit of conventional pulsed Doppler. Often the high PRF mode is automatically enabled when the Doppler velocity range is increased.

Doppler Velocity Instrument Controls

Pulsed and continuous-wave Doppler instrument controls typically include:

❐ Power output—the electrical energy transmitted to the transducer
❐ Receiver gain—the degree of amplification of returning signals
❐ "Wall" or high-pass filters—elimination of low-frequency Doppler shifts due to motion of myocardium and valves (allowing only the higher frequencies to pass the filter)
❐ Baseline shift—moves the zero line toward the top or bottom of the display
❐ Velocity range—expands or compresses the scale (within the limits for each Doppler modality, as discussed above)
❐ Dynamic range—compression of the signal amplitude into shades of gray

In addition, pulsed Doppler controls include:
❐ Sample volume depth
❐ Sample volume length
❐ The number of sample volumes (high-PRF Doppler echo)

The Doppler modality may be integrated with 2D imaging for each of the three major Doppler modalities: continuous-wave, pulsed, and color Doppler flow imaging. However, while color Doppler flow imaging is nearly always conjoined with 2D imaging, pulsed Doppler signal quality is optimized when the 2D image is "frozen," and continuous-wave Doppler is optimized using a dedicated, small-footprint transducer with no 2D imaging.

Doppler Velocity Data Artifacts

Many Doppler artifacts are related to ultrasound physics and beam geometry, analogous to those seen with 2D imaging. Others are specific to Doppler echocardiography (Table 1–7).

Clinically, the most important potential artifact is *velocity underestimation* due to a nonparallel intercept angle between the ultrasound beam and the direction of blood flow (Fig. 1–27). Velocity underestimation can occur with either pulsed or continuous-wave Doppler techniques and is of most concern when measuring high-velocity jets due to valve stenosis, regurgitation, or other intracardiac abnormalities. Attention to technical details with interrogation of the flow signal from multiple acoustic windows and careful angulation is needed to avoid velocity underestimation.

With pulsed Doppler echo, *signal aliasing* limits the maximum measurable velocity. If the examiner recognizes that aliasing has occurred, appropriate steps can be taken to resolve the velocity data if needed. Again the examiner needs to recognize that aliasing can be due to nonlaminar disturbed flow, as well as to high-velocity laminar flow.

TABLE 1–7   Doppler Ultrasound Artifacts

Artifact	Result
Nonparallel intercept angle	Underestimation of velocity
Aliasing	Inability to measure maximum velocity
Range ambiguity	Doppler signals from more than one depth along the ultrasound beam are recorded.
Beam width	Overlap of Doppler signals from adjacent flows
Mirror image	Spectral display shows unidirectional flow both above and below the baseline.
Electronic interference	Bandlike interference signal obscures Doppler flow.
Transit-time effect	Change in the velocity of the ultrasound wave as it passes through a moving medium results in slight overestimation of Doppler shifts.

Range ambiguity is inherent to continuous-wave Doppler but can occur with pulsed Doppler as well. With a sample volume positioned close to the transducer, strong signals from twice (or three times) the depth of the sample volume will be received in the next "receive" phase and may be misinterpreted as originating from the set sample volume depth. For example, in an apical four-chamber view, placement of a sample volume in the LV apex at half the distance to the mitral annulus results in a spectral display showing the inflow signal across the mitral valve from the "second" sample volume depth. This phenomenon of range ambiguity is used constructively in the high-PRF Doppler mode.

Beam width (and side or grating lobes) affects the Doppler signal, as occurs with 2D imaging, resulting in superimposition of spatially adjacent flow signals on the spectral display. For example, LV outflow and inflow may be seen on the same recording, especially with continuous-wave Doppler. Similarly, the LV inflow signal may be seen superimposed on the aortic regurgitant jet (Fig. 1–28).

A mirror-image artifact is common with spectral analysis, appearing as a symmetric signal of somewhat less intensity than the actual flow signal in the opposite-direction flow channel (Fig. 1–29). Mirroring often can be reduced or eliminated by decreasing the power output or gain of the instrument. Interrogation of a flow signal from a near-perpendicular angle can result in flow signals on both sides of the baseline that must be distinguished from artifact.

Electronic interference appears as a band of signals across the spectral display that may obscure the flow signals. These artifacts are due to inadequate shielding of other electric instruments in the examination environment and are particularly common during studies in the intensive care unit or operating room.

The *transit-time effect* is the change in propagation speed that occurs as an ultrasound wave passes through a moving medium, such as blood. This phenomenon is separate from the Doppler effect (which affects the backscattered signal) and is the basis of volume flow measurement with a transit-time flow probe. On the spectral display, the transit-time effect may result in a slight broadening of the velocity range at a given time point ("blurring" on the vertical axis), which potentially can result in slight overestimation of velocity.

Color Doppler Flow Imaging

Principles

Color Doppler flow imaging is based on the principles of pulsed Doppler echocardiography. However, rather than one sample volume depth along the

Figure 1–27 The importance of a parallel intercept angle between the ultrasound beam and direction of blood flow is shown. The cosine function versus intercept angle (*horizontal axis*) varies from 1 at a parallel angle (0° and 180°) to 0 at a perpendicular angle (90°). The percentage error if cos is assumed to be 1 in the Doppler equation, but in fact the intercept angle is *not* parallel; it varies from only 6% at a 20° angle to 50% at a 60° angle and 100% for perpendicular flows. At a perpendicular (90°) intercept angle, no blood flow velocities are recorded.

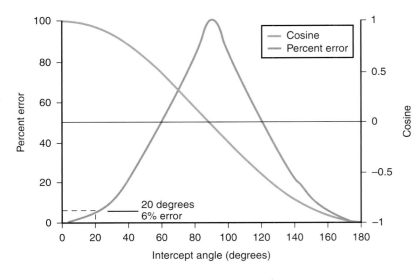

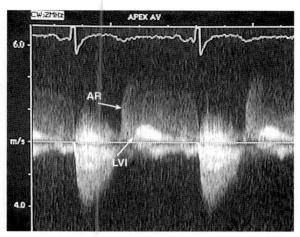

Figure 1–28 Doppler beam width artifact is demonstrated by the simultaneous display of superimposed aortic regurgitation (AR) and left ventricular inflow (LVI) curves.

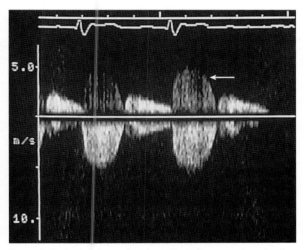

Figure 1–29 A mirror-image Doppler artifact with apparent weaker flow signals in the reverse channel (arrow).

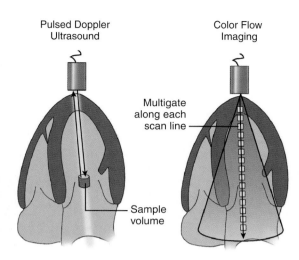

Figure 1–30 With pulsed Doppler the sample volume depth is determined by the time needed for ultrasound to travel to and from the depth of interest (left). With color flow imaging, multiple sample volume "gates" along each scan line are interrogated, with this process repeated for scan lines across the 2D image (right).

ultrasound beam, multiple sample volumes (or multigate) are evaluated along each sampling line (Fig. 1–30). By combining data from adjacent lines, a 2D image of intracardiac flow is generated.

Along each scan line, a pulse of ultrasound is transmitted, and then the backscattered signals are received from each "gate" or sample volume along that scan line (Table 1–8). In order to calculate accurate velocity data, several bursts along each scan line are used—typically eight—which is known as the burst length (Fig. 1–31). The PRF, as for conventional pulsed Doppler, is determined by the maximum depth of the Doppler signals. Signals from the eight sampling bursts at each position are analyzed to obtain mean velocity estimates for each sample volume along the scan line. Velocities are displayed using a color scale showing flow toward the transducer in red and flow away from the transducer in blue, with the shade of color indicating velocity up to the Nyquist limit. The option of displaying "variance" allows an additional color (usually green) to be added to indicate that the mean velocity for each of the eight bursts had excessive variability.

This process is repeated for each adjacent scan line across the image plane. Since each of these processes takes a finite amount of time depending on the speed of sound in tissue, the rapidity with which this image can be updated (the frame rate) depends on a combination of these factors.

Color Doppler Instrument Controls

The color flow display is dependent on each specific ultrasound instrument to some extent. However, many parameters are adjustable by the operator, so an optimal examination requires careful attention to instrument settings.

The color flow map usually can be varied in terms of:

❏ The color scale (assignment of colors to direction and velocity)
❏ Zero baseline position on the color scale
❏ The addition of variance to the color display

The specific color scale used is a matter of personal preference, with the diagnostic goal being to optimize the display and recognition of abnormal flow patterns.

The velocity range of the color flow map is determined by the Nyquist limit, and as for conventional pulsed Doppler, the range can be altered by shifting the zero baseline, changing the PRF, or altering the depth of the displayed image.

Color Doppler power output and gain are adjusted so that gain is just below the level at which random background noise appears. "Wall filters" can be

TABLE 1–8   Color Doppler Flow Imaging

	Definition	Examples	Clinical Implications
Sampling line	Doppler data are displayed from multiple sampling lines across the 2D image.	Instead of sampling backscattered signals from one depth (as in pulsed Doppler), signals from multiple depths along the beam are analyzed.	A greater number of sampling lines results in denser Doppler data but a slower frame rate.
Burst length	The number of ultrasound bursts along each sampling line	Mean velocity is estimated from the average of the backscattered signals from each burst.	A greater number of bursts results in more accurate mean velocity estimates but a slower frame rate.
Sector scan width	The width of the displayed 2D and color image	A greater sector width requires more sampling lines or less dense velocity data.	A narrower sector scan allows a greater sampling line density and faster frame rate.
Sector scan depth	The depth of the displayed color Doppler image	The maximum depth of the sector scan determines PRF (as with pulsed Doppler) and the Nyquist limit.	The minimum depth needed to display the flow of interest provides the optimal color display.
Color scale	Color display of Doppler velocity and flow direction	Most systems use shades of red for flow toward the transducer and blue for flow away from the transducer.	The color scale can be adjusted by shifting the baseline and adjusted the maximum velocity displayed (within the Nyquist limit).
Variance	The degree of variability in the mean velocity estimate at each depth along a sampling line	Variance typically is displayed as a green scale superimposed on the red-blue velocity scale. Variance can be turned on or off.	A variance display highlights flow disturbances and high-velocity flow, but even normal flows will be displayed as showing variance if velocity exceeds the Nyquist limit.

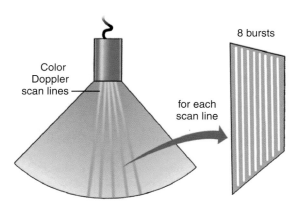

Figure 1–31 Along each color Doppler scan line, several (typically eight) bursts of ultrasound are transmitted and received to allow adequate velocity resolution.

varied to exclude low-velocity signals from the color flow display. In addition, many instruments allow variation in the assignment of a returning signal to 2D or Doppler display (depending on signal strength).

One approach to optimizing the color flow display is to reduce the 2D gain, since the instrument does not display flow data on top of "structures" even when the 2D signal is due to excessive gain.

Perhaps the most important technical factor in color flow imaging is optimization of *frame rate*. Color flow frame rate depends on sector width, depth, PRF, and the number of samples per sector line. The examiner optimizes frame rate by focusing on the flow of interest, narrowing the sector, and decreasing the depth as much as possible (Fig. 1–32). When frame rate remains inadequate for timing flow abnormalities, a color M-line through the area of interest may be helpful, for example, in assessment of aortic regurgitation.

Color Doppler Flow Imaging Artifacts

Color flow artifacts again relate to the physics of 2D and Doppler flow image generation (Table 1–9). *Shadowing* may be prominent distal to strong reflectors with absence of both 2D and flow data within the acoustic shadow.

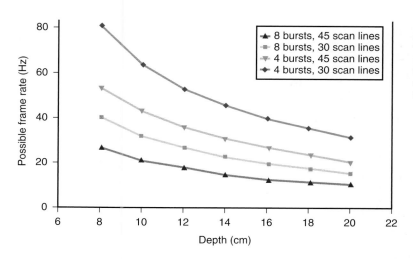

Figure 1–32 Graph of the maximum possible color Doppler frame rate (*y* axis) versus depth (*x* axis) for 8 or 4 bursts per scan line and 30 or 45 scan lines per frame. Note that at a depth of 16 cm a frame rate 20 or greater can be achieved only by decreasing the burst length to 4 or narrowing the sector to 30 scan lines.

Legend:
- ▲ 8 bursts, 45 scan lines
- ■ 8 bursts, 30 scan lines
- ▼ 4 bursts, 45 scan lines
- ◆ 4 bursts, 30 scan lines

TABLE 1–9	Color Doppler Artifacts
Artifact	**Appearance**
Shadowing	Absence of flow signal distal to strong reflector
Ghosting	Brief flashes of color that overlie anatomic structures and do not correlate with flow patterns
Background noise	Speckled color pattern over 2D sector due to excessive gain
Underestimation of flow signal	Loss of true flow signals due to inadequate gain
Intercept angle	Change in color (or absence at 90°) due to the angle between the flowstream and ultrasound beam across the image plane
Aliasing	"Wraparound" of color display resulting in a "variance" display even for laminar flow
Electronic interference	Linear or complex color patterns across the 2D image

Ghosting is the appearance of brief (usually one *or* two frames) large color patterns that overlay anatomic structures and do not correspond to underlying flow patterns. This artifact is caused by strong moving reflectors (such as prosthetic valve disks). Typically, this artifact is a uniform red or blue color, but it may be coded with a variance scale depending on the instrument. It is inconsistent from beat to beat.

Color Doppler gain settings have a dramatic effect on the color flow image. Extensive gain settings result in a uniform speckled pattern across the 2D image plane due to random *background noise*. Conversely, too low a gain setting results in a smaller displayed flow area than is actually present, an effect colloquially known as "dial-a-jet." Most experienced echocardiographers recommend setting the gain level just below the level of random background noise to optimize the flow signal.

As for any Doppler technique, the *intercept angle* between the ultrasound beam and direction of blood flow *for each scan line* affects the color display in terms of both direction and velocity. Thus, a uniform flow velocity traversing the image plane may appear red (toward the transducer) at one side of the sector and blue (away from the transducer) at the other edge of the sector, with a black area in the center where the flow direction is perpendicular to the ultrasound beam (Fig. 1–33).

Flow velocities that exceed the Nyquist limit at any given depth result in *signal aliasing*. Aliasing on color flow results in "wraparound" of the velocity signal, similar to that seen on a spectral display, so that an aliased velocity toward the transducer (should be red) will appear to be traveling away from the transducer (displayed in blue). Aliasing on color flow images is very common; for example, the LV inflow stream appears red and then blue (due to aliasing) in the apical view (Fig. 1–34). Color aliasing can be used to advantage to quantitate flow based on the proximal isovelocity surface area method described in Chapter 12. In some cases, aliasing results in a variance display (due to an apparent range of velocities at that site), emphasizing that a variance display does not always indicate disturbed flow.

Electronic interference on color flow displays is instrument dependent. As with other electric interference artifacts, it is most likely to occur in settings where numerous other instruments or devices are in use (e.g., operating room, intensive-care unit). Sometimes it appears as a linear multicolored band on the image along a few scan lines; sometimes more complex patterns are seen. Caution is needed in that sometimes electronic interference results in suppression of the

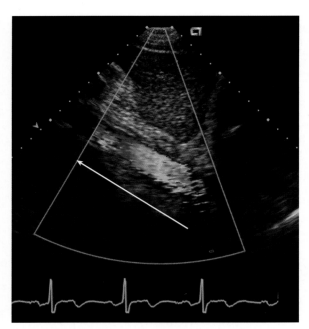

Figure 1–33 Color flow in the proximal abdominal aorta showing the importance of intercept angle on the color display. Although flow in systole goes from right to left across the image plane as shown by the *arrow*, flow on the right side of the image appears blue (because flow is directed toward the transducer but exceeds the Nyquist limit and thus has aliased to blue), and flow on the left side of the image appears red (because a larger intercept angle results in underestimation of velocity, which now is below the Nyquist limit).

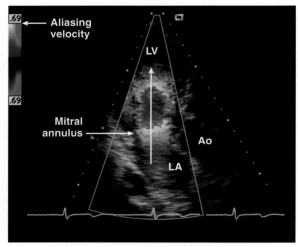

Figure 1–34 A normal left ventricular (LV) inflow signal (*top*) shows aliasing from red to blue at the mitral annulus level, because the velocity exceeds the Nyquist limit of 69 cm/s.

color flow signal. This artifact can be recognized by the absence of normal antegrade flow patterns.

Tissue Doppler

The Doppler principle also can be used to measure motion of the myocardium using either pulsed Doppler with a sample volume at a specific site in the myocardium or color Doppler to display myocardium motion in the entire image plane. The basic principles of Doppler ultrasound also apply to tissue Doppler. Tissue Doppler signals are very high amplitude, so power output and gain settings are low, whereas tissue Doppler velocities are very low, so the velocity range is small.

Both pulsed and color tissue Doppler velocities are angle dependent, showing motion toward and away from the transducer. Pulsed tissue Doppler uses a spectral display, allowing accurate measurement of velocity data. The color tissue Doppler display, like other color Doppler images, displays mean velocities for the component of motion toward and away from the transducer. The derivation of strain rate and strain from tissue Doppler data is discussed in Chapter 4.

BIOEFFECTS AND SAFETY

The use of ultrasound for diagnostic cardiac imaging has no known adverse biologic effects. However, ultrasound waves do have the potential to cause significant bioeffects depending on the intensity of exposure. Thus, the physician and cardiac sonographer must be aware of potential bioeffects in assessing the overall safety of the procedure.

Bioeffects

Ultrasound bioeffects (Table 1–10) can be divided into three basic categories:

- ❏ Thermal effects
- ❏ Cavitation
- ❏ Other (such as torque forces and micro streaming)

Thermal effects predominate with diagnostic ultrasound examinations. As the ultrasound wave passes through a tissue, heating occurs due to absorption of the mechanical energy of the sound wave. The rate of increase in temperature dT/dt depends on the absorption coefficient of the tissue for a given frequency α, the density ρ, and specific heat C_m of the tissue and the intensity I of ultrasound exposure:

$$dT/dt = 2\alpha I/\rho C_m \qquad (1\text{–}10)$$

Increases in temperature due to ultrasound exposure are offset by heat loss due to blood flow through the tissue (convective loss) and heat diffusion. More dense tissues (such as bone) heat more rapidly than less dense tissue (such as fat). However, the actual elevation in temperature for a specific tissue is difficult to predict both because of the complexity of the entire biologic system and because it is difficult to assess accurately the intensity of exposure. In addition, the actual degree of tissue heating depends on transducer frequency, focus, power output, depth, perfusion, and tissue density.

TABLE 1-10	Ultrasound Safety		
	Definition	**Examples**	**Clinical Implications**
Exposure intensity (*I*)	Ultrasound exposure depends on power and area: $I = power/area = W/cm^2$	Common measures of intensity are the SPTA or the SPPA.	Transducer output and tissue exposure affect the total ultrasound exposure of the patient.
Thermal bioeffects	Heating of tissue due to absorption of ultrasound energy described by the thermal index (TI)	The degree of tissue heating is affected by tissue density and blood flow. TI is the ratio of transmitted acoustic power to the power needed to increase temperature by 1°C. TI is most important with Doppler and color flow imaging.	Total ultrasound exposure depends on transducer frequency, power output, focus, depth, and exam duration. When the TI exceeds 1, the benefits of the study should be balanced against potential biologic effects.
Cavitation	Creation or vibration of small gas-filled bodies by the ultrasound wave	Mechanical index (MI) is the ratio of peak rarefactional pressure to the square root of the transducer frequency. MI is most important with 2D imaging.	Cavitation or vibration of microbubbles occurs with higher intensity exposure. Power output and exposure time should be monitored.

Cavitation is the creation or vibration of small gas-filled bodies by the ultrasound beam. Cavitation tends to occur only with higher intensity exposures. Microbubbles resonate (expand and decrease in size) depending on their dimension in relation to the sound wave with a resonance frequency F_0 defined by the radius of the microbubble (R_0 in microns):

$$F_0 = 3260/R_0 \qquad (1-11)$$

Microbubbles also can be created by ultrasound by expansion of small cavitation nuclei. Cavitation has not been shown to occur with ultrasound exposure due to diagnostic ultrasound systems. However, this effect may be more important when gas-filled bodies are introduced into the ultrasound field, such as with the use of contrast echocardiography.

Other ultrasound bioeffects occur only with much higher exposures than occur with diagnostic ultrasound. These effects include micro streaming, torque forces, and other complex biologic effects.

Safety

The intensity *I* of ultrasound exposure can be expressed in several ways. The most commonly used unit of measure of intensity is power per area, where power is energy over a specific time interval:

$$I = power/area = W/cm^2 \qquad (1-12)$$

The maximum overall intensity is then described as the highest exposure within the beam (spatial peak) averaged over the period of exposure (temporal average) and is known as the *spatial peak temporal average (SPTA) intensity*. Another common measure is the *spatial peak pulse average*, defined as the average pulse intensity at the spatial location where the pulse intensity is maximum. The FDA provides two maximum allowed limits for I_{SPTA} for cardiac applications: a regulated application-specific limit of 430 mW/cm^2 and an output display standard of 720 mW/cm^2, which allows the echocardiographer to balance the potential risks of ultrasound exposure with the benefit of the diagnostic test.

A major limitation of measuring the intensity of ultrasound exposure is that while measuring the *output* of the transducer is straightforward (e.g., in a water bath), estimating the actual tissue *exposure* is more difficult due to attenuation and other interactions with the tissue. Furthermore, tissue exposure is limited only to transmission periods and the time the ultrasound beam dwells at a specific point, both of which are considerably shorter than the total examination time. Other indices that incorporate these factors have been developed to better define the exposure levels with diagnostic ultrasound. These measures include the thermal index (TI) and the mechanical index (MI).

The soft tissue TI is based on the ratio of transmitted acoustic power to the power needed to raise tissue temperature by 1°C:

Figure 1–35 The potential bioeffects from ultra-sound. Safe and potentially harmful regions are delineated according to ultrasound intensity levels and exposure time. The *dashed line* shows the upper limit of intensities typically encountered in diagnostic ultrasound applications. *(From Bushberg JT, Seibert JA, Leidholdt EM, Boone JM: The Essential Physics of Medical Imaging. Philadelphia: Lippincott Williams & Wilkins, 2002.)*

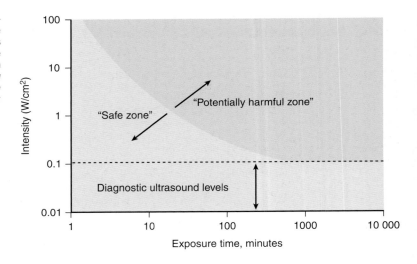

$$TI = W_{p}/W_{deg} \qquad (1\text{--}13)$$

where W_{p} is a power parameter calculated from output power and acoustic attenuation, and W_{deg} is the estimated power needed to increase the tissue temperature by 1°C. There are different thermal indexes for bone and cranial bone that are less relevant for cardiac ultrasound.

The MI describes the nonthermal effects of ultrasound (cavitation and other effects) as the ratio of peak rarefactional pressure and the square root of transducer frequency, with the specific definition:

$$MI = [\rho_{r.3}/(f_{c}^{1/2})]/C_{MI} \qquad (1\text{--}14)$$

where C_{MI} equals 1 Mpa $MHz^{-1/2}$, $\rho_{r.3}$ is the attenuated peak-rarefactional pressure in Mpa, and f_{c} is the center frequency of the transducer in MHz.

An MI or TI less than 1 is generally considered safe; higher numbers indicate a higher probability of a biologic effect. These indexes are displayed only on instruments capable of exceeding a MI or TI of 1. With a higher index the potential risks of ultrasound exposure must be balanced against the benefits of the diagnostic examination (Fig. 1–35). The TI is most important with Doppler and color flow imaging, whereas the MI is most important with 2D imaging.

While any biologic effect is likely to be small, a prudent approach is to proceed as follows:

❑ Perform echocardiography only when indicated clinically (see Chapter 5), as part of an approved research protocol or in appropriate teaching settings.
❑ Know the power output and exposure intensity of different modalities (imaging and Doppler) of each instrument.
❑ Limit the power output and exposure time as much as possible within the constraints of acquiring the necessary information.
❑ Keep up to date on any new scientific findings or data relating to possible adverse effects.

SUGGESTED READING

1. Bushberg JT, Seibert JA, Leidholdt EM, et al: The Essential Physics of Medical Imaging, 2nd ed. Philadelphia: Lippincott Williams & Wilkins, 2002, pp 469–554.
   Concise but detailed summary of ultrasound physics for the physician. Sections include characteristics of sound, interaction with tissue, transducer design and beam properties, resolution, image acquisition, artifacts, Doppler ultrasound, and bioeffects.
2. Kremkau FW: Diagnostic Ultrasound: Principles and Instruments, 7th ed. Philadelphia: Elsevier/Saunders, 2006.

Basic textbook, primarily for cardiac sonographers, with chapters on ultrasound, transducers, imaging instruments, Doppler effect, spectral instrumentation, color Doppler instrumentation, artifacts, and safety. Each chapter has a review section with multiple-choice questions. A comprehensive examination (with answers) is included.
3. Geiser EA: Echocardiography: physics and instrumentation. In Skorton DJ, Schelbert HR, Wolf GL, Brundage BH (eds): Marcus Cardiac Imaging: A Companion to Braunwald's Heart Disease, 2nd ed. Philadelphia: WB Saunders, 1996, pp 273–291.

Advanced chapter on echocardiographic instrumentation with excellent diagrams.
4. Bosch JG: Echocardiographic digital image processing and approaches to automated border detection. In Otto CM (ed): The Practice of Clinical Echocardiography, 3rd ed. Philadelphia: Elsevier/Saunders, 2007, pp 262–282.
   Advanced-level discussion of digital image procession, data compression and storage, and approaches to automated border detection. 88 references.
5. Zagzebski JA: Essentials of Ultrasound Physics. St Louis: Mosby, 1996.

Review of ultrasound physics for the beginning student. Concise text with clear schematic illustrations and tables. Topics covered include physics of diagnostic ultrasound, image storage and display, Doppler instrumentation, and bioeffects. Questions for review included with each chapter. Additional suggested readings.

6. Powis RL, Schwartz RA: Practical Doppler Ultrasound for the Clinician. Baltimore: Williams & Wilkins, 1991.
   Detailed but understandable book describing Doppler ultrasound techniques. An introduction to basic ultrasound principles and basic fluid dynamics also is provided.

7. Thomas JD, Rubin DN: Tissue harmonic imaging: why does it work? J Am Soc Echocardiogr 11:803–808, 1998.
   Discussion with clear illustrations of the physical basis of tissue harmonic imaging. Contrast harmonic imaging is based on generation of harmonic frequencies by vibrating microbubbles. Tissue harmonics are generated by the nonlinear effects of ultrasound wave propagation through tissue. Instrumentation factors critical to generation of tissue harmonic images include a wide dynamic range, a narrow transmit spectrum, and a sharp receiver filter.

8. Turner SP, Monaghan MJ: Tissue harmonic imaging for standard left ventricular measurements: fundamentally flawed? Eur J Echocardiogr 7:9–15, 2006.
   Tissue harmonic imaging improves signal-to-noise ratio but reduces the axial resolution of the ultrasound image. This review summarizes the physics of tissue harmonic imaging and discusses the potential impact on accuracy of ultrasound measurements.

9. Harris RA, Follett DH, Halliwell M, et al: Ultimate limits in ultrasonic imaging resolution. Ultrasound Med Biol 17:547–558, 1991.
   Detailed review on ultrasound image resolution for readers interested in the technical details of this problem; 61 references.

10. Thomas JD, Adams DB, DeVries S, et al: Guidelines and Recommendations for Digital Echocardiography: A report from the digital echocardiography committee of the American Society of Echocardiography. J Am Soc Echocardiogr 18:287–297, 2005.
    Summary and review including discussion of DICCOM standard, terminology, digital compression, components of the digital echocardiography laboratory, image acquisition protocols and pitfalls, image storage, and implementation issues.

11. Skorton DJ, Collins SM, Greenleaf JF, et al: Ultrasound bioeffects and regulatory issues: an introduction for the echocardiographer. J Am Soc Echocardiogr 1:240–251, 1988.
    A brief overview of bioeffects and safety prepared by the ASE Committee on Physics and Instrumentation.

12. O'Brien WD: Ultrasound-biophysics mechanisms. Prog Biophys Mol Biol 93:212–255, 2007.
    A detailed discussion, including mathematical principles, of ultrasound bioeffects including ultrasound waves, acoustic propagation, impedance, and attenuation; interactions with tissues; and the mechanisms and magnitude of thermal and nonthermal bioeffects. 285 references.

13. Meltzer RS: Food and Drug Administration ultrasound device regulation: the output display standard, the "mechanical index" and ultrasound safety [editorial]. J Am Soc Echocardiogr 9:216–220, 1996.
    Brief review of ultrasound bioeffects and cavitation-related bioeffects with a discussion of the potential impact, advantages, and disadvantages of regulation of ultrasound instrument output.

14. Fowlkes JB, Holland CK: Mechanical bioeffects from diagnostic ultrasound: AIUM consensus statements. American Institute of Ultrasound in Medicine. J Ultrasound Med 19:69–72, 2000.
    Section 1: Conclusions and recommendations, pp 73–76.
    Section 2: Definitions and description of nonthermal mechanisms, pp 77–84.
    Section 3: Selected biological properties of tissues: potential determinants of susceptibility to ultrasound-induced bioeffects, pp 85–96.
    Section 4: Bioeffects in tissues with gas bodies, pp 97–108.
    Section 5: Nonthermal bioeffects in the absence of well-defined gas bodies, pp 109–119.
    Section 6, Mechanical bioeffects in the presence of gas-carrier ultrasound contrast agents, pp 120–142.
    Section 7, Discussion of the mechanical index and other exposure parameters, pp 143–148.
    Section 8: Clinical relevance. References, pp 149–168.
    AIUM Consensus Development Conferences on ultrasound safety and bioeffects. Detailed document with eight sections as listed above.

15. Frizzell LA: Conclusions regarding biological effects of ultrasound for diagnostically relevant exposures. J Ultrasound Med 13:69–72, 1994.
    Summary of AIUM conference held in 1992 on the Bioeffects and Safety of Diagnostic Ultrasound including definitions of the mechanical index (MI) and tissue thermal index (TTI). Updated clinical statements are available at the AIUM web site (http://www.aium.org).

16. Miller DL: Update on safety of diagnostic ultrasonography. J Clin Ultrasound 19:531–540, 1991.
    Readable review of ultrasound bioeffects; 39 references.

17. AMA Council on Scientific Affairs: Medical diagnostic ultrasound instrumentation and clinical interpretation: report of the Ultrasonography Task Force. JAMA 265:1155–1159, 1991.
    AMA Council on Scientific Affairs' report on diagnostic ultrasound. Review of basic principles of ultrasound with emphasis on ultrasound artifacts.

18. Barnett SB, Kossoff G, Edwards MJ: Is diagnostic ultrasound safe? Current international consensus on the thermal mechanism. Med J Aust 160:33–37, 1994.
    Review of the thermal effects of diagnostic ultrasound that concludes that there is no evidence of adverse effects for exposures resulting in temperatures less than $38.5°C$.

19. Abbott JG: Rationale and derivation of the MI and TI: a review. Ultrasound Med Biol 3:341–441, 1999.
    Summary of the measurements, calculations, and clinical implications of the MI and TI for use in the output display standard on ultrasound instruments.

20. Barnett SB, Haar GR, Ziskin MC, et al: International recommendations and guidelines for the safe use of diagnostic ultrasound in medicine. Ultrasound Med Biol 26:355–366, 2000.
    Review article based on symposium sponsored by the World Federation for Ultrasound in Medicine and Biology (WFUMB) comparing national and international recommendations on the safe use of diagnostic ultrasound. Includes summary of US Food and Drug Administration (FDA) regulation by application-specific limits on acoustic power and the newer approach of user responsibility for appropriate use based on real-time display of safety indices.

2

Normal Anatomy and Flow Patterns on Transthoracic Echocardiography

BASIC IMAGING PRINCIPLES

Tomographic Imaging

Echocardiography provides tomographic images of cardiac structures and blood flow, analogous to a thin "slice" through the heart. Two-dimensional (2D) echocardiographic images provide detailed anatomic data in a given image plane, but complete evaluation of the cardiac chambers and valves requires integration of information from multiple image planes. Small structures that traverse numerous tomographic planes (such as the coronary arteries) are difficult to evaluate fully. In addition, structures may move in and out of the imaging plane as a result of motion due to cardiac contraction or respiratory movement of the heart within the chest. Respiratory variation in cardiac location is recognized easily by its timing, but movement of the heart during the cardiac cycle is more problematic because it may not be obvious on the 2D image. Cardiac motion relative to surrounding structures is described in three dimensions as:

❐ Translation (movement of the heart as a whole in the chest)

❑ Rotation (circular motion around the long axis of the left ventricle [LV])

❑ Torsion (unequal rotational motion at the apex versus the base of the LV)

Even if the 2D image plane is fixed in position, the location of underlying structures may vary between systole and diastole. For example, in the apical four-chamber view, adjacent segments (which may be supplied by different coronary arteries) of the LV may be seen in systole versus diastole.

Nomenclature of Standard Views

Each tomographic image is defined by its acoustic *window* (the position of the transducer) and *view* (the image plane) (Table 2–1). Standard echocardiographic image planes are determined by the axis of the heart itself (with the LV as the major point of reference) rather than by skeletal or external body landmarks (Fig. 2–1). The primary reference points on the heart are the apex, defined as the tip of the LV, and the base, defined as the valve annulus region. The four standard image planes then are:

❑ *Long-axis plane:* Parallel to the long axis of the LV, defined as an imaginary line drawn through the LV apex and the center of the LV base, with the image plane intersecting the center of the aortic valve

❑ *Short-axis plane:* Perpendicular to the long axis of the ventricle, resulting in circular cross-sectional views of the LV

❑ *Four-chamber plane:* Perpendicular to the short-axis plane and rotated about 60° from the long-axis plane, intersecting the major axis of the mitral and tricuspid valve annulus

❑ *Two-chamber plane:* Perpendicular to the short-axis plane, midway between the long-axis and

four-chamber views, intersecting the left ventricle, mitral valve, and left atrium (LA)

The other standard directional terms are medial versus lateral (the horizontal axis in a short-axis or four-chamber view) and anterior versus posterior (the vertical axis in a short-axis or long-axis view). This standard terminology also applies to other cardiac tomographic imaging techniques and to visualization of cardiac anatomy with three-dimensional (3D) echocardiography.

Acoustic windows are transducer positions that allow ultrasound access to the cardiac structures. The bony thoracic cage and adjacent air-filled lung limit the possible acoustic windows, making patient positioning and sonographer experience critical factors in obtaining diagnostic images. Transthoracic images typically are obtained from parasternal, apical, subcostal, and suprasternal notch acoustic windows. The transducer motions used to obtain the desired view are described as follows (Fig. 2–2):

❑ *Move* the transducer to a different position on the chest.

❑ *Tilt or point* the transducer tip with a rocking motion to image different structures in the same tomographic plane.

❑ *Angle* the transducer from side to side to obtain different tomographic planes somewhat parallel to the original image plane.

❑ *Rotate* the image plane at a single position to obtain intersecting tomographic planes.

Image Orientation

Most laboratories follow the American Society of Echocardiography (ASE) guidelines for image orientation in adults, although many pediatric cardiologists use alternate formats. The recommended orientation is with the transducer position (narrowest portion of the sector scan) at the top of the screen so that structures nearer to the transducer are at the top and structures farther from the transducer are at the bottom of the image. Thus, a transthoracic four-chamber view is displayed with the apex at the top of the image (because it is closest to the transducer), whereas a transesophageal (TEE) four-chamber view is displayed with the apex at the bottom of the image (because it is most distant from the transducer). This orientation aids in prompt recognition of ultrasound artifacts, shadowing, and reverberations, because the display of the origin of the ultrasound signal is the same for all acoustic windows and image planes.

The lateral (in short-axis views) and basal (in long-axis views) cardiac structures are displayed on the right side of the screen, which is similar to the format used for other tomographic imaging techniques. Short-axis views can be thought of as the observer looking from the apex toward the cardiac base;

TABLE 2–1	Transthoracic Echo Image Orientation Nomenclature

Window (Transducer Location)

Parasternal
Apical
Subcostal
Suprasternal

Image Planes

Short-axis
Long-axis
Four-chamber
Two-chamber

Reference Points

Apex versus base
Lateral versus medial
Anterior versus posterior

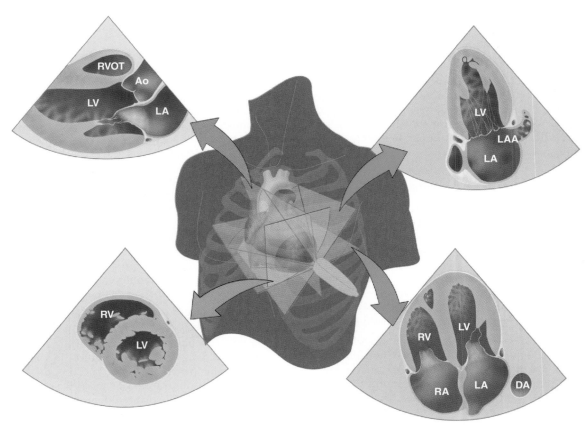

Figure 2–1 The four basic image planes used in transthoracic echocardiography. The long-axis view (*purple arrow*) extends from the LV apex through the aortic valve plane. The short-axis view is perpendicular to the long-axis view resulting in a circular view of the LV (*red arrow*). The two-chamber (*blue arrow*) and four-chamber views (*green arrow*) are each about 60° rotation from the long-axis view, and both are perpendicular to the short-axis view. The four-chamber view includes both ventricles and both atria. The two-chamber view includes the LV and LA; sometimes the atrial appendage is visualized. LAA, left atrial appendage.

long-axis views, as the observer looking from the left toward the right side of the heart. The four-chamber (horizontal long-axis) plane is displayed with lateral structures on the right side of the screen and medial structures on the left side (as for the short-axis view).

Examination Technique

The echocardiographic examination is performed by the physician or by a trained cardiac sonographer under the supervision of a qualified physician. Guidelines and recommendations for education and training in echocardiography for both sonographers and physicians have been published, as referenced in Chapter 5.

At the time of a transthoracic echocardiographic examination, relevant clinical data, prior imaging studies, and the indication for the study are reviewed. Blood pressure is recorded along with age, height, and weight. Then the patient is positioned comfortably for each view in either a left lateral decubitus or supine position. Electrocardiographic (ECG) electrodes are attached for display of a single lead (usually lead II) on the instrument display to aid in timing cardiac events. Specially

designed echocardiographic examination stretchers provide apical cutouts for optimal transducer positioning at the apex. The transducer is applied to the chest and upper abdomen using a water-soluble gel to obtain good contact without intervening air. The time needed to perform an echocardiographic examination depends on the specific clinical situation—from a few minutes in a critically ill patient to document cardiac tamponade to more than 1 hour to quantitate multiple lesions in a patient with complex valvular or congenital heart disease.

Technical Quality

Image quality depends on the degree of ultrasound tissue penetration, transducer frequency, instrument settings, and the sonographer's skill. Ultrasound tissue penetration or "acoustic access" to the cardiac structures is largely determined by body habitus, specifically how the heart is positioned in the chest relative to the lungs and chest wall. Conditions that increase the separation between the transducer and the cardiac structures (e.g., adipose tissue), decrease ultrasound

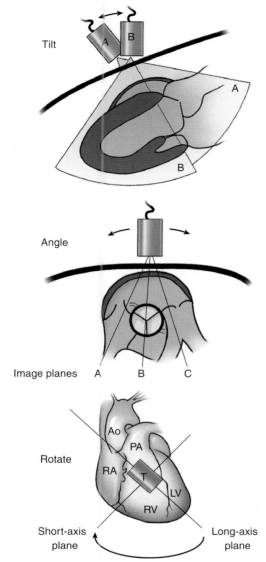

Tilt

Angle

Image planes   A   B   C

Rotate

Ao
PA
RA
T
LV
RV

Short-axis   Long-axis
plane   plane

Figure 2–2 Transducer motion at a given acoustic window using the example of a left parasternal transducer position. *Tilt:* The transducer is "rocked" to provide images (A or B) in the same tomographic plane. *Angle:* Different image planes (perpendicular to the plane of the figure at lines A, B, and C) are obtained by angulation of the transducer. *Rotation:* The transducer is "twisted" with a circular motion to provide a different image plane while maintaining the same orientation between the transducer itself and the chest wall.

structures against the chest wall. In addition, respiratory variation can be used to the sonographer's advantage by having the patient suspend respiration briefly in whatever phase of the respiratory cycle yields the best image quality. Unfortunately, even with careful attention to examination technique, echocardiographic images remain suboptimal in some patients.

Echocardiographic Image Interpretation

The physician uses the tomographic 2D echocardiographic images to build a mental 3D reconstruction of the cardiac chambers and valves, or uses a 3D echocardiographic dataset to examine anatomy in specific image planes (see Chapter 4). To do this, an understanding of image planes and orientation and the technical aspects of image acquisition (e.g., in recognizing artifacts) is needed, along with a detailed knowledge of cardiac anatomy. A list of anatomic terminology is shown in Table 2–2. Recording images as the tomographic plane is moved between standard image planes is important for this analysis and ensures that abnormalities that lie outside or between our arbitrary "standard" views are not missed. In complex cases, the physician may need to perform part of the study to appreciate the 3D relationship of the different image planes. Information obtained from anatomic 2D imaging then is integrated with physiologic Doppler data and clinical information in the final echocardiographic interpretation.

TRANSTHORACIC TOMOGRAPHIC VIEWS

The normal anatomy as seen on echocardiography is described below for each tomographic view. The best views for specific cardiac structures are indicated in Table 2–3.

Parasternal Window

Long-axis Views

With the patient in a left lateral decubitus position and the transducer in the left third or fourth intercostal space, adjacent to the sternum, a long-axis view of the heart is obtained that bisects the long axis of both aortic and mitral valves (Figs. 2–3 and 2–4). The patient's position may need adjustment between a steep left lateral and nearly supine position based on the images obtained in each subject. The *aortic root*, sinuses of Valsalva, sinotubular junction, and proximal 3 to 4 cm of the ascending aorta are seen in long axis. Further segments of the ascending aorta may be visualized by moving the transducer cephalad one or two interspaces. The upper limit of normal for aortic root end-diastolic dimension in adults is 1.6 cm/m^2 at the annulus and 2.1 cm/m^2 at the sinuses.

penetration (e.g., scar tissue), or interpose air-containing tissues between the transducer and the heart (e.g., chronic lung disease, recent cardiac surgery) lead to poor image quality. TEE images tend to show better structure definition because of greater ultrasound penetration given the shorter distance between the transducer and the cardiac structures, the use of a higher frequency transducer, and the absence of interposed lung. On transthoracic studies, optimal patient positioning for each acoustic window brings the cardiac

TABLE 2–2	Terminology for Normal Echocardiographic Anatomy
Location	**Term**
Aortic root	Sinuses of Valsalva Sinotubular junction Coronary ostia
Aortic valve	Right, left, and noncoronary cusps Nodules of Arantius Lambl's excrescences
Mitral valve	Anterior and posterior leaflets Posterior leaflet scallops (lateral, central, medial) Chordae (primary, secondary, tertiary; basal, and marginal) Commissures (medial and lateral)
Left ventricle	Wall segments (see Chapter 8) Septum, free wall Base, apex Medial and lateral papillary muscles
Right ventricle	Inflow segment Moderator band Outflow tract (conus) Supraventricular crest Anterior, posterior, and conus papillary muscles
Tricuspid value	Anterior, septal, and posterior leaflets Chordae Commissures
Right atrium	Right atrial appendage SVC, IVC junctions Valve of IVC (Chiari network) Crista terminalis Fossa ovalis Patent foramen ovale
Left atrium	LAA Superior and inferior left pulmonary veins Superior and inferior right pulmonary veins Ridge at junction of LAA and left superior pulmonary vein
Pericardium	Oblique sinus Transverse sinus

IVC, inferior vena cava; LAA, left atrial appendage; SVC, superior vena cava.

TABLE 2–3	Transthoracic Echo: Views for Specific Cardiac Structures
Anatomic Structures	**Best Views**
Aortic valve	PLAX PSAX Apical long-axis Anteriorly angulated A4C
Mitral valve	PLAX PSAX (MV level) A4C Apical long-axis
Pulmonic valve	PSAX (aortic valve level) RV outflow Subcostal short-axis (aortic valve level)
Tricuspid valve	RV inflow A4C Subcostal four-chamber and short-axis
Left ventricle	PLAX PSAX A4C, A2C, long-axis Subcostal four-chamber and short-axis
Right ventricle	PLAX (RVOT only) RV inflow PSAX (MV and LV levels) A4C Subcostal four-chamber
Left atrium	PLAX PSAX A4C, A2C, long-axis Subcostal four-chamber
Right atrium	PSAX (aortic valve level) A4C Subcostal four-chamber and short-axis

Aorta
  Ascending
 	
  Arch
  Descending
    thoracic
	PLAX (standard and up an interspace)
	SSN
	SSN
	Parasternal with angulation
	Modified A2C
	Subcostal

Interatrial septum	PSAX Subcostal four-chamber
Coronary sinus	PLAX to RV inflow view (sweep) Posterior angulation from A4C

A2C, apical two-chamber; A4C, apical four-chamber; MV, mitral valve; PLAX, parasternal long-axis; PSAX, parasternal short-axis; SSN, suprasternal notch.

In the long-axis view, the right coronary cusp of the *aortic valve* is anterior and the noncoronary cusp is posterior (the left coronary cusp is lateral to the image plane). In systole, the thin aortic leaflets open widely, assuming a parallel orientation to the aortic walls. In diastole, the leaflets are closed, with a small obtuse

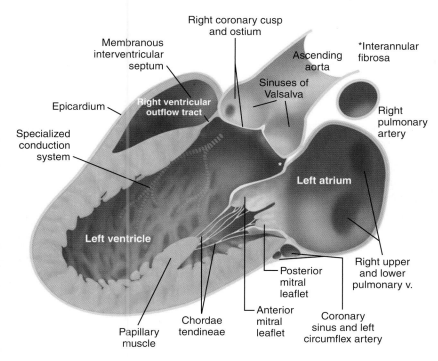

Right coronary cusp and ostium

Membranous interventricular septum

Ascending aorta

*Interannular fibrosa

Sinuses of Valsalva

Epicardium

Right ventricular outflow tract

Right pulmonary artery

Specialized conduction system

Left atrium

Left ventricle

Papillary muscle

Chordae tendineae

Posterior mitral leaflet

Anterior mitral leaflet

Right upper and lower pulmonary v.

Coronary sinus and left circumflex artery

Figure 2–3 Cardiac anatomy as seen in parasternal long-axis views in diastole showing the aortic root (Ao) anterior to the LA and mitral valve (MV). With an echocardiographic sector scan, typically only the basal segments of the LV are seen. The proximal ascending aorta usually can be imaged beyond the level of the sinotubular junction. The aortic valve is closed with the right coronary and non-coronary cusps visualized. The anterior and posterior leaflets of the open MV are seen. The segments of the LV imaged are the basal and midventricular segments of the anterior septum and posterior wall. The medial papillary muscle has been shown for reference, although slight medial angulation is needed to visualize this structure in the long-axis view. The right ventricular outflow tract is anterior, while the coronary sinus is in the atrioventricular groove. *(From Otto CM: Echocardiographic evaluation of valvular heart disease. In Otto CM, Bonow R [eds]: Valvular Heart Disease: A Companion to Braunwald's Heart Disease. Philadelphia: Elsevier/Saunders, 2009.)*

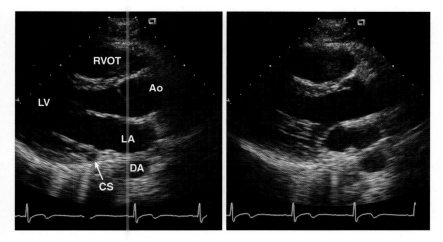

Figure 2–4 Normal parasternal long-axis 2D echo images at end-diastole (*left*) and end-systole (*right*) show the anatomic features seen in Figure 2-3. In addition, the descending thoracic aorta (DA) is seen posterior to the left atrium. CS, coronary sinus.

closure angle between the two leaflets. The leaflets appear linear from the closure line to the aortic annulus due to the hemicylindrical shape of the closed leaflets (linear along the length of the cylinder, curved along its short axis). In normal young individuals, the leaflets are so thin that only the apposed portions at the leaflets' closure line may be seen. The 3D anatomy of the attachment line of the aortic leaflets to the aortic root is shaped like a crown with the three commissures attached near the tops of the sinuses of Valsalva and the midportion of each leaflet attached near the base of each sinus (Fig. 2–5). This attachment line often is referred to as the aortic "annulus," although there are no distinct tissue characteristics of this attachment zone. Note that there is fibrous continuity between the aortic root and the anterior mitral leaflet. The absence of intervening myocardium between aortic and mitral valves helps identify the anatomic LV in complex congenital disease.

The anterior and posterior *mitral valve* leaflets appear thin and uniform in echogenicity, with chordal attachments leading toward the medial (or posteromedial) papillary muscle seen in the long-axis view, although the papillary muscle itself is slightly medial to the long-axis plane. The anterior mitral leaflet is longer than the posterior leaflet but has a smaller annular length so that the surface areas of the two leaflets are similar (Fig. 2–6). As the mitral leaflets open in diastole, the tips separate and the anterior leaflet touches or comes very close to the

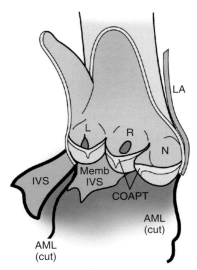

Figure 2–5 Schematic diagram of normal Ao valve anatomy shown in a frontal view with the Ao root "opened" between the left (L) and noncoronary (N) cusps by cutting through the anterior mitral leaflet (AML) to demonstrate the crown-shaped "annulus." The commissures are near the top of each sinus, and each leaflet has a hemicylindrical shape so that the closed leaflets appear as a straight line in the long-axis view. Each Ao leaflet has a coaptation zone (COAPT), with overlap between adjacent leaflets and a thicker region, the nodule of Arantius at the center of each cusp. The close anatomic relationships of the Ao valve to the interventricular septum (IVS), membranous septum (Memb IVS), mitral valve, and LA can be appreciated.

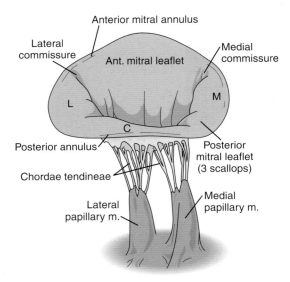

Figure 2–6 The mitral valve apparatus includes the leaflet, annulus, chordae, and papillary muscles. The anterior mitral leaflet attaches to a smaller portion of the circumference of the annulus than the posterior mitral leaflet but the anterior leaflet is longer. The posterior leaflet consists of three segments designated the lateral (L or P1), central (C or P2), and medial (M or P3) scallops. Both leaflets attach to both the medial and lateral papillary muscles.

ventricular septum. In systole, the leaflets coapt, with some overlap between the leaflets (apposition zone) and a slightly obtuse (>180°) angle relative to the mitral annulus plane. The chordae normally remain posterior to the plane of leaflet coaptation in systole. However, some normal individuals have systolic anterior motion of the chordae, due to mild redundancy of chordal tissue that is not associated with hemodynamic abnormalities. This must be distinguished from the pathologic systolic anterior motion of the mitral leaflets seen in hypertrophic obstructive cardiomyopathy. The mitral annulus (the attachment between the mitral leaflets, left atrium [LA], and LV) is an anatomically well-defined fibrous structure with an elliptical shape. The long-axis view bisects the minor axis of the mitral annulus. (The major axis is seen in the apical four-chamber view.)

The *left atrium* is seen posterior to the aortic root with a similar anteroposterior dimension as the aortic root. The *right pulmonary artery* lies between the aortic root and superior aspect of the LA but may not be well seen on transthoracic images. The *coronary sinus* is seen in the atrioventricular groove posterior to the mitral annulus. Dilation of the coronary sinus due to a persistent left superior vena cava (which can be confirmed by echo-contrast injection in a left arm vein) is an occasional incidental finding of no clinical significance that can mimic an LA mass.

Posterior to the LA, the *descending thoracic aorta* is seen in cross-section. A long-axis view of the descending thoracic aorta can be obtained from this window by rotating the transducer counterclockwise. Note that the oblique sinus of the pericardium lies between the LA and the descending thoracic aorta so that a pericardial effusion can be seen between these two structures, while a pleural effusion will be seen only posterior to the descending thoracic aorta.

The *LV* septum and posterior wall are seen at the base and midventricular level in the long-axis view, allowing assessment of wall thickness, chamber dimensions, endocardial motion, and wall thickening of these myocardial segments. LV end-diastolic and end-systolic measurements of wall thickness and internal dimensions are made in the long-axis view on 2D images from the septal to posterior wall tissue blood interface or using a 2D-guided M-mode recording (see below and Chapter 6). From the parasternal window the LV apex is not seen; the apparent "apex" usually is an oblique image plane through the anterolateral wall.

A portion of the muscular *right ventricular outflow tract* is seen anteriorly. Unlike the symmetric prolate ellipsoid shape of the LV, the right ventricle (RV) does not have an easily defined long or short axis. In effect, the RV is "wrapped around" the LV, with an inflow region, an apical region, and an outflow region forming a somewhat anteroposteriorly flattened U-shaped structure. Most standard image planes result in oblique tomographic sections of the

RV, so RV size and systolic function are best evaluated from multiple views, as discussed more fully in Chapter 6.

Right Ventricular Inflow and Outflow Views

In the long-axis plane the transducer is moved apically and then is angulated medially to obtain a view of the *right atrium, tricuspid valve,* and *right ventricle* (Fig. 2–7). In this RV inflow view, the septal and anterior leaflets of the tricuspid valve are well seen. The RV apex is heavily trabeculated, while the outflow tract (supracristal region) has a smoother endocardial surface. The moderator band, a prominent muscle trabeculation that traverses the RV apex obliquely and contains the

right bundle branch, may be seen in both parasternal and apical views (Fig. 2–8). The papillary muscles are more difficult to identify in the RV than in the LV. Typically, there are two principal papillary muscles (anterior and posterior) with a smaller supracristal (or conus) papillary muscle. The moderator band attaches near the base of the anterior RV papillary muscle.

The *coronary sinus* is identified as it enters the RA adjacent to the tricuspid annulus. By slowly scanning back to an LV long-axis view, the coronary sinus can be followed along its length.

Another normal anatomic feature of the RA (Fig. 2–9) that may be appreciated on echocardiographic imaging is the *crista terminalis,* a muscular ridge that courses anteriorly from the superior to

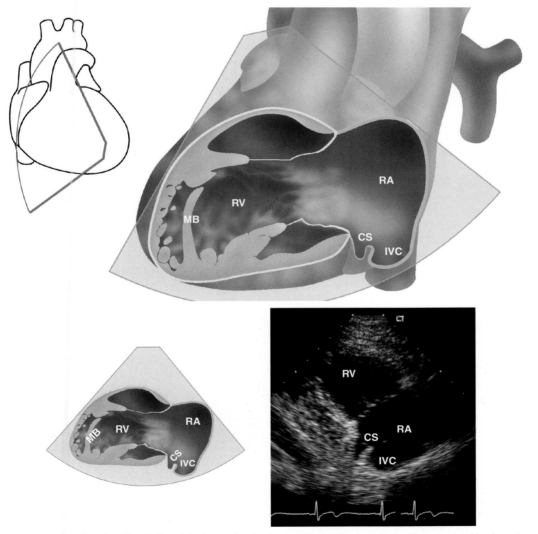

Figure 2–7 RV inflow view. The position of the image plane is shown on the line drawing with the 3D heart rotated to shown the anatomic details (*top*). The 2D image (*below left*) and tomographic plane (*below right*), shown in the standard orientation, show the RV and RA, tricuspid valve (TV), and ostia of the coronary sinus (CS) and inferior vena cava (IVC). In this view, two tricuspid leaflets are seen, typically the anterior and septal leaflets, but the posterior leaflet may be seen depending on the exact image plane and individual variation. MB, moderator band.

Figure 2–8 The interior of the RV. The crista supraventricularis separates the inflow part of the ventricle from the infundibulum, or conus arteriosus. Note the great distance between the septal leaflet of the TV and the pulmonary valve. *(From Rosse C, Gaddum-Rosse P: Hollinshead's Textbook of Anatomy, 5th ed. Philadelphia: Lippincott-Raven, 1997, p 473. Used with permission.)*

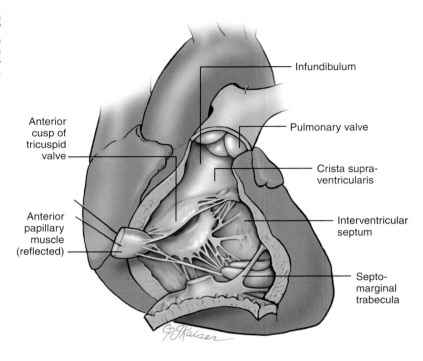

Figure 2–9 The interior of the RA seen from the right side. The view is toward the interatrial septum. *(From Rosse C, Gaddum-Rosse P: Hollinshead's Textbook of Anatomy, 5th ed. Philadelphia: Lippincott-Raven, 1997, p 473. Used with permission.)*

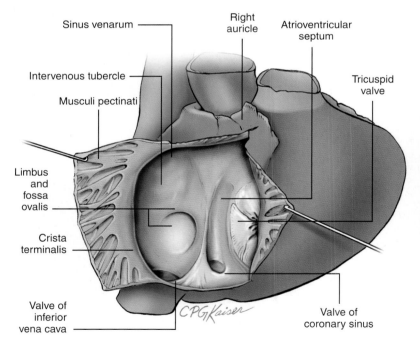

inferior vena cava and divides the trabeculated anterior portion of the RA from the posterior, smooth-walled sinus venosus segment. The RA appendage is rarely seen on transthoracic imaging but is a trabeculated protrusion of the RA extending anterior to the RA free wall and base of the aorta.

The *inferior vena cava* is seen entering the RA inferior to the coronary sinus. In some individuals a prominent Eustachian valve is seen at the junction of the inferior vena cava and RA both in this view and from the subcostal window. When a more extensive fenestrated valve is present, it forms a Chiari network extending from the inferior to superior vena cava, attached to the crista terminalis posteriorly and the fossa ovalis medially, with a netlike structure that appears as mobile echos in the RA. Both these findings are considered normal variants of no known clinical significance.

The interatrial septum is not well seen in the RV inflow view, being just inferior and parallel to the image plane. However, careful angulation between the long axis and RV inflow views allows examination of the atrial septum with recognition of the thick primum septum at its junction with the central fibrous body, the thin fossa ovalis in the central portion of the atrial septum, the ridgelike limbus located superior to the fossa, and the ridge adjacent to the junction with the coronary sinus.

Moving the transducer toward the base and then angulating laterally, a long-axis view of the RV outflow tract, *pulmonic valve*, and pulmonary artery is obtained. This view is particularly useful for recording flow velocities in the RV outflow tract and pulmonary artery.

Short-axis Views

Short-axis views are obtained from the parasternal window by rotating the transducer clockwise 90° and then angulating the transducer superiorly or inferiorly to obtain specific image planes.

At the *aortic valve* level (Figs. 2–10 and 2–11), the short-axis view demonstrates all three aortic valve leaflets—right, left, and noncoronary cusps. In systole the aortic leaflets open to a near-circular orifice. In diastole, the typical Y-shaped arrangement of the coaptation lines of the leaflets is seen. Identification of the number of aortic valve leaflets is made most accurately in systole, since a bicuspid valve may appear trileaflet in diastole due to a raphe in the position of a normal commissure. Normally, the aortic valve leaflets are thin at the base with an area of thickening on the ventricular aspect in the middle of

the free edge of each cusp, which serves to fill the space at the center of the closed valve. These nodules normally enlarge with age (nodules of Arantius) and can have small mobile filaments attached on the ventricular surface (Lambl's excrescences). These small but normal structures may be seen when echocardiographic images are of high quality and should not be mistaken for pathologic conditions. The origins of the left main and right coronary arteries often can be identified in this view.

The aortic and pulmonic valve planes normally lie perpendicular to each other. Thus, when the aortic valve is seen in short axis, the pulmonic valve is seen in long axis. In adults, evaluation of the leaflets of the pulmonic valve is limited; usually only one or two leaflets are seen well, and a short-axis view often is not obtainable. The close relationship between the aortic valve and other intracardiac structures is apparent in an anatomic view (Fig. 2–12). In addition to the pulmonic valve and RV outflow tract, which are seen anterolaterally adjacent to the left coronary cusp, portions of the tricuspid valve are seen anteriorly and slightly medially, adjacent to the right coronary cusp. The two leaflets of the tricuspid valve seen in this view are the septal and anterior leaflets.

Posteriorly, the RA, interatrial septum, and LA lie in proximity to the noncoronary cusp of the aortic valve. The LA appendage can be better imaged from this view by a slight lateral angulation and superior rotation of the transducer. The central location of the aortic valve illustrates how disease processes can extend from the aortic valve or root into the RV outflow tract, RA, or LA. Extension of disease processes into the ventricular septum or anterior mitral leaflet also is possible, as evident in the long-axis view.

At the *mitral valve* short-axis level (Fig. 2–13), the thin anterior and posterior mitral leaflets are seen as they open nearly to the full cross-sectional area of the LV in diastole and close in systole. The posterior leaflet consists of three major scallops—lateral, central, and medial (also called P1, P2, and P3)—although there is considerable individual variability. The two mitral commissures—the points on the annulus where the anterior and posterior leaflets meet—are located medially and laterally. Note that this parallels the arrangement of the papillary muscles so that chordae from the medial aspects of both anterior and posterior leaflets attach to the medial (or posteromedial) papillary muscle and chordae from the lateral aspects of both leaflets attach to the lateral (or anterolateral) papillary muscle. Chordae branch at three levels (primary, secondary, and tertiary) between the papillary muscle tip and mitral leaflet with a progressive decrease in chordal diameter and increase in the number of chordae from approximately 12 at the papillary muscle to 120 at the mitral leaflet. Most chordae attach at the free edge of the leaflets (called *marginal chordae*), but some (called *basal chordae*) attach to the LV surface of

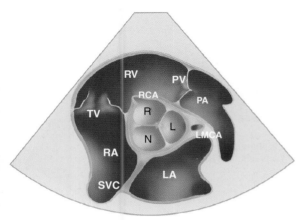

Figure 2–10 Parasternal short-axis view at the Ao valve level showing the relationship between the three cusps of the Ao valve—right coronary cusp (R), noncoronary cusp (N), left coronary cusp (L)—and the LA, RA, RVOT, and the PA with right and left branches. The positions of the right coronary artery (RCA), left main coronary artery (LMCA), superior vena cava (SVC), pulmonic valve (PV), and tricuspid valve (TV) are shown.

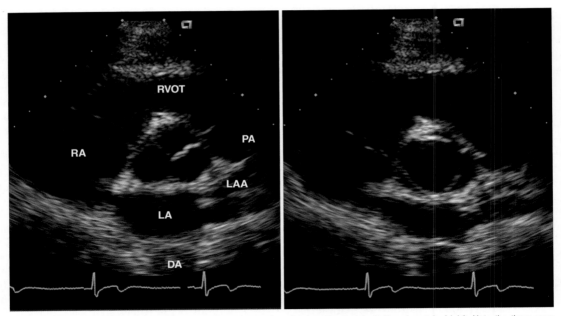

Figure 2–11 Two-dimensional echocardiographic images at the Ao valve level in diastole (*left*) and systole (*right*). Note the three open leaflets of the Ao valve in systole and the normal perpendicular relationship of aortic and pulmonic valves. LAA, left atrial appendage.

Figure 2–12 An anatomic view of the cardiac base looking toward the apex in a surgeon's view demonstrates the close relationships among the four cardiac valves. The Ao and pulmonic valve planes are perpendicular to each other. *(From Otto CM: Echocardiographic evaluation of valvular heart disease. In Otto CM, Bonow R [eds]: Valvular Heart Disease: A Companion to Braunwald's Heart Disease. Philadelphia: Elsevier/Saunders, 2009.)*

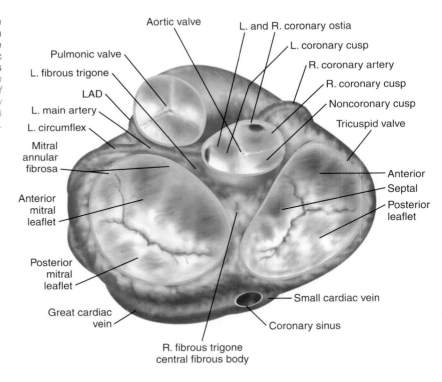

the leaflet. Occasionally, aberrant chordae to the ventricular septum or other structures are seen in an otherwise normal individual.

At the midventricular (or *papillary muscle*) level (Fig. 2–14), the normal LV is circular in the short-axis view. An elliptic appearance of the chamber usually is due to a nonperpendicular orientation relative to the long axis of the LV. Moving the transducer superiorly with apical angulation resolves this problem. Actual distortion of the circular cross section may be seen in patients with ischemic cardiac disease, prior myocardial infarction, and aneurysm formation. Although

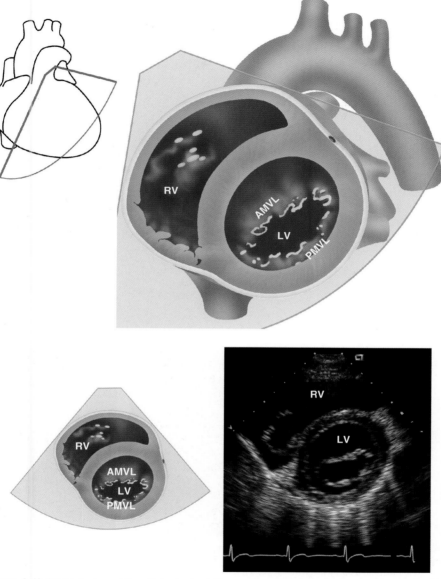

Figure 2–13 Short-axis plane at the mitral valve level. The position of the short-axis plane is shown on the line drawing. The 3D view is shown by tilting the apex up to show the cross-section of the RV and LV with the anterior and posterior mitral valve leaflets (AMVL and PMVL). The tomographic plane has been rotated with the apex of the sector at the top (*bottom left*) to correspond to the 2D echocardiographic image (*bottom right*).

chamber dimension measurements are made in the long-axis view, rotating the transducer between the long- and short-axis views at this level ensures that the short-axis measurement is both centered in the chamber and perpendicular to the long axis. Oblique measurements will result in overestimation of wall thickness and ventricular dimensions.

This view also allows assessment of segmental endocardial motion and wall thickening at the midventricular level. The nomenclature of LV myocardial segments is based on coronary anatomy as discussed in Chapter 8. Basically, the ventricle is divided into anterior (septum and free wall), anterolateral, inferolateral (also called posterior), and inferior (free wall and septum) segments for consistent descriptors of the location of abnormalities (Fig. 2–15). The segments are further defined by their location along the length of the ventricle as basal, midventricular, or apical. Ventricular septal motion may reflect abnormalities other than coronary disease, including RV volume and/or pressure overload, conduction abnormalities, and the post–cardiac surgery state (see Fig. 6–18).

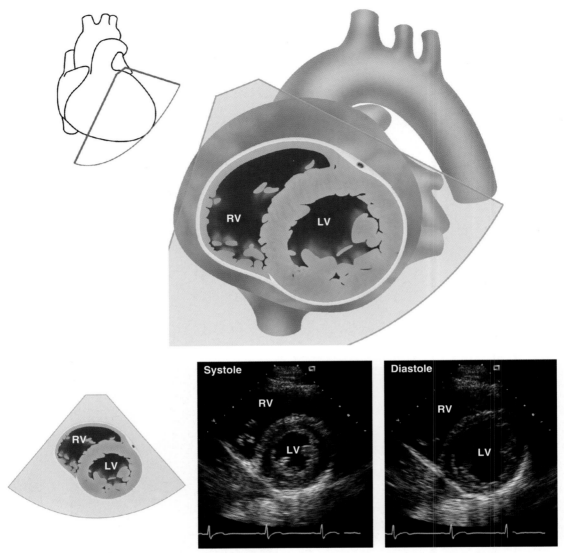

Figure 2–14 Short-axis plane at the papillary muscle level. The position of the short-axis plane is shown on the line drawing. The 3D view is shown by tilting the apex up to show the cross-section of the RV and LV with the medial and lateral papillary muscles. The tomographic plane has been rotated with the apex of the sector at the top (*bottom left*) to correspond to the 2D echocardiographic images in systole and diastole (*bottom right*). Note the circular shape of the LV with symmetric wall thickening and inward endocardial motion with contraction.

The medial and lateral papillary muscles are seen in this short-axis plane and serve as landmarks identifying the midventricular level. Rarely, one of the papillary muscles may be bifid, resulting in an appearance of three separate papillary muscles. Note that the apical segments of the LV myocardium are not seen in standard parasternal views. However, in some patients a short-axis view of the LV near the apex can be obtained by moving the transducer laterally and angling medially.

Apical Window

The apical window is identified initially by palpation of the LV apex with the patient in a steep left lateral decubitus position. An apical "cutout" in the examination stretcher allows optimal patient positioning and placement of the transducer on the apical impulse. Transducer position then is adjusted as needed to obtain optimal images. The relationship between the three basic apical views and the short-axis plane is shown in Figure 2–15.

Four-chamber View

In the apical four-chamber view, the length of the *LV* is seen in a plane perpendicular to both the short-axis and long-axis planes (Figs. 2–16 and 2–17). The anterolateral wall, apex, and inferior septum lie in this

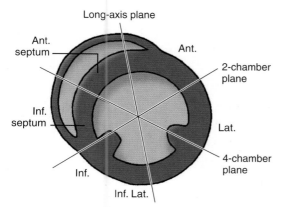

Figure 2–15 Relationship between the short-axis plane with LV wall segments indicated, and the apical four-chamber, two-chamber (also called vertical long axis), and long-axis image planes (perpendicular to the short-axis plane).

tomographic plane. The LV appears as a truncated ellipse with a longer length than width and a tapered but rounded apex. If the transducer is not positioned at the true apex, the LV will appear foreshortened, with a spherical shape and little tapering of the apex. Foreshortening of the long-axis plane must be distinguished from disease processes, such as chronic aortic

regurgitation, which result in increased sphericity of the ventricle. Although the RV is more trabeculated than the LV, prominent trabeculation also can be seen at the LV apex and must be distinguished from apical thrombus. When aberrant LV trabeculae transverse the ventricular chamber, a "chord" or "web" is seen on 2D echo.

Medially, the *right ventricle* is triangular in shape with a cavity about half the area of the LV. The RV apex is less round and more basal than the LV apex. The moderator band often is seen traversing the RV near the apex. The RV can be further evaluated by moving the transducer medially over the RV apex. Considerable individual variability in the shape and wall motion of the RV, particularly at the apex, is seen in normal individuals, so caution is needed in diagnosing an abnormal RV from any single tomographic plane.

The four-chamber view also shows the mitral annulus in its major dimension, the anterior mitral valve leaflet (located adjacent to the septum), and the posterior mitral valve leaflet (adjacent to the lateral wall), along with chordae and attachments to the lateral papillary muscle. The mitral leaflet tips separate widely in diastole, and in systole the closure plane of the leaflets may appear "flat" (a 180° closure angle) due to the nonplanar "saddle" shape of the annulus, with the

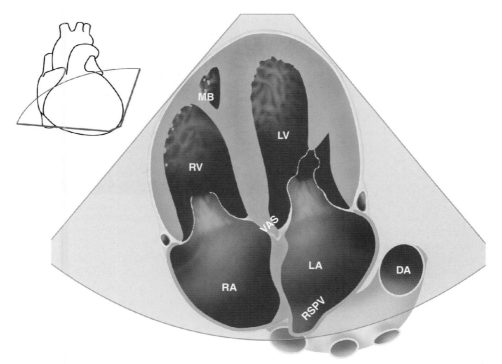

Figure 2–16 Apical four-chamber view. The apical four-chamber view shows the relationships of the LV and RV and the LA and RA. In the LV, the papillary muscle, chordae, and anterior and posterior mitral leaflets are seen. The descending artery (DA) is seen in partial cross-section lateral to the LA, while the right superior pulmonary vein (RSPV) drains into the left atrium adjacent to the interatrial septum. In the RV, the moderator band (MB) and the anterior and septal TV leaflets are seen. Note the ventricular atrial septum (VAS) separating the LV from the RA in association with the normal, slightly more apical position of the tricuspid compared with the mitral valve annulus.

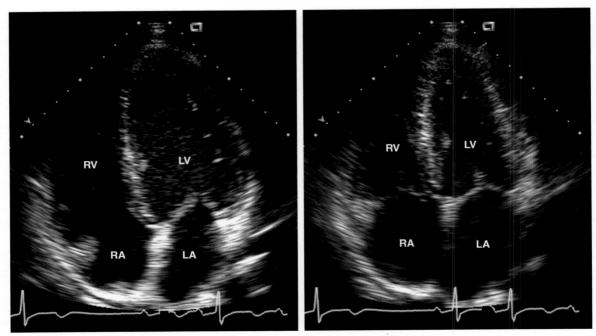

Figure 2–17 Two-dimensional echo images in an apical four-chamber view at end-diastole (*left*) and end-systole (*right*).

four-chamber view bisecting the annulus at its most apical position compared to the more basal annulus segments seen in a long-axis view. However, significant displacement of the leaflets beyond the plane of the mitral annulus is not seen unless the view is foreshortened or mitral valve disease is present.

The tricuspid annulus lies slightly (≤ 1.0 cm) closer to the apex than the mitral annulus. The tricuspid leaflets show a wide diastolic opening; thin, uniformly echogenic leaflets; and normal coaptation in systole. The septal leaflet is imaged adjacent to the septum. The tricuspid leaflet adjacent to the free wall may be either the anterior or posterior leaflet, depending on the exact rotation and angulation of the image plane.

The left and right atria are distal from the apical transducer position. Although a general assessment of size and shape can be made, ultrasound resolution at this depth is poor, and detailed evaluation of atrial tumors or clots often is not possible. The interatrial septum lies parallel to the ultrasound beam in this view, so "dropout"—absence of reflected signal—from the region of the fossa ovalis is common. This should not be mistaken for an atrial septal defect. Measurement of LA volume may be helpful when accurate evaluation of LA size is clinically indicated (Fig. 2–18).

The descending thoracic aorta can be seen lateral to the LA. The pulmonary veins enter the LA posteriorly but may be difficult to image at this depth in adults. If the transducer is angulated posteriorly from the four-chamber view, more posterior portions of the lateral and inferior septal myocardium are seen.

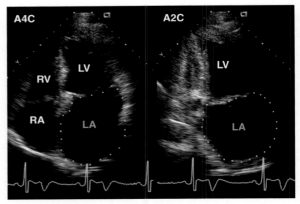

Figure 2–18 LA volume can be calculated by tracing the LA border in systole in the apical four-chamber and two-chamber views.

In addition, the length of the coronary sinus comes into view in the atrioventricular groove.

Angulating the transducer anteriorly, the aortic valve and root are seen in an oblique long-axis view. This view is sometimes referred to as the apical "five-chamber" view. More anterior portions of the septum and lateral wall are seen, especially at the base, as the transducer is angulated anteriorly. This view of the anterior mitral leaflet, LV outflow tract, and aortic valve is at an angle approximately 60° to 90° from the standard long-axis view. In some adults, further anterior angulation of the transducer allows visualization of the pulmonary artery arising from the RV. A view of the pulmonic valve from the apical window is more easily obtained in young adults and children.

Two-chamber View

From the four-chamber view, the transducer is rotated counterclockwise about 60° to obtain the two-chamber view of the LV, mitral valve, and LA (Fig. 2–19). The apical two-chamber view is used for evaluation of the anterior LV wall (seen to the right of the screen) and the posterior or inferolateral wall (seen on the left). Fine adjustments in transducer position may be needed to visualize the anterior wall endocardium due to interference from adjacent lung tissue. To ensure that the proper rotation has been made for a two-chamber view, the transducer is angled posteriorly to intersect both papillary muscles symmetrically. Then the transducer is angled slightly anteriorly so

that neither papillary muscle is seen in its long axis in this view. The anterior mitral leaflet is seen en face, so the apparent closure plane of the leaflet relative to the annulus can be misleading. The LA appendage may be visualized adjacent to the anterior wall. A long-axis view of the descending thoracic aorta can be obtained by angulating posteriorly and rotating counterclockwise from the two-chamber view.

Long-axis View

Rotating the transducer another 60° from the two-chamber view (120° from the four-chamber view) yields a long-axis view similar to the parasternal long-axis view. (Fig. 2–20) The aortic valve, LV outflow tract, and mitral valve are seen in long axis. The LV walls visualized in this view are the anterior septum (on the right side of the screen) and posterior

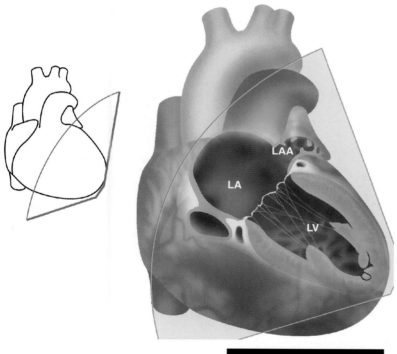

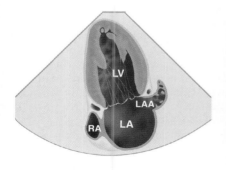

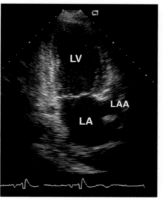

Figure 2–19 Apical two-chamber view. The position of the image plane is shown on the line drawing. The 3D view shows the cross-section of the LA and LV with the left atrial appendage (LAA), coronary sinus (CS) in the atrioventricular groove, and the mitral valve. In the apical two-chamber view, small portions of the posterior mitral leaflet are seen laterally and medially with the anterior leaflet filling most of the annulus area. Part of a papillary muscle has been shown for orientation, but the papillary muscles are located symmetrically posterior to the image plane. The tomographic plane has been rotated with the apex of the sector at the top (*bottom left*) to correspond to the 2D echocardiographic image (*bottom right*). In this view the inferior and anterior LV walls are seen.

Figure 2–20 Apical long-axis view. The position of the image plane is shown on the line drawing. The 3D view shows the cross-section of the Ao root, LV, LA, and RVOT. In the long- axis view the anterior and posterior mitral valve leaflets are seen. The tomographic plane has been rotated with the apex of the sector at the top (*bottom left*) to correspond to the 2D echocadiographic image (*bottom right*). In this view the anterior septum and posterior (inferolateral) LV walls are seen.

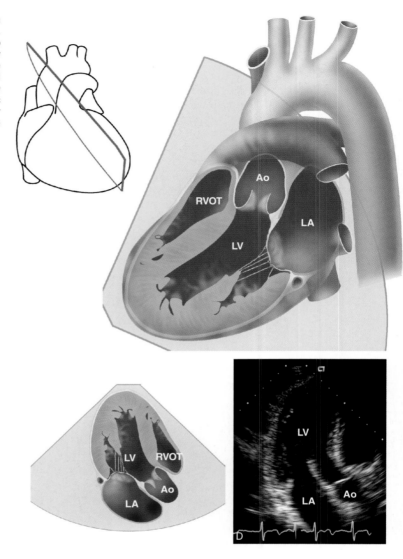

or inferolateral wall (on the left). Compared with the parasternal long-axis view, the LV apex now is seen, but the aortic and mitral valves are at a greater image depth (with consequent poorer image resolution).

Other Apical Views

Nonstandard short-axis views of the LV apex using a higher frequency transducer (5 or 7.5 MHz) are helpful if an LV apical thrombus is suspected. One useful view is obtained by sliding the transducer laterally from the LV apex and then angulating medially.

Subcostal Window

With the patient supine and the legs bent at the knees (if necessary) to relax the abdominal wall musculature, subcostal images of the cardiac structures are obtained. A view of all four chambers shows the RV free wall, the midsection of the interventricular septum, and the anterolateral LV wall (Fig. 2–21). In this view, the interatrial septum is perpendicular to the direction of the ultrasound beam, allowing evaluation of atrial septal defects.

A subcostal short-axis view of the LV allows measurements of LV wall thickness and dimensions that are comparable with dimensions obtained from a parasternal short-axis view, albeit at a greater depth and through different myocardial segments. The subcostal window provides a useful alternative for qualitative and quantitative evaluation of the LV when the parasternal window is inadequate.

Rotating the transducer inferiorly from the subcostal four-chamber view, a long-axis view of the inferior vena cava is obtained as it enters the right atrium (see Fig. 6–23). The size of the inferior vena cava (1–2 cm

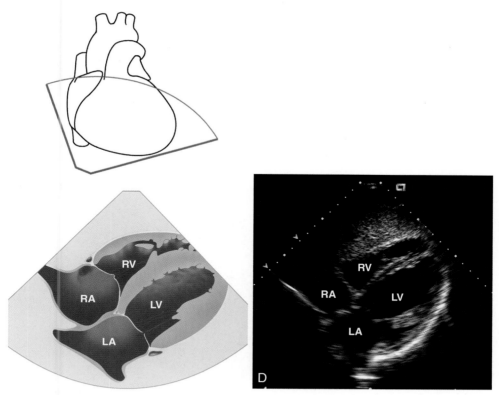

Figure 2–21 Subcostal four-chamber view. The position of the image plane (*left*), tomographic view rotated with apex of the sector scan at the top of the image (*center*), and corresponding 2D (*right*) subcostal view. The interatrial septum is perpendicular to the ultrasound beam from this window, allowing evaluation for atrial septal defects.

from the RA junction) at rest and changes in size with respiration are used to estimate RA pressure (see Table 6–7). The hepatic veins (particularly the central hepatic vein, which courses parallel to the ultrasound beam in this view) are helpful in assessing RA pressure and for recording RA Doppler filling patterns. The proximal abdominal aorta is imaged in long axis medial to the inferior vena cava.

Suprasternal Notch Window

With the patient supine and the neck extended, the transducer is positioned in the suprasternal notch or right supraclavicular position to obtain a view of the aortic arch in long and short-axis. The long-axis view (with respect to the aortic arch) shows the ascending aorta, arch, proximal descending thoracic aorta, and the origins of the right brachiocephalic and left common carotid and subclavian arteries (Fig. 2–22). The corresponding veins lie superior to the aortic arch, with the superior vena cava lying adjacent to the ascending aorta. The right pulmonary artery is seen "under" the curve of the aortic arch and can be followed to its branch point by rotating the transducer medially.

The short-axis view shows the aortic arch in cross-section. The left pulmonary artery can be imaged by rotating slightly laterally. The LA lies inferior to the pulmonary arteries in both long- and short-axis views, so it may be possible to evaluate atrial pathology or flow disturbances from this window.

Other Acoustic Windows

In specific cases, other acoustic windows may be needed. For example, a dextropositioned heart would necessitate mirror-image acoustic windows. When a large pleural effusion is present, good-quality images may be obtained in some cases by imaging from the posterior chest wall through the effusion with the patient in a sitting position.

M-MODE RECORDINGS

Although M-mode recordings have largely been replaced by 2D imaging, M-mode recordings still have an important role in evaluation of rapid motion of cardiac structures, since the sampling rate is 1800 frames per second rather than the 30 to 60 frames per second used for 2D imaging. The rapid sampling rate also makes identification of thin moving structures, such as the LV endocardium, more accurate

Figure 2–22 Suprasternal notch view. The position of the image plane is shown on the line drawing. The 3D view shows the cross-section of the ascending Ao, arch, and proximal descending Ao with the origins of the left carotid and subclavian arteries. The RPA lies immediately inferior to the arch, with the LA and Ao valve sometimes seen from this window.

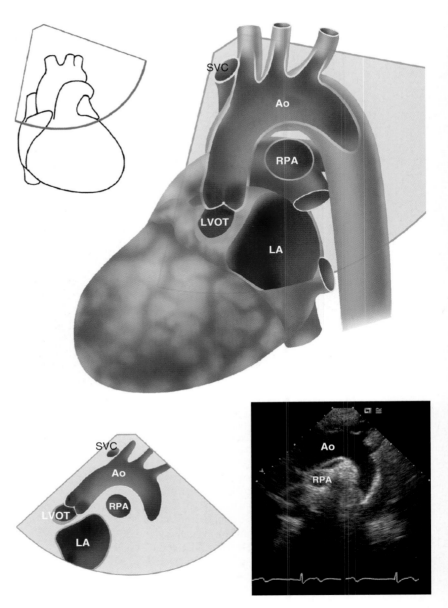

and reproducible by showing motion as well as depth of the structure of interest. The potential disadvantage of M-mode data—a nonperpendicular orientation to the structure of interest—can be avoided by using the 2D image in two orthogonal planes to position the M-mode sampling line.

Use of the M-mode feature is most helpful when guided by the 2D image and used for:

☐ timing of rapid cardiac motions,
☐ precise measurements of cardiac dimensions, or
☐ further evaluation of structures seen on 2D imaging (such as suspected vegetations) to aid in their identification.

Aortic Valve and Left Atrium

An M-mode recording through the aortic valve at the leaflet tip level shows the parallel walls of the aorta moving anteriorly in systole and posteriorly in diastole (Fig. 2–23). The LA is posterior to the aortic root and shows filling in atrial diastole (ventricular systole) and emptying in atrial systole (ventricular diastole). LA filling is largely responsible for the anterior displacement of the aortic root, so aortic root "motion" on M-mode reflects LA dimensions. Increased aortic root motion is seen when there is increased LA filling and emptying (e.g., with mitral regurgitation). Decreased aortic root motion is seen in states of low

Aortic Valve and Left Atrial M-Mode

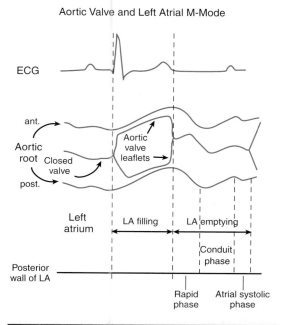

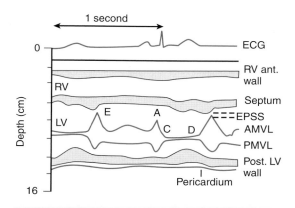

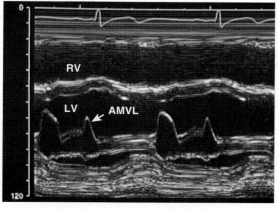

Figure 2–24 Schematic (*top*) and M-mode tracing (*bottom*) of a normal mitral valve.

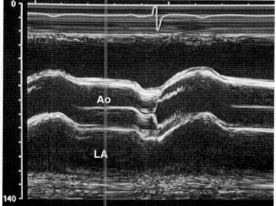

Figure 2–23 Schematic (*top*) and M-mode tracing (*bottom*) of a normal Ao valve and LA.

cardiac output, with corresponding low volumes of atrial filling and emptying.

The aortic leaflet coaptation point is seen as a thin line in diastole. In systole, the leaflets separate rapidly and completely, forming a boxlike appearance on the M-mode recording. Fine systolic fluttering of the aortic valve leaflets may be seen in normal individuals.

Mitral Valve

An M-mode recording at the mitral valve level intercepts the anterior RV wall and chamber, the interventricular septum, the anterior and posterior mitral leaflets, the posterior LV wall, and the pericardium (Fig. 2–24). The coaptation point of the mitral leaflets in systole is seen as a thin line that moves slightly anteriorly during systole, paralleling the motion of the

posterior wall. In early diastole, the leaflets separate widely, with the maximum early diastolic motion of the anterior leaflet termed the *E point*. Normally, there is only a small distance between the E point and the maximal posterior motion of the ventricular septum— *E-point septal separation (EPSS)*. In the absence of mitral stenosis an increased EPSS indicates LV dilation, systolic dysfunction, or aortic regurgitation.

The leaflets move toward each other in mid-diastole (diastasis) and then separate again with atrial systole, resulting in the late-diastolic peak, the *A point*. The slope of anterior mitral leaflet closure from the A point to the closure point *(C)* is linear unless LV end-diastolic pressure is elevated when a "*B* bump" or "*A–C* shoulder" may be seen on the M-mode recording of mitral valve motion. Fine fluttering of the anterior mitral leaflet is not seen in normal individuals and usually indicates aortic regurgitation.

Left Ventricle

A 2D-guided M-mode recording perpendicular to the long axis of and through the center of the LV at the papillary muscle level provides standard measurements of systolic and diastolic wall thickness and chamber dimensions (Fig. 2–25). These measurements are

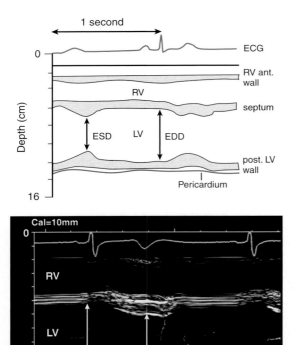

Figure 2–25 Schematic (*top*) and M-mode tracing (*bottom*) at the LV papillary muscle level. EDD, end-diastolic dimension; ESD, end-systolic dimension.

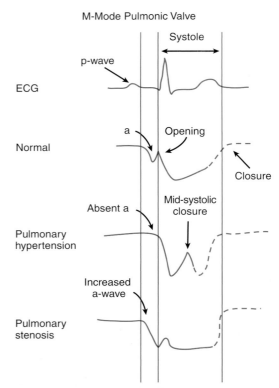

Figure 2–26 Patterns of pulmonic valve motion.

limited in that they represent only a single line through the LV and thus do not accurately describe the LV when the disease process is asymmetric, such as with prior myocardial infarction. However, many disease processes do result in symmetric changes in the LV (volume overload, hypertrophy), and the accuracy and reproducibility of these measurements make them useful in patient management. Examples of their utility include sequential evaluations of LV end-systolic dimension in patients with chronic asymptomatic aortic regurgitation or assessment of LV hypertrophy in hypertensive patients.

The posterior wall endocardium is identified as the continuous line with the steepest upslope in early systole, taking care to distinguish the endocardium from reflections due to overlying mitral chordal structures. Similarly, the endocardium of the septum is identified as a continuous line with systolic inward motion. Measurements are made from the leading edge of the septal endocardial echo to the leading edge of the posterior wall endocardium.

An M-mode recording at this level also may be helpful in timing the motion of the RV free wall

when cardiac tamponade is suspected or for detection of a small posterior pericardial effusion.

Other M-Mode Recordings

An M-mode recording through the pulmonic valve is similar to an aortic valve M-mode recording except that usually only one leaflet can be recorded in adults. The slight displacement of the leaflet in diastole (after atrial contraction) is called the A wave and is increased (>7 mm) when pulmonic stenosis is present and decreased (<2 mm) when pulmonary hypertension is present. Transient midsystolic closure (or "notching") of the pulmonic valve on M-mode may be seen when pulmonary hypertension is present (Fig. 2–26). An M-mode recording through the tricuspid valve is analogous to a mitral valve recording but rarely is useful clinically.

NORMAL INTRACARDIAC FLOW PATTERNS

Basic Principles

Laminar versus Disturbed Flow

Normal intracardiac flow patterns are characterized by laminar flow. *Laminar flow* is defined as movement of fluid along well-defined parallel stream lines with uniform flow velocities (Fig. 2–27). In three dimensions,

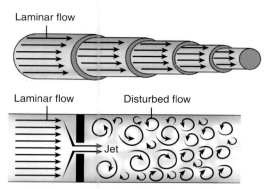

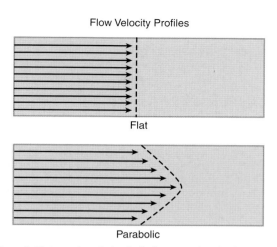

Figure 2–27 Laminar flow is characterized by parallel stream lines at uniform velocities with concentric layers of flow, each with a predictable and uniform direction and velocity (*top*). Disturbed flow occurs downstream from areas of narrowing (stenotic orifice, regurgitant orifice, or intracardiac shunt) with blood flow in multiple directions and velocities (*bottom*). In the orifice itself, a laminar high-velocity jet occurs.

Figure 2–28 In a schematic longitudinal cross-section of a flow stream, with the length of each arrow proportional to velocity, the difference between a flat and a parabolic flow velocity profile is shown.

laminar flow consists of concentric layers (or lamina) of flow, each with a predictable and uniform direction and velocity.

Steady laminar flow becomes disturbed when the dimensionless Reynolds number exceeds 2000 to 2500. The Reynolds number (R_e) is directly related to blood flow velocity V, lumen diameter d, and blood density ρ, and inversely related to viscosity γ:

$$R_e = (Vd\rho)/\gamma \qquad (2\text{-}1)$$

When blood flow patterns are disturbed, blood cells move in multiple directions at multiple velocities rather than along uniform, parallel stream lines. *Turbulence*, in fluid dynamic terms, refers to the specific situation in which the flow pattern of a particular fluid element is no longer predictable. While intracardiac flow disturbances rarely show true turbulence, this term is used clinically to denote nonlaminar flow.

Flow-Velocity Profiles

The spatial distribution of velocities in cross section at a specific intracardiac location and at a specific time point in the cardiac cycle is known as the *flow-velocity profile* (Fig. 2–28). If all the parallel stream lines in a laminar flow pattern have the same velocity, then the flow-velocity profile is "flat." If velocity is higher in the center of the vessel and lower at the walls of the vessel, the flow profile is "curved" (usually parabolic). While normal flow in peripheral vessels has a curved flow-velocity profile, many intracardiac flows have a relatively flat flow-velocity profile. Factors that tend to equalize the velocity distribution across the cross-sectional area of flow include tapering of the flow stream, acceleration of flow, and an inlet-type geometry. Thus, the proximal aorta and pulmonary artery and the mitral and tricuspid annuli have reasonably flat flow-velocity profiles. Downstream, the spatial

distribution of flow changes. For example, in the ascending aorta the flow profile becomes skewed, with higher velocity flow along the inside curve of the aortic arch and lower velocities along the outer curve. Many Doppler quantitative methods make assumptions about the spatial flow profile at a particular intracardiac site. In some cases these assumptions can be verified by careful pulsed or color Doppler evaluation.

Clinical Quantitative Doppler Methods

There are three basic principles common to the clinical use of Doppler ultrasound in evaluation of cardiac disease. These will be presented briefly here and in more detail, including technical aspects and potential pitfalls, in subsequent chapters as follows:

❒ Measurement of volume flow in Chapter 6
❒ The relationship between velocity and pressure gradients in Chapter 11
❒ The spatial flow pattern through a small orifice (e.g., regurgitant valve) in Chapter 12

Measurement of Volume Flow

When blood flow is laminar with a flat flow-velocity profile, it is intuitive that the instantaneous flow rate can be calculated as cross-sectional area or *CSA* (in cm^2) times flow velocity (in cm/s). Similarly, by integrating flow velocity over the duration of flow, stroke volume, *SV* (in cm^3) can be calculated as:

$$SV(\text{cm}^3) = CSA(\text{cm}^2) \times VTI(\text{cm}) \qquad (2\text{-}2)$$

where *VTI* is the velocity-time integral (cm) of the Doppler velocity curve. This method is used clinically to measure SV and cardiac output at rest or after physiologic or pharmacologic interventions, to evaluate the severity of valvular regurgitation, as a component in the equation for valve area calculations, and to quantitate the ratio of pulmonary to systemic blood flow in patients with intracardiac shunts.

Velocity-Pressure Relationships

At any area of significant narrowing in the flow stream—whether a stenotic valve, a ventricular septal defect, or a regurgitant orifice—flow velocity increases in relation to the degree of narrowing; the narrower the opening, the higher is the velocity for a given volume flow rate. In most clinical situations the velocity in this narrow "jet" through the narrowed orifice is related quantitatively to the pressure gradient across the narrowing, as stated in the simplified Bernoulli equation:

$$\Delta P = 4v^2 \qquad (2\text{-}3)$$

where ΔP is the instantaneous pressure gradient (mm Hg) and v is the instantaneous velocity (m/s). This relationship between pressure gradient and velocity is important for quantitation of valve stenosis severity, noninvasive determination of pulmonary artery pressures, and evaluation of other intracardiac hemodynamics (see Table 2–8) using continuous-wave Doppler ultrasound.

Spatial Pattern of Flow

Flow through a small orifice is characterized by a:

- ❑ Proximal flow convergence region
- ❑ Narrow flow stream through the orifice, called the vena contracta
- ❑ Downstream flow disturbance

Each of these components of the spatial flow pattern can be evaluated with color flow imaging, which allows real-time demonstrations of flow patterns in each tomographic plane, for example, with valve regurgitation. The proximal flow convergence region allows calculation of volume flow rates. The vena contracta provides a simple measure of regurgitant severity. The downstream flow disturbance allows detection of valvular regurgitation and intracardiac shunts, and determination of the anatomic level of RV or LV outflow obstruction. In addition, the 3D shape of the flow disturbance may provide clues as to the etiology of regurgitation.

Normal Antegrade Intracardiac Flows

Normal antegrade intracardiac flows can be evaluated with either pulsed or continuous-wave Doppler ultrasound (Tables 2–4 and 2–5). Accurate measurement of antegrade flow velocities is dependent on several technical factors. Most important is a parallel alignment between the ultrasound beam and the

TABLE 2–4 Transthoracic Views for Normal Antegrade Flow Velocities

Antegrade Flow	View
LVOT	A4C (angulated anterior) Apical long-axis
Aorta (ascending)	LV-apex SSN
Descending aorta Thoracic Proximal abdominal	SSN SC
LV inflow (mitral)	A4C or long-axis
RVOT	PSAX (aortic valve level) SC short-axis
RV inflow (tricuspid)	RV inflow A4C
LA inflow (pulmonary vein)	A4C
RA inflow	SC (central HV) SSN (SVC)

A4C, apical four-chamber; HV, hepatic vein; PSAX, parasternal short-axis; SC, subcostal; SSN, suprasternal notch; SVC, superior vena cava.

TABLE 2–5 Normal Antegrade Doppler Flow Velocities

	Normal Range (m/s)
Ascending Ao	1.0–1.7
LVOT	0.7–1.1
LV inflow	
E-velocity	0.6–1.3 (0.72 ± 0.14)
Deceleration slope	5.0±1.4 m/s
A-velocity	0.2–0.7 (0.47 ± 0.4)
PA	0.5–1.3
RV inflow	
E-velocity	0.3–0.7
RA filling (SVC, HV)	
Systole	0.32–0.69 (0.46 ± 0.08) m/s
Diastole	0.06–0.45 (0.27 ± 0.08) m/s
LA filling (PV)	
Systole	0.56 ± 0.13 m/s
Diastole	0.44 ± 0.16 m/s
Atrial reversal	0.32 ± 0.07 m/s

HV, hepatic vein; LVOT, left ventricular outflow tract; PV, pulmonary vein; SVC, superior vena cava.
Data sources: Wilson et al: Br Heart J 53:451, 1985; Hatle and Angelsen: Doppler Ultrasound in Cardiology, 2nd ed. Philadelphia: Lea & Febiger, 1985; Van Dam et al: Eur Heart J 8: 1221, 1987; 9:165, 1988; Jaffe et al: Am J Cardiol 68:550, 1991; Appleton et al: J Am Coll Cardiol 10:1032, 1987.

direction of blood flow. The ultrasound instrument measures Doppler frequency shifts. The displayed velocities are *calculated* with the Doppler equation based on transducer frequency, the speed of sound in blood, and the angle between the Doppler beam and flow of interest. For intracardiac flows, the 3D direction of flow is difficult to determine, particularly when flow is abnormal, and attempts to "correct" for the presumed intercept angle are likely to increase, rather than decrease, measurement error. Instead, the examiner positions the ultrasound beam as parallel as possible to the flow of interest based on obtaining the highest calculated velocity with careful transducer positioning and angulation. In the Doppler equation, $\cos \theta = 1$ (and therefore can be ignored) when flow is oriented directly away (intercept angle $= 0°$) or straight toward (intercept angle $= 180°$) the ultrasound transducer. Small deviations from a parallel intercept angle (up to 20°) result in only a small error (6%) in velocity calculations (see Fig. 1–27). While this approach generally results in accurate velocity data, the possibility of underestimation of intracardiac velocities due to a nonparallel intercept angle always must be considered in all echocardiographic examinations. This potential limitation becomes significant when recording high-velocity flows in valvular stenosis, regurgitation, or intracardiac shunts.

Other technical factors pertinent to recording antegrade flow velocities include the use of an appropriate velocity scale, wall filters, and gain settings. The standard velocity format is to display flows toward the transducer above and flows away from the transducer below the zero baseline. The baseline is shifted to maximize the flow of interest and the velocity scale adjusted so that the velocity curve uses the entire displayed range. Wall filters are set as low as possible, without resulting in excessive noise, to allow accurate measurement of time intervals. Gain settings are adjusted to show the peak velocity and velocity curve clearly without excessive background noise. A sample volume length of 5 to 10 mm typically is used to record antegrade flow velocities, because this length provides reasonable intracardiac localization with adequate signal strength.

Signal aliasing (as discussed in Chapter 1) occurs even with normal intracardiac flow velocities. Use of baseline shift can resolve this problem in most cases. If aliasing persists, use of high pulse repetition frequency or continuous-wave Doppler is needed for unambiguous display of the maximum velocity.

With appropriate instrument settings and attention to technical details, antegrade velocities with pulsed Doppler ultrasound appear as smooth envelopes with a well-defined onset and end of flow, a well-defined maximum velocity, and a thin band of velocities at each time point. The area under the velocity curve is "clear," because the flow velocities at a specific intracardiac site are relatively uniform. Continuous-wave

Doppler recordings differ in that the curve is "filled in" due to inclusion of lower velocities along the entire length of the ultrasound beam.

Left Ventricular Outflow

An apical or suprasternal notch window is used to obtain a parallel intercept angle between the ultrasound beam and direction of blood flow in the LV outflow tract and ascending aorta. In general, LV outflow velocities are most accurately recorded from a transthoracic approach, since it is more difficult to obtain a parallel intercept angle from the TEE approach. In some cases, a transgastric "apical" approach may be useful, but potential underestimation of velocity, due to a nonparallel intercept angle, always should be considered.

With a pulsed Doppler sample volume positioned on the LV side of the aortic valve, an ejection velocity curve is recorded with a steep acceleration slope, a sharply peaked early-systolic maximum velocity, and a less steep deceleration slope (Figs. 2–29 and 2–30). Note the narrow band of velocities at any instant in time during acceleration, reflecting the uniformity of blood flow velocity in the outflow tract during acceleration. During deceleration the range of flow velocities at any instant is slightly wider (spectral broadening), since instability in the flow pattern during deceleration results in slight variation in flow velocities. The aortic valve closing click is seen immediately following end-ejection. Flow recordings with pulsed Doppler on the aortic side of the valve appear similar except that the aortic valve opening click is seen, instead of the closing click, and the maximum velocity is slightly higher, by

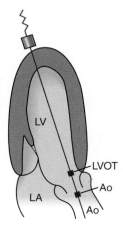

Figure 2–29 LV outflow velocity is recorded with pulsed Doppler from an anteriorly angulated apical four-chamber view or an apical long-axis view (as shown here) with the sample volume positioned just proximal to the Ao valve closure plane (LVOT). Sample volume position is adjusted based on the Doppler signal showing an Ao valve closing, but not opening click. The sample volume depth is increased to just beyond the tips of the open valve leaflets in systole for recording aortic flow velocity (Ao).

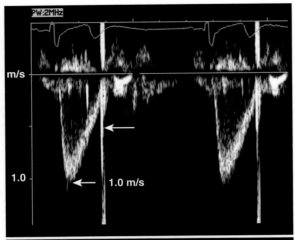

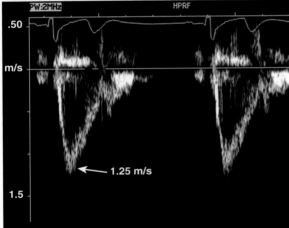

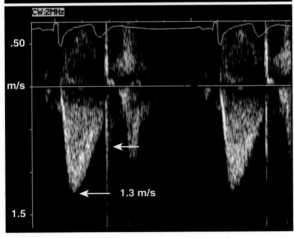

Figure 2–30 Normal LV, outflow recorded with pulsed Doppler proximal to the Ao valve (*top*) shows a smooth velocity curve with a well-defined peak of 1.0 m/s and a clear closing click. There is a very narrow velocity curve during acceleration with slight spectral broadening during deceleration due to differences in the uniformity of flow during acceleration and deceleration. Flow recorded using pulsed Doppler distal to the aortic valve (*center*) shows a higher velocity laminar flow with no visible valve click. Continuous-wave Doppler (*bottom*) recording of Ao flow shows both an opening and closing click and filling in of the velocity curve due to recording velocity along the entire length of the ultrasound beam.

0.2 to 0.4 m/s, than the outflow tract velocity due to slight narrowing of the cross-sectional area of flow at the aortic leaflet tips.

With continuous-wave Doppler interrogation of the aortic valve, both opening and closing clicks are recorded. The area under the velocity curve is filled in with lower velocity signals, because lower velocity blood flow signals that originate in the LV along the length of the ultrasound beam are displayed as well.

With a normal aortic valve, the area under the velocity curve (the *velocity-time integral*) reflects stroke volume, which can be calculated by multiplying by cross-sectional area. The normal antegrade maximum velocity across the valve is about 1 to 1.2 m/s and is the same whether measured by pulsed or continuous-wave Doppler methods. The normal outflow tract velocity typically is 0.8 to 1 m/s, corresponding to a velocity "step-up" across the valve or ratio of outflow tract to aortic velocity of 0.7 to 1.

The relationship between velocity and pressure gradients across *nonstenotic* valves is somewhat complex and is not fully described by the Bernoulli equation (which applies to areas of narrowing). The period of acceleration corresponds to a slight pressure gradient from the LV to the aorta, with the maximum pressure gradient corresponding to maximum acceleration. LV pressure falls below aortic pressure in mid-systole, and at this point, deceleration of flow occurs. Thus, for the normal valve, maximum velocity occurs at the pressure crossover point (see Fig. 6–1). During deceleration, aortic pressure remains slightly higher than LV pressure until flow decelerates to zero and the valve closes. At this point, LV pressure continues to decline rapidly.

Right Ventricular Outflow

The RV outflow tract and pulmonary artery velocities are recorded from a parasternal short-axis or RV outflow view (Fig. 2–31). In the normal individual the RV ejection curve is similar to the LV ejection curve except that peak velocity is slightly lower (0.8–1 m/s), the ejection period is longer, and the velocity curve is more rounded, with the maximum velocity occurring in mid-systole. The shapes of the RV and LV ejection curves appear to relate to the downstream vascular resistance. The low-resistance pulmonary vasculature results in a slower rate of acceleration of blood flow, with the maximum velocity (and pressure crossover) occurring later in the ejection cycle. When pulmonary vascular resistance is increased, the RV ejection curve resembles LV ejection more closely with a sharper velocity curve and earlier peak velocity.

Left Ventricular Inflow

Diastolic flow across the mitral valve shows two peaks: an early diastolic peak velocity (*E* wave) reflecting passive early-diastolic filling and a late

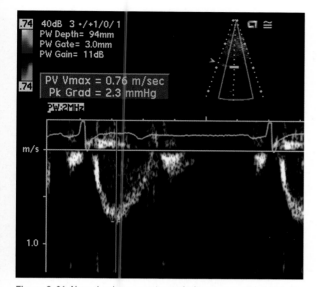

Figure 2–31 Normal pulmonary artery velocity curve recorded with the pulsed Doppler sample volume positioned in the mid–pulmonary artery from a parasternal short-axis view. The velocity curve is rounded with a peak in mid-systole and a maximum velocity of about 0.8 m/s. Compare the shape of this velocity curve with the LV outflow curve seen in Figure 2–30.

diastolic peak velocity due to atrial contraction (A wave) (Fig. 2–32). The normal E velocity in healthy young individuals is about 1 m/s, with an A velocity of 0.2 to 0.4 m/s, reflecting the normal small contribution of atrial contraction to LV diastolic filling. If diastole is long enough, a period of no flow, or diastasis, between the two flow curves is seen.

Even in normal individuals the pattern of LV diastolic filling varies with age, loading conditions, heart rate, and PR interval. With age, there is a gradual reduction in E velocity, prolongation in the rate of early diastolic deceleration, and increase in A velocity such that the ratio of E to A velocity changes from >1 in young individuals, to about 1 at ages 50 to 60, to <1 in older normal individuals.

Increased preload results in an increase in E velocity, while decreased preload has the opposite effect. When diastole is short (i.e., with a rapid heart rate), the A velocity becomes superimposed (or summated) onto the downslope of the E velocity, resulting in an apparent higher A velocity. At very high heart rates, only a single E/A peak may be seen. Prolongation of the PR interval has a similar effect. When atrial contraction occurs earlier in diastole, the A velocity

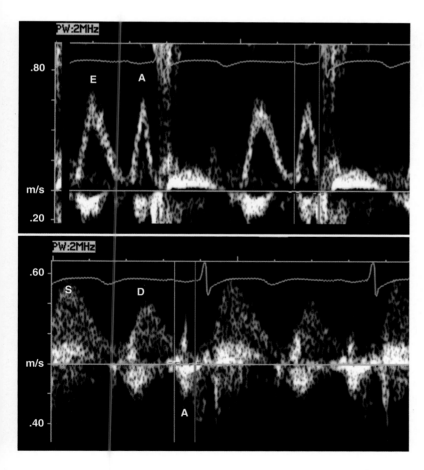

Figure 2–32 Normal LV inflow velocity curve (top) recorded with pulsed Doppler showing rapid early-diastolic filling (E) and the atrial (A) contribution to late-diastolic filling. LA filling (bottom) recorded on transthoracic echocardiography in the right superior pulmonary vein shows systolic (S) and diastolic (D) filling with a small atrial (A) reversal of flow.

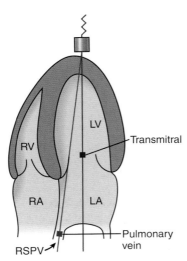

Figure 2–33 LV inflow is recorded from the apical view, usually in a four-chamber plane, with the sample volume positioned at the mitral leaflet tips in diastole (*blue*). Pulmonary vein (PV) flow is recorded in the right superior PV (RSPV) in the four-chamber view with the sample volume positioned about 1 cm into the PV (*red*).

is added to the downslope of the *E* velocity. These variations in the normal pattern of LV diastolic filling should be recognized to avoid an inappropriate interpretation of an "abnormality."

Typically, LV diastolic filling is recorded from an apical window on transthoracic studies (Fig. 2–33). In addition to the physiologic variability discussed above, the peak *E* velocity and the ratio of the *E* to *A* peaks may differ depending on whether the sample volume is placed at the mitral annulus or at the mitral leaflet tips. Appropriate positioning of the sample volume depends on whether the Doppler curve is used to evaluate diastolic filling of the LV (leaflet tips probably most useful) or transmitral stroke volume (mitral annular level most useful). Continuous-wave Doppler recordings show the highest velocities wherever they occur along the length of the ultrasound beam. LV diastolic filling is discussed in more detail in Chapter 7.

Right Ventricular Inflow

RV inflow can be recorded from an apical approach or from the parasternal RV inflow view. The pattern of RV diastolic filling is similar to LV filling, although peak flow velocities are slightly lower with a normal RV inflow *E* velocity of 0.3 to 0.7 m/s.

Left Atrial Filling

It is technically challenging to record LA filling from a transthoracic approach due to suboptimal signal strength at the depth of the pulmonary veins in many adults. However, with careful attention to technical details this flow curve is obtainable in the right superior pulmonary vein in an apical four-chamber view in

about 90% of patients (see Figs. 2–31 and 2–32). From a TEE approach, flow in both right and left pulmonary veins can be recorded, with the most laminar flow signals obtained from the left superior pulmonary vein.

Atrial contraction results in brief backflow in the pulmonary veins (*a* wave) followed by a biphasic filling pattern with prominent filling of the atrium (*x* descent) during ventricular systole, a second brief reversal of flow (*v* wave) following ventricular contraction, and a second atrial filling curve (*y* descent) during ventricular diastole (see Chapter 7). Abnormalities of LA filling can be seen in patients with mitral regurgitation (Chapter 12), constrictive pericarditis (Chapter 10), and restrictive cardiomyopathy (Chapter 9).

Right Atrial Filling

RA filling can be assessed from Doppler recordings of superior vena caval flow (from a suprasternal notch approach) or central hepatic vein flow (which lies parallel to the ultrasound beam from a subcostal window). The pattern of flow again is analogous to the pulsation pattern of the neck veins seen on clinical examination, with an *a* wave, an *x* descent reflecting systolic filling, a *v* wave, and a *y* descent reflecting diastolic filling of the RA (see Fig. 7–5).

Descending Aorta

Flow patterns in the descending aorta are important in the evaluation of cardiac disorders, because the downstream flow pattern depends on the presence and severity of specific cardiac lesions. Examples include aortic regurgitation, patent ductus arteriosus, and aortic coarctation. Descending thoracic aorta flow can be recorded from a suprasternal notch approach and shows antegrade flow with a systolic velocity curve, a peak velocity of about 1 m/s, and brief early-diastolic flow reversal. The proximal abdominal aorta recorded from a subcostal approach shows a similar flow pattern (see Figs. 16–8 and 16–10).

Normal Color Doppler Flow Patterns
Impact of Color Doppler Physics

While spectral Doppler (pulsed or continuous) is preferable for accurate measurement of specific intracardiac blood flow velocities, the overall pattern of intracardiac flow can be demonstrated with color flow imaging. Unfortunately, although in theory normal laminar flow should appear as a uniform red or blue color, in fact, color flow display instrumentation results in more complex patterns.

For example, flow in the LV outflow tract is a uniform red color from a parasternal long-axis view because the direction of flow is toward the transducer. The same flow is a uniform *blue* color from an apical

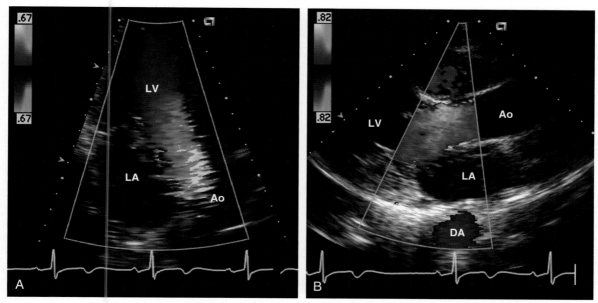

Figure 2–34 Flow in the left ventricular outflow tract recorded from an apical approach (**A**) is *blue* (away from the transducer), whereas the same flow from a parasternal position (**B**) is *red* (toward the transducer).

approach because now it is directed away from the transducer (Fig. 2–34). This same phenomenon can be seen with flows in a single image plane. For example, antegrade flow in the aortic arch from a suprasternal notch view appears red (toward the transducer) in the more proximal segment and blue (away from the transducer) more distally, with a small black area in the center of the image where the ultrasound beam is perpendicular to flow. Similarly, in the abdominal aorta from a subcostal approach, antegrade flow appears alternatively red and then blue as it transverses the image plane (see Fig. 1–33). In these examples, the change in color is due to a change in intercept angle between the ultrasound beam and blood flow at the left versus right edge of the sector, not to a change in the direction or velocity of blood flow.

Less dramatic changes in intercept angle across the 2D image also result in a complex color flow pattern for laminar normal flow. For example, evaluation of the LV outflow tract in an apical long-axis view may show an apparent higher systolic velocity along the ventricular septum than along the anterior mitral leaflet (Fig. 2–35). This appearance results from a more parallel intercept angle between the Doppler beam and blood flow along the septum than adjacent to the mitral valve. The same actual velocities across the outflow tract result in differing Doppler frequency shifts depending on this intercept angle. Since the instrument assumes that cos θ = 1 for each signal, a falsely low velocity is calculated for nonparallel intercept angles, with the resulting image showing an apparent increase in velocity across the image plane due to differing intercept angles.

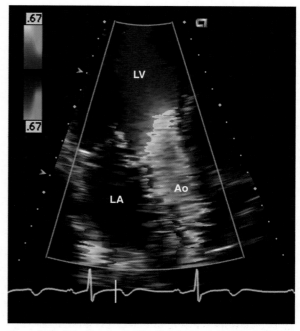

Figure 2–35 Color Doppler of LV outflow from an apical long-axis view shows aliasing proximal to the Ao valve, because the flow velocity (about 1 m/s) exceeds the Nyquist limit (0.67 m/s) at this depth. The change in color pattern across the outflow tract is due to a more parallel intercept angle between the ultrasound beam and flow along the septum versus near the mitral valve.

In addition to intercept angle, color flow images also are affected by the phenomenon of signal aliasing. The Nyquist limit, as displayed at the top and bottom of the color scale, typically is 60 to 80 cm/s with a

2- or 3-MHz transducer at depths used for transthoracic cardiac imaging. Since normal intracardiac flow velocities often exceed this limit, signal aliasing occurs. Flow toward the transducer is displayed in red at velocities less than the Nyquist limit, but once aliasing occurs, this same flow signal is displayed in blue. Thus, flow toward the transducer is red aliasing to blue, while flow away from the transducer is blue aliasing to red. In fact, multiple aliases can occur with high-velocity flows displayed sequentially as going from red to blue to red and so on. An example of normal aliasing is seen in the LV inflow pattern on the apical four-chamber view, where the red flow toward the apex turns blue as it exceeds the Nyquist limit (see Fig. 1–34). While confusing to a novice, patterns of signal aliasing can be used to advantage in quantitation of intracardiac flows using the proximal isovelocity surface area approach discussed in Chapter 12.

Another color image pattern seen even with normal intracardiac flows is *variance*, which often is encoded as green on the color display. While the concept of variance is that a single intracardiac site exhibits multiple flow velocities and directions (such as in a regurgitant jet), from the foregoing discussions of intercept angle and aliasing, it is apparent that a normal flow pattern might meet variance criteria. For example, in a region at the aliasing limit, the instrument may sequentially measure flow toward then away from the transducer due to aliasing and then assign variance to that color pixel. Awareness that a color variance pattern can occur with normal intracardiac flows avoids erroneous interpretations.

Normal Ventricular Outflow Patterns

Color flow imaging of LV outflow can be recorded from an apical approach in either an anteriorly angulated four-chamber view or a long-axis view. Flow is laminar, but aliasing typically occurs at this depth, resulting in a complex color pattern. While measurement of stroke volume proximal to the aortic valve, which assumes a flat flow velocity profile, has been validated, it remains controversial whether the appearance of aliasing along the ventricular septum in systole is due to a skewed flow profile or to variations in intercept angle across the color sector.

Note that while accurate measurements of antegrade velocities with pulsed or continuous-wave Doppler require a parallel intercept angle, with color flow imaging, the spatial pattern of flow is of interest rather than the absolute velocities. Thus, views with nonparallel intercept angles often are helpful. For example, LV outflow can be evaluated with color flow imaging in a parasternal long-axis view even though the flow direction is almost perpendicular to the ultrasound beam. As shown in Chapter 12, this view also is useful for evaluation of abnormal flows in the outflow tract, such as aortic regurgitation.

RV outflow can be visualized from a parasternal short-axis view, from the RV outflow view, or from a subcostal short-axis view. Since velocities are slightly lower and the depth of interrogation is less than for LV outflow, the flow pattern away from the transducer typically shows a uniform blue color.

Normal Ventricular Inflow Patterns

In the apical four-chamber view, LV inflow appears as a broad flow stream extending laterally across the mitral annulus and lengthwise to the LV apex. If the Nyquist limit is exceeded, signal aliasing occurs with a color shift at the aliasing velocity. In real time, the separate flows of early and late diastolic filling may be seen. When ultrasound penetration is optimal, diastolic flow extends from the pulmonary veins to the LV apex. In mid-diastole, the normal spatial pattern of LV inflow is directed toward the apex along the lateral LV wall, with simultaneous flow away from the transducer along the ventricular septum consistent with a "vortex" of flow in the LV in diastole (Fig. 2–36). Interestingly, this normal counterclockwise vortex often is reversed in patients after mitral valve replacement.

RV inflow patterns on color flow imaging are analogous to the patterns seen in the LV, although a diastolic "vortex" is not as prominent.

Normal Atrial Inflow Patterns

Inflow into the LA occurs via the four pulmonary veins. On transthoracic imaging, the right superior pulmonary vein is the easiest to visualize in the apical four-chamber

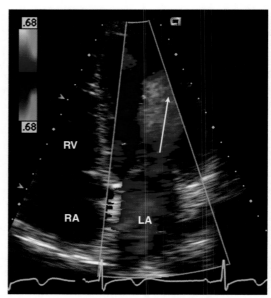

Figure 2–36 Normal pattern of LV filling in mid-diastole in an apical four-chamber view shows flow toward the apex (in red) along the lateral wall simultaneously with flow away from the transducer (in blue) along the septum.

view. Color flow imaging showing the biphasic red inflow from this vein allows correct placement of a pulsed Doppler sample volume for recording the spectral Doppler data. All four pulmonary veins can be visualized on TEE, but again, use of color flow imaging may facilitate identification of each vein. This approach is particularly helpful with right-sided veins, which may be difficult to recognize on 2D imaging alone.

Inflow into the RA occurs via the superior and inferior venae cavae and the coronary sinus. Evaluation may be complicated by some degree of tricuspid regurgitation (present in 80% to 90% of normal subjects and a higher percentage of patients), which typically is directed along the interatrial septum. Flow from the inferior vena cava and coronary sinus can be seen in the RV inflow view, as well as in the short-axis view at the aortic valve level and in the apical four-chamber view. Superior vena caval flow is seen from the suprasternal notch approach. In the RA, recognition of the several normal inflow patterns is important when an atrial septal defect is suspected. Note that 20% of normal subjects have a patent foramen ovale (demonstrable by intravenous echo contrast during a Valsalva maneuver), but color flow evidence for a patent foramen ovale is present in only about 5% of normal individuals.

Physiologic Valvular Regurgitation

With careful examination techniques a small amount of mitral and tricuspid regurgitation is detectable in between 50% and 80% of normal people. In addition, mild pulmonic regurgitation, appearing as a narrow red "flame" in diastole, is an incidental finding (present in 70% to 80% of normal individuals). These physiologic degrees of regurgitation are characterized by a localized signal that often is seen only briefly during the cardiac cycle. Small amounts of mitral, tricuspid, and pulmonic valvular regurgitation are of no apparent clinical significance. In contrast, aortic regurgitation is rarely seen in normal subjects (5% of individuals) on color flow imaging.

AGING CHANGES ON ECHOCARDIOGRAPHY

Between young adulthood and age 70, typical echocardiographic changes include an increase in LV wall thickness by about 2 mm with little change in chamber size, LV diastolic dysfunction with E-A reversal by about age 50 years, and progressive mild LA enlargement. Aortic dimensions also increase slightly, with about a 6% increase between the fourth and eighth decades of life. Calcific cardiac changes also are common, particularly mild aortic valve leaflet thickening without obstruction to outflow (e.g., aortic sclerosis), which is present in about 25% of adults over age 65 years, and calcification of the mitral annulus, seen in up to 50% of older adults. In many older adults, particularly with

a history of hypertension, there is a more acute angle between the aorta and ventricular septum, resulting in apparent basal septal thickening or a "septal knuckle." None of these findings may be strictly "normal," but they are seen in many older adults and should be interpreted in that context.

THE ECHOCARDIOGRAPHIC EXAMINATION

Core Elements

Although the echocardiographic examination should be directed toward the specific clinical question in each individual patient, it is important to use a systematic and consistent format for the examination. In some situations, only some parts of the standardized protocol may be needed; for example, a limited follow-up study in a patient with a recent, complete examination. In addition, as the study is in progress, additional imaging and data collection are needed to fully pursue the clinical question or any observed abnormalities.

Although the core echocardiographic elements may differ from laboratory to laboratory, the concept of a standardized examination sequence is critical to ensure that abnormalities are not missed. It is essential that blood pressure and the indication for echocardiography are reviewed prior to beginning the examination. An electrocardiographic lead should always be recorded to assist in evaluating timing of cardiac motion and Doppler flows. Measurements of the cardiac chambers, great vessels, and Doppler flow are made as appropriate for the clinical indication (Tables 2–6 to 2–8).

The Core Elements of the examination allow the physician to evaluate the following structures:

Left Ventricle
❏ Internal dimensions and wall thickness
❏ Segmental wall motion abnormalities
❏ Overall systolic function (including ejection fraction)
❏ Diastolic filling

Aortic Valve and Root
❏ Aortic root dimension and appearance
❏ Aortic valve anatomy
❏ Evidence for regurgitation or stenosis

Mitral Valve and Left Atrium
❏ Mitral valve anatomy and motion
❏ Evidence for stenosis or regurgitation
❏ LA size

Right Side of the Heart
❏ RV size and systolic function (qualitative)
❏ RA size
❏ Valve anatomy and function
❏ Estimated pulmonary artery pressure

Pericardium
❏ Evidence for thickening or effusion

TABLE 2–6   Clinical Echocardiographic Chamber and Great-Vessel Measurements*

Cardiac Structure	Basic Measurements	Additional Measurements	Technical Details
Left ventricle	ED dimension ES dimension ED wall thickness	ED volume ES volume 2D-stroke volume Ejection fraction Relative wall thickness LV mass	• 2D imaging is used to ensure measurements are centered and perpendicular to the long axis of the LV. • M-mode provides superior time resolution and more accurate identification of endocardial borders.
Left atrium	ES-AP diameter (PLAX)	LA area LA volume	• A left atrial AP dimension provides a quick screen but may underestimate LA size. • When LA size is important for clinical decision making, measurement of LA volume from apical views is helpful.
Right ventricle	Visual estimate of size	ED-RVOT diameter ED-RV length and diameter	• Quantitation of RV size by echo is challenging due to the complex 3D shape of the chamber.
Right atrium	Visual estimate of size		• RA size is usually compared to the left atrium in the A4C view.
Aorta	ED diameter at sinuses (PLAX)	• ED diameter indexed to expected dimension • Diameter at multiple sites in Ao	• With 2D echo, inner edge–to–inner-edge measurements are more reproducible. • Measurements at ES are about 2 mm greater than ED measurements
Pulmonary artery		ED diameter	

*2D measurements are made from the white-black interface on the image. M-mode measurements are made using the leading-edge–to–leading-edge convention.
A4C, apical four-chamber; AP, anterior-posterior; ED, end-diastole (onset of the QRS); ES, end-systole (minimum LV volume); PLAX, parasternal long-axis view.

TABLE 2–7   Normal Echocardiographic Valve Annulus and Great-Vessel Dimensions in Adults

	Range	Range (cm/m²) Indexed to BSA	Upper Limit of Normal
*Aorta (End-Diastole)**			
Annulus diameter (cm)	1.4–2.6	1.3 ± 0.1	<1.6
Diameter at leaflet tips (cm)	2.2–3.6	1.7 ± 0.2	<2.1
Ascending aorta diameter	2.1–3.4	1.5 ± 0.2	
Arch diameter (cm)	2.0–3.6		
Mitral Annulus			
ED (cm)	2.7 ± 0.4		
ES (cm)	2.9 ± 0.3		
Pulmonary Artery			
Annulus diameter (cm)	1.5–2.1		
Main PA (cm)	0.9–2.9		
Inferior Vena Cava Diameters			
1–2 cm from RA junction (cm)	Normal <1.7 cm		

*See Chapter 16 for a more detailed approach to normalization of aortic dimensions for age and body size.
ED, end-diastole; ES, end-systole.
Data sources: Roman et al: Am J Cardiol 64:507, 1989; Pini et al: Circulation 80:915, 1989; Schnittger et al: J Am Coll Cardiol 2:934, 1983; Kircher et al: Am J Cardiol 66:493, 1990.

TABLE 2–8 Reference Values for Echocardiographic Chamber Quantification

Chamber	Measurement	Normal Range Women	Men	Units
Left Ventricle				
	Diastolic diameter	3.9–5.3	4.2–5.9	cm
	Indexed to BSA	*2.4–3.2*	*2.2–3.1*	*cm/m²*
	Indexed to height	2.5–3.2	2.4–3.3	*cm/m*
	Diastolic volume	56–104	67–155	mL
	Indexed to BSA	*35–75*	*35–75*	*mL/m²*
	Systolic diameter	2.1–4.0		cm
	Indexed to BSA	*1.4–2.1*		*cm/m²*
	Systolic volume	19–49	22–58	mL
	Indexed to BSA	*12–30*	*12–30*	*mL/m²*
	Ejection fraction	≥55%	≥55%	
	Septal wall thickness	0.6–0.9	0.6–1.0	cm
	Posterior wall thickness	0.6–0.9	0.6–1.0	cm
	LV mass (2D method)	66–150	96–200	g
	Indexed to BSA	*44–88*	*50–102*	*g/m²*
	Relative wall thickness	0.22–0.42	0.24–0.42	
Left Atrium				
	AP diameter	2.7–3.8	3.0–4.0	cm
	Indexed to BSA	*1.5–2.3*	*1.5–2.3*	*cm/m²*
	LA area	≤20	≤20	cm²
	LA volume	22–52	18–52	mL
	Indexed to BSA	*22 ± 6*	*22 ± 6*	*mL/m²*
Right Ventricle				
	Diastolic wall thickness	<0.5		cm
	Mid-RV diastolic diameter	2.7–3.3		cm
	RV diastolic area (A4C)	11–28		cm²
	RV systolic area (A4C)	7.5–16		cm²
	Fractional area change	32%–60%		
	Tricuspid annular excursion	>1.5		cm
Right Atrium				
	RA dimension (A4C)	2.9–4.5		cm
	Indexed to BSA	*1.7–2.5*		*cm/m²*

A4C, apical four-chamber view; BSA, body surface area; AP, anterior-posterior.
Abstracted from Lang et al: J Am Soc Echo 2005; 18:1440–1463, 2005, with the addition of ES ventricular dimension data (not gender specific) from Pearlman et al: J Am Coll Cardiol 12:1432, 1988; Hahn et al: Z Kardiol 71:445, 1982; Erbel et al: Dtsch Med Wschr 107:1872, 1982; Schnittger et al: J Am Coll Cardiol 2:934, 1983.

Additional Components

Additional imaging and Doppler data are recorded as needed based on the clinical indications for the study and any abnormalities seen on the basic examination. The combination of Core Elements and Additional Components then constitutes a complete echocardiographic examination.

An example of findings on the Core Elements leading to additional data recording is when a calcified aortic valve is present. With this finding, attention is focused first on the precise valve anatomy—bicuspid, calcific, rheumatic—and then on the function of the valve. The degree of stenosis is quantitated from the maximum aortic jet velocity and calculation of valve area (see Chapter 11) and the degree of regurgitation is evaluated with color flow and continuous-wave Doppler techniques (see Chapter 12). Next, the LV response to the pressure load imposed by the abnormal aortic valve is assessed both for systolic function (see Chapter 6) and diastolic function (see Chapter 7).

Another example is evaluation of a patient after myocardial infarction. In this case attention is focused on the extent and distribution of LV segmental wall motion abnormalities (see Chapter 8). If apical akinesis or dyskinesis is noted, a diligent search for an apical thrombus is indicated (see Chapter 15). If the patient has a new murmur, careful evaluation is performed to evaluate the possibility of mitral regurgitation due to papillary muscle dysfunction or the possibility of a postinfarction ventricular septal defect. Overall LV systolic function is evaluated, as is RV function.

Even if no obvious abnormalities are noted during the basic examination, the study may be focused toward the specific clinical question in that patient. For example, if endocarditis is suspected (see Chapter 14), more attention to valvular anatomy is needed, with careful transducer angulation and nonstandard views to optimize visualization of possible valvular vegetations. Another example of how the clinical indication affects the examination is the patient referred

for heart failure symptoms. Even if the Core Elements are unremarkable, more complete evaluation of diastolic LV function may be helpful to evaluate for a cardiac cause of the patient's symptoms.

The need to focus the examination on the specific clinical question and at the same time ensure that significant abnormalities are not missed highlights the necessity for appropriate training of both the physician responsible for the examination and the sonographer performing the study, as well as for close interaction between these two individuals during the performance and interpretation of the study. Furthermore, interaction with the referring physician may be needed either before the examination is performed to clarify the differential diagnosis and clinical questions or after the examination to integrate the pretest likelihood with the echocardiographic findings and estimate the probability of any remaining diagnostic problems.

SUGGESTED READING

1. Lang RM, Bierig M, Devereux RB, et al: Recommendations for chamber quantitation: a report from the American Society of Echocardiography's Guidelines and Standards Committee and the Chamber Quantification Group, Developed in Conjunction with the European Association of Echocardiography, a branch of the European Society of Cardiology. J Am Soc Echocardiogr 18:1440–1463, 2005.
   Detailed discussion of methods for quantitation of left and right ventricular systolic function by 2D echocardiography and measurement of atrial size and aortic root dimensions. Technical details of image acquisition, diagrams illustrating quantitative methods, and tables of normal values are included.

2. Cerqueira MD, Weissman NJ, Dilsizian V, et al: Standardized myocardial segmentation and nomenclature for tomographic imaging of the heart: A statement for healthcare professionals from the Cardiac Imaging Committee of the Council on Clinical Cardiology of the American Heart Association. Circulation 105:539–542, 2002.
   Standards for defining cardiac image orientation and myocardial segments that can be used by all imaging modalities to enhance correlation between different approaches. The standard reference for cardiac displays is defined as the long axis of the LV. The names used for image planes are short-axis (90° to long axis), vertical long-axis, and horizontal long-axis (four-chamber plane). Myocardial segments are defined at the basal and midventricular level as (clockwise from the anterior septal insertion) as anterior, anterolateral, inferolateral, inferior,

   inferoseptal, and anteroseptal. There are four apical segments (anterior, septal, inferior, and lateral).

3. Quinones MA, Otto CM, Stoddard M, et al: Recommendations for quantification of Doppler echocardiography: A report from the Doppler quantification task force of the nomenclature and standards committee of the American Society of Echocardiography. J Am Soc Echocardiogr 15:167–184, 2002.
   Nomenclature standards for recording, measuring, and reporting Doppler data including pulsed, continuous, and color flow Doppler. Excellent review of normal flow patterns and basic Doppler principles for calculation of volume flow rate, pressure gradients, and regurgitant valve lesions. 77 references. Useful glossary of Doppler terms.

4. Sengupta PP, Krishnamoorthy VK, Korinek J, et al: Left ventricular form and function revisited: Applied translational science to cardiovascular ultrasound imaging. J Am Soc Echocardiogr. 20:539–551, 2007.
   This article reviews our current understanding of ventricular anatomy and function, with reference to implications for echocardiographic evaluation of ventricular function.

5. Lee KS, Abbas AE, Khandheria BK, et al: Echocardiographic assessment of right heart hemodynamic parameters. J Am Soc Echocardiogr 20:773–782, 2007.
   This review provides excellent illustrations and a practical approach to evaluation of right heart hemodynamics by echocardiography.

6. Barbieri A, Bursi F, Zanasi V, et al; Left atrium reclassified: Application of the American Society of Echocardiography/ European Society of Cardiology Cutoffs

   to unselected outpatients referred to the echocardiography laboratory. J Am Soc Echocardiogr 21:433–438, 2008.
   Detection of LA enlargement by the linear anterior-posterior diameter was compared to indexed LA volumes in a series of 578 patients undergoing echocardiography. Based on diameter measurement 49% had LA enlargement, whereas 76% meet criteria for enlargement based on indexed volumes. In those with an increased diameter measurement, 95% also had an increased volume index. However, of the 295 with a normal diameter, 59% had an increased volume index.

7. Lee KS, Appleton CP, Lester SJ, et al: Relation of electrocardiographic criteria for left atrial enlargement to two-dimensional echocardiographic left atrial volume measurements. Am J Cardiol 99:113–118, 2007.
   In a series of 261 echocardiographic studies, measurement of LA volumes by tracing apical biplane images of the atrium demonstrated atrial enlargement (LA volume > 32 mL/m2) in 43% of patients. Conventional ECG criteria for LA enlargement did not reliably correlate with measured LA volumes.

8. Schnittger I, Gordon EP, Fitzgerald PJ, et al: Standardized intracardiac measurements of two-dimensional echocardiography. J Am Coll Cardiol 2:934–938, 1983.
   Normal 2D echo intracardiac measurements are described in detail for 35 healthy adults.

9. Triulzi M, Gillam LD, Gentile F, et al: Normal adult cross-sectional echocardiographic values: Linear dimensions and chamber areas. Echocardiography 1:403–426, 1984.

Tabular presentation of normal echo dimensions in 72 normal adults.

10. Pearlman JD, Triulzi MO, King ME, et al: Limits of normal left ventricular dimensions in growth and development: Analysis of dimensions and variance in the two-dimensional echocardiograms of 268 normal healthy subjects. J Am Coll Cardiol 12:1432–1441, 1988.

    Graphic display of normal echo dimensions in 72 adults and 196 children showing relationship of each dimension to body surface area with mean and 90% tolerance limits.

11. Roman MJ, Devereux RB, Kramer-Fox R, et al: Two-dimensional echocardiographic aortic root dimensions in normal children and adults. Am J Cardiol 64:507–512, 1989.

    Derivation of gender-specific upper limits of normal (indexed to body size) for aortic root dimensions based on 135 adults and 52 children.

12. Benjamin EJ, Levy D, Anderson KM, et al: Determinants of Doppler indexes of left ventricular diastolic function in normal subjects (the Framingham Heart Study). Am J Cardiol 70:508–515, 1992.

    Detailed study of the relationship between age and Doppler measures of LV diastolic filling in the Framingham population after exclusion of subjects with hypertension, cardiac disease, or other organ system disease (n = 1485). E-velocity decreased from 0.71 ± 0.14 m/s at ages 20–29 years to 0.53 ± 0.17 m/s for those ~70 years of age. A-velocity increased from 0.35 ± 0.06 to 0.64 ± 0.14 m/s in the same groups. The E/A ratio was 1.03 ± 0.26 m/s at ages 60–69.

13. Appleton CP, Hatle LK, Popp RL: Superior vena cava and hepatic vein Doppler echocardiography in healthy adults. J Am Coll Cardiol 10: 1032–1039, 1987.

    Normal superior vena cava and hepatic vein Doppler flows show systolic and diastolic antegrade flow with a reduction or reversal in antegrade flow following atrial systole (A-wave). Variation with respiration is prominent in normal healthy adults.

14. Basnight MA, Gonzalez MS, Kershenovich SC, et al: Pulmonary venous flow velocity: Relation to hemodynamics, mitral flow velocity and left atrial volume, and ejection fraction. J Am Soc Echocardiogr 4:547–558, 1991.

15. Klein AL, Tajik AJ: Doppler assessment of pulmonary venous flow in healthy subjects and in patients with heart disease. J Am Soc Echocardiogr 4:379–392, 1991.

16. Bartzokis T, Lee R, Yeoh TK, et al: Transesophageal echo–Doppler echocardiographic assessment of pulmonary venous flow patterns. J Am Soc Echocardiogr 4:457–464, 1991.

    Each of these three references (14 to 16) provides detailed descriptions of normal pulmonary venous flow patterns and the physiologic variables that affect the flow pattern.

17. Chen MA: Aging changes seen on echocardiography. In Otto CM (ed): The Practice of Clinical Echocardiography, 3rd ed. Philadelphia: Elsevier/ Saunders, 2007, pp 952–976.

    Detailed review of the normal cardiac changes with aging as assessed by echocardiography including age-grouped tables of normal values for LV dimensions and function and Doppler flow velocities. The clinical utility of echocardiography and outcome data related to age are summarized. 133 references.

18. Gottdiener JS: Hypertension: impact of echocardiographic data on the mechanism of hypertension, treatment options, prognosis and assessment of therapy. In Otto CM (ed): The Practice of Clinical Echocardiography, 3rd ed.

Philadelphia: Elsevier/Saunders, 2007, pp 816–847.

    Cardiac changes in hypertensive heart disease and the prognostic implications of ventricular hypertrophy are reviewed. The use of echocardiography in clinical trials is discussed, including differences between field centers, sonographer training, reliability of measurements, and the potential impact of future studies on clinical care.

19. Stoddard MF: Echocardiography in the evaluation of cardiac disease resulting from endocrinopathies, renal disease, obesity and nutritional deficiencies. In Otto CM (ed): The Practice of Clinical Echocardiography, 3rd ed. Philadelphia: Elsevier/Saunders, 2007, pp 902–931.

    Typical cardiac changes seen in obese patients include both an increase in LV mass and chamber dimensions, combined with a decrease in systolic function. Diastolic function parameters also often are abnormal, LA size is increased, and the aortic root may be enlarged. Evaluation of echocardiographic findings in obese patients should be made in the context of these typical changes.

20. Gardin JM, Adams DB, Douglas PS, et al: Recommendations for a standardized report for adults transthoracic echocardiography: a report from the American Society of Echocardiography's Nomenclature and Standards Committee and Task Force for a Standardized Echocardiography Report. J Am Soc Echocardiogr 15:275–290, 2002.

    Recommendations for performing and reporting transthoracic echocardiography examinations in adults. An excellent resource for developing a standardized echocardiography examination in each laboratory.

3

Transesophageal Echocardiography

Transesophageal echocardiography (TEE) offers the advantages of improved image quality compared with transthoracic images, particularly of posterior structures, such as the pulmonary veins, left atrium (LA), and mitral valve. Image quality is improved both because of the decreased distance between the transducer and the structures of interest and because of the absence of intervening lung or bone tissue. A better signal-to-noise ratio and decreased image depth also allows use of higher frequency (5- and 7-MHz) transducers, which further enhances image quality.

However, TEE imaging is more risky than transthoracic imaging due to the insertion of the probe in the esophagus and the need for conscious sedation in most patients. Typically, a TEE examination provides additional information but does not replace a transthoracic examination, and in some situations transthoracic imaging provides better image quality and diagnostic Doppler data. For example, anterior structures, such as a prosthetic aortic valve, may be better imaged from the transthoracic approach. For Doppler velocity measurements, the transthoracic approach offers more acoustic windows with the ability to adjust transducer angle freely in both the transverse and elevational planes. In contrast, transducer position and angulation are constrained with the TEE approach by the relative positions of the esophagus and heart. The inability to align the

Doppler beam parallel to the flow of interest may result in substantial velocity underestimation. In addition, it often is more difficult to obtain standard anatomic measurements from the TEE approach due to oblique two-dimensional (2D) image planes. Thus, even when TEE imaging is necessary, data from the transthoracic examination are integrated into the final clinical interpretation.

In this chapter, the TEE procedure and risks are briefly outlined, followed by a description of the standard views obtained from each acoustic window (TEE, standard transgastric, transgastric apical, and descending aorta). Sections on the TEE 2D and Doppler evaluation of each cardiac valve and chamber are included to guide the reader to the optimal views for each anatomic structure. This chapter focuses on normal anatomy and flow patterns. Clinical indications for TEE imaging are discussed in Chapter 4 and pathologic images are integrated into subsequent chapters. The use of intraoperative TEE imaging is discussed in Chapter 18.

PROTOCOL AND RISKS

TEE is performed by a physician skilled in both echocardiography and the endoscopy procedure, as detailed in published guidelines for physician training. Typically a cardiac sonographer assists the physician, adjusting instrument settings for optimal image quality and data acquisition. Many physicians use mild conscious sedation, in addition to local anesthesia of the pharynx, to minimize patient discomfort and improve tolerance of the procedure. When conscious sedation is used, a designated, qualified individual (usually a nurse) monitors and documents the patient's blood pressure, heart rate, respiratory rate, arterial oxygen saturation, and level of consciousness throughout the procedure. In addition, the nurse ensures patency of the airway and provides suction of oral secretions as needed (see Suggested Reading 7). The specific protocols, medications used for conscious sedation, and monitoring procedures are dictated by the standards of each institution.

TEE has a very low incidence of complications when performed by trained individuals with appropriate patient selection and monitoring. However, this procedure does have known risks, which must be taken into consideration in deciding whether the potential information obtained justifies use of this procedure (Table 3–1). The rate of complications serious enough to interrupt the procedure is less than 1% with a reported mortality rate of fewer than 1 in 10,000 patients. Risks are higher in patients with a history of esophageal disease, impaired respiratory status, or sleep apnea. If the preprocedure history or physical examination suggests an increased risk for conscious sedation, appropriate consultation with anesthesiology is essential.

After sedation and local anesthesia of the pharynx, the probe is gently inserted via a bite block, positioned in the esophagus, and advanced as needed to obtain diagnostic images. If there is a history of esophageal disease or symptoms related to impaired swallowing, evaluation of the esophagus or gastroenterology consultation may be needed. In intubated patients, in the intensive care unit or operating room, care is needed to avoid compromise of the endotracheal tube position. Indwelling nasogastric or feeding tubes may limit probe motion or result in air between the transducer and heart, so often need to be removed for the TEE procedure.

The risk of aspiration is minimized by having the patient fast for several hours before the procedure, use of a left lateral decubitus position during probe insertion, and having the patient continue to fast after the procedure until recovery from the local anesthesia of the pharynx. Esophageal trauma or perforation is unlikely in the absence of a history of esophageal disease or swallowing difficulty, both of which can be ascertained by clinical history. Bleeding complications are rare and usually mild, and the procedure can be safely performed with therapeutic levels of systemic anticoagulation. Initial concern that TEE imaging might increase the risk of endocarditis has been alleviated by several studies showing the absence of bacteremia following this procedure, so that most physicians do not routinely use antibiotic prophylaxis.

TOMOGRAPHIC VIEWS

The exact views obtained on a TEE study vary depending on the relative positions of the heart, esophagus, and diaphragm in each patient (Fig. 3–1). Even though a multiplane probe allows full rotation of the scan plane, the fixed position of the transducer in the esophagus constrains the possible image planes that can be obtained, potentially resulting in oblique image orientations compared with the three-dimensional (3D) reference system used for standard echocardiographic views. The goal on TEE is to perform a systematic and comprehensive examination, using standard short-axis, long-axis, two-chamber, and four-chamber image planes whenever possible. Standard views then are supplemented with additional image planes to demonstrate the specific pathologic processes in each patient. 3D echocardiographic techniques can facilitate obtaining optimal views and display of spatial relationships, particularly for the atrial septum and mitral valve.

A recommended sequence of images composing a basic complete examination is shown in the Echo Exam section at the end of this chapter and in Chapter 18. The following sections describe views useful for evaluation of the valves and cardiac chambers that can be used to supplement the basic examination as determined by the specific clinical question.

The position of the tip of the probe is described as esophageal or transgastric and is referenced to the cardiac structures seen in each view. The absolute distance of the transducer from the patient's mouth will vary depending on body size and cardiac position. There also will be variability in the exact degree of rotation, tilt, and angulation needed to obtain the best

---

TABLE 3–1	Risks of Transesophageal Echocardiography

Risks of Esophageal Intubation

Dental trauma
Esophageal trauma or perforation
Bleeding
Aspiration
Dislodgement of endotracheal tube, especially on probe withdrawal
Displacement of nasogastric tubes

Risks of Conscious Sedation

Hypotension
Respiratory depression (hypoxia, respiratory arrest)
Arrhythmias
Bronchospasm
Death

Figure 3–1 Rotation of the image plane starting from the four-chamber view, with the LV apex centered in the image, allows a two-chamber view (see Fig. 3–7) at approximately 60° rotation and a long-axis view (see Fig. 3–9) at approximately 120° rotation. Slight repositioning and angulation of the transducer may be needed as the image plane is rotated to ensure inclusion of the LV apex in the image.

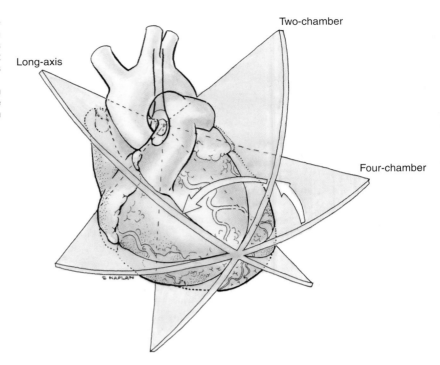

short-axis, long-axis, two-chamber, and four-chamber views. When standard views are obtained, the images correspond to the anatomy described for the equivalent transthoracic views, with the major difference being image orientation given the TEE transducer position.

For TEEs, transducer motions (Fig. 3–2) are referred to as:

❒ *Repositioning*, defined as movement of the probe up and down in the esophagus
❒ *Rotation*, defined as rotating the image plane from 0° to 180° using the multiplane control knob
❒ *Turning*, defined as moving the entire transducer in a rotational fashion in the esophagus to show a medial-lateral change in image plane

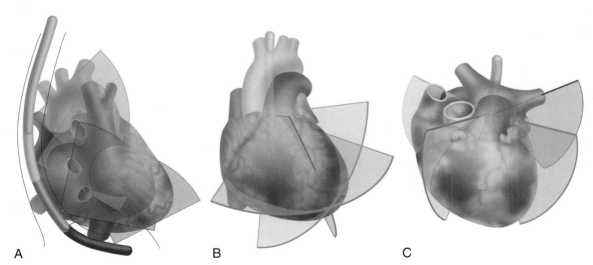

A   B   C

Figure 3–2 The position of the TEE transducer in the esophagus is illustrated (**A**) for a very high esophageal (*green*), high esophageal (*blue*), mid-esophageal (*purple*), and transgastric position (*magenta*), with the corresponding tomographic sector scan indicated for each probe position. Rotation of the image plane with the transducer in a midesophageal position (**B**), provides a four-chamber (green), two-chamber (blue), or long-axis (*purple*) image of the left ventricle. From a mid-esophageal position (**C**), turning the image plane from left to right provides images of the left pulmonary veins (*purple*), aorta and left ventricle (*blue*), right ventricle (*green*), and right atrium with superior and inferior vena cava (*yellow*).

□ *Angulation*, defined as bending and extending the probe so that the image plane is directed superiorly or inferiorly at an angle to the original image plane

□ *Tilt*, defined as lateral motion of the transducer tip to image different structures in the same image plane (although slight superior motion occurs as well)

From the TEE position, most image planes are achieved using repositioning, rotation, and turning of the transducer. The use of angulation is particularly important on transgastric views. A key principle in using a multiplane probe is that the anatomic area of interest should be centered in the image before rotation to a new view to ensure that the structure of interest remains in the image plane.

Esophageal Position

Four-chamber Plane

As the transducer is advanced into the esophagus from the mouth toward the stomach, acoustic access is limited by interposition of the air-filled trachea until the transducer passes the level of the carina. From a high TEE position, with the probe located posterior to the LA, a standard four-chamber view usually can be obtained in the 0° position with angulation of the transducer toward the left ventricular (LV) apex (Fig. 3–3). As with transthoracic imaging, slight changes in angulation allow imaging of the coronary sinus posteriorly and the LV outflow tract and aortic valve anteriorly (the "five-chamber" view) (Fig. 3–4). In the four-chamber view the lateral wall and inferior septal

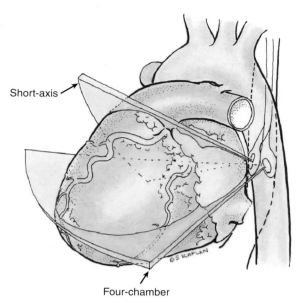

Short-axis

Four-chamber

Figure 3–4 Illustration of the use of angulation of the transducer from a high esophageal position with the probe at 0° rotation to obtain a four-chamber view (as shown in Fig. 3–3) or a short-axis view of the LA appendage (as shown in Fig. 3–8).

segments of the LV are seen. Care is needed to include as much of the full length of the ventricle as possible in this view. Typically, even with optimal positioning and angulation, TEE views are somewhat foreshortened compared with the true long axis of the ventricle, and the apparent apex may actually represent a more proximal segment of the anterior wall. The four-chamber

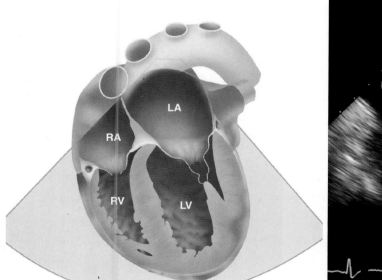
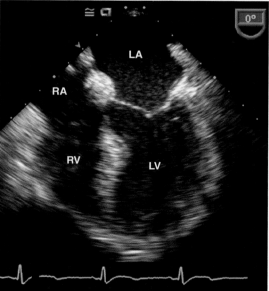

Figure 3–3 TEE four-chamber view. Drawing (*left*) and echocardiographic image (*right*) in a TEE four-chamber view is obtained from a high TEE position with the multiplane probe at 0° rotation. In this view the apparent apex may actually represent a segment of the anterior wall because of foreshortening of the long axis of the ventricle.

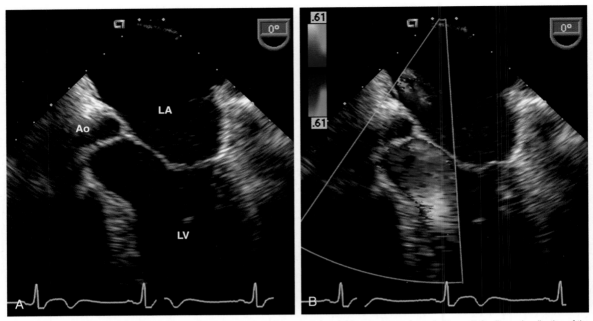

Figure 3–5 Slight anterior angulation from the four-chamber view, midway between the image planes shown in Figure 3–2, allows visualization of the aortic valve and LV outflow tract (**A**). Color flow shows normal systolic laminar flow in the outflow tract (**B**).

view is useful for evaluation of overall ventricular systolic function, regional wall motion (recognizing that the apex may be missed), and the pattern of septal motion. Biplane ejection fraction also can be calculated from traced endocardial borders at end-diastole and end-systole, although volumes may be underestimated due to foreshortening of the ventricular length.

When the transducer is positioned posterior to the center of the LA, the central portions of both the anterior and posterior leaflets of the mitral valve are well visualized in the 0° four-chamber view. Anterior angulation provides a view of the LV outflow tract and anterior mitral leaflet analogous to the apical five-chamber view (Fig. 3–5). Posterior angulation provides images of more lateral segments of the valve leaflets with the coronary sinus visualized on extreme posterior angulation.

While examining the LA in the four-chamber plane, it is helpful to slowly advance and withdraw the transducer to visualize the full superior and inferior extent or to slowly angulate the probe tip to provide sequential cross-sections of the LA. Because the LA is in the near field of the image, careful adjustment of imaging parameters is needed to avoid misinterpretation of near-field artifacts. For this reason, identification of a small thrombus along the posterior LA wall is problematic.

In the standard four-chamber TEE image, the size, shape, and systolic function of the right ventricle (RV) can be assessed by turning the probe toward the patient's right side. This view also provides visualization of the septal and anterior leaflets of the tricuspid valve and the right atrium (RA). The interatrial septum is well visualized with the fossa ovalis and primum septum region clearly identifiable (Fig. 3–6).

Two-chamber Plane

After the examiner ensures that the LV apex is in the center of the image in a four-chamber view, the image plane is slowly rotated to about 60° to obtain a two-chamber view. Because the apex often is not exactly centered in three dimensions, the position

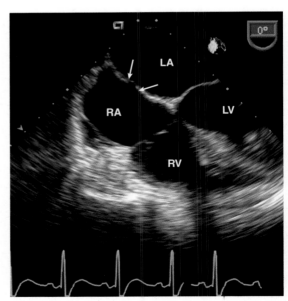

Figure 3–6 A view of the tricuspid valve and interatrial septum is obtained by turning the transducer from the four-chamber view toward the patient's right side. The thin central region of the interatrial septum known as the fossa ovalis is between the *arrowheads.*

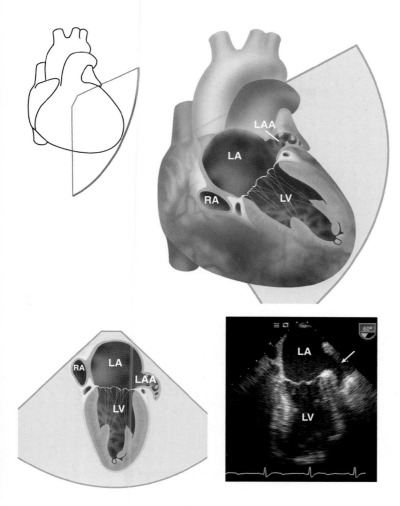

Figure 3–7 TEE two-chamber view. The position of the image plane is shown on the line drawing. This image plane is equivalent to the vertical long-axis plane with other tomographic imaging modalities. Typically, the image plane is rotated to approximately 60°, with adjustments to transducer position and flexion, although there is individual variation. The 3D view shows the cross-section of the LA and LV with the left atrial appendage (LAA), coronary sinus in the atrioventricular groove, and the mitral valve. In the two-chamber view, small portions of the posterior mitral valve leaflet are seen laterally and medially, with the anterior leaflet filling most of the annulus area. Part of a papillary muscle has been shown for orientation, but the papillary muscles are located symmetrically posterior to the image plane. The tomographic plane has been rotated with the apex of the sector at the top (*bottom left*) to correspond to the 2D echocardiographic image (*bottom right*).

and angulation of the transducer may need adjustment to obtain a two-chamber view that includes the full length of the LV (Fig. 3–7). In this view, the inferior and anterior LV walls of the LV are seen, allowing assessment of regional function and providing the orthogonal plane (along with the four-chamber view) for calculation of ejection fraction. In the two-chamber view typically only the anterior leaflet of the mitral valve is seen, so that it is difficult to evaluate leaflet prolapse in this view.

With further rotation to about 90°, the left atrial appendage is visualized in a view approximately perpendicular to that obtained in the transverse plane (Fig. 3–8). The left superior pulmonary vein can be seen entering the LA by slightly withdrawing and turning the probe laterally.

Long-axis Left Ventricular Plane

With the transducer positioned in the high esophagus, posterior to the LA, further rotation of the image plane to about 120° results in a long-axis view of the LV and aorta (Fig. 3–9). Again, slight adjustment of

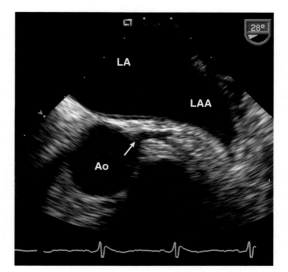

Figure 3–8 Left atrial appendage (LAA) and left main coronary artery seen at a rotation angle of about 30°. Starting in the four-chamber view the probe is slightly withdrawn and angulated anteriorly. Note the normal trabeculation in the LAA compared to the smooth LA wall. This image was obtained with a 7.0-MHz transducer to optimize detection of atrial appendage thrombus.

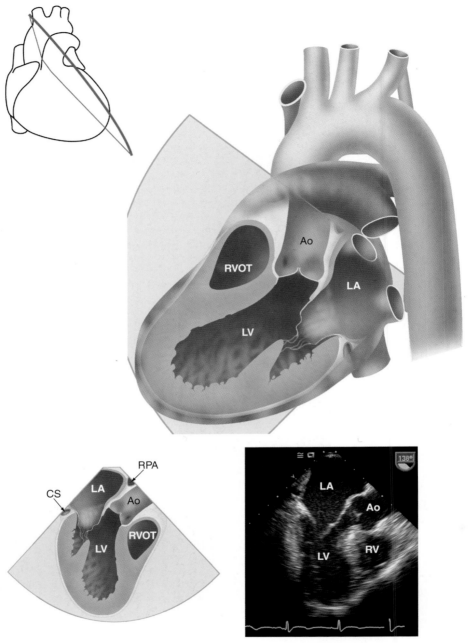

Figure 3–9 TEE long-axis view. The position of the image plane is shown on the line drawing. This view typically is obtained at approximately 120° rotation, but there is considerable individual variability in the exact image plane needed to show the Ao and LV in a long-axis orientation. The 3D view shows the cross-section of the Ao, LV, LA, and right ventricular outflow tract (RVOT). In the long-axis view, the anterior mitral valve leaflet (AMVL) and posterior mitral valve leaflet (PMVL) are seen. The tomographic plane has been rotated with the apex of the sector at the top (*bottom left*) to correspond to the 2D echocardiographic image (*bottom right*).

transducer position and angulation may be needed to obtain a view that includes the LV apex. Similar to a transthoracic long-axis view, the proximal ascending aorta, sinuses of Valsalva, and right and noncoronary leaflets of the aortic valve are well visualized.

Scanning between this view and the 90° image planes allows appreciation of the perpendicular relationship between aortic and pulmonic valve planes and the slightly more cephalad position of the pulmonic valve. Note that in the esophageal long-axis plane,

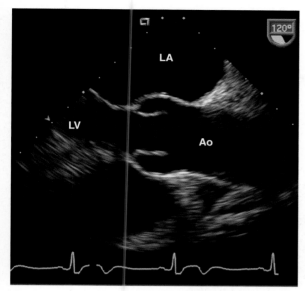

Figure 3–10 From the TEE long-axis view, further cephalad segments of the ascending Ao can be seen by slight withdrawal of the transducer in the esophagus.

withdrawing the transducer in the esophagus results in more cephalad images of the ascending aorta with the superior limit of imaging determined by the interposed air-filled bronchus (Fig. 3–10).

The anterior and posterior mitral leaflets are seen in a long-axis orientation, and the coronary sinus can be identified in cross-section in the atrioventricular groove. The right pulmonary artery is visualized posterior to the aortic root at the superior aspect of the LA. In the long-axis view the anterior septum and posterior wall of the LV are seen. In addition, a portion of the RV outflow tract is seen anterior to the aortic valve (in the far field of the image).

Other Long-axis Image Planes

At a rotation angle of 90°, the probe can be turned from the LV long-axis view toward the patient's left side to obtain a long-axis view of the pulmonic valve and RV outflow tract (Fig. 3–11). In this view, the pulmonic valve is in the far field of the image and may be shadowed by the aortic valve and root if calcification is present. Portions of the RV and tricuspid valve are seen, depending on the exact position of the heart relative to the esophagus in each patient.

At a 90° rotation with the probe turned toward the patient's right side, images of the RV and tricuspid valve in an inflow view are obtained. If the probe is turned further to the right, a long-axis view of the RA is obtained, with the superior vena cava entering from the right side of the screen and the inferior vena cava on the left (Fig. 3–12). In some individuals a

eustachian valve at the inferior caval-atrial junction is seen. The trabeculated RA appendage often can be seen with slight medial rotation from this view.

Minor changes in the rotation angle may be needed to optimize each view. As with the LV long-axis view, adjustment of transducer position (advancement and withdrawal) allows imaging of much of the cephalad-to-caudal extent of the cardiac structures in each of these tomographic planes.

Short-axis Plane

A short-axis view at the aortic valve level can be obtained by rotating the image plane to between 30° and 45° and withdrawing the probe in the esophagus to the level of the aortic valve. Visualization of aortic valve anatomy is excellent, showing the three leaflets and sinuses of Valsalva (Fig. 3–13). The origin of the left main coronary artery is easily identified after minor adjustments in the depth and tilt of the image plane. The right coronary artery is more difficult to visualize and is clearly identified in only a minority of patients. The interatrial septum is well seen, with the fossa ovalis clearly defined.

By turning the transducer laterally and angulating superiorly from the 0° esophageal position, the LA appendage and left superior pulmonary vein are seen (Fig. 3–14). Prominent features include normal trabeculation of the atrial appendage and a variably prominent ridge at the junction of the left superior pulmonary vein and the LA appendage. Compared to the left superior pulmonary vein, which enters the LA anteriorly with flow directed parallel to the ultrasound beam, the left inferior pulmonary vein enters the atrium with flow perpendicular to the ultrasound beam. The left inferior pulmonary vein can be seen by advancing the transducer and angulating slightly inferiorly. The right pulmonary veins can be imaged by rotating the transducer medially and withdrawing the transducer cephalad (to see the anteriorly directed right superior pulmonary vein) or by angulating the transducer inferiorly (to see the medially directed right inferior pulmonary vein). The pulmonary veins also can be identified in the 90° image plane, turning the transducer toward the patient's right to show the right pulmonary veins and to the left for the left pulmonary veins. Again, color flow imaging often facilitates identification of the pulmonary veins based on the characteristic venous inflow patterns.

In many patients, the pulmonary artery can be imaged in the 0° image plane by further withdrawing the probe in the esophagus to obtain a view straight down the main pulmonary artery from the bifurcation to the valve level. In some cases, this view is limited by the position of the air-filled bronchus, and some patients may find the probe uncomfortable when positioned at this level in the esophagus.

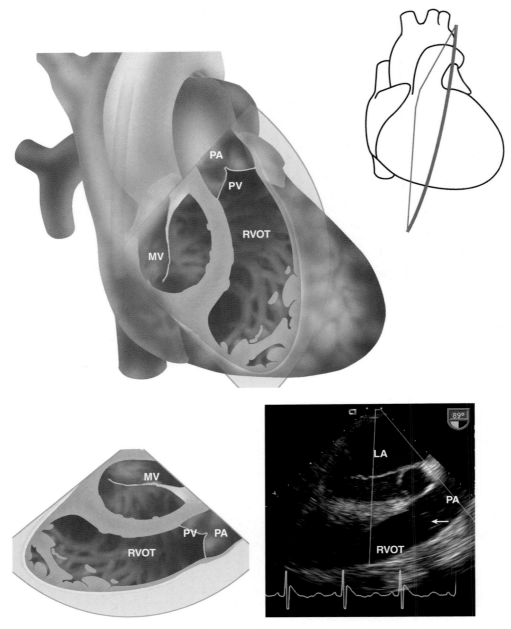

Figure 3–11 Transesophageal RV outflow tract (RVOT) view. In the 90° TEE image plane, the RVOT, pulmonic valve (*arrow*), and PA can be demonstrated with the probe turned toward the patient's left side (*top*). The tomographic plane has been rotated with the apex of the sector scan at the top (*bottom left*) to correspond to the echocardiographic image (*bottom right*).

Standard Transgastric Position

Short-axis Plane

As the transducer is passed into the stomach, slight resistance may be encountered at the gastroesophageal junction. With the probe tip in the stomach, superior angulation (flexing the scope) in the 0° image plane results in a short-axis view of the LV at the papillary muscle level (Fig. 3–15). In this view, global LV systolic function, LV dimensions and wall thickness, and regional LV function can be evaluated (Fig. 3–16).

Depending on the position of the patient's heart with respect to the diaphragm, a short-axis view at

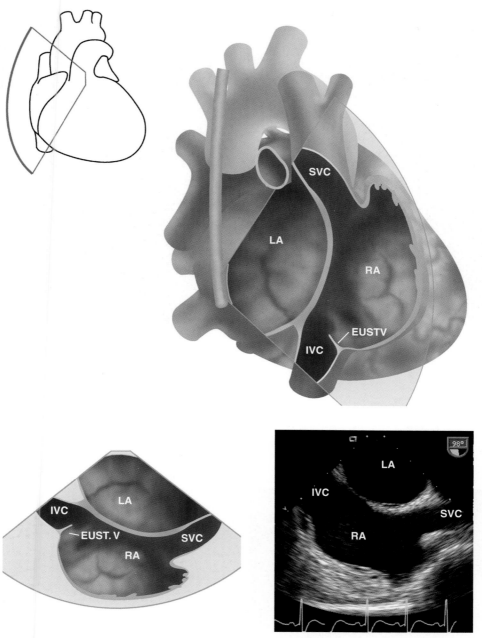

Figure 3–12 Transesophageal bicaval view. With the probe turned toward the patient's right side, the RA, superior vena cava (SVC), and inferior vena cava (IVC) can be visualized in the 90° TEE image plane as shown in the drawing *(top)* with visualization of the SVC and IVC, LA and RA. A eustachian valve (EUST.V) often is present at the IVC-RA junction. The tomographic plane has been rotated with the apex of the sector scan at the top *(bottom left)* to correspond to the echocardiographic image *(bottom right)*. Part of the trabeculated RA appendage is seen adjacent to the SVC.

the mitral valve level may be obtainable by slight withdrawal of the transducer toward the esophagus (Fig. 3–17). The transgastric short-axis view at the mitral valve level is helpful in precise definition of the mitral valve apparatus anatomy in patients with valve dysfunction.

Two-chamber Plane

A two-chamber view of the LV can be obtained from the transgastric position by rotating the image plane to the 90° position (Fig. 3–18). From this two-chamber view, turning the entire probe toward the

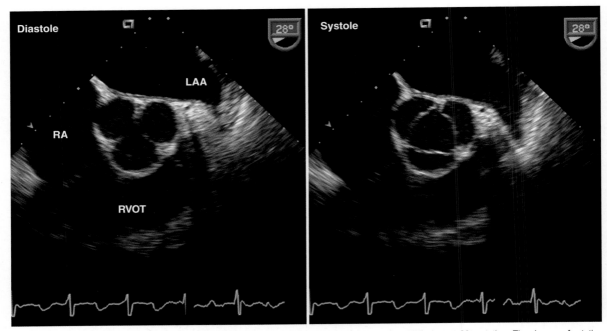

Figure 3–13 A short-axis view of the aortic valve in diastole (*left*) and systole (*right*) is seen in a TEE view at 28° rotation. The degree of rotation needed to obtain this short-axis view varies from approximately 30° to 50°; the images themselves should be used to ensure a true short-axis image. Oblique image planes may result in artifactual distortion of the valve apparatus.

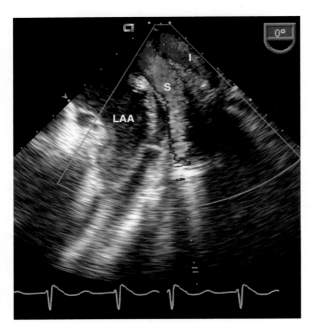

Figure 3–14 The left superior (S) and inferior pulmonary veins (I) are seen in the 0° plane with the probe at the level of the left atrial appendage (LAA). Color-flow imaging facilitates identification of the pulmonary views as they enter the LA.

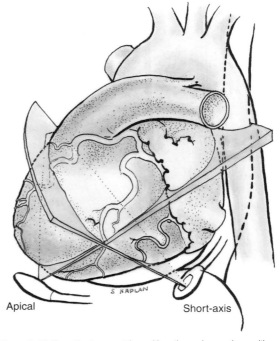

Figure 3–15 From the transgastric position, the probe can be positioned near the gastroesophageal junction to obtain a short-axis view of the LV or can be advanced into the stomach to obtain an "apical" view. Transgastric apical images may show a foreshortened LV because the true LV apex often does not lie on the diaphragm.

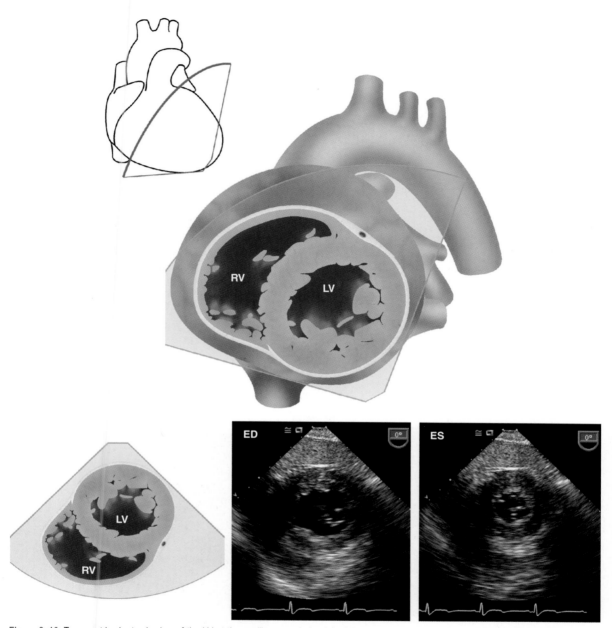

Figure 3–16 Transgastric short-axis view of the LV at the papillary muscle level (*top*) is obtained by retroflexion of the transducer from a transgastric position. This view is particularly valuable for intraoperative monitoring of LV size and global and regional systolic function. The tomographic plane has been rotated with the apex of the sector at the top (*bottom left*) to correspond to the ED and ES echocardiographic images (*bottom center and right*).

patient's right side results in a view of the RA, tricuspid valve, and RV similar to a transthoracic RV inflow view. In some individuals the RV outflow tract and pulmonic valve also can be visualized.

Transgastric Apical Position

Four-chamber Plane

From the transgastric short-axis view, the transducer is further advanced into the fundus of the stomach. In most individuals an "apical" four-chamber view

can be obtained using the 0° image plane of the probe if the LV lies on the diaphragm, without intervening lung. Note that the transducer may not be on the true LV apex, so this view typically is foreshortened. Anterior angulation shows the aortic valve in a view similar to the transthoracic five-chamber view.

Long-axis Plane

From the transgastric apical four-chamber plane, rotation of the image plane to 120° results in a

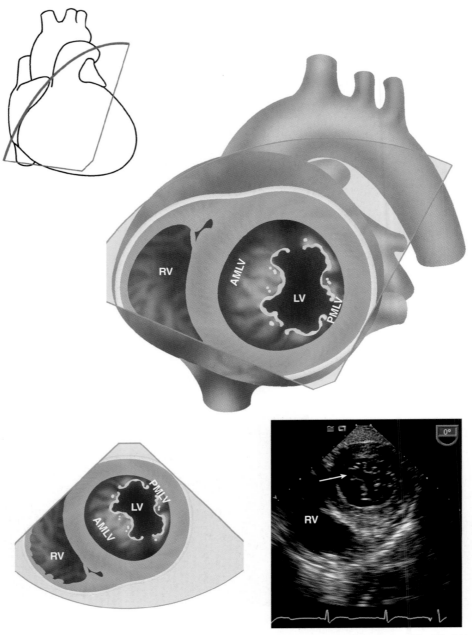

Figure 3–17 Transgastric short axis at the mitral valve (MV) level. From the transgastric short-axis view of the LV, slight withdrawal of the probe toward the gastroesophageal junction may allow a short-axis view of the MV with definition of the anterior MV leaflet (AMVL) and posterior MV leaflet (PMVL). The tomographic plane has been rotated with the apex of the sector scan at the top (*bottom left*) to correspond to the echocardiographic image (*bottom right*).

long-axis view of the LV outflow tract, providing a more parallel intercept angle for Doppler study of outflow tract and aortic velocities. However, this view cannot be obtained in all patients, particularly if the transducer is not on the true LV apex, because lung tissue is interposed between the transducer and cardiac structures as the image plane is rotated.

Descending Thoracic Aorta

From the TEE or transgastric position, the transducer is turned posteriorly until the image plane is directed slightly left of the patient's spine to obtain a short-axis view of the descending thoracic aorta. The aorta appears circular and shows normal systolic

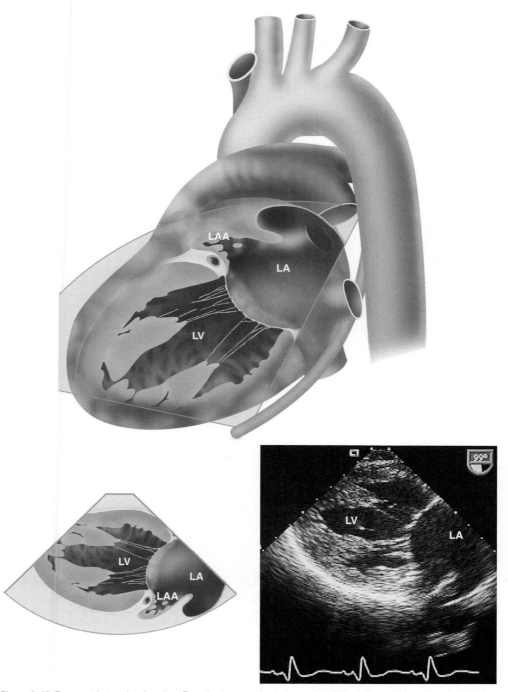

Figure 3–18 Transgastric two-chamber view. From the transgastric short-axis view, 90° rotation provides a two-chamber view of the LV, LA, and left atrial appendage (LAA) (*top*). The tomographic image plane has been rotated with the apex of the sector at the top to correspond with the echocardiographic image (*bottom right*). Turning the transducer toward the patient's right side from this view provides a two-chamber view of the RA and RV, analogous to a transthoracic RV inflow view.

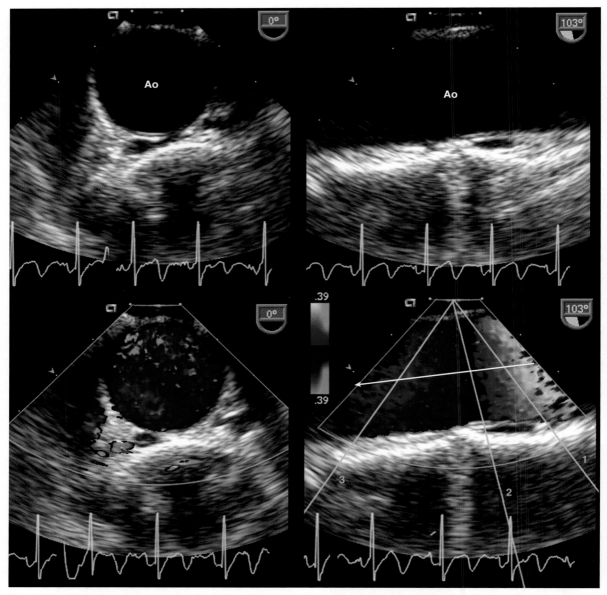

Figure 3–19 TEE 2D and color flow images of the descending thoracic Ao in short axis (*left*) (0° rotation) and long-axis (*right*) (90° rotation) views on 2D echo (*top*) and with color flow imaging (*bottom*). The short-axis view shows flow filling the Ao in systole. In the long-axis view, although the direction and velocity of flow are uniform (*white arrow*), the color displayed depends on the angle between the ultrasound beam and flow direction. Lines for three ultrasound beam angles are shown in cyan (1, 2, 3) illustrating how the color changes from red for flow directed toward the transducer (1), to black where flow is perpendicular to the ultrasound beam (2), and then to blue where flow is directed away from the transducer (3).

pulsations (Fig. 3–19). The descending thoracic aorta can be imaged in sequential short-axis views from its post-gastric position to the junction with the aortic arch as the probe is slowly withdrawn in the esophagus. When the transducer reaches the level of the arch, turning the transducer medially, with inferior angulation, allows a long-axis view of the arch itself. Imaging in the short-axis view as the probe is withdrawn along the length of the aorta ensures visualization of the entire aortic endothelium.

The long-axis view of the descending aorta, obtained by centering the aorta in the 2D sector and rotating the image plane to 90°, complements the short-axis view in evaluation of aortic dissections, aneurysms, and atheromas and improves the differentiation of ultrasound artifacts from anatomic abnormalities. The 90° image plane also allows identification of the origin of the left subclavian artery, which is important for describing the proximal extent of dissection and for placement of an intra-aortic balloon pump (see Chapter 16).

VALVE ANATOMY AND NORMAL DOPPLER FLOWS

Optimal evaluation of valve anatomy and function on TEE echocardiography includes the use of at least two standard orthogonal imaging planes (Table 3–2). This approach provides a reasonably complete evaluation of valve anatomy and aids recognition of ultrasound artifacts. Continuous-wave and pulsed Doppler velocities should be recorded with the ultrasound beam aligned parallel to the flow stream. However, a parallel intercept angle may be difficult to achieve given the constraints on transducer position from the TEE approach. As with transthoracic imaging, color Doppler is helpful for evaluation of abnormal flow patterns even at nonparallel intercept angles.

Left Ventricular Outflow and Aortic Valve

The aortic valve and LV outflow tract are imaged in long axis from the high TEE probe position with rotation of the image plane to about 120° (Fig. 3–20). A short-axis view of the aortic valve is obtained by rotating the image plane to about 45° (see Fig. 3–13). In the short-axis view, slight withdrawal of the probe shows the sinuses of Valsalva and left main coronary artery while slight advancement provides a short-axis

view of the LV outflow tract. In the 0° four-chamber view, the outflow and aortic valve also may be seen by anterior angulation of the image plane (see Fig. 3–5). In both the short- and long-axis views, image quality is optimized by use of a high transducer frequency and adjustment of the depth, or use of zoom mode, to maximize the valve image.

Color flow imaging in long and short-axis views of the valve allows evaluation for valvular regurgitation, including vena contracta width and the origin and direction of the regurgitant jet (see Chapter 12). A cross-sectional area of the aortic regurgitant jet can be obtained starting in a short-axis view of the aortic valve and slowly advancing the probe in the esophagus to obtain a short-axis view of the outflow tract.

Measurement of antegrade velocity across the aortic valve is limited by the nonparallel intercept angle between the ultrasound beam and the direction of blood flow from the TEE position. In some patients, a transgastric apical view allows recording of pulsed and continuous-wave Doppler flow velocities proximal to and across the aortic valve (Fig. 3–21). However, caution still is needed in interpretation of the Doppler data, since intercept angle may be oblique. If aortic valve pathology is present, transthoracic recording of antegrade velocities is more accurate and should be performed in all cases.

TABLE 3–2 Transesophageal Views for Cardiac Valves

Valve	View	Probe Position	Rotation Angle
Aortic	Long axis	High esophageal *or* Transgastric	~120°–130° ~90° (turn probe to visualize LVOT)
	Short axis	High esophageal	~30°–50°
	Five-chamber	High esophageal *or* Transgastric apical	0° (anteriorly angulated)
Mitral	Long axis	High esophageal Transgastric	~120°–130° 90°
	Short axis	Transgastric (at GE junction)	Can be obtained in some patients at 0° with probe flexed
	Four-chamber	High esophageal *or* Transgastric apical	0°
Pulmonic	Long axis	Very high esophageal	0° (looking straight down PA from bifurcation)
	Outflow view	High esophageal	~90° (turn probe to left)
Tricuspid	Four-chamber	High esophageal	0°
	RV inflow (esophageal)	High esophageal	~90° (turn probe to right)
	RV inflow (transgastric)	Transgastric	~90° (turn probe to right)

GE, gastroesophageal; LVOT, left ventricular outflow tract.

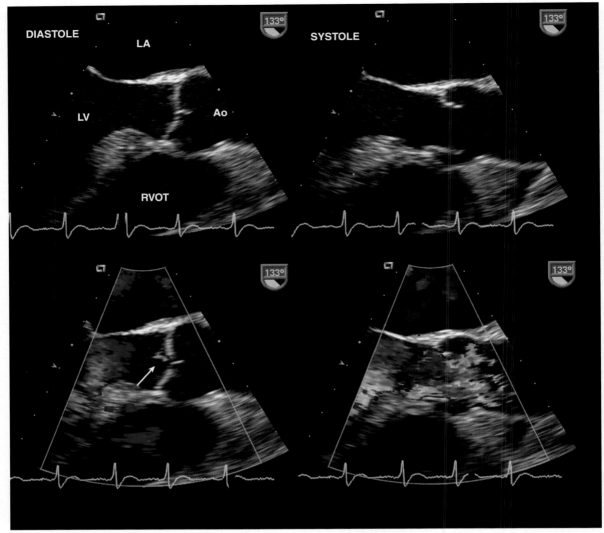

Figure 3–20 Long-axis images of the aortic valve with the depth adjusted to optimize evaluation of valve anatomy and motion. The 2D images (*top*) in diastole (*left*) and systole (*right*) show normal aortic and mitral opening and closure. The color flow images show trace aortic regurgitation (*arrow*) in diastole (*left*) and normal antegrade flow in the LVOT and aorta in systole (*right*).

Figure 3–21 Transgastric apical view angulated anteriorly to include the aortic root (*left*) with the line indicating the position of the Doppler beam and the sample volume depth for pulsed Doppler just proximal to the aortic valve. LVOT velocity with pulsed Doppler (*upper right*) and aortic jet velocity with 2D-guided CW Doppler ultrasound (*lower right*). When a high-velocity jet is suspected, careful angulation and positioning of the transducer is needed to obtain the highest velocity signal. Because of the constraints on transducer positioning and the lack of a view equivalent to the trans-thoracic SSN view, the possibility of velocity underestimation should be considered.

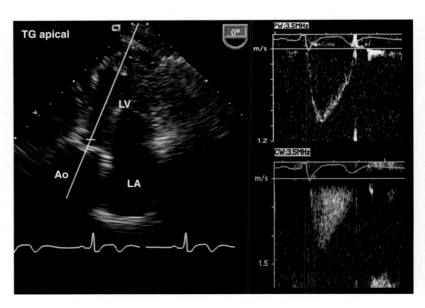

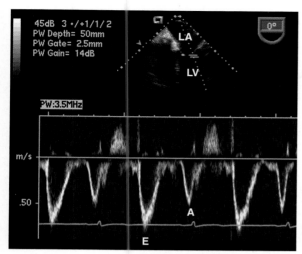

Figure 3–22 LV inflow recorded with pulsed Doppler with the sample volume positioned at the mitral leaflet tips from an anteriorly angulated transesophageal four-chamber view. The flow pattern is similar to a transthoracic recording of LV inflow, albeit inverted as the flow is directed away from the transducer.

Left Ventricular Inflow and Mitral Valve

The mitral valve is evaluated by slow rotation from the TEE four-chamber view to the long-axis view with image recording at about 30° increments. Transducer depth is decreased to include just the mitral valve, transducer frequency is increased to improve image

resolution, and the transducer position is centered relative to the valve annulus. The leaflets and subvalvular apparatus are usually well seen in these views unless there is valve calcification with shadowing of distal structures. If additional views are needed, transgastric short-axis and two-chamber views of the mitral valve may be helpful. The valve may be seen on the transgastric apical view, although image quality often is suboptimal at the depth of the mitral valve.

The pattern of antegrade flow across the mitral valve (LV diastolic filling) is recorded with pulsed Doppler in the four-chamber or long-axis view at a parallel intercept angle (Fig. 3–22). Since the flow is directed away from the transducer, the velocity curve with the typical early diastolic peak *(E)* and late diastolic peak *(A)* velocities is shown below the baseline. Transmitral flow also can be recorded from the transgastric apical approach, although signal strength is lower due to the greater depth of the mitral valve from this position.

Color Doppler is used to evaluate for mitral regurgitation as the image plane is slowly rotated from the four-chamber to two-chamber to long-axis view. The image plane that best shows the proximal jet geometry (proximal isovelocity acceleration and vena contracta) is used for quantitative measures of regurgitant severity as discussed in Chapter 12. Mitral regurgitation also is evaluated with continuous-wave Doppler from the high esophageal position, using the color flow signal to align the continuous-wave Doppler beam with the vena contracta of the regurgitant jet (Fig. 3–23).

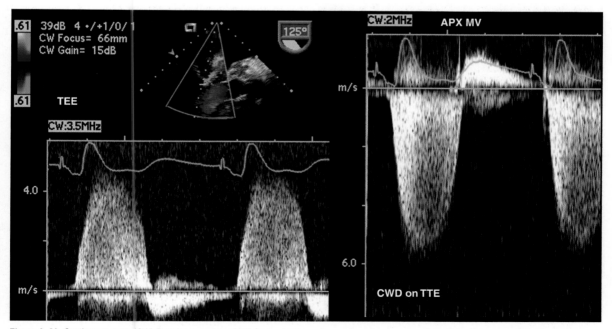

Figure 3–23 Continuous-wave (CW) Doppler recording of MR from a transesophageal four-chamber view (*left*). Color flow was used to identify the vena contracta of the regurgitant jet for the initial positioning of the CW Doppler beam. Transducer position and angulation then were modified as needed to obtain a clear signal with the highest flow velocity. Even so, a higher velocity was obtained with a transthoracic-dedicated CW Doppler transducer, immediately after the transesophageal examination (*right*).

Right Ventricular Outflow and Pulmonic Valve

The RV outflow tract is best imaged from a high esophageal position at 0° rotation with a long-axis view of the pulmonary artery from the valve plane to its bifurcation. Doppler velocities can be recorded from this position at a parallel intercept angle as flow is directed straight toward the transducer (Fig. 3–24). The pulmonic valve also may be visualized in the 90° long-axis plane with the pulmonic valve seen in its perpendicular relationship to the aortic valve in the far field of the image (see Fig. 3–11). However, velocities cannot be recorded from this approach due to a nonparallel intercept angle. In some patients the pulmonic valve also can be imaged from the transgastric position either in the 90° image plane including the tricuspid valve or in a very anteriorly angulated apical four-chamber view.

Right Ventricular Inflow and Tricuspid Valve

The tricuspid valve is well imaged in the standard four-chamber views, both from the TEE position and from the transgastric apical view. Other useful views include the TEE RV inflow view and the transgastric two-chamber view turned to show the right

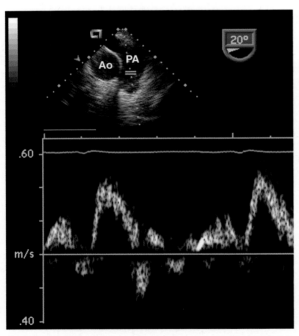

Figure 3–24 A very high transesophageal position provides a long-axis view (*top*) of the main PA and its bifurcation into right and left pulmonary branches. The ascending Ao is seen in short axis. This view allows recording of flow in the PA at a parallel intercept angle, because flow is directly toward the transducer (*bottom*).

heart structures. In a transgastric view obtained close to the diaphragm, the entry of the coronary sinus into the RA adjacent to the tricuspid valve can be seen. Further advancement of the transducer often allows a short-axis view of the tricuspid valve.

The tricuspid regurgitant jet may be recorded from either TEE or transgastric views; however, underestimation of velocity should be considered given the limited ability to vary transducer position to ensure a parallel intercept angle. If high pulmonary pressures are suspected, transthoracic continuous-wave Doppler recordings or invasive measures of pulmonary pressure should be obtained.

CHAMBER ANATOMY AND ATRIAL INFLOWS

Left Ventricle

Standard views of the LV are obtained from the TEE position in four-chamber, two-chamber, and long-axis views (Table 3–3). A standard short-axis view is obtained from the transgastric position. These views allow calculation of LV volumes and ejection fraction. Comparisons with radionuclide and contrast angiography have shown that TEE calculation of ejection fraction is both accurate and reproducible (Fig. 3–25). End-diastolic and end-systolic volumes often are underestimated because the image plane does not include the full long-axis of the ventricle. However, TEE remains accurate for evaluation of relative changes in ventricular volumes based on short-axis area changes in an individual patient. LV volume status can be assessed during surgery using a combination of these views, or using a single view, such as the transgastric short-axis view for continuous monitoring.

Standard views of the LV also allow evaluation of regional ventricular function for each myocardial segment with a high degree of interobserver reproducibility for grading of wall motion in standard segments. In the transgastric short-axis view the wall segments are the same as in a transthoracic short-axis view, *except* that the entire image has been rotated approximately 180° clockwise (if standard display format is used). Compared with a transthoracic subcostal short-axis view, the image is rotated 90° clockwise (see Fig. 8–6).

Left Atrium

The location and flow patterns of the pulmonary veins are readily assessed by TEE (Fig. 3–26). The flow pattern is most easily recorded in the left superior pulmonary vein where the typical systolic and diastolic antegrade flows and the reversal after atrial contraction can be appreciated (Fig. 3–27). Flow

TABLE 3–3 Transesophageal Views for Evaluation of Cardiac Chambers, Great Vessels, and Atrial Septum

Chamber	View	Probe Position	Rotation Angle
Left ventricle	Four-chamber	High esophageal	0°
	Two-chamber	High esophageal	60°
		Transgastric	90°
	Long-axis	High esophageal	120°
	Short-axis	Transgastric	0° with angulation of the probe tip
Left atrium	Four-chamber	High esophageal	0°
			Also allows assessment of all four pulmonary veins with medial and lateral turning and slight angulation of the transducer
	Two-chamber	High esophageal	60°
	Long-axis	High esophageal	120°
Right ventricle	Four-chamber	High esophageal	0°
	RV inflow view	High esophageal *or*	90° with probe turned toward patient's right side
		Transgastric	90° with probe turned toward patient's right side
Right atrium	Four-chamber	High esophageal	0° with posterior angulation to visualize coronary sinus
	RA view	High esophageal	90° with probe turned toward patient's right side
	Low atrial view	GE junction	0° to visualize entry of coronary sinus into right atrium
Atrial septum	Rotational view	High esophageal	Rotation from 0° to 120°, patent foramen ovale often best seen at 60° to 90°
Aorta	Long-axis	High esophageal	Long (120°) and short-axis views of aortic sinuses and ascending aorta
	Posterior view of aorta	Transgastric to high esophageal pullback	Short-axis view (0°) pullback along length of descending aorta
Pulmonary artery	RV outflow view	High esophageal	90°
	Long axis of PA to bifurcation	Very high esophageal	0°

GE, gastroesophageal.

patterns are in general similar in all four pulmonary veins although flow tends to be more laminar with a narrow band of velocities on the spectral display in the left superior pulmonary vein. However, exceptions do occur as, for example, when mitral regurgitation is present. In this situation the regurgitant jet may be directed eccentrically, altering flow patterns in some, but not all, pulmonary veins.

If LA thrombus is suspected, the atrial appendage should be examined in at least two orthogonal views. Recognition of low flow (spontaneous contrast) and appendage thrombi are enhanced by use of a high transducer frequency (7 MHz) and zoom mode. Care is needed to distinguish normal trabeculation from localized thrombus formation. Trabeculae tend to be more linear and are continuous with the atrial wall in more than one view. Thrombi typically protrude

into the appendage, often with independent motion (see Chapter 15).

The flow pattern in the LA appendage can be recorded with pulsed Doppler ultrasound with the sample volume positioned in the appendage, about 1 cm from the junction with the body of the LA. The normal flow pattern (see Fig. 15–21) is characterized by ejection of blood from the appendage following atrial contraction at a velocity >40 cm/s. Abnormal flow patterns are seen with atrial fibrillation, atrial flutter, and other tachyarrhythmias.

The interatrial septum is well seen in the standard four-chamber view and can be evaluated in detail by centering the septum in the image and then slowly rotating the image plane from 0° to 120°, keeping the septum centered in the image plane. The fossa ovalis and primum septum are clearly demarcated,

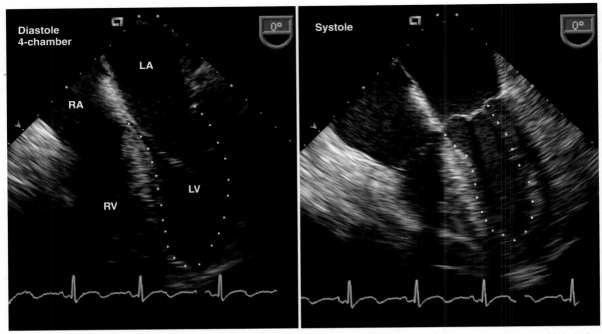

Figure 3–25 Examples of endocardial border tracings at end-diastole and end-systole in a TEE four-chamber view for calculation of LV ejection fraction. Borders are also traced in the two-chamber view at 60° of rotation.

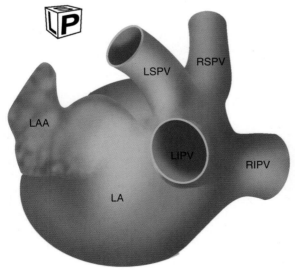

Figure 3–26 Drawing of 3D anatomy of the left atrium and pulmonary veins showing the orientation of the left and right superior pulmonary veins (LSPV and RSPV) with flow directly toward the TEE transducer and the more horizontally oriented left and right inferior pulmonary veins (LIPV and RIPV) with flow more perpendicular to the Doppler beam. The orientation cube indicates left (L), superior (S), and posterior (P).

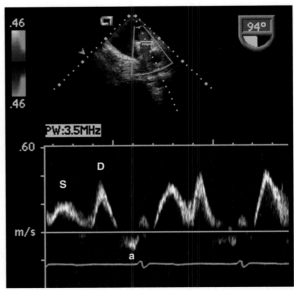

Figure 3–27 Pulsed Doppler recording of normal flow in the left superior pulmonary vein shows systolic (S) and diastolic (D) inflow with a small atrial (a) reversal signal.

and the "flap valve" of a patent foramen ovale often can be identified on 2D imaging, prior to confirmation with color Doppler or an intravenous contrast injection (see Fig. 4–12).

Right Ventricle

As with transthoracic echocardiography, quantitation of RV size and systolic function is difficult due to the complex geometry of this chamber. Qualitative assessment of size and function is made from the TEE four-chamber and transgastric short-axis views.

Right Atrium

The body of the RA is best imaged in the TEE four-chamber view. In addition, the TEE long axis view of the RA, obtained with the image plane at 90° and the probe rotated toward the patient's right, allows visualization of the atrial appendage (with normal trabeculation) and the entrances of the superior and inferior vena cavae. Movement of the probe up in the esophagus allows evaluation of the cephalad extent of the superior vena cava, while movement toward the stomach provides additional views of the inferior vena cava.

The coronary sinus can be identified in a posteriorly angled four-chamber view. The entry of the coronary sinus into the right atrium is best seen in the 0° image plane with the transducer positioned near the gastroesophageal junction and angulated superiorly (Fig. 3–28).

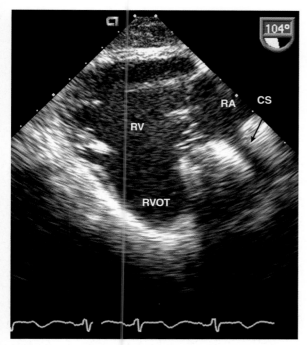

Figure 3–28 Low TEE view of the right heart showing the entry of the coronary sinus (CS) into the RA, the RV, and the RV outflow tract (RVOT).

THE TRANSESOPHAGEAL ECHOCARDIOGRAPHIC EXAMINATION

A standard structured sequence of image acquisition on TEE imaging ensures evaluation of all four cardiac chambers, all four valves, both great arteries and vena cavae, and the four pulmonary veins. Although this sequence may need to be modified to focus immediately on an acute process in unstable patients or may need to be abbreviated in patients who do not tolerate the study, the time needed for a standardized study is relatively short and these data can be acquired in most patients. A standardized examination ensures that unexpected findings are not missed and provides the data needed for subsequent review of findings in the patient.

The specific sequence used in each laboratory may vary, depending on patient populations and physician preferences. One suggested approach is shown in Table 3–4. This sequence starts with a high TEE view at enough depth to image the LV in four-chamber, two-chamber, and long-axis views. A two-beat cine loop of each view is recorded, so this sequence takes only about 1 minute, even with the time to adjust the probe position. In the long-axis view, the probe is pulled back to show a larger extent of the ascending aorta.

Depth is then decreased to focus on 2D imaging of the aortic and mitral valve in the long-axis view. The mitral valve is further evaluated by rotation from the long-axis view, back to the four-chamber view, recording images at 30° to 60° increments; the aortic valve short axis is obtained with rotation of the image plane to 30° to 50°. Each of these valves then is evaluated for regurgitation in the same views. Antegrade mitral flow and mitral regurgitant continuous-wave Doppler are recorded if needed.

Next the pulmonary veins are identified using a combination of 2D and color flow imaging at a rotation angle of either 0° or 90°, looking first at the left and then the right pulmonary veins. The atrial appendage is visualized by angulating superiorly from the 0° image plane and in the two-chamber plane, using a high-frequency transducer and magnified views. Flows in the pulmonary veins and atrial appendage are recorded, if needed. The atrial septum is examined by centering the septum in the four-chamber view, with identification of the fossa ovalis. Then the image plane is slowly rotated to 90°, keeping the septum centered in the image. Color flow imaging while rotating back to 0° allows identification of a patent foramen ovale.

The RV and tricuspid valve are examined in the four-chamber view turned toward the right side and in a low TEE view. Tricuspid regurgitation with color flow imaging is evaluated in these views and in a short-axis view. The superior and inferior vena cavae are seen in the 90° plane, which also may show the RA appendage. Visualization of the pulmonic

TABLE 3–4   The Basic TEE Exam

Probe Position	Rotation Angle	Views	Focus
High esophageal *Set depth to include LV apex.*	0° 60° 120°	Four-chamber Two-chamber Long-axis	• LV size, global and regional fx • RV size and systolic fx • LA and RA size
High esophageal ↓*Depth to optimize valves.*	120° 120° → 0° 120° 30–50° 0° 60° 90° 0° → 90° 0° 90° 0° 60° 90°	Long-axis Two-chamber Four-chamber Long-axis Short-axis Depth to show LAA and PVs Rotational scan Four-chamber SVC/IVC view Four-chamber Short-axis RV-outflow	• MV • Aortic valve • Aorta • LAA (resolution mode, 7 MHz) • PVs • Atrial septum • RV • RA • SVC and IVC • TV • Pulmonic valve and pulmonary artery
TG	0° 90°	Short-axis Long-axis	• LV wall motion, wall thickness, chamber dimensions • RV size and fx • LV and MV • Turn medially to image RV and TV
TG apical	0°	Four-chamber	• Useful for antegrade aortic flow but may still be nonparallel intercept angle
TG to high esophageal	0°	Short-axis DA	• Image aorta from the diaphragm to aortic arch

valve is more difficult, but images at 90° and a very high 0° TEE view may be helpful.

In patients who tolerate transgastric passage of the probe, short-axis and two-chamber views of the LV are obtained. Apical transgastric views are optional, depending on the clinical indication.

After checking with the other medical professionals assisting the examination (e.g., the nurse and sonographer) that all the needed data have been recorded, the probe is turned posteriorly to image the descending aorta in short axis. The probe is slowly withdrawn, keeping the descending aorta centered in the image plane, and turning the probe to look down the aortic arch just before probe withdrawal.

This basic examination may be supplemented with additional views and Doppler flows depending on the specific clinical question. For example, a study to evaluate for patent foramen ovale also would include a right-sided saline contrast study. The findings on these basic views also may mandate further evaluation. For example, in a patient with endocarditis, findings consistent with a para-aortic abscess would lead to detailed examination for valve dysfunction and any intracardiac shunts or fistula.

SUGGESTED READING

1. Burwash IG, Chan KW.: Transesophageal echocardiography. In Otto CM (ed): The Practice of Clinical Echocardiography, 3rd ed. Philadelphia: Elsevier/Saunders, 2007, pp 3–30. *Detailed chapter on performance of TEE, standard image planes, Doppler flows, and indications. 266 references.*
2. Oxorn D, Otto CM: Atlas of Intraoperative Echocardiography: Clinical, Surgical and Pathologic Correlation. Philadelphia: Elsevier/Saunders, 2007. *This text and CD-ROM includes over 100 intraoperative TEE cases with surgical photographs and video clips and examples of*

pathology, in addition to still images and video clips of the TEE examination. Each case is accompanied by a clinical vignette, brief discussion, and suggested reading.

3. Sidebotham S, Merry A, Leggett M, et al: Practical Perioperative Transoesophageal Echocardiography: Text with CD-ROM. Butterworth-Heinemann, 2003.
   This 288-page paperback book and CD-ROM provides a concise overview of TEE that is helpful for TEE imaging in all clinical settings, although cases are focused on the intraoperative setting.

4. Perrino AC, Reeves ST: A Practical Approach to Transesophageal Echocardiography, 2nd ed. Lippincott Williams & Wilkins, 2007.
   This 512-page paperback book includes a basic introduction to TEE and addresses specific clinical situations, especially in intensive care unit and perioperative patients. Multiple-choice questions accompany each chapter.

5. Flachskampf FA: The standard TEE examination: procedure, safety, typical cross-sections and anatomic correlations, and systematic analysis. Semin Cardiothorac Vasc Anesth 10:49–56, 2006.
   A brief review of the technical aspects and safety of TEE. A table with suggested views for a TEE examination is provided along with examples of more detailed examination protocols for specific clinical situations.

6. Daniel WG, Erbel R, Kasper W, et al: Safety of transesophageal echocardiography: A multicenter survey of 10,419 examinations. Circulation 83:817–821, 1991.
   In 10,419 TEE examinations performed at 15 European centers over 1 year, probe insertion was unsuccessful in only 2% of attempted studies and the procedure had to be interrupted in only 1% of cases. Reasons for interrupting the procedure included intolerance of the endoscope, pulmonary, cardiac, and bleeding complications. There was one death (1/10,000)

due to bleeding from a lung tumor with esophageal infiltration. Since nearly all these studies were performed without conscious sedation, the additional risk associated with sedative medications must be considered. The ratio of TEE to transthoracic studies in this registry averaged 9% but varied from 1.4% to 23.6% between institutions.

7. Practice guidelines for sedation and analgesia by non-anesthesiologists: A report by the American Society of Anesthesiologists Task Force on Sedation and Analgesia by Non-Anesthesiologists. Anesthesiology 84:459–471, 1996.
   Consensus statement detailing the clinical standards for conscious sedation including patient evaluation, preprocedure preparation, monitoring (level of consciousness, ventilation, oxygenation, and hemodynamics), data recording, and availability of emergency equipment. The importance of having a staff person dedicated solely to patient monitoring and safety is emphasized, and the appropriate training of personnel is discussed.

8. Ryan T, Burwash I, Lu J, : The agreement between ventricular volumes and ejection fraction by transesophageal echocardiography or a combined radionuclear and thermodilution technique in patients after coronary artery surgery. J Cardiothorac Vasc Anesth 10:323–328, 1996.
   Three sets of measurements of radionuclide and TEE echocardiographic measurement of LV volumes and ejection fraction were made after coronary artery bypass grafting surgery. Ejection fraction measured by TEE using Simpson's rule or the area-length method was accurate and reproducible. However, agreement for measurement of ventricular volumes was poor.

9. Smith MD, MacPhail B, Harrison MR, et al: Value and limitations of transesophageal echocardiography in determination of left ventricular volumes and ejection fraction. J Am Coll Cardiol 19:1213–1222, 1992.

In 36 patients undergoing left ventriculography, various TEE methods for calculation of LV ejection fraction and volumes were compared with ventriculography. Ejection fraction was most accurately evaluated with the biplane Simpson's rule method (r = 0.85). However, ventricular volumes and length were consistently underestimated by TEE, suggesting that foreshortening of the long axis of the ventricle occurs with transesophageal images.

10. Groban L, Dolinski SY: Transesophageal echocardiographic evaluation of diastolic function. Chest 128: 3652–3663, 2005.
    A very clear and concise review of the physiology of diastole and evaluation of diastolic function using TEE measurements of transmitral, pulmonary venous, and tissue Doppler velocity data.

11. Karski JM: Transesophageal echocardiography in the intensive care unit. Semin Cardiothorac Vasc Anesth 10:162–166, 2006.
    A short review of the clinical utility of TEE in intensive care unit patients. The most critical information provided by TEE is evaluation of intravascular volume status and myocardial dysfunction. Other diagnoses that can be made using TEE include dynamic LV outflow obstruction, cardiac tamponade, native or prosthetic valve dysfunction, aortic dissection and detection of intracardiac masses or shunt.

12. Porembka DT: Importance of transesophageal echocardiography in the critically ill and injured patient. Crit Care Med 35(8 Suppl):S414–S430, 2007.
    In intensive care unit patients, the diagnostic yield of TEE is 78%. The results of the TEE study change therapy in about 60% to 65% of intensive care unit patients. This is a detailed review of the literature with over 100 references, tables summarizing clinical studies, and illustrations of TEE views.

4

Advanced Echocardiographic Modalities

THREE-DIMENSIONAL
ECHOCARDIOGRAPHY
    Acquisition
    Display
    Clinical Utility

MYOCARDIAL MECHANICS
    Tissue Doppler Strain and Strain Rate
    Speckle Tracking Strain Imaging
    Dyssynchrony

CONTRAST ECHOCARDIOGRAPHY
    Contrast Agents
    Applications
    Limitations and Safety

INTRACARDIAC ECHOCARDIOGRAPHY
    Instrumentation
    Technique
    Applications
    Limitations and Safety

INTRAVASCULAR ULTRASOUND
    Instrumentation and Technique
    Applications

HAND-HELD ECHOCARDIOGRAPHY
    Instrumentation
    Applications
    Limitations

SUGGESTED READING

Transthoracic and transesophageal echocardiography (TEE) are standard clinical diagnostic modalities that are widely available and utilized by most cardiologists. In addition, other echocardiographic modalities in clinical practice include:

❏ Stress echocardiography
❏ Contrast echocardiography
❏ Three-dimensional (3D) echocardiography
❏ Strain and strain right imaging

Stress echocardiography now is a standard approach in most echocardiography laboratories. Contrast echocardiography is increasingly utilized, particularly at academic medical centers. Three dimensional echocardiography will become more widely available as simpler user interfaces become standard. Evaluation of myocardial mechanics is in development, using tissue Doppler or speckle tracking to measure myocardial strain and strain rate.

In addition, several newer applications of cardiac ultrasound are used in specific clinical settings by physicians with special expertise in areas other than echocardiography. In many cases these ultrasound examinations are performed as part of another diagnostic or therapeutic procedure, and the primary physician may be an anesthesiologist, an interventional cardiologist, an electrophysiologist, emergency room physician,

or general internist. These procedures include the following:

❏ Intraoperative TEE
❏ Intracardiac echocardiography (ICE)
❏ Intravascular ultrasound (IVUS)
❏ Hand-held echocardiography

As detailed in Chapter 5, appropriate education and training in cardiac ultrasound is needed by these physicians. However, the cardiac sonographer and physician often are involved in ensuring optimal data acquisition and interpretation of these examinations. This chapter provides an introduction to these other echocardiographic modalities. Intraoperative TEE is discussed in more detail in Chapter 18. Advanced echocardiographers will want to read further on these topics as indicated in the Suggested Reading.

THREE-DIMENSIONAL ECHOCARDIOGRAPHY

The term *3D echocardiography* refers broadly to several approaches for acquisition and display of cardiac ultrasound images. Different 3D approaches are similar in that cardiac structures are shown in relationship to each other in all three spatial dimensions and in that structures can be rotated or viewed from different orientations, even after image acquisition. One of the challenges of 3D echocardiography is ensuring adequate image resolution in all three dimensions, given the constraints of ultrasound physics and transducer design. Another challenge is ensuring temporal, as well as spatial, resolution.

Acquisition

There are two basic approaches to acquisition of echocardiographic data in a 3D format:

❏ Volumetric ultrasound imaging
❏ Two-dimensional (2D) imaging in multiple planes with a known 3D location

Volumetric imaging utilizes a complex multiarray transducer that simultaneously acquires ultrasound data from a 3D pyramidal volume. Rapid parallel-image processing provides ultrasound images that can be viewed in real time in any orientation on the screen (Fig. 4–1). Alternatively, a volumetric transducer allows simultaneous display of more than one tomographic image plane (Fig. 4–2) or a 3D image from a specific point of view, such as a view of the mitral valve from the left atrium (Fig. 4–3).

Advantages of volumetric ultrasound image acquisition include real-time image formation and rapid acquisition. The disadvantage of volumetric imaging is that it is difficult to optimize image quality for all structures in the 3D volume simultaneously. Even when technical issues related to beam focusing and image display are resolved, the direction of the ultrasound beam relative to the structure of interest affects image quality; this is because resolution still depends on the orientation of the ultrasound beam relative to the specular reflector, with optimal resolution in the axial direction for structures perpendicular to the ultrasound beam. In addition, ultrasound artifacts such as shadowing, reverberations, and poor penetration may affect the image, as with any ultrasound modality.

Three-dimensional echocardiography also can be performed with image acquisition in multiple 2D image planes, as long as the position of each image plane in 3D space is known and linked to the 2D image. This approach can be used with rotational image acquisition, such as on TEE, from a single transducer location. Alternatively, images can be acquired from multiple transducer positions when combined with a locator system that records the position and angle of each image plane (Fig. 4–4). The advantages of 2D acquisition for 3D images are that image quality can be optimized in each image plane and data from multiple transducer locations can be combined to produce a fuller dataset than from a single volumetric transducer location. Disadvantages include misregistration of images if the transducer (with rotational scanning) or the patient (with multiple

transducer locations) moves during the acquisition period, and the time needed to reconstruct the 3D image from nonsimultaneous 2D image planes.

Display

There are three basic approaches to display of 3D echocardiographic data:

❏ Real-time "3D" display
❏ Simultaneous 2D image planes
❏ Border reconstructions

The most intuitive display format for 3D echocardiography is a 3D image that can be rotated and viewed from multiple perspectives in real time. Current display formats suffer from attempting to show 3D images on 2D displays; this limitation should be resolved as 3D display systems become more widely available. The real-time 3D display also can be "cropped" to show different views of the interior structures of the heart. For example, the mitral valve can be viewed from the perspective of the LA; this provides a compelling view of prolapsing segments of the valve in patients with myxomatous mitral valve disease. The image can then be rotated and re-cropped to show a long axis–type image of the mitral valve. Similarly, the aortic valve can be viewed en face from the perspective of the aorta, a view that correlates closely with the surgical view of valve anatomy, from the left ventricular (LV) side of the valve or in a long-axis orientation (Fig. 4–5). As 3D display systems improve, it may be possible to "travel" through the heart, for example following the path of blood flow in a patient with complex congenital heart disease.

The 3D echocardiographic dataset also can be used to generate multiple 2D image planes. Volumetric scanning allows simultaneous display of multiple image planes (Fig. 4–6). The ability to acquire LV images in multiple planes simultaneously should speed image acquisition during stress echocardiography, potentially improving diagnostic accuracy. In addition, the ability to "move through" a 3D dataset in any 2D image plane will allow better appreciation of cardiac anatomy in patients with complex structural heart disease and allow precise localization of abnormalities. The ability to interrogate the 3D volumetric dataset after image acquisition will facilitate diagnosis in complex cases.

As with 2D echocardiography, quantitation from 3D data requires identification of cardiac borders. Border tracing of 2D images, which are then reconstructed into a 3D volume, provides very accurate LV volume measurements. Semiautomated border tracing algorithms aid in rapid analysis of multiple tomographic images. 3D reconstructions of the LV also allow detailed assessment of ventricular shape, regional ventricular function, and 3D strain rate and strain measurements. In addition, right ventricle

Figure 4–1 A 3D echocardiographic acquisition from an apical view is cropped to visualize structures within the 3D ultrasound volume. **A,** On the schematic drawing, standard image planes in short-axis (*purple*), long-axis (*red*), and four-chamber (*green*) planes are shown; however, any 3D cropping plane can be created. The full volume ultrasound (**B1**) is shown. Cropping in the transverse plane in blue (**B2**) yields a short-axis view (**B3**); the sagittal plane in red (**B4**) yields either an apical two-chamber (**B5**) or long axis view depending on depth and angle of the cropping plane; and the coronal plane in green (**B6**) yields an apical four-chamber view (**B7**). *(From Picard MH: Three-dimensional echocardiography. In Otto CM [ed]: The Practice of Clinical Echocardiography, 3rd ed. Philadelphia: Elsevier/ Saunders, 2007, Figure 4–5, p 91.)*

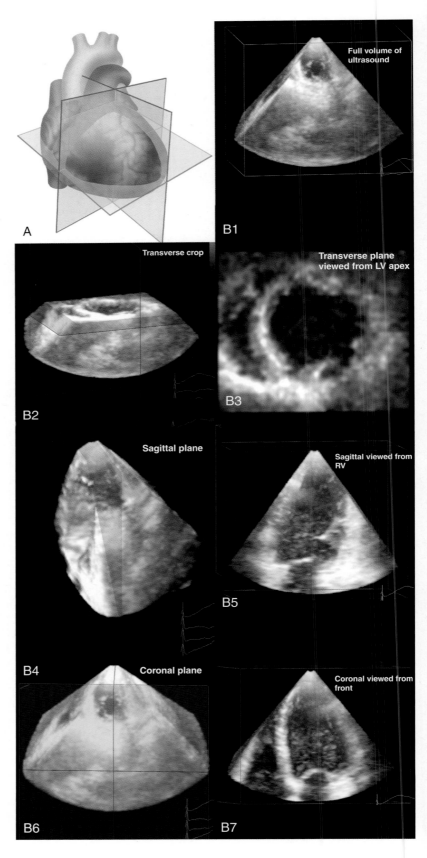

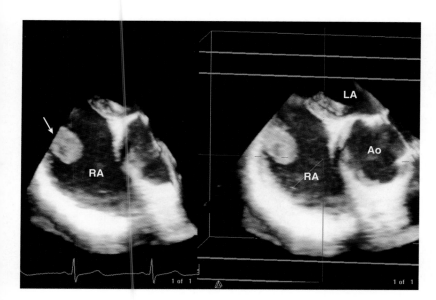

Figure 4–2 Three-dimensional imaging of a RA mass (*arrow*) using a volumetric real-time 3D transesophageal transducer. The volume of image data (*right*) can be cropped and rotated as needed to show the structure of interest in the final image (*left*).

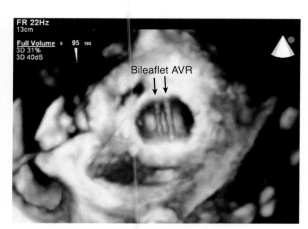

Figure 4–3 Real-time 3D transesophageal imaging of a bileaflet mechanical aortic valve replacement (AVR) with the leaflets open during systole, with the 3D dataset cropped and rotated so the viewer is looking at the valve from the aortic side.

(RV) size and function can be quantitated by 3D echocardiography. Quantitative 3D measurements of the mitral valve apparatus have provided insight into the mechanisms of mitral regurgitation (Fig. 4–7).

Clinical Utility

The clinical role of 3D echocardiography will continue to evolve as this technology matures. In addition to providing more detailed anatomic relationships and more accurate quantitation, 3D images are more intuitive than 2D images, allowing quicker appreciation of cardiac anatomy by more health care providers. Potentially, 3D echocardiography could be faster than 2D scanning and could reduce variability

in image acquisition. However, because instrumentation is in development, 3D echocardiography is not yet a routine part of the clinical examination in most laboratories and standardized approaches to a complete 3D examination are in evolution. One immediate application of real-time 3D echocardiography (RT3DE) is rapid acquisition of a volumetric image of the LV from the apical approach, with display of simultaneous apical four-chamber, two-chamber, and long-axis views along with multiple parallel short-axis views. This approach may be particularly useful for evaluation of regional LV function during stress echocardiography. Quantitating LV volumes and ejection fraction from RT3DE also is likely to have widespread clinical utility. In addition, some specialized centers use 3D echocardiography to supplement the standard 2D and Doppler examination, when complex structural disease is present. For example, real-time 3D TEE images of the mitral valve are helpful in patients undergoing mitral valve repair for mitral prolapse. In adults with an atrial septal defect, 3D TEE images of the size and shape of the defect can assist in choosing the optimal closure device.

MYOCARDIAL MECHANICS

LV function is a complex event that is only partially described by clinical measures of ejection fraction, qualitative changes in regional wall motion, and measures of diastolic filling. Ventricular contraction occurs in the longitudinal direction (the base moves toward the apex), in the radial direction (walls thicken), and in the circumferential direction (cavity size decreases perpendicular to the long axis of the chamber). In addition,

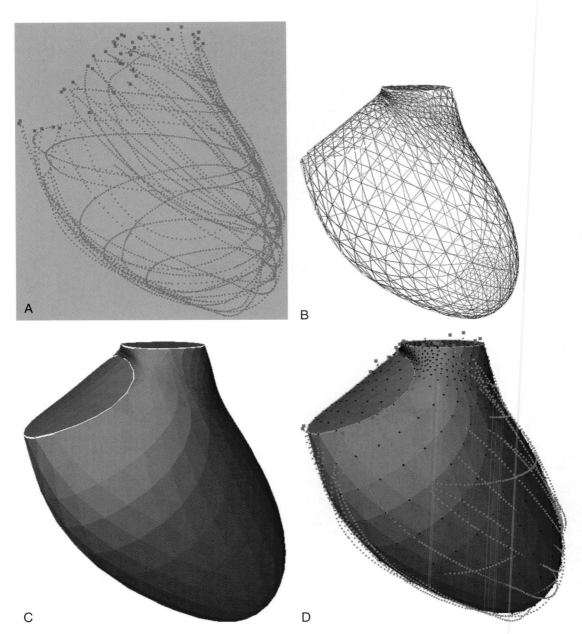

Figure 4–4 In vivo reconstruction of the LV cavity at end-diastole. **A,** Traced borders using freehand transthoracic scanning from multiple acoustic windows including short axis and apical rotation view, registered in 3D using a magnetic locator system. The aortic annulus is indicated in red and the mitral annulus in green points. **B,** Using the piece-wise smooth subdivision method for 3D reconstruction, the second-subdivision mesh (520 faces) is fit to the traced border points with reconstruction of the aortic and mitral annulus. **C,** Final reconstructed surface of the LV at end-diastole. **D,** Superimposed actual traced borders and points on the reconstructed surface. *(Courtesy of Florence Sheehan, MD.)*

the apex and base rotate in opposite directions during contraction, resulting in a twisting motion called torsion. There are several promising approaches to a more complete and quantitative description of myocardial function including strain rate and strain, derived from tissue Doppler or speckle tracing data, and descriptors of myocardial dyssynchrony, derived from imaging or tissue Doppler data.

Tissue Doppler Strain and Strain Rate

Doppler blood flow velocity measurements are based on backscatter of low amplitude, high velocity signals from moving blood cells. Conversely, Doppler tissue velocity measurements are based on the high amplitude, low velocity signals reflected from the myocardium. Thus, these signals are easily separated by

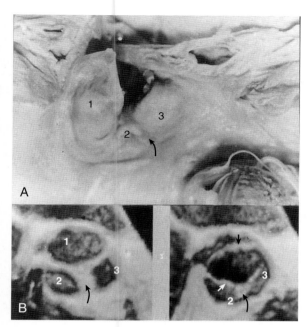

Figure 4–5 Pathologic specimen showing the ventricular side of a bicuspid aortic valve with fusion of leaflets 2 and 3 (**A**), corresponding closely with images obtained by 3D echocardiography in diastole and systole (**B**). *(From Espinola-Zavaleta N, Muñoz-Castellanos L, Attié F, et al: Anatomic three-dimensional echocardiographic correlation of bicuspid aortic valve. J Am Soc Echocardiogr 16:46–53, 2003.)*

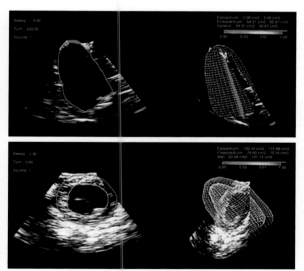

Figure 4–6 The use of an interactively aided algorithm for calculation of LV volume and mass. The slice view is shown on the *left* for a long-axis image (*top*) and short-axis image (*bottom*), with the operator-traced endocardial and epicardial borders shown. Using these operator-traced borders, the computer instantly generates a meshlike cast of the ventricle that is superimposed on the image (*right*). These images can be freely rotated to allow the operator to evaluate, and modify as needed, the correspondence between the computer-generated cast and the LV surface. *(From Schmidt MA, Freidlin RZ, Ohazama CJ, et al: Anatomic validation of a novel method for left ventricular volume and mass measurements with use of real-time 3-dimensional echocardiography. J Am Soc Echocardiogr 14:1–10, 2001, Fig. 1.)*

adjusting the gain, wall filters, and velocity scale of the Doppler spectral or color display.

Tissue Doppler velocity recording at a specific intracardiac site is analogous to pulsed Doppler blood flow velocities. Tissue velocity measurements depend on a parallel alignment between the ultrasound beam and direction of myocardial motion; in other words, motion is measured only in the direction toward and away from the transducer. For example, a component in evaluation of diastolic function is the tissue Doppler signal recorded in the apical four-chamber view with a 2-mm sample volume positioned about 1 cm apical from the septal side of the mitral annulus (Fig. 4–8). The spectral display is recorded at a velocity range of ± 0.2 m/s, using a very low gain and wall filter setting. The Doppler velocities show systolic motion of the myocardium toward the apex, corresponding to the apical motion of the annulus in systole seen on 2D imaging. In diastole there is an early diastolic motion of the myocardium (m) away from the apex (E_m, also called E'), corresponding to the early phase of LV filling, and a late diastolic motion away from the apex (A_m), corresponding to the atrial phase of ventricular filling. The utility of tissue Doppler for diastolic function evaluation is discussed further in Chapter 7.

Strain rate imaging is based on the difference in tissue Doppler velocity (V) between sample volumes divided by the distance (D) between them (Fig. 4–9) or the rate of change in myocardial length, normalized to the original length. Strain rate (SR) then is:

$$SR = (V_2 - V_1)/D$$

The units of strain are seconds^{-1} (or /s), because the velocity measured in centimeters per second (cm/s) is divided by the distance in centimeters. Typically, strain rate is measured in the base to apex direction, in the apical four-chamber view with three sample volumes placed in the septal or lateral wall myocardium about 12 mm apart. The tissue Doppler mean velocity curves are examined to ensure a clear signal without excessive noise, lack of aliasing, and avoidance of blood pool signals. The instrument calculates strain rate from these velocity curves for each time point and displays strain rate in seconds^{-1} as a function of time. The strain rate curve looks like a mirror image across the baseline of the velocity curve, because myocardial shortening is a negative strain and lengthening is a positive strain. Strain rate provides data on relative timing of myocardial motion and measurement of peak systolic and diastolic strain rates. Peak systolic strain rate is a measure of ventricular contractile function that is insensitive to changes in loading conditions.

Strain is a measure of deformation of a material, defined as the difference between the final length (l) and the original length (l_o), divided by the original length. Thus, strain can be thought of as the percentage change in length.

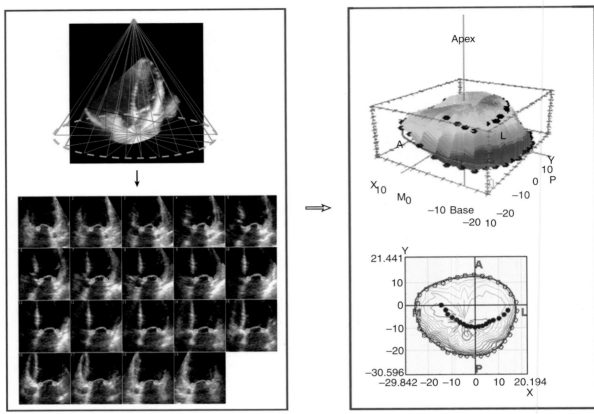

Figure 4–7 Three-dimensional reconstruction of the mitral valve apparatus by using real-time 3D echocardiography and a novel software system for mitral valve quantification (REAL VIEW, YD, Ltd). *Left panel,* The 3D volumetric image is automatically cropped into 18 equally spaced radial planes. The mitral annulus and leaflets are traced in each cropped plane. From these data, 3D images of the mitral leaflets and annulus are reconstructed. *Right upper panel,* Reconstructed 3D image that shows the actual configuration of the curved annulus and leaflets with surface colorations. In this case with ischemic MR, the mitral annulus flattened with apparent tenting of the mitral leaflets, which were tethered into the LV, showing mountain-shape leaflet bulging. *Right lower panel,* Mitral leaflet configuration is represented in contour to appreciate the degree of tenting in the vertical view from the LV. Blue dots indicate coaptation line. *(Courtesy of Nozomi Watanabe, MD, Kawasaki University, Okayama, Japan.)*

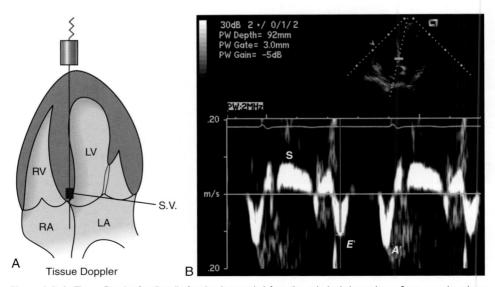

Figure 4–8 A, Tissue Doppler for diastolic function is recorded from the apical window using a 2-mm sample volume positioned in the myocardium about 1 cm from the mitral annulus. **B,** A tissue Doppler signal showing that in systole (S) the myocardium moves toward the apex. In diastole the myocardial velocity is directed away from the transducer first with early diastolic filling (E') and then with atrial contraction (A'). Myocardial velocities are higher at the base than the apex.

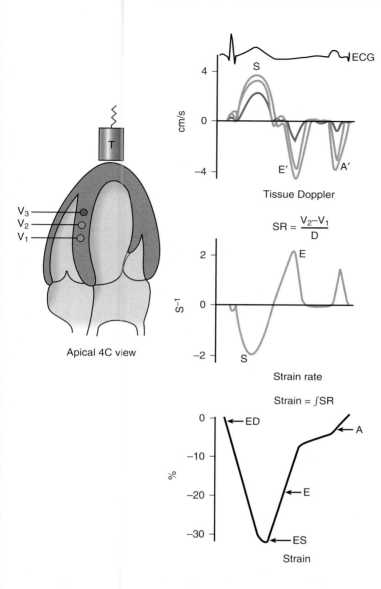

Figure 4–9 Schematic diagram of the derivation of strain rate and strain from myocardial tissue velocities. From the apical view at least three Doppler sample volumes are positioned in the myocardium about 12 mm apart. The three graphs on the *right* show one cardiac cycle, matched for timing as shown by the ECG at the top. The tissue Doppler tracings show mean velocity versus time with the line colors corresponding to each sample volume position. Strain rate is calculated for each time point at the change in velocity (V) between each two sample volume positions, divided by the distance (D) between them. Strain is determined by integration of the strain rate to generate a curve similar to an LV volume curve with a rapid decrease in strain during ejection (ED to ES) and a rapid increase in strain in early diastole (E) with another increase in late diastole after atrial contraction (A).

$$\text{Strain} = [(l - l_o)/l_o] \times 100\%$$

Strain can be estimated from the tissue Doppler strain rate by integrating the curve over time.

Thus, strain is analogous to ejection fraction (i.e., change in volume normalized to initial volume), with the advantages that spatial and temporal localization is possible. In fact, a graph of strain over the cardiac cycle (Fig. 4–9) looks similar to a ventricular volume curve. Because strain is relative to the baseline length, end-diastole is considered zero strain. During systole strain decreases rapidly until end-systole is reached. Isovolumetric relaxation and contraction result in a slight flattening of the curve just before and after systole. In diastole there is a rapid increase in strain during the early phase of diastolic filling (E), followed by

a plateau during diastasis and then another increase with atrial contraction (A) back to the baseline at end-diastole. Peak systolic strain is a measure of regional ventricular function. However, like ejection fraction, strain varies with preload.

Doppler strain rate and strain imaging have been shown to be more sensitive than conventional echocardiographic measurements for detection of early myocardial involvement in amyloidosis, diabetes, and hypertrophic cardiomyopathy. The sensitivity and specificity of this approach for detection of subclinical cardiac involvement awaits further validation. Strain and strain rate have also been proposed as potentially useful for detection of myocardial ischemia during stress testing and for diagnosis of myocardial viability but is not currently part of a standard stress echocardiographic study.

Accurate measurement of strain rate and strain requires careful attention to technical aspects of data recording. The sample volumes must fit within the myocardium at an adequate distance from each other. In addition, velocity is only measured in the direction toward and away from the transducer. Signal quality is enhanced by use of harmonic imaging, an adequate pulse repetition frequency, a high frame rate, and tracking the sample volume to the ventricular wall. The Suggested Reading provides further details about data acquisition and interpretation.

Speckle Tracking Strain Imaging

As its name implies, this approach is based on tracking the motion of small bright spots in the myocardium (speckles) on the gray-scale image as they move during the cardiac cycle. Speckles are natural acoustic markers due to interference patterns caused by backscattered signals from small structures (less than a wavelength) in the myocardium. The advantages of speckle tracking over Doppler tissue velocities are (1) simpler data acquisition, (2) lack of angle dependence, (3) direct measurement of strain, (4) multiple simultaneous measurements in the image plane, and (5) the ability to do the analysis after image acquisition. The ultrasound system tracks speckles and determines the distance between two markers in a defined myocardial region and then plots this distance over the cardiac cycle (Fig. 4–10). Thus, speckle tracking provides a direct measure of strain—the change in length of the myocardium relative to the original length. In addition, circumferential strain can be measured from short-axis views, radial strain in multiple segments, and longitudinal strain in long-axis views. Strain rate is the first derivative, or slope, of the graph of strain over the cardiac cycle. The clinical utility of speckle tracking strain imaging is under evaluation.

Dyssynchrony

The term *dyssynchrony* describes a pattern of ventricular contraction in which some areas contract before other areas in an irregular spatial and temporal pattern. Dyssynchrony is primarily seen in patients with a reduced ejection fraction, either from a cardiomyopathy or due to ischemic disease, and may be appreciated on 2D imaging in some cases. Attempts to measure the amount of dyssynchrony have utilized imaging, conventional Doppler, and tissue Doppler approaches. M-mode echocardiography has been used to measure the time interval from the QRS on the electrocardiogram (ECG) to maximum inward motion of the ventricular wall, comparing the septum to the posterior wall. This approach is limited by the many other causes of changes in septal motion. Interventricular dyssynchrony has been measured at the difference between LV and RV pre-ejection periods, measured from the QRS complex to onset of aortic or pulmonic flow, respectively, with abnormal defined as a difference in these measurements >40 ms.

With pulsed tissue Doppler, the variation in time to peak systolic velocity at different locations in the myocardium also provides a measure of dyssynchrony. Tissue Doppler mean velocity data displayed using a color scale superimposed on the 2D image is analogous to color Doppler flow imaging. With a normal pattern of ventricular contraction there is a uniform pattern of red in systole and blue in diastole.

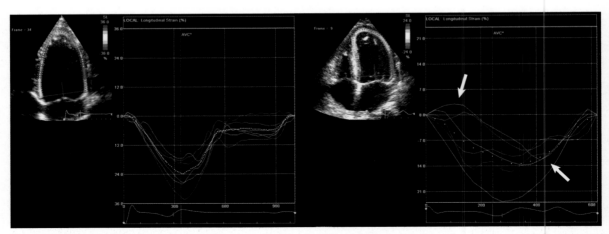

Figure 4–10 Speckle tracking echocardiography showing long-axis strains. The *left panel* shows typical strain pattern from a normal LV. The *right panel* shows recordings from a patient with an anterior myocardial infarction. In the apical LV segments (*arrows*) there is lengthening during early systole and there is post-systolic shortening (*arrows*). *(From Smiseth OA, Edvardsen T: Tissue Doppler and speckle tracking echocardiography. In Otto CM [ed]: The Practice of Clinical Echocardiography, 3rd ed. Philadelphia: Elsevier/Saunders, 2007, p 123, Fig. 5–11.)*

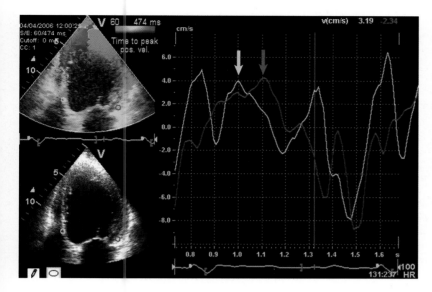

Figure 4–11 Measurement of intraventricular dyssynchrony: A4C view of the LV. The tissue Doppler traces from the apical part of the septum (*yellow*) show delayed ejection velocity (*yellow arrow*) compared to the corresponding ejection velocity from the apical part of the lateral wall (*white arrow*). The delay is 170 ms. Note the large post-systolic velocity from the septum (*red arrow*). A4C, apical four-chamber. *(From Smiseth OA, Edvardsen T: Tissue Doppler and speckle tracking echocardiography. In Otto CM [ed]: The Practice of Clinical Echocardiography, 3rd ed. Philadelphia: Elsevier-Saunders, 2007, p 132, Fig. 5–25.)*

Dyssynchrony results in a chaotic pattern of red-blue as different areas of the myocardium contract at different times and rates. Tissue Doppler data also can be displayed as a graph of tissue velocity versus time with separate colored lines for each myocardial region of interest (Fig. 4–11).

Simultaneous recording of tissue Doppler velocity curves from several sites allows measurement of the differences in time from the QRS to peak tissue velocity. For example, the standard deviation of measurements from 12 different segments has been proposed as a predictor of the response to pacemaker-based resynchronization therapy for heart failure. However, there is no consensus on the optimal approach to evaluation of ventricular dyssynchrony, and the exact role in clinical decision making remains unclear. Approaches to 3D echocardiographic evaluation of dyssynchrony also are in development.

According to the ASE Guidelines (see Suggested Reading 8), useful measures of dyssynchrony are:

1. A difference of 65 ms in the tissue Doppler *S*-wave peaks between opposing LV walls in the apical four-chamber or long-axis view
2. A difference of 40 ms in the interval from the QRS to onset of flow (pulsed Doppler) in the RV versus LV outflow tract
3. A difference of 130 ms in the septal to posterior wall delay, measured by M-mode or by speckle tracking radial strain

After biventricular pacer implantation for cardiac resynchronization therapy (CRT), echocardiography can be used to optimize the atrioventricular (AV) delay. The recommended approach is:

1. Ensure an optimal ECG signal on the echocardiography instrument.
2. Record pulsed Doppler LV inflow velocities with the sample volume at the mitral annulus level, with a low wall filter and high sweep speed and a clear mitral closure click.
3. AV delay is optimized when the *E* and *A* waves are not merged and the *A* wave ends at least 40 ms before the mitral closure click (or QRS onset).

When the AV delay is too short, the *A* wave is absent or truncated; an excessive AV delay results in superimposition of the *A* wave on the *E* wave, with a single diastolic filling curve.

CONTRAST ECHOCARDIOGRAPHY

Contrast echocardiography refers to the injection into the bloodstream of an agent that results in increased echogenicity of the blood or myocardium on ultrasound imaging, producing opacification of the cardiac chambers or an increase in echo-density of the myocardium. Ultrasound "contrast" is generated by the presence of microbubbles in the ultrasound field. At low ultrasound power outputs, microbubbles scatter ultrasound at the gas/liquid interface, resulting in detection of a strong signal by the transducer. Fundamental ultrasound imaging is based on detection of this signal reflected from the fluid/gas interface. In addition, ultrasound causes compression and expansion (e.g., oscillation) of microbubbles, with the resonant frequency of a microbubble inversely related to its diameter. Harmonic imaging detects this nonlinear resonant signal. However, at higher power outputs ultrasound results in microbubble destruction. Thus, careful adjustment of instrument power outputs is needed during contrast imaging.

Contrast Agents

There are two types of echo-contrast agents, those that opacify the:

☐ right heart or
☐ left heart and myocardium

Depending on the size of the microbubbles relative to the lung capillary diameter, the microbubbles are trapped in the pulmonary capillaries so that no contrast material is seen in the left side of the heart in the absence of an intracardiac right to left communication (Fig. 4–12). Microbubbles in the 1- to 5-μm size range will traverse the pulmonary bed and microbubbles in this size range resonate at a frequency of 1.5 to 7 MHz, corresponding to clinical transducer frequencies.

The most widely used agent for right heart contrast is agitated saline. A simple approach is to rapidly push 5 mL of sterile saline, with a small amount (about 0.2 mL) of air between two syringes connected with a three-way stopcock. This results in the production of large microbubbles that do not pass through the pulmonary vascular bed. When the saline appears opaque, it is injected rapidly into a peripheral vein during echocardiographic imaging, with the total volume and rate of injection adjusted based on image

quality. The contrast effect may be enhanced by following the contrast injection with 10 mL of nonagitated saline. Care is taken to ensure that there is no visible free air in the injection system. In addition, agitated saline should not be used in patients with known significant right to left shunts.

Commercially available left heart contrast agents consist of air or low solubility fluorocarbon gas in stabilized microbubbles encapsulated with denatured albumin, monosaccharides, or other formulations. These agents typically are prepared just before injection, with specific directions for preparation and use of each agent. Some require resuspension before each bolus intravenous injection. Others are diluted and given as a continuous infusion. Microbubbles are fragile, so careful handling and infusion techniques are needed for diagnostic results. The optimal volume and rate of infusion depend on the specific contrast agent used, with the objectives being to provide full opacification while minimizing attenuation due to excess microbubble density.

Instrument settings are adjusted to optimize image quality during contrast opacification of the LV including a decrease in the overall power output (usually to a mechanical index of about 0.5), a focal depth setting at the middle or near field, a lower transducer frequency, and an increase in overall gain and dynamic range.

Applications

Contrast echocardiography has four proposed diagnostic applications:

☐ Detection of intracardiac shunts
☐ Enhancement of Doppler signals
☐ LV opacification
☐ Myocardial perfusion

Right heart contrast allows detection of right to left intracardiac shunts by the appearance of contrast in the left heart within 1 to 2 beats of contrast appearance in the right heart. With a patent foramen ovale, right to left shunting may be present only after Valsalva maneuver because of the transient increase in right atrial (RA), compared with LA, pressure (see Chapter 15). Even with predominant left to right shunts (e.g., with an atrial septal defect) there usually is a small amount of right to left shunting when the pressures on both sides of the defect are similar, allowing detection of shunting with right heart contrast. Other examples of the utility of right heart contrast include identification of a persistent left superior vena cava or identification of the systemic venous inflow pathway in complex congenital heart disease.

Contrast has been used at some centers to increase Doppler signal strength, for example, the tricuspid

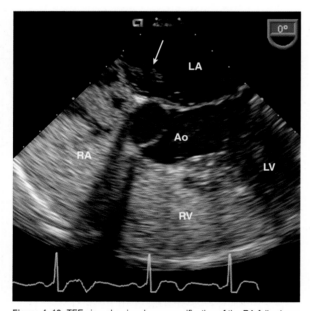

Figure 4–12 TEE view showing dense opacification of the RA following a peripheral venous injection of agitated saline solution, which does not pass through the pulmonary vascular bed. A small amount of contrast (*arrow*) has entered the LA via a patent foramen ovale.

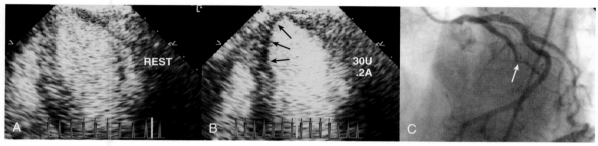

Figure 4–13 An example of an inducible septal and apical perfusion defect during dobutamine stress echocardiography using contrast echocardiography. **A,** The ventricular chamber is bright due to contrast filling the chamber. The myocardium also shows increased echogenicity in all segments, because myocardial perfusion is normal at rest. **B,** During stress the apical segment of the septum becomes akinetic, and the *arrows* depict a subendocardial perfusion defect that corresponds with the coronary angiogram (**C**) showing an occluded left anterior descending coronary artery (*arrow*). *(From Porter TR, Xie F: Contrast ultrasound imaging: methods, analysis and applications. In Otto CM [ed]: The Practice of Clinical Echocardiography, 3rd ed. Philadelphia: Elsevier/Saunders, 2007, p 73, Fig. 3–10.)*

regurgitant jet. However, the effect of contrast on the Doppler signal varies with instrument parameters, and this approach has not gained widespread use.

LV opacification in patients with poor image quality either on resting studies or during stress echocardiography enhances recognition of segmental wall motion abnormalities and overall LV systolic function (see Chapter 8). Contrast enhancement improves the accuracy of echocardiographic stress studies when endocardial definition is suboptimal (Fig. 4–13).

Assessment of myocardial perfusion with contrast echocardiography is technically challenging. Only about 6% of the stroke volume perfuses the myocardium, so the relative number of microbubbles in the coronary circulation is small. Mechanical and ultrasound destruction of microbubbles further limits the contrast effect. Thus, special imaging modes such as intermittent imaging, pulse inversion, or power modulation imaging are needed for myocardial contrast imaging. Myocardial contrast perfusion imaging may improve detection of coronary disease on stress studies and may allow identification of impaired coronary perfusion at rest. However, other approaches for evaluation of myocardial perfusion, including nuclear perfusion imaging, positron emission tomography, and cardiac magnetic resonance imaging, are superior and are the current clinical standard.

Limitations and Safety

Right heart contrast to detect large intracardiac shunts is needed infrequently, given the sensitivity and specificity of color Doppler and TEE imaging. The primary use of right heart contrast is for detection of a patent foramen ovale. A small ventricular septal defect usually will not be detected with a right heart contrast injection, since there is little right to left shunting.

The use of left heart contrast requires considerable experience to judge the infusion rate and volume needed to optimally opacify the LV. When the microbubble density is too high, an excessive contrast effect at the apex results in attenuation of the signal or "shadowing" of the rest of the LV. A swirling appearance may be seen with too little contrast or in low flow states. Bubble destruction due to a high mechanical index also results in a swirling pattern with inadequate ventricular opacification.

The addition of a contrast injection to the echocardiographic examination increases the cost and risk of the procedure. In addition the added time and personnel needed for placement of an intravenous line during a standard echocardiographic examination or exercise stress study make this approach impractical in many laboratories. Although major adverse reactions to left-sided contrast agents are rare, patients may experience nausea/vomiting, headache, flushing, or dizziness. Hypersensitivity reactions can occur.

Recently, the US Food and Drug Administration (FDA) added a "black box" warning for the use of pharmacologic ultrasound contrast because of patient deaths and other adverse effects temporally related to a contrast study. Contraindications to the use of perflutren contrast agents are a known right-to-left or bidirectional shunt, or a history of hypersensitivity to perflutren, and this contrast agent should not be injected intra-arterially. The use of pharmacologic contrast requires a physician order, is restricted to studies where improved endocardial definition is necessary, and should be avoided in high-risk patients. Blood pressure, arterial oxygen saturation, and ECG monitoring for 30 min after the contrast injection are recommended in high-risk patients, including those with pulmonary hypertension or unstable cardiopulmonary conditions. Resuscitation equipment and trained personnel should be available in the event of an adverse reaction.

INTRACARDIAC ECHOCARDIOGRAPHY

Instrumentation

Intracardiac echocardiography (ICE) uses a catheter-like ultrasound probe that is passed into the right heart chambers from the femoral vein (Fig. 4–14). The transducer frequency is variable from 5 to 10 MHz to provide adequate penetration to image structures at distances up to 10 cm from the transducer and to provide optimal image resolution. Current devices provide single-plane imaging, pulsed and color Doppler, with a steerable probe connected to a standard ultrasound imaging system.

Technique

Typically, the 10 French 90-cm-long disposable probe is inserted via a venous sheath as part of an invasive cardiac procedure in the cardiac catheterization or electrophysiology laboratory. The physician performing the interventional or electrophysiologic procedure also acquires the cardiac images, since expertise in intracardiac manipulation of catheters is needed for this procedure. Fluoroscopy is used for placement of the probe, because it does not accommodate a guidewire. The tip of the probe can be tilted and flexed using dials at the base of the probe, and the image plane also can be adjusted by advancing, withdrawing, or rotating the probe, similar to a single-plane TEE transducer. The transducer can be positioned in the:

- ❑ inferior vena cava,
- ❑ right atrium (RA), or
- ❑ right ventricle (RV),

with the RA location most useful for monitoring invasive procedures.

From the inferior vena cava the transducer is turned to visualize the abdominal aorta. From the RA position the following views are obtained:

- ❑ Short-axis aortic valve
- ❑ Tricuspid valve and RV
- ❑ Mitral valve and LV
- ❑ Interatrial septum
- ❑ LA and left pulmonary veins

The interatrial septum is visualized from an RA position with the catheter retroflexed to show the fossa ovalis, septum primum, and RA and LA. The aortic valve is visualized by straightening and slightly anteflexing the probe, and turning it toward the aorta (Fig. 4–15). The tricuspid valve and RV are best visualized by anteflexing the probe after positioning the tip superiorly in the RA. From this position, turning the probe posteriorly allows visualization of the mitral valve and LV. The left pulmonary veins are visualized by angulation from the atrial septal view inferiorly to image the LA appendage, and then the pulmonary views (Fig. 4–16). From this position the probe is turned clockwise and advanced superiorly in the atrium to visualize the two right pulmonary veins. These views allow diameter measurements and pulsed and color Doppler interrogation of all four pulmonary veins (Fig. 4–17).

From the RV, a view of the outflow tract and pulmonary artery can be obtained. The LV also can be evaluated, but care in interpretation of wall motion is needed if the catheter is moving in the RV.

Applications

ICE is primarily utilized for monitoring invasive procedures, although the diagnostic potential of this modality has not been fully evaluated. In a patient undergoing an invasive cardiac procedure, image quality is usually inadequate on transthoracic imaging, and TEE imaging typically requires general anesthesia, given the length of the procedure. ICE is well tolerated, provides accurate information, and provides continuous imaging data to the physician performing the procedure.

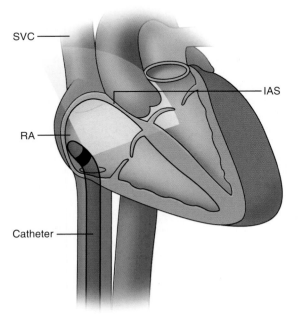

Figure 4–14 ICE is performed by advancing the probe from the IVC to the RA. The probe is retroflexed to image the IAS. *(From Bartel T, Muller S, Caspari G, et al: Intracardiac and intraluminal echocardiography: indications and standard approaches. Ultrasound Med Biol 28:997–1003, 2002.)*

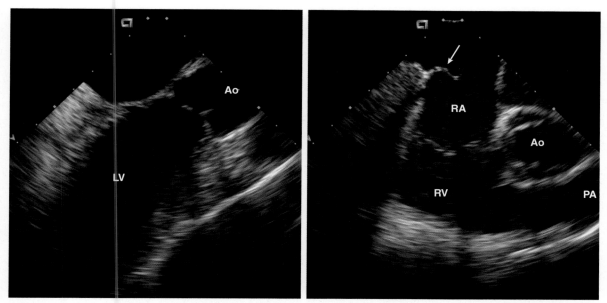

Figure 4–15 Intracardiac view of the aortic valve in a short-axis (*left*) and long-axis (*right*) orientation obtained with the transducer tip in the RA.

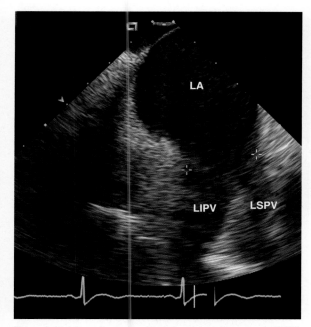

Figure 4–16 Intracardiac image of the left superior pulmonary vein (LSPV) and left inferior pulmonary vein (LIPV) during an electrophysiology ablation procedure with measurement of the diameter of the PV orifice.

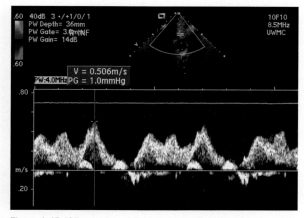

Figure 4–17 ICE recording of PV flow using pulsed Doppler ultrasound.

The primary applications of ICE in the cardiac catheterization laboratory are:

❑ Percutaneous defect closures
❑ Catheter mitral balloon valvotomy
❑ Percutaneous aortic valve replacement
❑ Other percutaneous interventions for structural heart disease

ICE at baseline before closure of an atrial septal defect allows evaluation of the atrial septal defect size and position, and identification of adjacent structures including the pulmonary veins and coronary sinus. During the procedure, intracardiac imaging allows optimal positioning of the device at each stage of the procedure (Fig. 4–18). After the device is deployed, color flow intracardiac imaging allows evaluation for any residual shunt.

For electrophysiology procedures, ICE is used to monitor the:

❑ Trans-septal puncture
❑ Detailed evaluation of LA and pulmonary vein anatomy

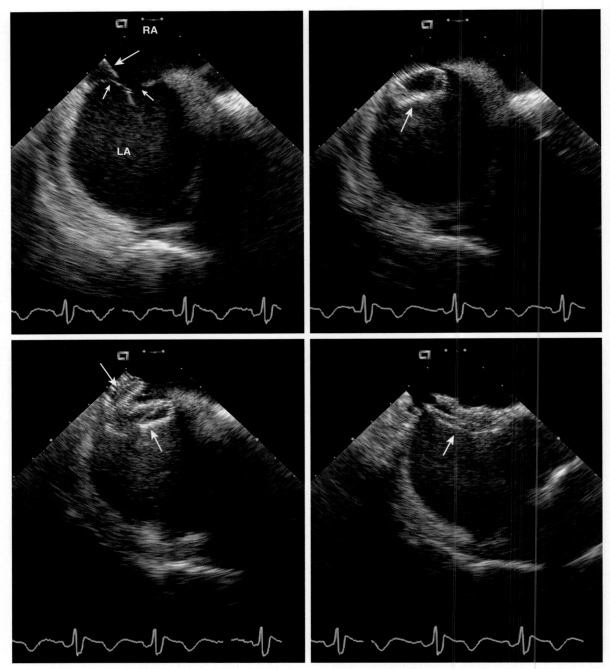

Figure 4–18 ICE guidance during placement of an Amplatzer atrial septal closure device. The catheter is guided across the atrial septal defect (*top left*), and the LA side of the device is deployed first (*top right*), followed by deployment of the RA side of the device (*bottom left*). When the device is correctly positioned, the guiding catheter is detached with flattening the two sides of the device to close the atrial septal defect (*bottom right*). *(Images courtesy of Steve Goldberg, MD.)*

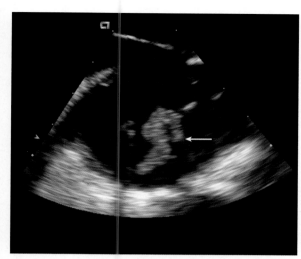

Figure 4–19 ICE allowed the rapid recognition of thrombus associated with a catheter in the RA during an electrophysiologic procedure. The patient was promptly treated with increased anticoagulation and catheter removal of the thrombus with no clinical complications. *(Image courtesy of Robert Rho, MD.)*

□ Placement of the radiofrequency ablation probe with optimal probe-tissue contact
□ Development of spontaneous contrast during the ablation
□ Detection of any complications of the procedure

The trans-septal catheter produces "tenting" of the atrial septum when correctly positioned, improving the safety of this procedure. Potential complications that can be detected immediately with ICE include intracardiac thrombus formation (Fig. 4–19), pericardial effusion, and pulmonary vein obstruction.

Limitations and Safety

The major limitations of ICE are cost and the risks of an invasive procedure. However, because most patients undergo ICE as part of an invasive therapeutic procedure, there is little additional risk. The current cost of the disposable catheter is substantial, which limits use of this technology for diagnostic purposes. The single-plane probe design is adequate, but a biplane or multiplane probe would improve image acquisition.

INTRAVASCULAR ULTRASOUND

Instrumentation and Technique

Intravascular ultrasound (IVUS) utilizes a 30- to 50-MHz transducer on a steerable catheter that is positioned within the coronary arteries during interventional coronary procedures. This transducer provides an image depth of 2 to 3 cm with high resolution of the vessel wall and atherosclerotic plaques (Fig. 4–20). Catheter positioning and image acquisition are performed by the interventional cardiologist as part of the therapeutic procedure. Image acquisition typically is performed with a small dedicated ultrasound system.

Applications

Intravascular ultrasound is used when standard angiographic and pressure data are inadequate to evaluate the

□ Length and severity of coronary artery narrowing
□ Composition of the atherosclerotic plaque

These data then are used to guide the therapeutic approach by the interventional cardiologist.

HAND-HELD ECHOCARDIOGRAPHY

Instrumentation

The term *hand-held echocardiography* refers to the bedside use of small lightweight ultrasound systems. Some of these systems are very small ("pocket-size") and have only limited capabilities, whereas others have nearly all the features of a standard ultrasound system and are still easily carried in one hand (Fig. 4–21).

Applications

These ultrasound systems are useful for rapid triage of patients in the emergency department and intensive care unit as they allow evaluation for

□ Pericardial effusion
□ Overall LV and RV systolic function
□ Segmental wall motion abnormalities

In addition, they may identify valve abnormalities such as aortic valve calcification on 2D imaging or mitral regurgitation on color flow imaging. However, in general, evaluation of valve disease, diastolic function, suspected aortic dissection, and congenital heart disease requires a full echocardiographic examination with a standard ultrasound system. An example of the utility of hand-held ultrasound includes the patient with chest pain and a nondiagnostic ECG; an akinetic anterior wall indicates coronary disease, whereas a pericardial effusion suggests pericarditis. Another example is the hypotensive patient; severe global LV hypokinesis indicates heart failure, while

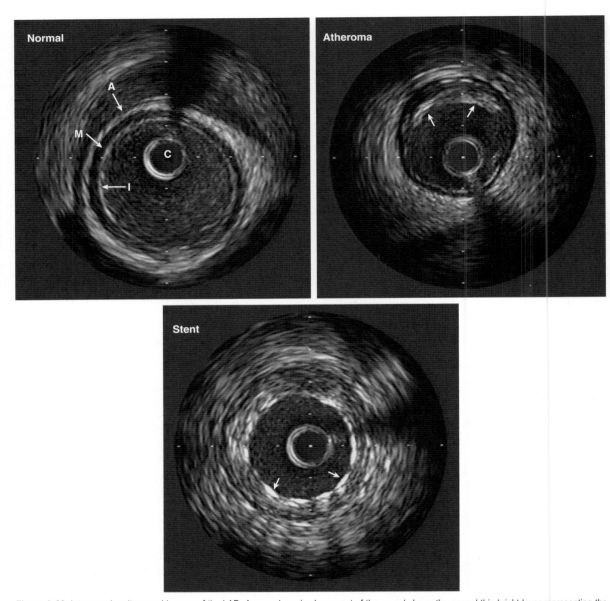

Figure 4–20 Intravascular ultrasound images of the LAD. A normal proximal segment of the vessel shows the normal thin bright layer representing the intima (I), the darker region corresponding to the media (M), and the adventia (A) surrounding the artery wall. In a more distal segment of the vessel (note the smaller vessel diameter) an atheroma is present, with the typical eccentric crescent-shaped lesions extending from 10 o'clock to 2 o'clock (*arrows*) in the artery. A region with a stent shows the close apposition between the stent (*arrows*) and vessel wall.

a small hyperdynamic LV suggests an alternate diagnosis, such as septic shock.

Limitations

Accurate use of these imaging devices requires appropriate training and experience in cardiac ultrasound. The greatest limitation of these instruments is a missed diagnosis due to an inexperienced operator or suboptimal image quality. Whenever hand-held images suggest a new cardiac diagnosis or when diagnostic images cannot be obtained, a complete echocardiographic examination is needed. Most hand-held systems provide only limited or no recording capacity, so the only record is the physician's notes describing the images, similar to reporting of physical examination findings.

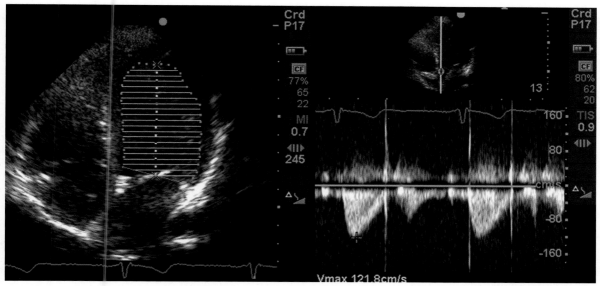

Figure 4–21 A hand-held echocardiography system was used to acquire an apical four-chamber view for calculation of EF (*left*). Continuous-wave Doppler ultrasound from an apical approach was used to measure aortic velocity (*right*).

SUGGESTED READING

3D Echocardiography

1. Picard MH: Three-dimensional echocardiography. In Otto CM (ed): The Practice of Clinical Echocardiography, 3rd ed. Philadelphia: Elsevier/Saunders, 2007, pp 86–114.
   Detailed review of the modes of 3D image acquisition, display, and quantitative analysis of 3D data. Summary of current clinical applications. 164 references.

2. Mor-Avi V, Sugeng L, Lang RM: Real-time 3-dimensional echocardiography: An integral component of the routine echocardiographic examination in adult patients? Circulation 119:314–329, 2009.
   State-of-the-art review of real-time 3D Echocardiography (RT3DE) with discussion of quantification of LV and RV volumes and ejection fraction, contrast-enhanced RT3DE, and evaluation of valvular heart disease. 115 references.

3. Hung J, Lang R, Flachskampf F, et al: 3D echocardiography: a review of the current status and future directions. J Am Soc Echocardiogr 20:213–233, 2007.
   Position paper from the American Society of Echocardiography summarizing methodology of reconstructed and real-time 3D gray-scale and color images. Detailed tables list studies on accuracy and reproducibility of 3D left and right ventricular volumes and ejection fraction.

4. Tsukiji M, Watanabe N, Yamaura Y, et al: Three-dimensional quantitation of mitral valve coaptation by a novel software system with transthoracic real-time three-dimensional echocardiography. J Am Soc Echocardiogr 21:43–46, 2008.
   Reconstruction of the mitral leaflets using custom software with real-time 3D imaging allows assessment of the mechanism of regurgitation. The degree of leaflet tenting at the onset and at maximal mitral valve closure allows calculation of coaptation area, which is reduced in patients with dilated cardiomyopathy compared with normal subjects.

5. Matsumura Y, Fukuda S, Tran H, et al: Geometry of the proximal isovelocity surface area in mitral regurgitation by 3-dimensional color Doppler echocardiography: Difference between functional mitral regurgitation and prolapse regurgitation. Am Heart J 155:231–238, 2008.
   Real-time 3D color Doppler demonstrated that the shape of the proximal isovelocity surface area (PISA) is flattened, with a longer horizontal length and shorter radius, in patients with functional mitral regurgitation, leading to underestimation of regurgitant severity by about 24%.

Myocardial Strain Rate, Strain, and Dyssynchrony

6. Smiseth OA, Edvardsen T: Tissue Doppler and speckle tracing echocardiography. In Otto CM (ed): The Practice of Clinical Echocardiography, 3rd ed. Philadelphia: Elsevier/Saunders, 2007, pp 115–137.
   Detailed explanations of the principles of tissue Doppler echocardiography and the physiology of ventricular contraction. The clinical applications of strain rate and strain imaging in myocardial ischemia and diastolic dysfunction are reviewed. Approaches to measurement of ventricular dyssynchrony are summarized and illustrated. 148 references.

7. Marwick TH: Measurement of strain and strain rate by echocardiography: Ready for prime time? J Am Coll Cardiol 47:1313–1327, 2006.
   A very understandable, but sophisticated, explanation of strain rate and strain with nice illustrations. The technical aspects of data recording, potential pitfalls, and artifacts are discussed in detail. Highly recommended for tips on how to acquire diagnostic data.

8. Gorcsan J, Abraham T, Agler DA, et al: American Society of Echocardiography Dyssynchrony Writing Group: Echocardiography for cardiac resynchronization therapy: Recommendations for performance and reporting—a report from the American Society of Echocardiography Dyssynchrony Writing Group endorsed by the Heart Rhythm Society. J Am Soc Echocardiogr 21:191–213, 2008.
   This consensus document reviews echocardiographic approaches and makes specific recommendations for Doppler optimization of the atrioventricular delay after cardiac resynchronization therapy (CRT). Approaches to

evaluation of ventricular dyssynchrony are reviewed in detail, with recommendations on the cutoff values and best approaches for clinical use. However, based on the literature thus far, the Writing Group does not recommend that CRT therapy be withheld based on an echocardiographic dyssynchrony study in patients who meet standard criteria for CRT, and dyssynchrony reporting should not include therapeutic recommendations. 92 references.

9. Abraham TP, Dimaano VL, Liang HY: Role of tissue Doppler and strain echocardiography in current clinical practice. Circulation 116:2597–2609, 2007.

   Review focused on the clinical applications on strain analysis in evaluation of global and regional ventricular function, cardiomyopathies, dyssynchrony analysis, and diastolic function. Newer approaches to evaluation of RV and RA function are also discussed. An excellent section on "cautions" reviews acquisition and data analysis issues that affect diagnostic utility.

10. Perk G, Tunick P, Kronzon I: Non-Doppler two-dimensional strain imaging by echocardiography: From technical consideration to clinical applications. J Am Soc Echocardiogr 20:234–243, 2007.

    Concepts of strain rate and strain are discussed, followed by the general principles of non-Doppler 2D strain imaging (speckle tracking). Details of the technique for acquisition and analysis of speckle tracking data are included, along with a summary of the validation studies for this approach.

11. Mullens W, Tang WH, Grimm RA: Using echocardiography in cardiac resynchronization therapy. Am Heart J 154:1011–1020, 2007.

    This article provides a detailed review of all the approaches to evaluation of dyssynchrony including details of data acquisition and analysis and clinical implications. There are several clear illustrations that demonstrate details of the measurements. There also is a concise summary of the clinical trials thus far using dyssynchrony measures. 42 references.

12. Kass DA: An epidemic of dyssynchrony: But what does it mean? J Am Coll Cardiol 51:12–17, 2008.

    A viewpoint and commentary on the clinical significance of dyssynchrony, what the measurements mean, and approaches to therapy.

13. Anderson LJ, Miyazaki C, Sutherland GR, et al: Patient selection and echocardiographic assessment of dyssynchrony in cardiac resynchronization therapy. Circulation 117:2009–2023, 2008.

    A review of echocardiographic approaches to resynchronization therapy with extensive tables summarizing the literature and clear illustrations of the methodology. The authors currently do not recommend routine use of echocardiographic dyssynchrony measurements in selection of patients for CRT. As a research tool, dyssynchrony measures may provide further insight into the mechanism of benefit with biventricular pacing for heart failure.

Contrast Echocardiography

14. Porter TR, Xie F: Myocardial contrast echocardiography: Methods, analysis, and applications. In Otto CM (ed): The Practice of Clinical Echocardiography, 3rd ed. Philadelphia: Elsevier/Saunders, 2007, pp 62–85.

    Review of the methods for performing and analyzing contrast echocardiography plus a review of the current and potential clinical applications of this technique. 164 references.

15. Stewart MJ: Contrast echocardiography. Heart 89:342–348, 2003.

    Review of the principles of contrast echocardiography, indications for right heart contrast, LV opacification, and myocardial perfusion imaging. 20 annotated references. Clear illustrations.

16. Bhatia VK, Senior R: Contrast echocardiography: Evidence for clinical use. J Am Soc Echocardiogr 21:409–416, 2008.

    This review article (supported by Bristol-Myers Squibb Medical Imaging) summarizes the characteristics of the ideal contrast agent, current clinical applications, clinical safety, and technical issues is the use of contrast echocardiography. The accuracy of myocardial contrast echocardiography for diagnosis of coronary in stable patients is emphasized. Contrast agents should be avoided in the setting of an acute myocardial infarction.

17. U.S. Food and Drug Administration prescribing information for perflutren (Definity; Bristol-Myers Squibb, New York, New York) approved 10 October 2007 (http://www.fda.gov/cder/foi/label/2007/021064s007lbl.pdf) and current updates at http://www.fda.gov/cder/drug/infopage/microbubble/default.htm. Accessed 28 February 2009.

    The FDA statement on perflutren ultrasound contrast agents is provided on their official web site and will be updated if there are any changes from the current drug labeling.

18. Main ML, Goldman JH, Grayburn PA: Thinking outside the "box"—the ultrasound contrast controversy. J Am Coll Cardiol 50:2434–2437, 2007.

    A contrasting point of view on the safety of ultrasound contrast with a concise summary of the literature and key references.

19. Mulvagh SL, Rakowski H, Vannan MA, et al: American Society of Echocardiography Consensus Statement on the Clinical Applications of Ultrasonic Contrast Agents in Echocardiography. J Am Soc Echocardiogr 21:1179–1220, 2008.

    These guidelines recommend ultrasonic contrast agents to improve evaluation of LV regional and global function when image quality is suboptimal, particularly during stress testing; to better define LV structural abnormalities, including apical thrombus, ventricular noncompaction and apical hypertrophic cardiomyopathy; and for diagnosis of complications of acute myocardial infarction including aneurysm, pseudo-aneurysm, and myocardial rupture.

Intracardiac Echocardiography

20. Bartel T, Müller S, Konorza T, et al: Intracardiac echocardiography. In Otto CM (ed): The Practice of Clinical Echocardiography, 3rd ed. Philadelphia: Elsevier/Saunders, 2007, pp 138–151.

    This chapter reviews the instrument and imaging approach to ICE. The use of ICE in monitoring procedures is described and illustrated, including atrial septal defect and patent foramen ovale closure, LA appendage closure, radiofrequency pulmonary vein ablation, myocardial septal ablation, percutaneous mitral valve procedures, and perioperative imaging of the aortic valve and aorta.

21. Mullen MJ, Dias BF, Walker F, et al: Intracardiac echocardiography guided device closure of atrial septal defects. J Am Coll Cardiol 41:285–292, 2003.

    Both ICE and TEE were performed in 24 patients undergoing percutaneous atrial septal defect closure. ICE was feasible and provided all the needed images in 96% of cases.

22. Bartel T, Konorza T, Arjumand J, et al: Intracardiac echocardiography is superior to conventional monitoring for guiding device closure of interatrial communications. Circulation 107:795–797, 2003.

    In a randomized study of TEE versus ICE in 44 patients undergoing percutaneous atrial septal defect or patent foramen ovale closure, there were no complications in either group. However, fluoroscopy and procedure time were shorter and general anesthesia was not needed in the ICE ultrasound group.

Intravascular Echocardiography

23. Weissman NJ, Mintz GS: Intravascular ultrasound: Principles and clinical applications. In Otto CM (ed): The Practice of Clinical Echocardiography, 3rd ed. Philadelphia: Elsevier/Saunders, 2007, pp 152–171.

    Review of the special characteristics of intravascular ultrasound (IVUS) imaging, catheter design, and clinical implications of IVUS images for patient management.

Hand-held Echocardiography

24. Goldman ME, Croft LB: Hand-carried ultrasound. In Otto CM (ed): The Practice of Clinical Echocardiography, 3rd ed. Philadelphia: Elsevier-Saunders, 2007, pp 172–184.

    This chapter reviews the concept of the "echo stethoscope" for bedside examination and the use of hand-held echo by noncardiologists and in screening populations for heart disease.

25. Seward JB, Douglas PS, Erbel R, et al: Hand-carried cardiac ultrasound (HCU) device: recommendations regarding new technology. A report from the Echocardiography Task Force on New Technology of the Nomenclature and Standards Committee of the American Society of Echocardiography. J Am Soc Echocardiogr 15:369–373, 2002.

    The ASE recommends that hand-held ultrasound as an extension of the physical examination should be performed only by health professionals with at least level 1 training (see Chapter 5) in echocardiography.

Clinical Indications and Quality Assurance

APPROACH TO THE DIAGNOSTIC USE OF ECHOCARDIOGRAPHY

Reliability of a Diagnostic Test

The reliability of a diagnostic test includes two components: accuracy and precision. Accuracy is the ability of the test to make a correct numerical measurement—for example, left ventricular (LV) volume—or to correctly diagnose the presence or absence of a condition (for example, coronary artery disease, CAD). Precision reflects the agreement of repeated evaluations, including acquisition, measurement, and interpretation of data. The combination of accuracy and precision determines the value of echocardiography in different clinical situations.

Accuracy

The accuracy of a numerical measurement, such as wall thickness, aortic jet velocity, or aortic diameter, is expressed as the agreement between the echocardiographic measurement and a reference standard. These measurements reflect continuous variables; there is a continuous range of values from the smallest to largest seen in clinical practice. For example, aortic jet velocity ranges from <1 m/s to as high as 6 m/s. The numerical reference standard may be an anatomic measurement at surgery or autopsy, direct measurements in an experimental model, or comparison of echocardiography to other imaging techniques or hemodynamic recordings. Published data on accuracy of echocardiographic data is shown in tables in each chapter of this book and typically is expressed by a correlation coefficient and regression equation with standard errors. Alternatively, an approach called Bland-Altman analysis is used that compares the deviation of each measurement (echocardiography and the reference standard) from the mean of both measurements.

For echocardiographic diagnosis that are either present or absent (called categorical variables), accuracy reflects the certainty with which a specific diagnosis can be confirmed or excluded based on the test results (Fig. 5–1). An example is echocardiography for the diagnosis of endocarditis: the patient either has or does not have endocarditis, there is no

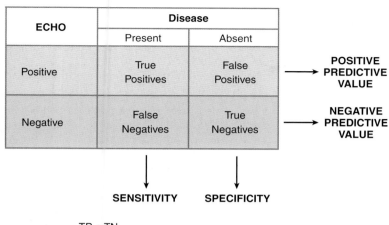

ECHO	Disease	
	Present	Absent
Positive	True Positives	False Positives
Negative	False Negatives	True Negatives

→ POSITIVE PREDICTIVE VALUE

→ NEGATIVE PREDICTIVE VALUE

SENSITIVITY   SPECIFICITY

$$\text{ACCURACY} = \frac{\text{TP} + \text{TN}}{\text{All Tests}}$$

Figure 5–1 Sensitivity and specificity in comparison with positive and negative predictive value. Note that predictive values are dependent on the prevalence of the disease in the study population and thus cannot be extrapolated to other patient groups TN, true negative; TP, true positive.

range of values. Accuracy for this type of test is described in terms of sensitivity and specificity. The sensitivity of a test is the degree to which it identifies all patients with the disease (i.e., true positives [TP] plus false negatives [FN]); specificity is the degree to which a test identifies all patients without the disease (i.e., true negatives [TN] plus false positives [FP]).

❏ Sensitivity = "true-positive" tests/all patients with the disease
= TP/(TP + FN)
❏ Specificity = "true-negative" tests/all patients without the disease
= TN/(TN + FP)

Accuracy indicates the percentage of patients in whom the test results are correct in identifying the presence or absence of disease.

❏ Accuracy = true positives plus true negatives/total number of tests
= (TP + TN)/all tests

Using a diagnostic test to determine if a disease is present or absent depends on the "cutoff" value or breakpoint used to define the test as abnormal. Sensitivity and specificity are related inversely to each other; in general, the higher the sensitivity, the lower the specificity, and vice versa. Whether a higher sensitivity is preferable to a higher specificity depends on the clinical question. If the goal of the test is identification of all patients with the disease, a high sensitivity is preferable. If the goal is confirmation of the diagnosis in an individual patient, a high specificity is preferable.

The relationship between sensitivity and specificity can be evaluated quantitatively for any given diagnostic test by graphing the sensitivity (y axis) versus 1 – specificity (x axis), with each point on the curve representing a different breakpoint defining the test as abnormal. The area under the curve reflects the

clinical value of the test, with a larger area indicating a more reliable diagnostic test. The point on the receiver-operator curve, where sensitivity and specificity are maximized indicates an appropriate breakpoint (Fig. 5–2).

Precision

The reproducibility of echocardiographic imaging and Doppler data is affected by variability in:

❏ Recording
❏ Measurement
❏ Interpretation

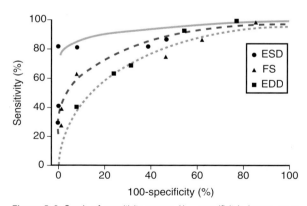

Figure 5–2 Graph of sensitivity versus (1 – specificity), known as a receiver-operator curve. LV contractility was determined in a series of patients with chronic severe mitral regurgitation by measurement of elastance (E_{max}). The clinical value of echocardiographic LV EDD, ESD, and fractional shortening (FS) for identification of impaired contractility is shown using receiver-operator curves. An LV ESD of 40 mm had the best sensitivity (82%) and specificity (100%) for prediction of impaired contractility, defined by reduced elastance. *(From Flemming MA, Oral H, Rothman ED, et al: Echocardiographic markers for mitral valve surgery to preserve left ventricular performance in mitral regurgitation. Am Heart J 140:476–482, 2000.)*

In addition, variability can occur both when the same person repeats the data acquisition or measurement at a different time (intraobserver variability) and when data acquisition or measurement is performed by different people (interobserver variability). These sources of imprecision are a major limitation of echocardiography in clinical practice. There are several approaches to improving precision, and thus reliability, of echocardiographic data. Appropriate training and experience help ensure correct acquisition of data, including correctly aligned image planes and Doppler recordings, optimization of instrument parameters, and standardized study protocols. Measurement precision is improved with adherence to published standards, quality control in each laboratory, and comparison with reference standards when possible. Interpretation variability is minimized by using standard terminology and diagnostic criteria, developing a consensus approach to reporting in each laboratory, and comparing images and Doppler data to previous recordings in that patient whenever possible; that is, the report should specify whether there is a change from previous studies based on direct comparison of the recorded data, with side-by-side measurements as needed. Measurement variability is reported in each chapter when this information is available.

Expertise

The quality of an echocardiographic examination is highly dependent on the expertise of the sonographer performing the study, the physician interpreting the data, and the expertise of the laboratory. Optimal acquisition of image and Doppler data require experience, in addition to education and training. Physician interpretation is affected both by the data acquired (e.g., if images of a ventricular thrombus are not recorded, the physician will not see it) and by the education, training, and experience of the physician. Laboratory expertise affects data quality in terms of study protocols, time allocation and efficiency, instrumentation, and the group expertise of the sonographers and physicians. Thus, echocardiographic studies performed in different laboratories are not always comparable, and published studies on the accuracy of echocardiographic diagnosis may not apply to all diagnostic examinations.

Integration of Clinical Data and Test Results

Predictive Value

A major limitation of applying sensitivity/specificity data to an individual patient is the problem of whether a particular patient has a "true" or a "false" test result. Predictive values indicate the percentage of patients with a positive test result who have the suspected disease and the percentage with a negative test result that do not have the suspected disease.

❑ Positive predictive value = true positives divided by all positives
❑ Negative predictive value = true negatives divided by all negatives

However, predictive values are determined by the prevalence of disease in the population studied as well as by the sensitivity and specificity of the test. Intuitively, this is obvious comparing the use of echocardiography to "screen" healthy young subjects for endocarditis (many false-positive results due to ultrasound imaging artifacts) versus the same test in patients who have a new murmur, fever, and positive blood cultures, with a high prevalence of disease. The finding of valvular vegetation on echocardiography in the latter group has a much higher predictive value for a diagnosis of endocarditis than in the healthy subjects, even though the sensitivity and specificity of echocardiography for diagnosing endocarditis are the same in both groups. Thus, the positive or negative predictive value of a test reflects disease prevalence as well as test accuracy.

Likelihood Ratio

The likelihood ratio indicates the relative likelihood of disease in an individual patient, based on a positive or negative test result. The likelihood ratio for a positive test result is calculated as:

$$+\text{Likelihood ratio} = \text{Sensitivity}/(1 - \text{specificity})$$

or

$$+\text{Likelihood ratio} = \frac{\text{true-positive rate}}{\text{false-positive rate}}$$

A positive likelihood ratio >10 indicates an excellent test, and 5–10 indicates a good test.

The likelihood ratio for a negative test result is calculated as:

$$-\text{Likelihood ratio} = (1 - \text{sensitivity})/\text{Specificity}$$

or

$$-\text{Likelihood ratio} = \frac{\text{false-negative rate}}{\text{true-negative rate}}$$

A negative likelihood ratio <0.1 indicates an excellent test, and a ratio of 0.1 to 0.2 indicates a reasonably good test.

For example, diagnosis of LV thrombus by echocardiography, assuming a sensitivity of 95% and a specificity of 88%, has a positive likelihood of 7.9 (a good diagnostic test) and a negative likelihood ratio of 0.06 (an excellent diagnostic test). The positive likelihood is not excellent, because ultrasound artifacts may be mistaken for a ventricular thrombus.

The excellent negative likelihood depends on a high-quality echocardiographic study and the expertise of the sonographer to ensure that an apical thrombus is not missed by echocardiographic imaging.

Pre- and Post-test Probability

Another approach to the use of sensitivity/specificity data in patient management is to consider relevant clinical data along with the test result. The value of a diagnostic test increases when the pre-test likelihood of disease is integrated with the test results to derive a post-test likelihood of disease. This approach is known as Bayesian analysis. For example, the pre-test likelihood of severe aortic stenosis in an asymptomatic 30-year-old woman with no systolic murmur on careful auscultation is very low. An echocardiogram purporting to show severe aortic stenosis most likely is an erroneous interpretation (a false-positive test result). In this setting, the result does not increase the post-test likelihood of disease very much. In contrast, in an elderly man with a 4/6 aortic stenosis murmur and symptoms of angina, syncope, and heart failure, the diagnosis of severe valvular aortic stenosis can be made with a high level of certainty even before any test is performed. The echocardiogram serves only to confirm the diagnosis and define the severity of obstruction. In general, diagnostic tests are most helpful when the pre-test likelihood of disease is intermediate so that the test result will substantially change the post-test likelihood of disease (Fig. 5–3).

The most comprehensive approach to evaluation of a diagnostic test is clinical decision analysis. Clinical decision analysis incorporates several rigorous approaches to the problem of clinical prediction, with the method most applicable to a diagnostic test, such as echocardiography, being the threshold approach. The basic tenet of clinical decision analysis as applied to a diagnostic test is that the test results should have an impact on patient care by either

❑ prompting a change in therapy or
❑ leading to a change in the subsequent diagnostic strategy in that patient.

This basic assumption is formalized in the threshold model of decision analysis. In this approach two disease probability thresholds are defined for the diagnostic test:

❑ A lower threshold below which the risk of the test is greater than the risk of not treating the patient
❑ An upper threshold above which treating the patient is a lower risk than performing the test

The intermediate range—where the risk of treating or not treating the patient is greater than the risk of the diagnostic test—is known as the test zone (Fig. 5–4). For any specific indication the test zone for echocardiography generally is wide because of the low risk and high accuracy of this technique. However, both an upper and lower threshold still are definable for echocardiography. The upper threshold is reached in situations in which the diagnosis is clear, and echocardiographic examination would only delay appropriate treatment. For example, a patient with a classic presentation of an ascending aortic dissection (chest pain, wide mediastinum, peripheral pulse loss) requires prompt surgery. Any delay due to unnecessary diagnostic testing could result in additional morbidity or mortality.

It is tempting to assume that there is no lower end to the test zone for echocardiography given the absence of known adverse biologic effects of this procedure. However, the risk of the test also includes the risks of additional diagnostic tests or even erroneous treatment choices resulting from a false-positive or false-negative echocardiographic finding. For example, an echocardiogram is not indicated to evaluate for aortic dissection

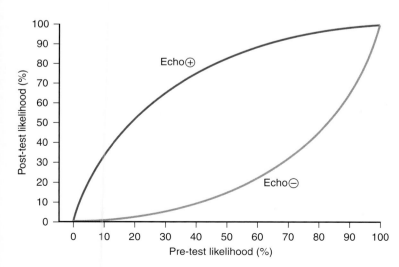

Figure 5–3 Bayesian analysis of the pre-test and post-test likelihood of CAD when the exercise echocardiogram shows inducible ischemia (+Echo) or is normal (−Echo). These curves were generated based on a sensitivity of 85% and a specificity of 82% of exercise echocardiography for diagnosis of significant (>70% luminal narrowing) coronary artery disease. In clinical practice the pre-test likelihood is based on the patient's clinical history, age, and gender. The post-test likelihood then depends on the result of the exercise echocardiogram. For example, if the pre-test likelihood is 50%, an exercise echocardiogram showing inducible ischemia indicates an 83% likelihood of coronary disease, whereas a negative test indicates only a 15% likelihood of coronary disease.

Threshold Approach to Clinical Decision Making

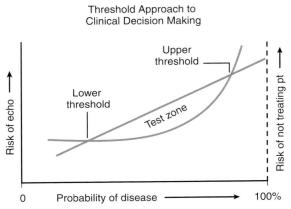

Figure 5–4 Diagram illustrating the threshold approach to clinical decision making. The risk of the diagnostic test—in this case, echocardiography—is shown in the blue line (left y axis) with the risk of not treating the patient for the suspected disease shown in the gray line (right y axis). The probability of disease based on the clinical presentation is shown from 0 to 100% on the x axis. The lower threshold is the point at which the risk of echocardiography is lower than the risk of not treating the patient. The upper threshold is the point at which the risk of echocardiography (including false-negative results, delay in treatment) is greater than the risk of treating the patient. The test zone is the pre-test likelihood of disease between these two thresholds.

in a young patient with atypical chest pain and a normal physical examination, electrocardiogram (ECG), and chest roentgenogram. If a false-positive echocardiographic diagnosis leads to further evaluation with cardiac catheterization, any complications from the invasive procedure ultimately can be considered a consequence of the echocardiographic results. Thus, a lower limit to the test zone does exist for echocardiography and can be defined for each specific diagnostic indication by applying decision analysis techniques. Other clinical decision analysis approaches have been applied to specific clinical problems that use echocardiographic data as a branch point in the decision analysis tree.

Cost-Effectiveness

An additional consideration in medical practice is the cost-effectiveness of a diagnostic procedure. Note that this term includes not only the cost of the test (echocardiography compares favorably with other cardiac diagnostic tests) but also the effectiveness of the test—that is, test accuracy and its impact on patient management. This type of analysis has been applied to some echocardiographic diagnostic issues, but more widespread use of this approach is needed.

Clinical Outcomes

The most important measure of the value of a diagnostic test is its impact on subsequent clinical outcome (Fig. 5–5). While the first step in evaluation of the clinical utility of a test includes various measures of diagnostic accuracy in comparison to some accepted standard, the more important assessment is whether the diagnostic test changes the subsequent diagnostic or therapeutic plan in each patient. Finally, the clinical utility of the test depends on its ability to predict prognosis; for example, survival in patients with dilated cardiomyopathy, timing of valve surgery in patients with chronic regurgitation, or the rate of hemodynamic progression in patients with valvular stenosis. Echocardiographic data are increasingly used in clinical outcome studies, as referenced in the Suggested Readings throughout this textbook.

Indications and Appropriateness Criteria

The indications for echocardiography are based on the reliability of this approach for diagnosis in a wide range of cardiovascular disease and are summarized in consensus guidelines developed by the American Heart Association and American College of Cardiology. In

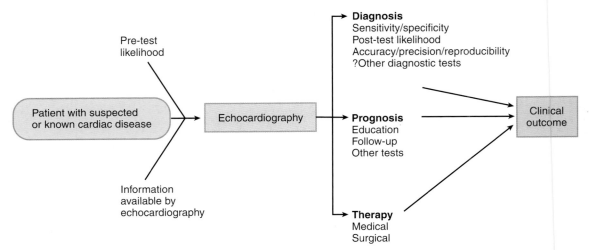

Figure 5–5 Flow chart illustrating the importance of the impact of the echocardiographic results on diagnosis, prognosis, and therapy. Ultimately, the effect of the echocardiographic examination on clinical outcome is the best measure of the usefulness of the test result.

addition, specific recommendations on the use of echocardiography often are included in disease-specific guidelines, for example, guidelines for management of valvular heart disease and for heart failure.

Appropriateness criteria go beyond indications to consider the clinical setting in which a diagnostic test is appropriate. For example, exercise echocardiography is sensitive and specific for diagnosis of coronary artery disease (CAD) but should not be used as a routine screening test in all patients. Appropriateness criteria have been developed by the American College of Cardiology in collaboration with other organizations that provide helpful guidance. However, these guidelines do not include all possible clinical situations, since only a relatively short list of possible indications was considered.

Ideally, the echocardiogram request should indicate an appropriate clinical question (not "evaluate heart") and, when possible, an estimate of the probability of the diagnosis in that patient. Next, the reliability of echocardiography for that diagnosis and the likelihood that the echocardiographic results will alter patient management are considered prior to performing the study. Often it is helpful to consider the specific branch point in the diagnostic/therapeutic plans that the echocardiographic results will be applied to in the clinical decision process.

With these considerations in mind, there are certain situations in which the use of echocardiography clearly changes patient management:

❐ Making the correct anatomic diagnosis. For example, differentiating a primary valvular problem from systolic LV dysfunction in a patient with heart failure symptoms.
❐ Providing important prognostic data in a patient with a known anatomic diagnosis. For example, stenosis severity in valve disease or LV ejection fraction in cardiomyopathy.
❐ Identifying complications of a known diagnosis— for example, paravalvular abscess in endocarditis or LV thrombus in cardiomyopathy.

In addition, there are numerous other settings in which echocardiography is considered to be clinically appropriate.

Throughout this text the accuracy (sensitivity and specificity) of echocardiography for each specific diagnosis will be indicated, if known. The clinician then should integrate these data with the pre-test likelihood of disease in each patient. Critical evaluations of the diagnostic utility of echocardiography in specific patient populations and clinical settings will be highlighted, including evaluation of chest pain in the emergency room (Chapter 8), decision making in adults with aortic stenosis (Chapter 11) and aortic regurgitation (Chapter 12), the diagnosis and prognosis of endocarditis (Chapter 14), and intraoperative assessment of mitral valve repair (Chapter 18).

TRANSTHORACIC ECHOCARDIOGRAPHY

Appropriate Indications

By Clinical Signs and Symptoms

An echocardiogram often is requested to evaluate a specific clinical sign or symptom such as chest pain, heart failure symptoms (Fig. 5–6), a murmur, or cardiomegaly on chest radiography (Fig. 5–7). When the echocardiographer evaluates a patient with one of these indications, it is important that the differential diagnosis be considered and each possibility excluded or confirmed during the course of the examination. For example, a patient with a systolic murmur may have valvular aortic stenosis, a subaortic membrane, hypertrophic cardiomyopathy, mitral regurgitation, a ventricular septal defect, pulmonic stenosis, or tricuspid regurgitation. With two-dimensional (2D) imaging and Doppler evaluation, each of these possible diagnoses can be evaluated. If a careful examination reveals none of these abnormalities, it may be concluded that the murmur is a benign "flow" murmur (Fig. 5–8).

Similarly, in the echocardiographic examination of a patient with chest pain, even if the referring physician has made a presumptive diagnosis of CAD, the echocardiographer should be alert to any findings suggesting other causes for chest pain such as LV outflow obstruction (valvular aortic stenosis or hypertrophic cardiomyopathy), aortic dissection, or pericarditis. The echocardiographic differential diagnosis for common symptoms is shown in Table 5–1 and for common physical signs in Table 5–2. These examples are not meant to be an exhaustive list of the possibilities but rather represent an illustration of the types of conditions the echocardiographer should consider in performing and interpreting the examination.

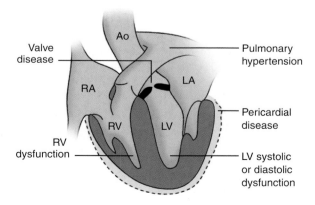

Figure 5–6 Diagram illustrating some of the more common causes of heart failure that should be actively excluded or confirmed during echocardiographic examination.

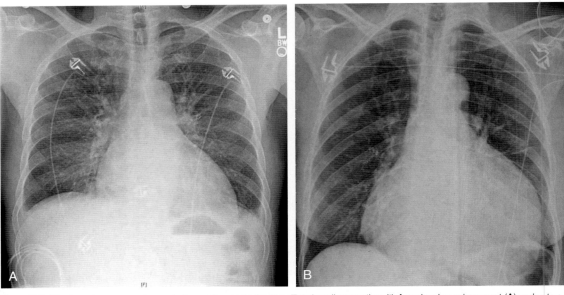

Figure 5–7 Chest roentgenograms demonstrating cardiomegaly due to a dilated cardiomyopathy with four-chamber enlargement (**A**) or due to a large pericardial effusion (**B**). Echocardiography reliably identifies the cause of an enlarged cardiac silhouette.

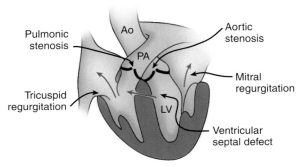

Figure 5–8 Diagram illustrating the most common etiologies for a systolic murmur. If an echocardiogram is requested for this indication, the sonographer should focus the examination toward confirmation or exclusion of each of these possibilities.

TABLE 5–1	Differential Diagnosis for the Echocardiographer: Common Symptoms
Reason for Echo	**Differential Diagnosis**
Chest pain	Coronary artery disease Aortic dissection Pericarditis Valvular aortic stenosis Hypertrophic cardiomyopathy
Heart failure	LV systolic dysfunction (global or segmental) Valvular heart disease LV diastolic dysfunction Pericardial disease RV dysfunction
Palpitations	LV systolic dysfunction Mitral valve disease Congenital heart disease (e.g., atrial septal defect, Ebstein anomaly) Pericarditis No structural cardiac disease

By Anatomic Diagnosis

In many patients referred for echocardiography, a definite or presumptive anatomic diagnosis has been made (Tables 5–3 and 5–4). In these patients the echocardiographer needs to be aware of the information that can be obtained by echocardiography, the limitations of echocardiography, and alternative diagnostic approaches.

For example, in a patient with a systolic murmur known to be due to valvular aortic stenosis, the echocardiogram may be requested to evaluate the severity of obstruction, the degree of coexisting aortic regurgitation, the presence of LV hypertrophy, and the status of LV systolic function, as well as to detect any associated valvular abnormalities (e.g., mitral regurgitation). Usually echocardiography provides all the needed information for clinical decision making other than coronary artery anatomy, but the echocardiographer must acknowledge that stenosis severity may have been underestimated if there was a nonparallel intercept angle between the direction of the aortic jet and the ultrasound beam. In cases where the echocardiographic results appear to be discordant with the clinical impression, additional diagnostic tests may be needed.

TABLE 5–2 Differential Diagnosis for the Echocardiographer: Common Signs

Reason for Echo	Differential Diagnosis
Cardiac murmur Systolic	Flow murmur (no valve abnormality) Aortic stenosis, subaortic obstruction, hypertrophic obstructive cardiomyopathy Mitral regurgitation Ventricular septal defect Pulmonic stenosis Tricuspid regurgitation
Diastolic	Mitral stenosis Aortic regurgitation Pulmonic regurgitation Tricuspid stenosis Patent ductus arteriosus (continuous murmur)
Cardiomegaly on chest radiography	Pericardial effusion Dilated cardiomyopathy Specific chamber enlargement (e.g., LV in chronic AR)
Systemic embolic event	Decreased LV systolic function LV aneurysm LV thrombus Prosthetic heart valve Atrial fibrillation LA thrombus Patent foramen ovale Intracardiac tumor

AR, aortic regurgitation.

TABLE 5–3 Appropriate Indications for Echocardiography in Patients with Valvular Heart Disease

Abnormal Cardiac Murmur

Initial diagnosis

Value Regurgitation

Suspected MV prolapse
Initial evaluation of known or suspected valvular regurgitation
Routine (yearly) re-evaluation for asymptomatic severe valvular regurgitation
Re-evaluation for a change in clinical status

Valve Stenosis

Initial evaluation of known or suspected native valvular stenosis
Routine (yearly) evaluation for asymptomatic severe valvular stenosis
Re-evaluation for a change in clinical status

Prosthetic Valves

Initial evaluation of prosthetic valve as a baseline study
Re-evaluation for suspected dysfunction, thrombosis, or a change in clinical status

Endocarditis

Initial evaluation of suspected infective endocarditis (native or prosthetic valve) with positive blood cultures or a new murmur
Re-evaluation of infective endocarditis in high-risk patients—virulent organism, severe hemodynamic lesion, aortic involvement, persistent bacteremia, a change in clinical status, or symptomatic deterioration

Abstracted from Suggested Reading 17.

Echocardiography in a patient with endocarditis is a second, more complex example. On one hand, echocardiography can detect valvular vegetations, identify the specific valves involved, evaluate the presence and degree of valve dysfunction, and measure associated chamber enlargement. Both left and right ventricular systolic function can be qualitatively and quantitatively evaluated. In addition, abscess formation may be identified. While the potential prognostic value of measuring vegetation size remains controversial, many clinicians find this information of clinical value. On the other hand, a definite diagnosis of endocarditis requires the presence of both echocardiographic and bacteriologic criteria. When echocardiographic findings are atypical, additional clinical criteria must be present to make the diagnosis. The sensitivity of echocardiography for detection of valvular vegetations varies with image quality; conversely, healed valvular vegetations may persist after a previous episode of endocarditis. Transesophageal echocardiography (TEE) is more sensitive for diagnosing valvular vegetations and should be considered if the clinical suspicion of endocarditis is moderate to high and the transthoracic (TTE) study does not show typical vegetations. TEE also is much more sensitive for the diagnosis of paravalvular abscesses and for evaluation of prosthetic valve endocarditis.

In the Echo Exam section at the end of this book, the key echocardiographic findings, limitations of echocardiography, and alternate diagnostic approaches for several anatomic diagnoses are indicated. Each of these topics is covered in detail in subsequent chapters.

By Clinical Setting

The third category of indications for echocardiography is the examination requested because the patient is a member of a clinical group in whom "routine" echocardiographic studies are thought to be clinically valuable. These examinations fall into one of four categories (see Table 5–3):

TABLE 5–4   Appropriate Indications for Echocardiography in Patients with Heart Failure, Cardiomyopathies, and Hypertensive and Pulmonary Heart Disease

Heart Failure

Initial evaluation of known or suspected heart failure (systolic or diastolic)
Re-evaluation of known heart failure (systolic or diastolic) to guide therapy
Evaluation for dyssynchrony in a patient being considered for cardiac resynchronization therapy
Patient with implanted pacing device with symptoms possibly due to suboptimal device settings
Baseline and serial re-evaluations in patients undergoing therapy with cardiotoxic agents

Cardiomyopathies

Initial evaluation of known or suspected hypertrophic cardiomyopathy
Re-evaluation of known hypertrophic cardiomyopathy in a patient with a change in clinical status
Evaluation of suspected restrictive, infiltrative, or genetic cardiomyopathy
Screening study for structure and function in first-degree relatives of patients with inherited cardiomyopathy

Hypertensive Heart Disease

Initial evaluation of suspected hypertensive heart disease

Pulmonary Heart Disease

Respiratory failure with suspected cardiac etiology
Known or suspected acute pulmonary embolism
Known or suspected pulmonary hypertension

Abstracted from Suggested Reading 17.

TABLE 5–5   Other Appropriate Indications for Echocardiography

General

Symptoms that may be due to a cardiac cause
Other testing suggesting cardiac disease (such as ECG, CXR, BNP)
Hypotension or hemodynamic instability of uncertain or suspected cardiac etiology

Ischemic Cardiac Disease

Acute chest pain with suspected myocardial ischemia in patients with nondiagnostic laboratory markers and ECG
Initial evaluation of LV function following acute MI
Suspected complication of myocardial ischemia/infarction
Re-evaluation of LV function following MI when results will guide therapy

Other

Adult congenital heart disease
Sustained or nonsustained SVT or VT
Possible cardiovascular source of embolic event
Cardiac masses (suspected tumor or thrombus)
Pericardial disease
Marfan syndrome and related inherited connective tissue disorders

BNP, brain natriuretic peptide (a serum marker for heart failure); CXR, chest radiography; ECG, electrocardiogram; MI, myocardial infarction; SVT, supraventricular tachycardia; VT, ventricular tachycardia.
Abstracted from Suggested Reading 17.

❏ Screening examinations to detect cardiac abnormalities in a group of patients with a high prevalence of disease
❏ Monitoring examinations performed as part of a therapeutic procedure
❏ Evaluation before and after a therapeutic intervention to assess the effect of the intervention and detect possible complications
❏ Baseline studies performed in patients at risk for subsequent cardiac disease or progression of preexisting cardiac disease

Screening examinations are performed in first-degree family members of patients with genetically transmitted cardiac diseases, such as Marfan syndrome or hypertrophic cardiomyopathy, to detect possible cardiac involvement in those individuals. In patients with positive blood cultures and/or a fever of unexplained etiology, an echocardiogram may be ordered to detect possible endocarditis. Similarly, in patients with cerebrovascular events that may be embolic in origin, an echocardiogram is requested to identify any potential cardiac sources of emboli (Table 5–5).

Monitoring examinations may be performed sequentially over brief or prolonged periods of time. Intraoperative monitoring of LV size and systolic function by TEE is useful in cardiac patients undergoing noncardiac surgery to optimize ventricular preload and for early identification of ischemia, thus preventing perioperative myocardial infarction. Monitoring of LV size and systolic function over many years is performed in patients with chronic valvular regurgitation to determine the optimal timing of surgical intervention. In hypertensive patients, monitoring of LV wall thickness and mass allows assessment of the effect of long-term antihypertensive therapy on end-organ damage (in this case, the LV).

Preintervention and postintervention echocardiography may be used to detect possible procedural complications (e.g., pericardial effusion after electrophysiologic catheter studies or after endomyocardial biopsy). In addition, echocardiography may be used to assess the effect of the intervention by comparing preprocedure and postprocedure studies (e.g., in patients undergoing coronary revascularization procedures, percutaneous mitral balloon commissurotomy, or surgical mitral valve repair). The effects of pharmacologic therapy on a specific endpoint of interest also may be evaluated. Examples include the changes in stroke volume with medical therapy for dilated cardiomyopathy or changes in the pattern of LV diastolic filling after beta blockade for hypertrophic cardiomyopathy.

Baseline echocardiographic studies serve as a reference point in patients with a high likelihood of subsequent cardiac dysfunction. In a patient with a prosthetic valve, a baseline study performed when the patient is asymptomatic and clinically stable provides the normal antegrade velocity across the valve in that individual; the degree of normal prosthetic valve regurgitation; the state of the LV with respect to residual dilation, hypertrophy, or systolic dysfunction; and an estimate of postoperative pulmonary artery pressure. If the patient subsequently presents with suspected valve dysfunction, a more complete and sensitive assessment is possible by comparison with the baseline study than if no previous examination were available. Another example of the value of a baseline study is assessment of LV systolic function prior to starting a potentially cardiotoxic chemotherapeutic regimen. A baseline study allows differentiation of subtle early systolic dysfunction due to chemotherapy from mild dysfunction that may be at the lower limits of the normal range.

TRANSESOPHAGEAL ECHOCARDIOGRAPHY

The indications for TEE are based on its superior image quality compared with transthoracic imaging, particularly of posterior cardiac structures. In many cases, TEE is performed after a complete transthoracic examination. However, there are some clinical situations wherein it is appropriate to begin with a TEE examination (Table 5–6). Some echocardiographers advocate the use of TEE imaging whenever transthoracic images are nondiagnostic. However, given that the threshold approach to clinical testing predicts a narrower test window as the risk of the test increases, it is appropriate to consider TEE studies somewhat more critically. The indications for a TEE study should be discussed with the referring physician on a case-by-case basis to determine if the information potentially obtainable justifies the slight but real risk of the TEE approach.

Several definite indications for TEE are apparent when the limitations of transthoracic imaging are considered. The improved sensitivity of TEE versus transthoracic for detection of paravalvular abscess in patients with endocarditis has been demonstrated convincingly (Chapter 14). TEE clearly is indicated for evaluation of prosthetic mitral valve dysfunction, since the shadows and reverberations from the prosthetic valve no longer obscure the left atrium (LA) from this approach as they do on transthoracic images (Fig. 5–9) (see also Chapter 13). Abnormalities of the posterior

TABLE 5–6	Appropriate Indications for Use of Transesophageal Echocardiography as the Initial Test

- Suspected acute aortic pathology including dissection/transsection
- Guidance of percutaneous noncoronary cardiac interventions including but not limited to septal ablation, mitral valvuloplasty, PFO/ASD closure, radiofrequency ablation
- Severe MR to determine the mechanism of regurgitation and suitability of valve repair
- Suspected prosthetic mitral valve dysfunction*
- Suspected endocarditis with a moderate or high pre-test probability (e.g., bacteremia, especially staphcylococcal bacteremia or fungemia)
- Suspected complications of endocarditis (e.g., abscess, fistula)*
- Persistent fever in patient with intracardiac device
- Evaluation of posterior structure (e.g., atrial baffles) in patients with congenital heart disease*
- Evaluation of patients with atrial fibrillation/flutter to facilitate clinical decision making with regard to anticoagulation and/or cardioversion and/or radiofrequency ablation

*Not considered in the Appropriateness Guidelines Document but generally accepted as appropriate indications for TEE as the initial approach.
ASD, atrial septal defect; MR, mitral regurgitation; MV, mitral valve; PFO, patent foramen ovale.
Abstracted from Suggested Reading 17 with modification.

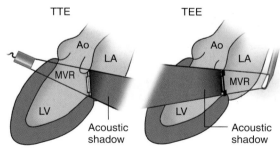

Figure 5–9 Diagram illustrating the problem of acoustic shadowing from a prosthetic MV. On the left, with transthoracic echocardiography (TTE), the acoustic shadow obscures the LA, limiting assessment of valvular incompetence by Doppler techniques. On the right, with TEE, the LA now can be evaluated for valvular incompetence. However, the acoustic shadow now obscures the left ventricular outflow tract.

aspect of a prosthetic aortic valve also will be seen well with the TEE approach, although the anterior portion of the paravalvular region will be shadowed by the posterior aspect of the prosthetic valve.

Improved evaluation of mitral valve anatomy and the degree of mitral regurgitation are especially useful in the perioperative evaluation of patients undergoing surgical mitral valve repair (Chapter 18). In patients with congenital heart disease, TEE imaging improves diagnostic certainty, particularly in evaluation of posterior structures such as an interatrial baffle surgical repair or a sinus venosus atrial septal defect. The sensitivity of TEE for detection of LA thrombus far exceeds transthoracic imaging. Finally, excellent images of the thoracic aorta, arch, and ascending aorta allow accurate diagnosis of aortic dissection by TEE. Other indications for TEE include evaluation for a patent foramen ovale in patients with a systemic embolic event, and exclusion of endocarditis when this diagnosis is a possibility.

TABLE 5–7 Appropriate Indications for Exercise or Pharmacologic Stress Echocardiography*

Low Pre-test Probability of CAD (10-Year Risk <10%) with:

Angina or equivalent and an uninterruptable ECG or inability to exercise

Intermediate (10-Year Risk 10% to 20%) to High (10-Year Risk >20%) Probability of CAD with:

Angina or equivalent
Acute chest pain without diagnostic ECG changes or elevated cardiac enzymes
New-onset heart failure
New-onset atrial fibrillation
Nonsustained ventricular tachycardia

Prior Abnormal Test Results

Abnormal catheterization or stress study with worsening symptoms on medical therapy
Coronary calcium score (Agatston) ≥400
Coronary stenosis of unclear significance by invasive or CT angiography

Risk Assessment

Before noncardiac surgery with poor exercise tolerance (<4 METs)
Following acute coronary syndrome when early catheterization not planned
Recurrent chest pain late after coronary revascularization

Other

Assessment of myocardial viability with known CAD eligible for revascularization
Evaluation of low output AS
Symptomatic patients with mild MS at rest
Asymptomatic severe AR or MR with LV size not meeting surgical criteria
Contrast is appropriate when one or more contiguous segments are not seen on noncontrast images

*The stress modality is exercise, unless the patient is unable to exercise.
AS, aortic stenosis; AR, aortic regurgitation; CAD, coronary artery disease; CT, computed tomography; ECG, electrocardiogram; MET, metabolic equivalent; MR, mitral regurgitation; MS, mitral stenosis.
These indications are abstracted from Suggested Reading 18.

STRESS ECHOCARDIOGRAPHY

In many cardiac conditions, abnormalities of cardiac function are manifested only when increased oxygen consumption results in increased cardiac demands that cannot be met by the usual compensatory changes (Table 5–7). This basic concept has led to the widespread use of stress testing in patients with cardiovascular disease. Increased cardiac demand can be induced by exercise or with appropriate pharmacologic interventions. The risk of this approach is related to the risk of stress testing with no significant additive effect of echocardiographic imaging.

Exercise echocardiography is performed by recording images of the LV immediately before and immediately after treadmill exercise testing or by recording images during supine or upright bicycle exercise. The most common indication for exercise echocardiography is suspected or known CAD. At rest, LV endocardial motion and wall thickening are normal, even if significant coronary disease is present, unless there has been prior myocardial infarction. Increased myocardial oxygen demands, such as with exercise, result in ischemia when significant stenosis of an epicardial coronary artery is present. This results sequentially in myocardial metabolic changes, decreased wall thickening and endocardial motion, electrocardiographic changes, and angina, in that order. Echocardiographic images recorded during ischemia show abnormalities of wall motion, allowing detection of significant CAD. The specific coronary arteries involved can be identified by the anatomic pattern of induced wall motion abnormalities. Exercise echocardiography, as discussed in detail in Chapter 8, has been found to be more sensitive than exercise ECG (and as sensitive as nuclear perfusion imaging) for detection of significant CAD. Exercise echocardiography is particularly helpful in patients with an abnormal resting ECG (such as bundle branch block or LV hypertrophy). It also has been used to assess the extent of disease, to document functional improvement after revascularization, and to detect restenosis after angioplasty.

In addition to changes in segmental wall motion with exercise stress testing, parameters of global ventricular function, including ventricular volumes, ejection fraction, and the Doppler LV ejection velocity curve, can be evaluated. Other Doppler parameters may be helpful in specific settings. For example, a patient with mitral stenosis will show an excessive rise in pulmonary artery systolic pressure (estimated from the tricuspid regurgitant jet) with exercise. In a patient with aortic coarctation, the increase in gradient across the coarctation with exercise can be demonstrated with Doppler recordings.

Pharmacologic stress echocardiography replaces exercise testing when the patient is unable to exercise (e.g., peripheral vascular disease, musculoskeletal limitation). In addition, pharmacologic stress testing allows monitoring by echocardiography as the dose is increased, providing data at sequential stress levels. Pharmacologic stress testing most often is performed using a beta-agonist such as dobutamine, which increases myocardial contractility, myocardial oxygen demands, and the degree of peripheral vasodilation. An alternate pharmacologic agent is adenosine, which vasodilates coronary vessels, resulting in relative inequalities in blood flow between myocardium supplied by normal versus stenosed coronary arteries.

OTHER MODALITIES

Contrast Echocardiography

Contrast studies with agitated saline to opacify the right heart are performed to document an atrial septal defect (Chapter 17), patent foramen ovale (Chapter 15) or persistent left superior vena cava (Chapter 15) (Table 5–8). Commercially available contrast agents provide smaller microbubbles (4 to 10 μm in diameter) that are injected intravenously but traverse the pulmonary capillary bed. These microbubbles provide opacification of the LV chamber, which enhances endocardial definition for evaluation of global and regional ventricular function. Contrast enhancement is indicated on both resting and stress echocardiographic studies when image quality is suboptimal and evaluation of ventricular function is needed. Radiocontrast agents can be injected directly into a coronary artery to define the area perfused by that vessel, for example, at the time of percutaneous septal ablation for hypertrophic cardiomyopathy.

Three-dimensional Echocardiography

Three-dimensional (3D) echocardiographic techniques are likely to become more widely used as the technology becomes easier to use and is integrated into standard ultrasound systems. Voxel reconstructions are most useful for demonstrating complex intracardiac 3D relationships, particularly in cases of valvular and congenital heart disease. Disadvantages of gray-scale voxel reconstructions are that the data are only qualitative and optimal display is dependent on the operator's choice of image plane, thus requiring considerable experience both with the 3D technique and with the anatomy of complex cardiac abnormalities.

Three-dimensional reconstructions based on tracing intracardiac borders allow highly accurate measurements of ventricular volumes and systolic function, as discussed in Chapter 6. This approach will become more widely used in the clinical setting as more reliable methods for automatic edge detection become available.

Hand-held Ultrasound

Small, relatively inexpensive, portable or "hand-held" echocardiography instruments are of great clinical utility in the emergency department, coronary care unit, and cardiology clinic for triage of acutely ill patients. Indications for hand-held ultrasound are still evolving, but these instruments appear to be most useful for evaluation of overall and regional ventricular function and detection of pericardial fluid. For example, a hand-held echocardiogram in a patient with chest pain and a nondiagnostic ECG that shows akinesis of the anterior wall indicates the need for prompt coronary intervention. Conversely, the finding of a large pericardial effusion leads to a different diagnostic and therapeutic pathway. However, caution is needed in the use of these instruments. As with any ultrasound imaging technique, accurate diagnosis depends on the training and experience of the examiner. In addition, image quality and instrument functions are limited on these small devices as compared with standard ultrasound systems. Each medical center will need to carefully evaluate the use of these devices and monitor diagnostic accuracy.

IMAGE AND DOPPLER DATA STORAGE

There are several reasons to record the echocardiographic examination, including:

- ❏ Later review and/or quantitation
- ❏ Documentation
- ❏ Communication with the patient, referring physician, and other consultants
- ❏ Comparison with any future studies in that patient
- ❏ Clinical research

TABLE 5–8	Indications for Contrast Echocardiography
Right Heart Contrast (Agitated Saline)	
Detection of atrial septal defects and patent foramen ovale	
Documentation of persistent left superior vena cava	
Left Heart Contrast (Intravenous Agents with Transpulmonary Passage)	
Enhancement of contrast between LV chamber and endocardium (improved border recognition)	
Myocardial perfusion	
Improved visualization of LV structural abnormalities (thrombus, noncompaction, aneurysm, etc.)	
Improved detection of cardiac masses	
Intracoronary Contrast (Radiocontrast Agents)	
Opacification of myocardium perfused by injected vessel (e.g., during catheter ablation for hypertrophic cardiomyopathy)	

Since the entire examination may be quite lengthy, depending on the specific findings in each patient, only selected segments of the examination are recorded.

The current standard is digital recording and storage of cine loop images and still-frame Doppler data. Echocardiographic images and color Doppler are captured in a cine loop format triggered by the QRS signal on the ECG with the cardiac cycle recorded from end-diastole to end-diastole. Doppler signals are recorded as stills from images of the spectral tracing. Images and Doppler data are saved in the standardized Digital Imaging and Communication in Medicine (DICOM) format, which uses data compression methods that allow retention of image quality but result in an acceptable storage size. The overall size of the study also is controlled by storing only 1 to 2 cardiac cycles for each view and storing only selected views. Thus, digital image storage of echocardiographic studies requires:

❒ A clear ECG signal for timing of acquisition
❒ Acquisition of representative image and Doppler data by the sonographer
❒ A laboratory protocol for the specific data to be recorded
❒ Appropriate computer networking and storage facilities

Attention to the ECG signal at the time of recording is essential to ensure correct cine loop capture. A noisy signal or a small amplitude QRS signal may result in capture of only part of the cardiac cycle. When there is an irregular cardiac rhythm, such as atrial fibrillation, additional beats for each cine loop may be needed. Other situations where additional cardiac cycles (or backup videotape recording) may be needed include saline contrast studies and situations wherein a longer sweep from view to view is needed. Transient events may be difficult to capture in a digital format.

QUALITY ASSURANCE IN ECHOCARDIOGRAPHY

There are several steps to ensuring that high quality echocardiographic studies are provided to our patients (Fig. 5-10). These include documentation of sonographer and physician competency, appropriate laboratory standards and procedures, and continuous quality improvement measures. Documentation of competency typically is based on:

❒ Accreditation—endorsement of a training program or laboratory by a recognized national accreditation agency
❒ Certification—documentation of appropriate training and successful completion of an examination in the area of expertise by each physician and sonographer
❒ Credentialing—standards set by each health care organization for health care professionals providing patient care at that institution

In addition, innovative approaches to quality assurance based on statistical analysis of physician or laboratory performance have been proposed. Statistical database approaches will be increasingly useful as medical record systems are computerized.

Sonographer Education and Training

The sonographer must be familiar with patterns of disease in clinical cardiology, as well as with the technical aspects of performing the examination. Thus, sonographer education and training must include a knowledge base of cardiac anatomy and physiology, cardiac pathology, and clinical cardiology, in addition to ultrasound physics and the echocardiographic examination. Training also includes patient interaction skills, basic medical procedures (such as sterile technique), patient privacy, and so forth.

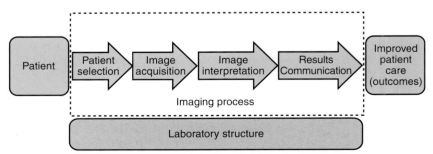

Figure 5-10 Dimensions of care framework for evaluating quality of cardiovascular imaging. The quality of an imaging study depends on multiple processes, as well as appropriately educated and trained sonographers and physicians and high-quality imaging systems. The value of clinical imaging depends on appropriate patient selection, optimal image acquisition, correct interpretation, and clear communication of results. *(From Douglas P, Iskandrian AE, Krumholz HM, et al: Achieving quality in cardiovascular imaging. Proceedings from the American College of Cardiology–Duke University Medical Center Think Tank on Quality in Cardiovascular Imaging. J Am Coll Cardiol 48:2141–2151, 2006.)*

Guidelines for education and training of cardiac sonographers have been published by the American Society of Echocardiography (ASE) and are periodically updated. Education and training in an accredited program is recommended, with accreditation for cardiac sonographer programs provided by two Joint Review Commissions (JRCs) under the auspices of the Commission on Accreditation of Allied Health Educational Programs: the JRC–Diagnostic Medical Sonography (JRC-DMS) and the JRC–Cardiovascular Technology (JRC-CVT). Education and training include acquisition of both cognitive and technical skills with demonstration of competency in each area. After completion of training, sonographers can be credentialed by the American Registry of Diagnostic Medical Sonographers (ARDMS), with separate examinations for adult and pediatric echocardiography, or by Cardiovascular Credentialing International (CCI). Cardiac sonographers must attend formal continuing medical education meetings to maintain these credentials.

Physician Education and Training

The physician must have expertise in the technical aspects of the examination, as well as the expected findings in each disease state, in order to guide the sonographer in optimizing data quality and to interpret the recorded data correctly. Details such as transducer frequency, gain controls, processing curves, and depth settings significantly affect image quality. The appropriate choice of Doppler modality for the flow of interest—pulsed, color flow, or continuous-wave Doppler—determines data quality. Factors such as wall filters, gain, sample volume size, and color sector width also significantly affect data collection. Knowledge of how these factors impact data quality and knowledge of which views and approaches yield optimal data allow the physician to assess the reliability of recorded data, to suspect abnormalities that may not have been noted explicitly during the examination, to recognize imaging and flow artifacts, and to direct the sonographer in optimal data acquisition.

Physician education and training in echocardiography most often takes place during Cardiology Fellowship Training, in a program accredited by the American Council of Graduate Medical Education (ACGME). In addition, specific recommendations for training in echocardiography have been published, and are periodically updated, by the American College of Cardiology and American Heart Association (ACC/AHA). These recommendations divide training into three levels of expertise:

Level 1: Basic introduction to echocardiography needed by all cardiologists
Level 2: Qualified to independently interpret echocardiographic studies
Level 3: Additional qualifications to supervise an echocardiography laboratory

It is recommended that Level 2 training in TTE be achieved before training in advanced procedures, including TEE and stress echocardiography. Recommended numbers of procedures during training are indicated in Table 5–9.

Most physicians completing a 3- or 4-year program in Cardiology will have achieved Level 2 training. Successful completion of the American Board of Internal Medicine examination in Cardiovascular Disease, in conjunction with at least Level 2 training as documented by the program director, provides verification of competence in TTE.

Other physicians may achieve competency in echocardiography based on the same training guidelines recommended for cardiology trainees. Physicians who receive echocardiography training outside of cardiology fellowship programs have the option of taking the examination provided by the National Board of Echocardiography (NBE) to document competency. In addition, specific guidelines for training of cardiovascular anesthesiologists in echocardiography have been published by the ASE focusing on expertise in TEE and intraoperative echocardiography. The NBE offers a special examination for cardiovascular anesthesiology.

In order to maintain competency in echocardiography, physicians should document Continuing

TABLE 5–9	Summary of ACC/AHA Recommendations for Training in Echocardiography			
Level of Expertise	Cumulative Duration (Months)	Cumulative Number of Studies Performed	Cumulative Number of Studies Interpreted	Annual Studies to Maintain Competence
1	3	75	150	
2	6	150	300	300
3	12	300	750	500
Stress echo		100		100
TEE		50		25–50

Medical Education and should interpret a minimum of 300 studies per year for Level 2 and 500 studies per year for Level 3, with performance of some studies recommended. For maintaining competency in TEE, 25 to 50 studies should be performed and interpreted annually, with 100 studies per year recommended for stress echocardiography.

Echocardiography Reporting

It is essential that sonographers relay technical concerns to the physician and direct attention to abnormalities noted during the examination. Conversely, the physician should give feedback to the sonographer about the completeness and quality of data recorded and offer suggestions for future patient studies. The physician review also may indicate that additional echocardiographic recordings are needed, either before the patient leaves the laboratory or at a later examination.

The echocardiographic report serves at least two purposes: (1) it conveys the results of the test to the referring physician, and (2) it serves as a narrative summary of the echocardiographic examination for comparison with future studies. Given the wide variety of views and flows that can be recorded, it is helpful for the report to document the structures imaged (even if normal), the flow signals recorded, the different Doppler modalities used, and the overall quality of the study. Any areas of limitation in the study are noted.

In each patient, the various echocardiographic findings then are integrated with each other in the final interpretation. For example, a report describing mitral regurgitation also would include a clear description of valve anatomy with an indication of the most likely etiology of regurgitation or the differential diagnosis if the etiology were unclear. Mitral regurgitant severity is estimated and the method(s) used to generate this estimate are indicated. In addition, the degrees of LA and LV dilation are described, with attention to serial changes if previous studies are available. LV systolic function is quantitated, and the degree of pulmonary hypertension is estimated. All these findings fit together physiologically and thus can be reported in a logical integration of the data. For example, significant mitral regurgitation results in LV and LA enlargement due to volume overload, while the chronically elevated LA pressure leads to pulmonary hypertension.

Finally, these findings are reviewed in the context of the patient's clinical presentation, potential implications of the findings are discussed with the referring physician, and additional diagnostic tests or follow-up studies are recommended as clinically indicated. If principles of clinical decision analysis are being used in patient management, the pre-test and post-test likelihood of disease can be estimated. Ideally, the overall impact of the echocardiographic findings on the patient's therapy or subsequent diagnostic evaluation is reviewed with the referring physician both before and after the examination. Specific comments about timing of periodic echocardiography or consideration of referral to a cardiologist also may be appropriate. Of course, any unexpected or serious findings on echocardiography should promptly be relayed to the referring physician. In some cases, the echocardiography attending physician may need to assume immediate care of the patient, for example, with persistent abnormalities after stress testing or with the unexpected finding of an aortic dissection.

Echocardiography Laboratory Accreditation

Accreditation of echocardiography laboratories is available through the Inter-Societal Commission for the Accreditation of Echocardiography Laboratories (ICAEL). This accreditation process reviews all aspects of the echocardiographic examination including:

❐ Physician training and experience
❐ Sonographer training and experience
❐ Continuing medical education of physicians and sonongraphers
❐ Physical facilities (instruments, exam area, etc.)
❐ Echocardiography performance
❐ Laboratory procedures and protocols
❐ Echocardiographic reporting and data storage
❐ Quality assurance measures

The detailed recommendations of the ICAEL provide a useful starting point for laboratory policies and procedures that then can be modified as needed for each institution. The recommendations also include the essential components of TTE, TEE, and stress echocardiography examinations.

SUGGESTED READING

Diagnostic Testing Principles

1. Sox HC Jr, Blatt MA, Higgins MC, et al: Medical Decision Making. Stoneham, MA, Butterworth Heinemann, 1988.

A readable, concise textbook summarizing the entire spectrum of medical decision making from sensitivity/specificity to cost-benefit analysis.

2. Diamond GA, Forrester JS: Analysis of probability as an aid in the clinical diagnosis of coronary-artery disease. N Engl J Med 300:1350–1358, 1979.

Classic article on use of Bayes' theorem to determine post-test likelihood based on pretest likelihood and test results using the example of exercise ECG for diagnosis of CAD.

3. Wasson JH, Sox HC, Neff RK, et al: Clinical prediction rules. Applications and methodological standards. N Engl J Med 313:793–799, 1985.

Defines approach to developing and validating new clinical prediction rules. This article will be of particular value to individuals proposing new diagnostic approaches based on echocardiographic data.

4. Pauker SG, Kassirer JP: The threshold approach to clinical decision making. N Engl J Med 302:1109–1117, 1980.

Clear and concise discussion of the concepts of decision analysis focusing on the threshold approach.

5. Pauker SG, Kassirer JP: Decision analysis. N Engl J Med 316:250–258, 1987.

Review of decision analysis including Bayes' rule, decision trees, and outcome measures. 52 references.

6. Gill CJ, Sabin L, Schmid CH: Why clinicians are natural Bayesians. BMJ 330:1080–1083, 2005.

This short review provides an elegant discussion with examples of how clinical decision making tends to follow a Bayesian approach. The principles of clinical decision making as detailed here are directly applicable to echocardiographic diagnosis.

7. Detsky AS, Naglie IG: A clinician's guide to cost-effectiveness analysis. Ann Intern Med 113:147–154, 1990.

Outlines simplified models for cost-effectiveness analysis that should be applicable to comparisons of the use of different diagnostic tests in a specific clinical setting. Provides guidelines for setting priorities within a health care organization based on cost-effectiveness analysis.

8. Akobeng K: Understanding diagnostic tests 2: Likelihood ratios, pre- and post-test probabilities and their use in clinical practice. Acta Paediatrica 96:487–491, 2007.

A review of approaches to using the results of a diagnostic test such as echocardiography in clinical practice. The use of likelihood ratios in clinical decision making in individual patients is emphasized.

Medical Imaging

9. Douglas PS: Improving imaging: our professional imperative. J Am Coll Cardiol 48:2152–2155, 2006.

A thoughtful review and position paper stating the view that we need to expand the evidence base demonstrating that echocardiographic diagnosis positively affects clinical outcome. In addition, improvements in the quality of image acquisition, interpretation, and echocardiography reporting are needed for optimal clinical care.

10. Douglas P, Iskandrian AE, Krumholz HM, et al: Achieving quality in cardiovascular imaging. Proceedings from the American College of Cardiology–Duke University Medical Center Think Tank on Quality in Cardiovascular Imaging. J Am Coll Cardiol 48:2141–2151, 2006.

This consensus document provides a framework for improving the quality of diagnostic imaging. In addition to laboratory structure, this review emphasizes the importance of appropriate patient selection, quality of acquired images, variability in data acquisition and interpretation, and the importance of communicating results in a clear, definitive, complete, and timely fashion.

11. Patel MR, Spertus JA, Brindis RG, et al: ACCF proposed method for evaluating the appropriateness of cardiovascular imaging. J Am Coll Cardiol 46:1606–1613, 2005.

Appropriateness criteria are developed starting with a literature review followed by synthesis of the evidence, and review of proposed indications. Then an expert panel rates a list of indications in two rounds—first independently, then after a group discussion. A score from 1 (inappropriate) to 9 (most appropriate) is assigned each clinical indication, with a score of 7–9 considered appropriate. These criteria can be further validated by retrospective review of clinical records and prospectively in clinical decision making.

12. Iglehart JK: The new era of medical imaging—progress and pitfalls. N Engl J Med 354:2822–2828, 2006.

A summary of the rapid increase in the number of medical imaging procedures performed in Medicare patients and the potential measures to limit this expansion or reduce the overall cost to the health care system.

Guidelines for Education and Training

13. Quinones MA, Douglas, PA, Foster E, et al: American College of Cardiology/American Heart Association Clinical Competence Statement on Echocardiography: A report of the American College of Cardiology/American Heart Association/American College of Physicians–American Society of Internal Medicine Task Force on Clinical Competence. Circulation 107:1068–1089, 2003.

Detailed recommendations for physician education and training and maintenance of competency in echocardiography. This document includes sections on TTE, TEE, perioperative echocardiography, stress echocardiography, congenital heart disease, fetal echocardiography, and new technologies (hand-held devices, contrast, intracoronary, and intracardiac ultrasound).

14. Ryan T, Armstrong WF, Khandheria BK: Task force 4: Training in echocardiography endorsed by the American Society of Echocardiography. J Am Coll Cardiol 51:361–367, 2008.

Recommendations for training in echocardiography as a component of a 3-year Fellowship Program in Cardiovascular Disease.

15. Ehler D, Carney DK, Dempsey AL, et al: Guidelines for cardiac sonographer education: recommendations of the American Society of Echocardiography Sonographer Training and Education Committee. J Am Soc Echocardiogr 14:77–84, 2001.

Detailed summary of the educational requirements for education in cardiac sonography. A useful outline for training programs for curriculum development. Physicians should review these guidelines to ensure appropriate education of sonographers performing studies under their supervision.

Guidelines for Indications and Appropriateness of Echocardiography

16. Thomas JD, Zoghbi WA, Beller GA, et al: ACCF 2008 training statement on multimodality noninvasive cardiovascular imaging: A report of the American College of Cardiology Foundation/American Heart Association/American College of Physicians Task Force on Clinical Competence and Training. J Am Coll Cardiol 53:125–148, 2009.

This guideline document outlines recommended training for physicians in integrated noninvasive cardiovascular imaging, including echocardiography, nuclear cardiology, computed tomographic (CT) and cardiac magnetic resonance (CMR) imaging. The appendix provides a concise summary of the curriculum content needed for understanding basic imaging physics, common principles of imaging and clinical applications of these modalites.

17. Cheitlin MD, Alpert JS, Armstrong WF, et al: ACC/AHA/ASE 2003 Guidelines update for the clinical application of echocardiography: Summary article. A report of the American College of Cardiology/American Heart Association Task Force on Practice Guidelines. Circulation 108: 1146–1162, 2003.

Task force guidelines on indications for echocardiography divided into class I indications (general agreement that echocardiography is important), class II (divergence of opinions), and class III (not appropriate).

18. Douglas PS, Khandheria B, Stainback RF, et al: ACCF/ASE/ACEP/ASNC/SCAI/SCCT/SCMR 2007 appropriateness criteria for transthoracic and transesophageal echocardiography. J Am Coll Cardiol 50:187–204, 2007.

The appropriateness of echocardiography as a diagnostic test was ascertained for 59 clinical situations by a panel of experts grading each clinical situation on a 1 (inappropriate) to 9 (definitely appropriate) scale. Echocardiography was considered appropriate for 44 of these clinical situations (score 7–9), inappropriate (scale 1–3) for 14 clinical situations, and of uncertain appropriateness in 1 situation (use of TEE to evaluate for cardiac source of embolus when TTE imaging and ECG are normal and there is no history of atrial arrhythmias).

19. Douglas PS, Khandheria B, Stainback RF, et al: ACCF/ASE/ACEP/AHA/ ASNC/SCAI/SCCT/SCMR 2008 appropriateness criteria for stress echocardiography. Circulation 117:1478–1497, 2008.

   This expert panel considered 51 potential indications for stress echocardiography. First, each expert provided a score from 1 to 9 where 7–9 indicate an appropriate indication, 1–3 indicates an inappropriate indication, and 4–6 are uncertain indications. After a meeting to discuss these indications with blinded access to the other reviewers' scores, each expert rescored the indications to provide final recommendations. The use of stress echocardiography before and after organ transplantation was not considered in this document.

USEFUL WEB SITES

Professional Organizations

American College of Cardiology (ACC): http://www.acc.org.
American Heart Association (AHA): http:// www.americanheart.org.
Society for Diagnostic Medical Sonography (SDMS): http://www.sdms.org.
American Society of Echocardiography (ASE): http://www.asecho.org.
European Society of Cardiology (ESC): http://www.escardio.org.
Society of Cardiovascular Anesthesiologists (SCA): http://www.scahq.org.

   All of these professional organizations have guidelines for training and education and for the indications for echocardiography that are posted on the web sites and periodically updated.

Accreditation

Accreditation Council on Graduate Medical Education (ACGME): http://www.acgme. org.

   Provides the requirements and procedures for accreditation of physician training programs, including Fellowship in Cardiovascular Disease, with details of required training in echocardiography.

Commission on Accreditation of Allied Health Education Programs (CAAHEP): http://www.caahep.org.

   Includes essentials and guidelines for accreditation of programs in cardiac sonography by the Joint Review Commission for Diagnostic Medical Sonography (JRC-DMS) and the Joint Review Commission for Cardiovascular Technology (JRC-CVT). Also includes lists of accredited programs. Currently the JRC-DMS provides accreditation to a total of 153 programs, with 51 echocardiography programs. The JRC-CVT provides accreditation to a total of 34 programs, with 24 noninvasive cardiology programs.

Inter-Societal Commission for Accreditation of Echocardiography Laboratories (ICAEL): http://www.icael.org.

   Details of the requirements and procedures for accreditation of echocardiography laboratories. This web site has a wealth of detail that will be useful to any laboratory seeking to establish protocols and procedures.

Certification

American Registry of Diagnostic Medical Sonography (ARDMS): http:// www.ardms.org.

   The ARDMS offers four credentials, one of which is Registered Diagnostic Cardiac Sonographer (RDCS), with examination options in adult and pediatric echocardiography.

Cardiovascular Credentialing International (CCI): http://www.cci-online.org.

   CCI offers five examinations, one of which is echocardiography leading to credentialing as a Registered Cardiac Sonographer (RCS).

American Board of Internal Medicine (ABIM): http://www.abim.org.

   Policies for physician credentialing in internal medicine and its subspecialities, including cardiovascular disease, with examination dates and registration. An index provides verification of physician status on these examinations.

National Board of Echocardiography (NBE): http://www.echoboards.org.

   The NBE offers two examinations: Examination of Special Competency in Adult Echocardiography (ASCeXAM) and Examination of Special Competency in Perioperative Transesophageal Echocardiography (PTEeXAM), along with recertification examinations in both areas. Certification is based on documentation of training and experience and passing the examination.

6

Left and Right Ventricular Systolic Function

T he degree of ventricular systolic dysfunction is a potent predictor of clinical outcome for a wide range of cardiovascular disease, including ischemic cardiac disease, cardiomyopathies, valvular heart disease, and congenital heart disease. Echocardiography provides both qualitative and quantitative measures of systolic function. Visual estimates of global and regional function from echocardiographic images, quantitative ventricular volumes and ejection fractions (EFs) based on endocardial border tracing, and Doppler echocardiographic ejection phase indices all are valuable clinical tools.

Evaluation of ventricular systolic function is the most important application of echocardiography, so that even when evaluation of ventricular systolic function is not the focus of the examination, it plays a key role in every study. For research applications, echocardiographic measures of left ventricular (LV) systolic function provide important baseline data on disease severity. In addition, these data can serve as a sensitive and reliable surrogate endpoint for intervention trials in patients with ventricular dysfunction.

BASIC PRINCIPLES

Cardiac Cycle

Systole typically is defined as the segment of the cardiac cycle from mitral valve closure to aortic valve closure (Fig. 6–1). The onset of systole is defined by the electrocardiogram (ECG) as ventricular depolarization

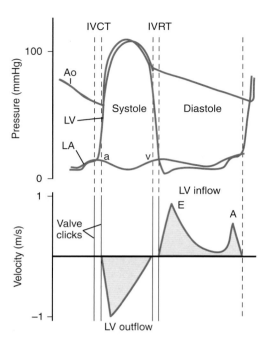

Figure 6–1 The cardiac cycle. LV, Ao, and LA pressures are shown with the corresponding Doppler LV outflow and inflow velocity curves. The isovolumic contraction time (IVCT) represents the time between MV closure and Ao valve opening, while the isovolumic relaxation time (IVRT) represents the time between Ao valve closure and MV opening.

(onset of the QRS complex), with the end of systole occurring after repolarization (end of T wave). In terms of ventricular pressure and volume curves over time, systole begins when LV pressure exceeds left atrial pressure, resulting in closure of the mitral valve. Mitral valve closure is followed by isovolumic contraction, during which the cardiac muscle depolarizes, calcium influx and myosin-actin shortening occur, and ventricular pressure rises rapidly at a constant ventricular volume (although shape changes may occur). When ventricular pressure exceeds aortic pressure, the aortic valve opens. During ejection (aortic valve opening to closing), LV volume falls rapidly as blood flows from the LV to the aorta. LV pressure exceeds aortic pressure for approximately the first half of systole, corresponding to rapid acceleration of blood flow and a small pressure difference from the ventricle to the aorta. In the normal heart, pressure crossover occurs in midsystole, so during the second half of systole, aortic pressure exceeds LV pressure, resulting in continued forward blood flow but at progressively slower velocities (deceleration). Aortic valve closure occurs at the dicrotic notch of the aortic pressure tracing, immediately following end-ejection. In sum, systole includes isovolumic contraction and ventricular ejection (acceleration and deceleration phases). Ventricular volume ranges from a maximum at end-diastole (or onset of systole) to a minimum at end-systole.

Physiology of Systolic Function

During systole, ventricular myocardial fibers contract circumferentially and longitudinally, resulting in myocardial wall thickening and inward motion of the endocardium. The simultaneous decrease in ventricular size and increase in pressure results in ejection of a volume of blood (stroke volume, SV) from the ventricle. Stroke volume reflects the *pump performance* of the heart. The decrease in chamber volume relative to end-diastolic volume (EDV), or EF, reflects overall *ventricular function*. Ventricular function and pump performance depend on:

- ❏ Contractility (the basic ability of the myocardium to contract)
- ❏ Preload (initial ventricular volume or pressure)
- ❏ Afterload (aortic resistance or end-systolic wall stress)
- ❏ Ventricular geometry

Contractility is the intrinsic ability of the myocardium to contract, independent of loading conditions or geometry. Evaluation of contractility itself thus requires measurement of ventricular ejection performance under different loading conditions. Experimentally, contractility often is described by the slope of the end-systolic pressure-volume relationship (E_{max}). To derive this value, LV pressure is graphed on the vertical axis, with volume on the horizontal axis, rather than graphing each individually as a function of time (Fig. 6–2). This pressure-volume "loop" then represents a single cardiac cycle, with different pressure-volume loops for the same ventricle representing different loading conditions (such as increasing or decreasing ventricular EDV or

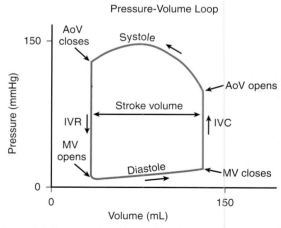

Figure 6–2 Pressure-volume loop. LV volume is graphed on the horizontal axis, with pressure on the vertical axis. The temporal direction of pressure-volume changes is shown by the *arrows*. During diastole, volume increases with little rise in pressure. After MV closure, isovolumic contraction (IVC) results in a rapid rise in pressure with no change in volume. At the onset of ejection, the aortic valve (AoV) opens with a rapid decrease in LV volume during systole. AoV closure is followed by isovolumic relaxation (IVR).

changing afterload). E_{max} is the slope of the line that intersects the end-systolic pressure-volume point for each curve. A decrease in contractility results in a decrease in stroke volume and larger LV volumes (Fig. 6–3). Contractility itself can be affected by several physiologic parameters including heart rate, coupling interval, and metabolic factors, as well as by disease processes and pharmacologic agents.

The effect of preload on ventricular ejection performance is summarized by the Frank-Starling curve showing ventricular end-diastolic volume (or pressure) on the horizontal axis and stroke volume on the vertical axis (Fig. 6–4A). For a given degree of contractility there is a curvilinear relationship between these variables such that increasing EDV results in a greater stroke volume. An increase in contractility results in a greater increase in stroke volume for a given increase in preload; a decrease in contractility has the opposite effect.

Afterload, defined by resistance or impedance, has an inverse relationship with myocardial fiber shortening such that increasing vascular resistance results in a decreased stroke volume (see Fig. 6–4). An increase in contractility allows maintenance of a normal stroke volume with a higher afterload. With a decrease in contractility, even slight increases in afterload further decrease myocardial fiber shortening and stroke volume.

Measurement of LV systolic function independent of loading conditions is difficult using echocardiographic

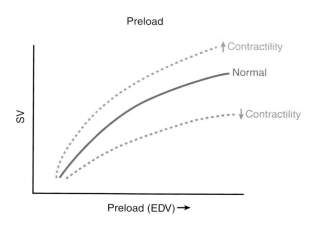

Preload

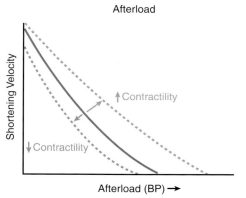

Afterload

Figure 6–4 *Top,* The relationship between preload, often defined by end-diastolic volume (EDV) and stroke volume (SV), is shown for a normal (*blue*) LV. With increased contractility there is a greater increase in SV for an increase in EDV (*pink*); with decreased contractility, there is a smaller increase in SV for an increase in EDV (*green*). *Bottom,* The inverse relationship between afterload, approximated by blood pressure (BP) or systemic vascular resistance, and LV myocardial shortening velocity is shown for a normal ventricle (*blue*). With increased contractility, shortening velocity (and SV) can be maintained at higher afterloads (*pink*); with decreased contractility, shortening velocity is lower for any given afterload (*green*).

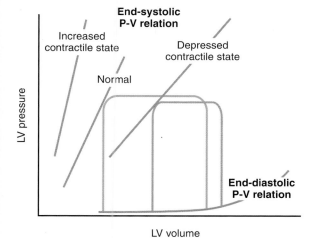

Figure 6–3 LV pressure-volume (P-V) loops with a normal ventricle shown in yellow and an acute decrease in contractile state shown in pink. The slope of the line intersecting the end-systolic (ES) pressure volume points at different loading conditions, shown as a green line for each P-V loop, is a measure of contractility known as elastance (E_{max}), which is insensitive to changes in loading conditions. With decreased contractility, the P-V loop is displaced to the right and the ES P-V line shifts downward and to the right. The effect of an acute increase in contractile state is illustrated by the line on the left; the slope of the ES P-V line is increased (the corresponding loop is not shown). *(From Aurigemma GP, Gaasch WH, Villegas B, et al: Noninvasive assessment of left ventricular mass, chamber volume, and contractile function. Curr Probl Cardiol 20:418, 1995.)*

or other clinical approaches. It rarely is possible to construct pressure-volume loops under different loading conditions due to the problem of measuring instantaneous LV volumes and the potential risk of altering loading conditions in ill patients. Thus, clinical evaluation of ventricular function has focused on measurements of cardiac output, EF, and end-systolic dimension or volume, even though the load dependence of these measures is a clearly acknowledged limitation. Wall stress measurements are complex but may become more widely utilized with technologic advances.

Ventricular Volumes and Geometry

The normal shape of the LV is symmetric with two relatively equal short axes and with the long axis running from the base (mitral annulus) to the apex.

In long-axis views, the apex is slightly rounded, so the apical half of the ventricle resembles a hemiellipse. The basal half of the ventricle is more cylindrical, so the ventricle appears circular in short-axis views. Various assumptions about LV shape have been used to derive formulas for calculating ventricular volumes from linear dimensions (M-mode), cross-sectional areas (CSAs; two-dimensional [2D] echo) or three-dimensional (3D) volumes. Formulas using linear or cross-sectional measurements are simplifications to greater or lesser degrees, and there is variability among patients in the shape of the ventricle.

While instantaneous ventricular volumes throughout the cardiac cycle are of interest, usually only EDV and end-systolic volume (ESV) are measured in the clinical setting. EF is:

$$EF(\%) = (SV/EDV) \times 100\% \qquad (6\text{--}1)$$

where stroke volume (SV) is calculated as

$$SV = EDV - ESV \qquad (6\text{--}2)$$

with cardiac output obtained by multiplying SV by heart rate

Other useful parameters of ventricular function include (1) wall stress and (2) LV mass.

Cardiac Output

The basic function of the heart is as a pump, so that measurements of cardiac output are useful in routine day-to-day patient management. Cardiac output is the volume of blood pumped by the heart per minute, with stroke volume being the amount pumped on a single beat. While cardiac output can be derived from ventricular volumes, as described above, a variety of other approaches to measurement are available, including right heart catheterization with indicator dilation methods (Fick, thermodilution); angiographic, radionuclide, or cardiac magnetic resonance (CMR) ventricular volumes; and CMR or Doppler flow velocity methods.

Response to Exercise

Ventricular systolic function and cardiac output are dynamic, responding rapidly to the metabolic demands of the individual. Cardiac output increases from a mean of 6 L/min at rest to 18 L/min with exercise in young, healthy adults. Most of this increase in cardiac output is mediated by an increase in heart rate. With supine exercise, there is only a minimal increase in stroke volume (about 10%), whereas with upright exercise, the increase in stroke volume is approximately 20% to 35%. With exercise, EDV is unchanged or slightly decreased, but EF increases and ESV decreases. With imaging techniques, endocardial motion and myocardial wall thickening are augmented with an appearance of "hypercontractility" during and immediately following exercise.

IMAGING OF THE LEFT VENTRICLE

Qualitative Evaluation of Systolic Function

Both global and regional ventricular function can be evaluated with 2D echocardiography on a semiquantitative scale by an experienced observer. On transthoracic (TTE) imaging, overall LV systolic function is evaluated best from multiple tomographic planes, typically:

- ❐ Parasternal long-axis view
- ❐ Parasternal short-axis view
- ❐ Apical four-chamber view
- ❐ Apical two-chamber view
- ❐ Apical long-axis view

On transesophageal (TEE) imaging equivalent views from a high TEE and transgastric position are used. Attention to image acquisition is needed to obtain adequate endocardial definition. The echocardiographer then integrates the degree of endocardial motion and wall thickening from these views to classify overall systolic function as normal, mildly reduced, moderately reduced, or severely reduced. Some experienced observers can estimate EF visually from 2D images with a reasonable correlation with EFs measured quantitatively by echocardiography or other techniques. Typically, EF is estimated in intervals of 5% to 10% (i.e., 20%, 30%, 40%, and so on), or an estimated EF range is reported (e.g., 20% to 30%).

There are several other imaging parameters that provide a qualitative measure of LV systolic function. M-mode signs include:

- ❐ The separation between the maximum anterior motion of the anterior mitral leaflet and maximum posterior motion of the ventricular septum (E point septal separation)
- ❐ The degree of anteroposterior motion of the aortic root

With normal systolic function the anterior mitral leaflet opens to nearly fill the ventricular chamber resulting in little (0–5 mm) E point septal separation. With systolic dysfunction this distance is increased due to a combination of LV dilation and reduced motion of the mitral valve as a result of low transmitral volume flow. Similarly, LV systolic dysfunction results in reduced LA filling and emptying (low cardiac output), seen on M-mode as reduced anteroposterior motion of the aortic root.

On 2D echocardiography the mitral annulus moves toward the ventricular apex in systole, with the magnitude of this motion proportional to the extent of shortening in ventricular length—a useful measure of overall LV systolic function. Normal subjects have motion of the mitral annulus toward the apex ≥ 8 mm, with a mean value of 12 ± 2 mm in both four- and two-chamber views. The sensitivity of mitral annulus motion <8 mm is 98% with a specificity of 82% for identification of an EF <50%.

Qualitative evaluation of overall systolic function is a simple and highly predictive index that is of great clinical utility. On the other hand, several factors can limit the usefulness of this evaluation. First, the accuracy of the estimated EF is dependent on the experience of each observer. Second, inadequate endocardial definition can result in incorrect estimates of systolic function. Third, integration of data from multiple tomographic images can be difficult when the pattern of contraction is asynchronous (with conduction defects, pacers, postoperative septal motion) or when the pattern of contraction is asymmetric (with prior myocardial infarction or with ischemia), especially when dyskinesis is present. To some extent these limitations are minimized by an experienced observer, optimal endocardial definition, and integration of data from multiple views. However, when possible it is preferable to avoid the limitations of estimates of systolic function by performing quantitative measurements.

Regional ventricular function also can be evaluated by imaging in multiple tomographic planes on TTE or TEE imaging. Regional function is evaluated qualitatively by dividing the ventricle into segments corresponding to the coronary artery anatomy and then grading wall motion on a 1 to 4+ scale as normal (score = 1), hypokinetic (score = 2), akinetic (score = 3), or dyskinetic (score = 4). In some cases, hyperkinesis— that is, a compensatory increase in wall motion in regions remote from an acute myocardial infarction or the normal increase seen with exercise—also is scored. Evaluation of segmental wall motion is discussed in detail in Chapter 8.

Quantitative Evaluation of Left Ventricular Systolic Function

Linear Dimensions

LV internal dimensions and wall thickness are routinely made using 2D echocardiography, although 2D-guided M-mode measurements are recommended in some specific situations, such as serial evaluation for valvular heart disease, particularly when identification of the endocardium is suboptimal on the 2D freeze-frame image (Table 6–1). Measurements of LV size are most accurate when the ultrasound beam is perpendicular to the blood/endocardium interface because of the precision of axial, compared with lateral, resolution.

On a standard examination ventricular size is measured in the parasternal long-axis view, at the level of the mitral leaflet tips (mitral chordal level), perpendicular to the long-axis of the ventricle (Fig. 6–5). Biplane imaging or scanning between the long- and short-axis views is helpful to ensure the

measurements are centered in the short-axis plane, as well. TEE measurements of LV internal dimensions are made in a transgastric two-chamber view at the junction between the basal third and apical third of the ventricle. Wall thickness is measured in the transgastric short-axis view. On 2D images, LV internal dimensions are measured at end-diastole and end-systole from the tissue/blood interface (white-black transition). End-diastole is defined as the onset of the QRS, the first frame after mitral valve closure or maximum ventricular volume. End-systole is defined as the smallest ventricular volume or the frame just before mitral valve opening.

When 2D-guided M-mode measurements are used, the transducer often must be moved cephalad to obtain a perpendicular angle between the M-line and the long axis of the ventricle. If only an oblique orientation is possible, correctly aligned measurements should be made from the 2D image instead. The major advantage of M-mode echocardiography is high time resolution, which facilitates recognition of endocardial motion and thus a more accurate measurement of ventricular internal dimensions. On M-mode, the LV posterior wall endocardium is the most continuous line with the steepest systolic motion. The posterior wall epicardium is identified as the echo reflection immediately anterior to the pericardium. The septal endocardium also shows the steepest slope in systole with a continuous reflection through the cycle. On the right ventricular (RV) side of the septum, it is important to exclude any reflections due to RV trabeculations. Conversely, a dark "mid-septal" stripe often is noted and should not be confused with the endocardial borders. LV wall thickness and dimensions are measured from the leading edge to leading edge of each interface of interest for optimal measurement accuracy. For example, ventricular internal dimensions are measured from the leading edge of the septal endocardium to the leading edge of the posterior wall endocardium (Fig. 6–6). Normal values for these measurements are indicated in Table 2–8.

In addition to LV wall thickness and internal dimensions (LVIDs) at end-diastole and end-systole, endocardial fractional shortening (FS) can be calculated as:

$$FS(\%) = (LVID_d - LVID_s)/LVID_d \times 100\% \quad (6–3)$$

Fractional shortening is a rough measurement of LV systolic function, with the normal range being about 25% to 45% (95% confidence limits). Instead of endocardial fractional shortening, as shown in Equation 6–3, midwall fractional shortening is a better reflector of contractility, because it reflects both the inward motion of the endocardium and the degree of wall thickening. However, midwall shortening calculations are rarely used in clinical practice because 2D measures of ventricular systolic function are more robust.

TABLE 6–1 Left Ventricular Dimension Measurements

	TTE–2D	TTE–2D Guided M-mode	TEE
Transducer position	Parasternal	Parasternal	Transgastric (TG)
Image plane	Long axis	Long axis	Two-chamber view (rotation angle 60°–90°)
Measurement position in LV chamber	Perpendicular to LV long axis in the center of the LV Biplane imaging or rotation between long- and short-axis views helps ensure a centered measurement.	Perpendicular to LV long axis in the center of the LV Correct M-line orientation often requires moving the transducer up an interspace.	Perpendicular to LV long axis in the center of the LV Ensuring a centered measurement is more difficult on TEE.
Measurement site along LV length	Just apical to the mitral leaflet tips (chordal level)	Just apical to the mitral leaflet tips (chordal level)	At the junction of the basal one third and apical two thirds of the LV
Measurement technique	White/black interface	Leading edge to leading edge	White/black interface
Timing in cardiac cycle End-diastole End-systole	Onset of QRS frame just before MV closure, or maximum LV volume Minimum LV volume or frame just before aortic valve closure	Onset of QRS frame just before MV closure, or maximum LV volume Minimum LV volume or frame just before aortic valve closure	Onset of QRS frame just before MV closure, or maximum LV volume Minimum LV volume or frame just before aortic valve closure
Advantages	Feasible in most patients Measurements can be made perpendicular to LV long axis.	High sampling rate facilitates identification of endocardium. Reproducible	Data can be obtained intra-operatively to monitor preload. Ultrasound beam is perpendicular to endocardium from TG view, improving border recognition.
Disadvantages	Endocardial and epicardial borders may be difficult to accurately identify. Slow frame rate compared with M-mode	M-line measurements should only be made if a perpendicular LV measurement is possible. Requires more attention to transducer and M-line position.	Image plane may be oblique. Wall thickness is measured in a TG short axis view.

Ventricular Volumes

Two-dimensional echocardiographic calculation of ventricular volumes is based on endocardial border tracing at end-diastole and end-systole in one or more tomographic planes on TTE or TEE images (Table 6–2). Prerequisites for quantitative evaluation by 2D echocardiography are:

❏ Nonoblique standard image planes or image planes of known orientation relative to the long and short axis of the LV
❏ Inclusion of the apex of the ventricle
❏ Adequate endocardial definition
❏ Accurate identification of the endocardial borders

In some patients image quality is inadequate for endocardial definition. Even when image quality is adequate, endocardial borders must be traced manually by an experienced physician or sonographer for accurate quantitation of LV systolic function by echocardiography. Since 2D echocardiography is a tomographic technique, LV volume calculations are based on geometric assumptions about the shape of the LV. By convention, the papillary muscles are included in the ventricular chamber, with endocardial borders extrapolated along the base of the papillary muscle, following the expected curvature of the ventricular wall. Obviously, accuracy in individual patients will be highest with methods that have the fewest geometric assumptions and that use data from multiple tomographic images.

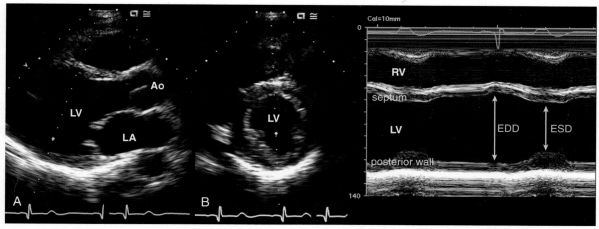

Figure 6–5 LV end-diastolic and end-systolic dimensions are measured from the parasternal window. 2D measurements are made for the white/black interface of the septum to the posterior wall, taking care to measure perpendicular to the long axis of the ventricle (**A**) and centered in the short axis (**B**). Similarly, 2D- guided M-mode measurements are made after verifying the M-line is centered in the LV in the short-axis view and perpendicular to the long axis of the LV in the long-axis view. The transducer should be in a high intercostal space to ensure the M-line is not oblique. The high sampling rate of the M-mode recording allows more precise identification of the endocardium.

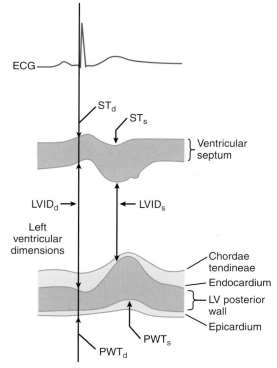

Figure 6–6 Schematic of an M-mode echocardiogram obtained using 2D echocardiographic guidance. Diastolic measurements are made coincident with the Q wave of the simultaneous ECG. D, diastole; LVID, left ventricular internal dimension; PWT, posterior wall thickness; S, systole; ST, septal thickness. *(From Aurigemma GP, Gaasch WH, Villegas B, et al: Noninvasive assessment of left ventricular mass, chamber volume, and contractile function. Curr Probl Cardiol 20:381, 1995.)*

The greatest accuracy would be expected with 3D reconstructions that use data from multiple tomographic images of known orientation and make no geometric assumptions (Table 6–3). Real-time 3D volumetric datasets provide the promise of rapid measurement of LV volumes, without geometric assumptions. However, this approach typically still requires manual identification of the endocardial border or several points on the endocardium. Further validation is needed to ensure that semi-automated volume measurements are precise enough for clinical decision making (see Suggested Reading 7–9). Simpler methods, based on one to three image planes, provide reasonably accurate information with less time-consuming data collection. These simpler methods are the current clinical standard.

Several approaches for calculation of LV volumes from tomographic data, based on different geometric assumptions, have been proposed, ranging from a simple ellipsoid shape to complex hemicylindrical hemiellipsoid shapes (Fig. 6–7). The most robust and practical method for clinical use is Simpson's rule or *method of disks*, which calculates ventricular volume as the sum of a series of parallel "slices" from apex to base.

$$\text{LV volume} = \sum_{i}^{n} A_i T \qquad (6\text{–}4)$$

Where A is the area and T is the thickness of each of n slices. For example, if 20 disks are summated, LV volume is:

$$\text{LV volume} = \sum_{n=20} [A_i \times L/20] \qquad (6\text{–}5)$$

This approach is accurate even when ventricular geometry is distorted and is the approach recommended in consensus guidelines. The apical biplane approach requires tracing of endocardial borders at end-diastole and end-systole in both four-chamber and two-chamber views, from either TTE or TEE

TABLE 6-2   Selected Studies Validating 2D-Echocardiographic LV Volume Measurements

First Author and Year	Volume/Method	n	r	Regression Equation	SEE	Standard of Reference
Teicholz 1974	Ejection fraction $V = [7.0/(2.4 + D)] \times D^3$	25	0.87	Echo = 0.61 angio + 0.01 mL		Biplane LV-angio
Schiller 1979	Modified Simpson's rule Diastolic volume Systolic volume Ejection fraction	30	0.80 0.90 0.87	Echo = 0.7 angio −1 mL Echo = 0.7 angio − 2 mL Echo = angio + 5%	15 mL 8.5 mL 7.6%	
Folland 1979	Modified Simpson's rule Ejection fraction Ejection fraction	35	0.78 0.75	Angio = 1.01 echo + 0.04 Radionuclide = 0.75 echo + 0.07	9.7% 8.7%	Single-plane angio Radionuclide
Parisi 1979	Modified Simpson's rule Diastolic volume Systolic volume Ejection fraction	50	0.82 0.90 0.80	Angio = 1.08 echo + 30 mL	39 mL 29 mL 9%	Single-plane angio
Gueret 1980	Modified Simpson's rule Diastolic volume Systolic volume Ejection fraction	11	0.89 0.86 0.92	Cine = 0.88 echo + 22 mL Cine = 0.95 echo + 11 mL Cine = 1.13 echo − 7.5%	10 mL 9 mL 5%	Cineangiography in closed-chest dogs 1 hr after LAD occlusion
Silverman 1980	Biplane area-length Diastolic volume Systolic volume Ejection fraction	20	0.96 0.91 0.82	Echo = 1.05 angio − 3.64 Echo = 1.37 angio − 1.37 Echo = 9.87 angio + 0		Biplane angio
Wyatt 1980	Modified Simpson's rule 2/3 area length Area-length (cylinder) Hemiellipsoid (bullet)	21	0.98 0.97 0.97 0.97	Echo = 1.0x − 0.7 mL Echo = 1.0x − 8.9 mL Echo = 1.49x − 13.4 mL Echo = 1.25x − 11.1 mL	6.6 mL 8.6 mL 12.8 mL 10.9 mL	Directly measured fluid volume in fixed hearts
Starling 1981	Simpson's rule Diastolic rule Systolic volume Ejection fraction	70	0.80 0.88 0.90	Echo = 0.66 angio + 42 mL Echo = 0.72 angio + 18 mL Echo = 0.76 angio + 12%	34 mL 27 mL 7%	Single or biplane (n = 30) LV angio

Author/Year	Method / Parameter	n	r	Regression equation	SEE/error	Technique
Quinones 1981	Simplified method	55				
	Ejection fraction		0.93		6.7%	Radionuclide
			0.91		7.4%	Angio
Tortoledo 1983	Simplified method	52				Single-plane angio
	Diastolic volume		0.88	Angio = 1.07 echo – 7.3 mL	28 mL	
	Systolic volume		0.94	Angio = 1.0 echo + 1.3 mL	19 mL	
	Ejection fraction		0.92	Angio = 0.93 echo + 3%	7%	
Weiss 1983	Modified Simpson's rule (15–19 "slices")	52	0.97		6.6% (mean % error)	Direct volume measurement in isolated ejecting dog hearts
Erbel 1985	Simpson's rule	46				Single-plane LV angio
	Diastolic volume		0.91	Echo = 0.66 angio + 0.8 mL	26 mL	
	Systolic volume		0.94	Echo = 0.57 angio + 18 mL	19 mL	
	Ejection fraction		0.80	Echo = 0.61 angio + 13%	9%	
Zoghbi 1990	Echo-tilt method	24				Biplane angio
	Diastolic volume		0.92	Angio = 0.80 echo + 37 mL	23 mL	
	Systolic volume		0.96	Angio = 0.97 echo – 1 mL	16 mL	
	Ejection fraction		0.82	Angio = 1.17 echo – 4%	10%	
Smith 1992	TEE Simpson's rule	36				LV angio (single-plane)
	Diastolic volume		0.85	Echo = 0.75 angio + 0.2 mL	42 mL	
	Systolic volume		0.94	Echo = 0.78 angio – 3.5 mL	22 mL	
	Ejection fraction		0.85	Echo = 0.82 angio + 9%	8%	
Zile 1992	Prolate ellipsoid using constant long axis–to–short axis ratio	25				LV angio in dog model
	Diastolic volume		0.96	Echo = 1.0 angio – 1.8 mL		
	Systolic volume		0.95	Echo = 0.98 angio – 0.65 mL		

LAD, left anterior descending coronary artery.

Data sources: Teichholz et al: N Engl J Med, 291:1220–1226, 1974; Schiller et al: Circulation 60:547–555, 1979; Folland et al: Circulation 60:760–766, 1979; Parisi et al: Clin Cardiol 2:257–263, 1979; Gueret et al: Circulation 62:1308–1318, 1980; Silverman et al: Circulation 62:548–557, 1980; Wyatt et al: Circulation 61:1119–1125, 1980; Kan et al: Eur Heart J 2:337, 1981; Starling et al: Circulation 63:1075–1084, 1981; Quinones et al: Circulation 64:744–753, 1981; Tortoledo et al: Circulation 67:579–584, 1983; Weiss et al: Circulation 67:889–895, 1983; Erbel et al: Circulation 67:205–215, 1983; Zoghbi et al: J Am Coll Cardiol 15:610–617, 1990; Smith et al: J Am Coll Cardiol 19:1213–1222, 1992; Zile et al: J Am Coll Cardiol 20:986–993, 1992.

TABLE 6-3   Selected Studies Validating 3D-Echocardiographic LV Volume Measurements

First Author and Year	Method	n	r	Regression Equation	SEE	Standard of Reference
Nessly 1991	Canine model	33	0.86	Echo = 0.83 RNA + 4 mL	6 mL	RNA
Kuroda 1991	In vitro phantom					
	Pullback reconstruction		0.99	Echo = 1.1x − 10 mL	5.8 mL	True volume by weight
	Rotational reconstruction		0.99	Echo = 1.0x − 7 mL	6.5 mL	
Handschumacher 1993	Ventricular phantoms		0.99	Echo = 0.96x + 2.2 mL	2.7 mL	Direct volumes
	Gel-filled excised ventricles		0.99	Echo = 0.99x + 0.11 mL	5.9 mL	
Gopal 1993	Normal adults	15	EDV 0.92	Echo = 0.84 MRI + 22 mL	7 mL	MRI
			ESV 0.81	Echo = 0.51 MRI + 18 mL	4 mL	
Sapin 1993	Excised porcine hearts	25	0.99	y = 1.02 echo + 3.7 mL	7.1 mL	Direct volumes
Sapin 1994	Patients (mean age 48 yrs)	35	EDV 0.97		11.0 mL	LV angio
			ESV 0.98		10.2 mL	
Jiang 1995	In vitro phantoms	10	0.99		3.2–6.1 mL	Direct volumes
	Autopsy hearts with LV aneurysms	12	0.99		3.4–4.2 mL	
	Canine LV aneurysm model	19	EDV 0.99		4.3 mL	
			ESV 0.99		3.5 mL	
Gopal 1997	Patients with abnormal LV	30	EDV 0.90		31.8 mL	MRI
			ESV 0.93		24.1 mL	
Altmann 1997	Children	12	EDV 0.98		8.7 mL	MRI
			ESV 0.98		5.6 mL	
Leotta 1997	In vitro phantom	12	1.00	y = 1.00x − 0.6 mL	1.3 mL	Direct volumes
	In vitro heart	5	1.00	y = 1.02x − 1.3 mL	0.4 mL	Direct volumes
	In vivo (human)	20	0.99	3D-SV = 1.18 DOP − 17.9 mL	2.8 mL	Doppler SV

Study	Subjects	n	Correlation	Regression	Difference	Comparison
Kuehl 1998	Patients	24	EDV 0.9 ESV 0.94 EF 0.93	$y = 0.87x + 2.2$ $y = 0.96x - 0.6$ $y = 0.96x - 2.0$	23.9 17.2 7.0 mL	Angio
Mele 1998	Patients	50	EDV 0.95 ESV 0.96 EF 0.92	$y = 0.93x + 9.1$ $y = 0.94x + 4.3$ $y = 0.90x + 4.1$	15.2 11.4 6.2 mL	Angio, RNA, MRI
Nosir 1998	Patients	41	EF 0.99			RNA
Qin 2000	Patients (13 with LV aneurysms)	29	LV volumes $r = 0.97$		Mean difference −28 mL	MRI
Teupe 2001	Fixed pig hearts	20	LV volumes $r = 0.99$		3.0–5.5 mL	Anatomic volumes
Schmidt 2001	Explanted sheep hearts	11	LV volumes $r = 0.99$	$y = 0.98x + 1.31$	2.2 mL	Known volumes
Lee 2003	Patients	25	EDV 0.99 ESV 0.99 EF 0.92		11.3 mL 10.2 mL 6%	MRI
Kawai 2003	Patients	15	EDV 0.94 ESV 0.96 EF 0.93	$y = 0.82x + 5.1$	EDV 21.6 mL ESV 14.8 mL EF 7.6%	SPECT

Angio, contrast angiography; DOP, Doppler; EDV, end-diastolic volume; EF, ejection fraction; ESV, end-systolic volume; MRI, magnetic resonance imaging; RNA, radionuclide angiography; SPECT, single-photon emission computed tomography; SV, stroke volume.

Data sources: Nessly et al: J Cardiothorac Vasc Anesth 5:40–45, 1991; Kuroda et al: Echocardiography 4:475–484, 1991; Handschumacher et al: J Am Coll Cardiol 21:743–753, 1993; Gopal et al: J Am Coll Cardiol 22:258–270, 1993; Sapin et al: J Am Coll Cardiol 22:1530, 1993; Sapin et al: J Am Coll Cardiol 24:1054, 1994; Jiang et al: Circulation 91:222, 1995; Gopal et al: J Am Soc Echo 10:853, 1997; Leotta et al: J Am Soc Echo 10:830, 1997; Kuehl et al: Am Soc Echo 11:1113, 1998; Mele et al: 11:1001, 1998; Nosir et al: J Am Soc Echo 11:620, 1998; Qin et al: J Am Coll Cardiol 36:900–907, 2000; Teupe et al: Int J Cardiovasc Imaging 17:99–105, 2001; Schmidt et al: J Am Soc Echocardiogr 14:1–10, 2001; Lee et al: J Am Soc Echocardiogr 14:1001–1009, 2001; Kawai et al: J Am Soc Echo 2003; 16:110–115, 2003.

Biplane Apical

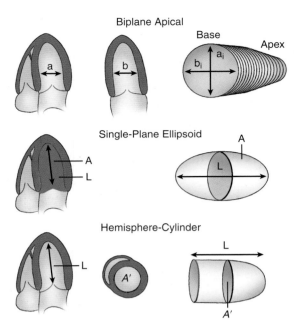

Single-Plane Ellipsoid

Hemisphere-Cylinder

Figure 6–7 Examples of three formulas for LV volume calculations showing the 2D echocardiographic views and measurements on the *left* and the geometric model on the *right*. For the biplane apical method, endocardial borders are traced in A4C and A2C views, which are used to define a series of orthogonal diameters (*a* and *b*). A "Simpson's rule" assumption based on stacked disks is used to calculate volume. The single-plane ellipsoid method uses the 2D area (*A*) and length (*L*) in a single (usually A4C) view. The hemisphere-cylinder method uses a short-axis endocardial area at the midventricular level (*A'*) and a long-axis length (*L*). For each method, both end-diastolic and end-systolic measurements are needed for calculation of end-diastolic and end-systolic volumes, respectively, and for ejection fraction determination.

images (Fig. 6–8). These borders are then used to calculate CSAs of a series of elliptical disks. End-diastolic volume is calculated from end-diastolic images and end-systolic volumes from end-systolic images. Stroke volume, then, is the difference between EDV and ESV (Eq. 6–2), while EF is calculated with Equation 6–1.

When only a four-chamber view is available, a single-plane EF can be calculated that summates a series of disks with a circular CSA. Another alternative is the area-length method, which assumes that the base of the ventricle is approximated by a cylinder and the apex by an ellipsoid, sometimes called the "bullet" formula using a long-axis length L and the area A_m of an orthogonal short-axis view at the midpapillary level:

$$\text{LV volume} = 5/6 \times A_m L \qquad (6\text{–}6)$$

In the presence of a distorted ventricular shape or regional wall motion abnormalities, these alternate methods will be less accurate, since if the region of abnormal wall motion is included in the dimension or area measurements, volumes will be overestimated and vice versa.

Left Ventricular Mass

LV mass is the total weight of the myocardium, derived by multiplying the volume of myocardium by the specific density of cardiac muscle. LV mass can be estimated from M-mode dimensions of septal thickness (ST), posterior wall thickness (PWT), and LVID_s at end-diastole as:

$$\begin{aligned} \text{LV mass} = 0.80 \\ \times [1.04(\text{ST}_d + \text{PWT}_d + \text{LVID}_d)^3 - \text{LVID}_d^3] \\ + 0.6 \text{ g} \end{aligned} \qquad (6\text{–}7)$$

On 2D or 3D echocardiography, LV mass theoretically can be determined by tracing epicardial borders to calculate the total ventricular volume (walls plus chamber), subtracting the volumes determined from endocardial border tracing, and then multiplying by the specific density of myocardium:

$$\text{LV mass} = 1.05 \text{ (total volume} - \text{chamber volume)} \qquad (6\text{–}8)$$

However, epicardial definition rarely is adequate for this approach. Instead, mean wall thickness is calculated from epicardial (A_1) and endocardial (A_2) areas in a short-axis view at the papillary muscle level (Fig. 6–9). LV mass measurements often are indexed for body size (either as body surface area or height) using gender-specific normal values (see Table 2–8).

Relative wall thickness (RWT) is a simpler measure of ventricular geometry in patients with hypertrophy that reflects the relative thickness of the walls compared to chamber size. RWT is calculated from PWT and LV internal dimension, both at end-diastole, as:

$$\text{RWT} = 2\text{PWT}_d/\text{LVID}_d \qquad (6\text{–}9)$$

Ventricular geometry can be classified based on RWT (normal < 0.42) and LV mass as:

Normal geometry—normal LV mass and normal RWT
Concentric hypertrophy—increased LV mass and increased RWT
Eccentric hypertrophy—increased LV mass with normal RWT
Concentric remodeling—normal LV mass with increased RWT

Concentric hypertrophy is typical of ventricular pressure overload due to aortic stenosis with a small chamber and thick walls, whereas eccentric hypertrophy is typical of chronic volume overload due to aortic regurgitation with a dilated chamber with normal wall thickness but an increased total weight of the ventricle. Hypertensive heart disease most often results in concentric remodeling with a normal total ventricular weight but walls that are relatively thick compared with the chamber size.

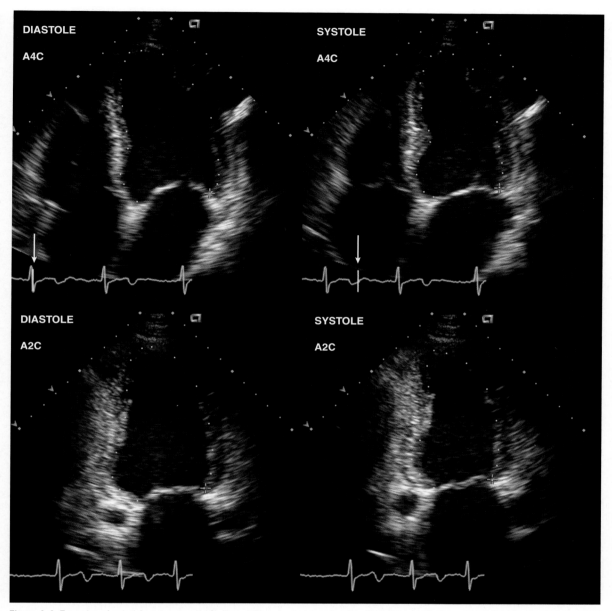

Figure 6–8 Examples of apical four-chamber (A4C) (**A** and **B**) and apical two-chamber (A2C) (**C** and **D**) views at end-diastole (onset of the QRS) (**A** and **C**) and end-systole (minimum LV area) (**B** and **D**), showing the traced endocardial borders for calculation of ventricular volumes.

Left Ventricular Wall Stress

Wall stress is the force per unit area exerted on the myocardium. Wall stress is dependent on

- Ventricular cavity radius (R)
- Pressure (P)
- Wall thickness (Th)

The basic equation for wall stress (σ) is:

$$\sigma = P \times R / 2\mathrm{Th} \qquad (6\text{--}10)$$

Wall stress can be described in three dimensions as circumferential, meridional (longitudinal), or radial (Fig. 6–10). End-systolic calculations of circumferential and meridional wall stress reflect ventricular afterload, whereas end-diastolic wall stress reflects preload. Both meridional and circumferential wall stress can be calculated from 2D echocardiographic measures of chamber size and wall thickness. Although the concept of wall stress is important in understanding ventricular function, especially in ventricular pressure or volume overall states (such as hypertension, aortic stenosis, aortic or mitral regurgitation), wall stress calculations are largely reserved for research applications as detailed in Suggested Reading 4.

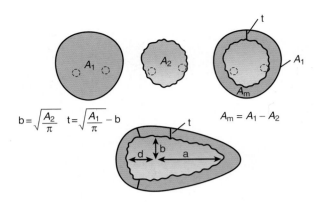

$$b = \sqrt{\frac{A_2}{\pi}} \quad t = \sqrt{\frac{A_1}{\pi}} - b \qquad A_m = A_1 - A_2$$

$$LV \; mass \; (AL) = 1.05 \; \{[{}^{5}\!/_{6} \, A_1 \, (a + d + t)] - [{}^{5}\!/_{6} \, A_2 \, (a + d)]\}$$

Figure 6–9 Schematic illustrating the technique used to calculate LV mass with the area-length method. Endocardial and epicardial borders are traced (and papillary muscles excluded). Mean wall thickness (*t*) is back-calculated from the LV cavity area (A_2) and total area (A_1), and minor axis radius (*b*). The sum *a* + *d* is equivalent to the diastolic LV cavity length, which is measured from the A4C view. *(From Otto CM: Practice of Clinical Echocardiography, 3rd ed. Philadelphia: Elsevier, 2008. Adapted from Schiller N, Shah P, Crawford M, et al: J Am Soc Echocardiogr 2:358–367, 1989.)*

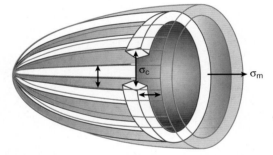

Figure 6–10 Schematic of the LV (represented as a truncated ellipsoid) illustrating the major stress vectors. Meridional stress (σ_m) is the force acting along the long axis of the LV; meridional stress opposes long axis shortening. Circumferential stress (σ_c) is the force acting in the equatorial direction; circumferential stress opposes circumferential fiber shortening, and circumferentially oriented fibers are located in the midwall of the LV. *(From Aurigemma GP, Gaasch WH, Villegas B, et al: Noninvasive assessment of left ventricular mass, chamber volume, and contractile function. Curr Probl Cardiol 20:375, 1995.)*

Technical Aspects

Endocardial Definition

Accurate identification of the ventricular endocardium is key in the echocardiographic evaluation of LV systolic function. Endocardial definition is affected by the physics of ultrasound instrumentation, by anatomic factors, and by technical factors, including the skill of the sonographer. The endocardial-ventricular cavity interface is curved from any imaging window, so the endocardium appears as a thin, bright line where it is perpendicular to the ultrasound beam (axial resolution) but as a broad, "blurred" line where the beam is parallel to the endocardial/ventricular cavity interface (lateral

resolution). As for other ultrasound targets, lateral resolution is depth dependent. In addition, there may be "dropout" of signals due to attenuation, a parallel intercept angle, acoustic shadowing, or reverberations.

Anatomically, the endocardium is not a smooth surface but has numerous trabeculations that are most prominent at the LV apex. The ultrasound beam is reflected from the inner edge of these trabeculations so that the "endocardium" identified by echocardiography differs from the "endocardium" identified by contrast ventriculography or CMR imaging, in which contrast fills these trabeculations, outlining their outer edge.

Several technical factors affect endocardial definition during image acquisition, and meticulous examination technique is needed for optimal image quality. First, acoustic access can be optimized by:

- Patient positioning
- Use of an echo stretcher with an apical cutout
- Having the patient suspend respiration
- Careful adjustment of transducer position

Instrument settings can dramatically affect image quality, including:

- Transducer frequency
- Gain
- Gray-scale settings
- Focal depth
- Tissue harmonic imaging

Endocardial borders are traced from digitally acquired images using the real-time motion of the images to aid in identification of the endocardial border during the tracing process. End-diastolic and end-systolic images are traced on the same cardiac cycle, with end-diastole defined as onset of the QRS complex and end-systole defined as minimal ventricular volume. For the apical biplane approach, the patient is positioned in a steep left lateral position, using a stretcher with an apical cutout, to avoid foreshortening the ventricular apex. A higher frequency transducer is used for optimal image quality, provided penetration is adequate, and when available the focal depth of the transducer is adjusted to the depth of interest. The sector depth and width are adjusted to maximize the size of the LV on the screen and to optimize frame rate. Tissue harmonic imaging improves endocardial definition in most patients. In addition, the patient is asked to suspend respiration, while avoiding a Valsalva maneuver, at the phase of respiration where image quality is optimal. Sometimes B-color imaging improves identification of the endocardium. When endocardial definition remains poor despite these measures, use of an intravenous contrast agent to opacify the LV may be considered.

The trained human observer remains the most accurate means for endocardial border tracing, limiting the wide application of quantitative methods because manual tracing of endocardial borders at end-diastole and end-systole in at least two views remains a tedious and time-consuming task. In many cases, identification of the endocardium requires analysis of the moving image using both the cine-loop and frame-by-frame features of the system to assist in identification of the border as the bright linear echo reflection that moves with the cardiac cycle and is spatially continuous. In the future, automatic edge detection programs or other approaches to determination of area changes may alleviate this problem.

Geometric Assumptions

In addition to the geometric assumptions of the mathematical formula, quantitation of LV volumes depends on accurate visualization of the endocardium along the entire length of the chamber. Two-dimensional views that foreshorten the LV will result in underestimation of LV length, which affects both TTE and TEE approaches. With TTE imaging, adequate apical views require a steep left lateral decubitus position with an apical cutout in the echo-stretcher mattress to visualize the true long axis of the chamber. On TEE imaging, even with adjustment of transducer position and angulation of the image plane it may not be possible to include the apex in the four-chamber and two-chamber views.

Respiratory motion and cardiac motion within the chest during the cardiac cycle further confound the geometric assumptions of LV volume calculations. The effect of respiratory motion of the heart relative to the transducer can be avoided by measuring beats at the same phase of respiration or by having the patient briefly suspend respiration during data acquisition. In some cases, optimal images are obtained when the patient suspends respiration after taking in a small breath, rather than at end-expiration. It is more difficult to correct for the motion of the heart itself using a tomographic imaging procedure. Cardiac translation (movement of the heart in the chest), rotation (movement around the long axis of the heart), and torsion (unequal rotational motion of the heart) can result in images of different segments of the LV during systole and diastole, even with a fixed image plane. While cardiac motion has only a limited effect on the accuracy of LV volume calculations, it can have a pronounced effect on quantitative evaluation of regional ventricular function, as discussed in Chapter 8.

Accuracy and Reproducibility

Qualitative comparison of LV systolic function from different studies on the same patient is facilitated by the digital cine-loop side-by-side format used in most laboratories. With this approach, a single high-quality beat is captured in digital format (either the entire cardiac cycle or just the systolic phase). The study to be compared is captured similarly with the same number of frames in the cine-loop so that when the images are played side by side, heart rates are "matched" temporally. The advantage of this approach is that the same view can be examined as long as is needed for careful qualitative (or quantitative) evaluation. This approach is particularly useful for evaluation of regional ventricular function. Of course, the influence of loading conditions on LV systolic function still must be considered when comparing studies performed at different time points in a patient's clinical course.

In most reported series intraobserver variability for LV volumes ranges from 5% to 10%. Interobserver variability is greater, ranging from 7% to 25% for ventricular volumes. Since EF is a calculated percentage, reproducibility is better, with variability of about 10%. These values are similar to reported variability for ventricular volumes and EF determined by contrast or radionuclide ventriculography. Note that variability between studies in an individual patient includes:

❐ Physiologic variability (loading condition, heart rate, volume states)
❐ Image acquisition variability (endocardial definition, image orientation)
❐ Measurement variability in tracing the endothelial borders

With optimal data a significant change between studies is a difference in EF >2%, EDV >2%, and ESV >5%.

DOPPLER EVALUATION OF LEFT VENTRICULAR SYSTOLIC FUNCTION

Stroke Volume Calculation

Doppler echocardiographic evaluation of LV systolic function usually is based on calculation of stroke volume and cardiac output (Table 6–4). Using Doppler and 2D echo data, stroke volume (in cm^3 or mL) is calculated as cross-sectional area (CSA, cm^2) of flow times the velocity-time integral (VTI in cm) of flow through that region:

$$SV = CSA \times VTI \qquad (6–11)$$

Conceptually, the LV ejects a volume of blood into the cylindrical aorta on each beat (Fig. 6–11). The base of this cylinder is the systolic CSA of the outflow tract, while its height is the distance the average blood cell traveled during ejection for that beat. This distance is expressed as the integral of the Doppler systolic velocity-time curve, since velocity is the first derivative of distance. Alternatively, this distance also can be thought of as mean velocity (cm/s) multiplied by ejection duration (seconds). Again, since the volume of a cylinder is base times height, stroke volume is CSA multiplied by the VTI.

TABLE 6–4   Selected Studies Validating Doppler Volume Flow Measurement

First Author and Year	Volume Flow Site and Method	n	r	Regression Equation	SEE	Standard of Reference
Huntsman 1983	Ascending aorta	100	0.94	DOP = 0.95x + 0.38	0.58 L/min	TD CO
Fisher 1983	Mitral leaflets	52	0.97	DOP = 0.98x + 0.02	0.23 L/min	Roller pump
Meijboom 1983	Mitral leaflets	26	0.99	DOP = 0.97x + 0.07	0.13 L/min	EM flow and roller pump
	RVOT	26	0.99	DOP = 0.96x + 0.11	0.16 L/min	Roller pump
Lewis 1984	Mitral annulus	35	0.96	TD = 0.91x + 5.1	5.9 mL	TD SV
	LVOT	39	0.95	TD = 0.91x + 7.8	6.4 mL	TD SV
Stewart 1985	Mitral leaflets	29	0.97	DOP = 0.98x + 0.3	0.3 L/min	Roller pump
	Aortic annulus	33	0.98	DOP = 1.06x + 0.2	0.3 L/min	Roller pump
	Pulmonary annulus	30	0.93	DOP = 0.89x + 0.4	0.5 L/min	Roller pump
Bouchard 1987	Aortic leaflets	41	0.95	DOP = 0.97x + 1.7	7 mL	TD SV
Dittmann 1987	Mitral annulus	40	0.86	DOP = 0.88 + 1.75	0.80 L/min	TD CO
	LVOT (M-mode)	40	0.93	DOP = 0.94x + 0.44	0.59 L/min	TD CO
DeZuttere 1988	Mitral orifice (instantaneous)	30	0.91	DOP = 0.92x + 0.35	0.53 L/min	TD CO
Hoit 1988	Mitral leaflets	48	0.93	DOP = 1.1x − 0.45	0.36 L/min	TD CO
Otto 1988	LVOT (proximal to aortic stenosis)	52	0.91	DOP = 1.0x + 0.03	0.25 L/min	EM flow and timed collection
Burwash 1993	LVOT (proximal to aortic stenosis)	75	0.86	CO = 0.92 DOP + 0.26	0.50 L/min	Transit-time flow probe
Lefrant 2000	Ascending aorta	58 patients (314 paired data)	0.84	DOP = 0.84 TD + 1.39		TD CO
Gentles 2001	Ascending aorta	20 children with complex CHD	0.96	DOP = 0.98 Fick − 0.08		Fick CO
Chandraratna 2002	Pulmonary artery (continuous)	50 ICU patients	0.92	DOP = 0.93 TD + 0.60	0.7 L/min	TD CO

CHD, congenital heart disease; CO, cardiac output; DOP, Doppler; EM, electromagnetic flowmeter; LVOT, left ventricular outflow tract; TD, thermodilution.

Data sources: Huntsman et al: Circulation 67:593–601, 1983; Fisher et al: Circulation 67:872–877, 1983; Meijboom et al: Circulation 68:437–445, 1983; Lewis et al: Circulation 70:425–431, 1984; Stewart et al: J Am Coll Cardiol 6:653–662, 1985; Bouchard et al: J Am Coll Cardiol 9:75–83, 1987; Dittman et al: J Am Coll Cardiol 10:818–823, 1987; DeZuttere et al: J Am Coll Cardiol 11:343–350, 1988; Hoit et al: Am J Cardiol 62:131–135, 1988; Otto et al: Circulation 78:435–441, 1988; Burwash et al: Am J Physiol 265 (Heart Circulation Physiol 34): 1734, 1993; Lefrant et al: Intensive Care Med 26:693–697, 2000; Gentles et al: J Ultrasound Med 20:365–370, 2001; Chandraratna et al: J Am Soc Echocardiogr 15:1381–1386, 2002.

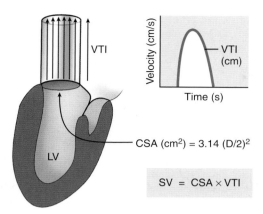

$$CSA\ (cm^2) = 3.14\ (D/2)^2$$

$$SV = CSA \times VTI$$

Figure 6–11 Doppler stroke volume (SV) calculation. The cross-sectional area (CSA) of flow is calculated as a circle based on a 2D echo diameter (D) measurement. The length of the cylinder of blood ejected through this CSA on a single beat is the velocity time integral (VTI) of the Doppler curve. Stroke volume (SV) then is calculated as CSA × VTI.

This approach to stroke volume calculation depends on several basic assumptions:

- ❒ Accurate cross-sectional flow area measurement
- ❒ Laminar flow with spatially "flat" flow velocity profile
- ❒ Parallel intercept angle between Doppler beam and direction of blood flow
- ❒ Velocity and diameter measurements made at the same anatomic site

First, the area must be measured accurately. Typically, diameter is measured and 2D area calculated as $\pi(D/2)^2$ based on the assumption of a circular geometry. Deviations from a circular geometry or changes in area during the flow period will result in inaccuracies unless appropriate corrections are included in the calculations. Of note, small errors in 2D diameter measurements become large errors in cross-sectional area because radius (half the diameter) is squared in the calculations. Using a transducer orientation and instrument settings that maximize image quality, performing measurements based on axial (rather than lateral) resolution, performing diameter measurements in two orthogonal planes (when possible), and averaging several beats can help minimize this source of error.

Second, the pattern of flow is assumed to be laminar, and the spatial flow profile across the flow stream is assumed to be relatively flat. These assumptions ensure that the velocity curve represents the spatial (as well as temporal) average flow in that region. The validity of the assumption of laminar flow in the great vessels and across normal cardiac valves is demonstrated by the narrow band of velocities and smooth spectral signal seen on pulsed Doppler echo recordings. A flat flow profile also is a reasonable assumption at the inlet to the great vessels and across the valve planes due to the effects of geometric convergence and acceleration. A flat flow

velocity profile can be confirmed by moving the sample volume across the flow stream in two orthogonal views to demonstrate uniform velocities at the center and the edges of the flow stream.

Third, the Doppler signal is assumed to have been recorded at a parallel intercept angle to flow, resulting in an accurate velocity measurement (based on a cos θ = 1 in the Doppler equation). In practical terms, the sonographer aligns the Doppler beam in the presumed direction of flow and then carefully moves the ultrasound beam across the image plane and in the elevational plane to obtain the highest velocity signal, indicating the most parallel alignment with flow. Note that the optimal window for Doppler interrogation is when the ultrasound beam and flow stream are parallel, while the optimal window for diameter measurement is when the ultrasound beam and tissue/blood interfaces are perpendicular.

Fourth, it is crucial that the diameter and velocity measurements be made at the same anatomic site, since the CSA and flow velocity curves must be temporally and spatially congruent for accurate volume flow rate calculations. As the CSA of flow narrows or expands, flow velocity will increase or decrease correspondingly so that conjoining information from two different anatomic sites will result in erroneous stroke volume data. Similarly, dynamic changes in stroke volume occur with changes in heart rate, loading conditions, exercise, etc. so that measurements made at disparate times cannot be combined. In clinical practice, diameter and velocity recordings are made in close sequence and are repeated if there is any question of an interval physiologic change.

Sites for Stroke Volume Measurement

Stroke volume can be measured by this approach at any intracardiac site where both area and the flow velocity integral can be recorded given the assumptions of laminar flow and a flat flow profile.

Left Ventricular Outflow

LV stroke volume can be measured in the aorta either at the aortic valve leaflet tips or in the ascending aorta. While some would argue which anatomic level (ascending aorta or leaflet tips) should be used, measurements at each of these levels can be accurate provided that diameter and flow velocity are measured at the same anatomic site. Ascending aortic diameter is measured from a parasternal long-axis view, and the flow velocity curve is recorded from either an apical or a suprasternal notch window. If continuous-wave Doppler ultrasound is used, the highest velocities along the path of the beam will be recorded, so the narrowest segment of the aorta (the sinotubular junction) is used for diameter measurements. Alternatively, a circular orifice area can be calculated from an M-mode diameter of aortic leaflet opening, and pulsed Doppler can be used to record the flow velocity in the aortic orifice itself. Note that if aortic valve disease is present, stroke volume measurement in the ascending aorta will be inaccurate due to nonlaminar flow distal to the valve.

Measurement of stroke volume in the LV outflow tract, at the aortic annulus just proximal to the valve leaflets, offers the advantages that (1) flow remains laminar proximal to a stenosis (allowing transaortic stroke volume calculations in patients with aortic valve disease) and (2) the needed data can be recorded in nearly all patients. LV outflow tract diameter is measured in a parasternal long-axis view parallel and immediately adjacent to the aortic valve, in midsystole, from the white/black edge of the septal endocardium to the black/white edge of the anterior mitral leaflet (Fig. 6–12). Pulsed Doppler is used from an apical approach to record the velocity curve, using the closing click of the aortic valve to ensure that the sample volume is located at the annulus (the same site as the diameter measurement). The small region of flow convergence proximal to the narrowed aortic valve is avoided by moving the sample volume slightly apically until a narrow spectral width is seen at the velocity peak.

On TEE imaging, outflow tract diameter is measured in a long-axis view with improved accuracy due to the higher resolution images on TEE. LV outflow velocity sometimes may be recorded from a transgastric apical view or, starting from a transgastric short-axis view, in a long-axis view just medial to the two-chamber view used for LV dimension measurements. However, it is difficult to ensure a parallel intercept angle between the ultrasound beam and LV outflow so that underestimation of stroke volume is likely.

Mitral Valve

Transmitral stroke volume calculations assume that the mitral annulus is the limiting cross-sectional flow area, with the leaflets moving passively in response to the flow stream. Transmitral stroke volume is calculated as the product of the cross-sectional annulus area and the VTI of flow recorded at the mitral annulus level. On TEE imaging, transmitral flow rate is accurately and easily measured in the four-chamber view with the pulsed Doppler sample volume placed at the annulus level and diameter measured from the 2D image (Fig. 6–13). Although the mitral annulus is most accurately described as a curved ellipse, with the major (and apical) axis seen in the four-chamber view and the minor (and basal) axis seen in the long-axis view, for most clinical applications the mitral annulus is assumed to be circular. The mitral annulus diameter can be measured in a parasternal long-axis view, which has the advantage of using axial resolution, which improves accuracy but the disadvantage of ambiguity in the correct site for measurement because the site of Doppler recording must be estimated. Alternatively, diameter can be measured in the apical four-chamber view, which has the advantage that diameter can be measured on the same image that displays the sample volume, ensuring a correct measurement site, but the disadvantage of lateral resolution, which limits the accuracy of the measurement.

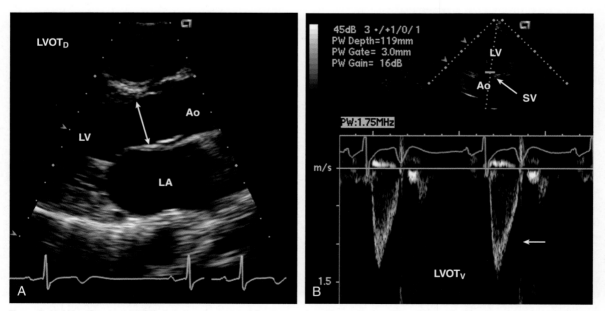

Figure 6–12 LV outflow tract (LVOT) diameter measurement from a parasternal long-axis view (**A**) and the pulsed Doppler recording of LV outflow just proximal to the aortic valve from an apical approach (**B**) for stroke volume calculation. The Ao valve closing click (*arrow*) on the outflow tract velocity recording ensures that the sample volume (SV) location is immediately adjacent to the valve, corresponding with the site of outflow tract diameter measurement.

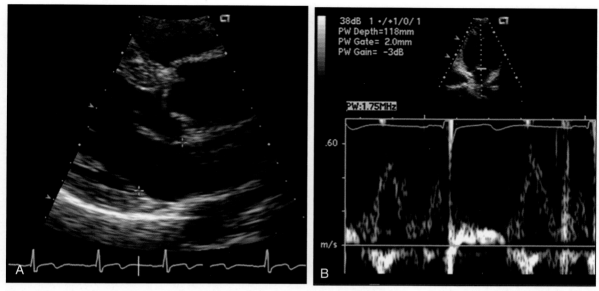

Figure 6–13 Transmitral stroke volume is calculated from mitral annulus area in diastole multiplied by the velocity time integral (VTI) of flow at the annulus. In this example, annulus diameter (*left*) is 3.4 cm, so the circular cross-sectional area is 9.1 cm^2. The VTI of transmitral flow is 9.8 cm yielding a stroke volume of 89 mL or a cardiac output of 6.7 L/min at a heart rate of 75 beats/min.

Right Side of the Heart

In the right side of the heart, stroke volume can be calculated by analogous methods in the pulmonary artery or across the tricuspid valve (Fig. 6–14). In adult patients, use of the pulmonary artery site on TTE imaging often is limited by poor image quality resulting in unobtainable or inaccurate pulmonary artery diameter measurements. However, from a TEE approach, pulmonary artery flow and diameter often can be measured using a very high transducer position looking from the pulmonary artery bifurcation toward the pulmonic valve.

Differences in Transvalvular Volume Flow Rates

In a normal heart, stroke volume across each of the four valves is equal, and measurement at more than one site only serves as an internal accuracy check. However, in the presence of valvular regurgitation or an intracardiac shunt, calculation of stroke volume at two intracardiac sites allows quantitation of the degree of regurgitation or pulmonic-to-systemic shunt ratio, as detailed in Chapters 12 and 17.

Other Doppler Measures of Left Ventricular Systolic Function

Ejection Acceleration Times

In addition to stroke volume calculations, the shape of the Doppler ejection curve may provide information about ventricular function. When systolic function is normal, the isovolumic contraction period is

short, and the rate of pressure rise in early systole is rapid. These features are reflected in the Doppler velocity curve, which shows a short isovolumic contraction time, a rapid acceleration of blood in early systole, and a short time interval from the onset of flow to maximum velocity. With impaired LV systolic function, the isovolumic contraction time (also known as the pre-ejection period) becomes progressively longer, the rate of acceleration diminishes, and the time to maximum velocity increases, with all these changes mirrored in the Doppler velocity curve. In addition to measuring these variables at rest, some centers have found evaluation of aortic ejection curves with exercise useful in detection of LV systolic dysfunction.

Rate of Ventricular Pressure Rise (dP/dt)

When mitral regurgitation is present, the continuous-wave Doppler velocity curve indicates the instantaneous pressure difference between the LV and the LA in systole, assuming a constant intercept angle between the mitral regurgitant jet and the ultrasound beam. Given the rapid rate of rise of LV pressure with normal systolic function (and the low LA pressure), mitral regurgitation typically shows a rapid rise to maximum velocity as per the Bernoulli equation. If the rate of rise in ventricular pressure is reduced due to LV systolic dysfunction, the rate of increase in velocity of the mitral regurgitant jet also is reduced. For example, in patients with premature ventricular beats, the altered contractility of the premature beat will be evidenced by a marked difference in the rate of velocity increase of the mitral regurgitant jet. The slope of the mitral regurgitant jet can be

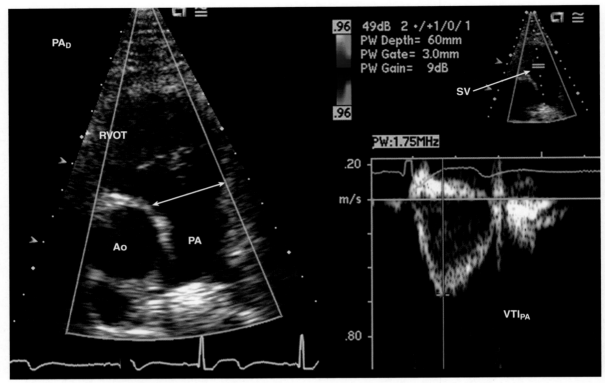

Figure 6–14 PA diameter measurement in a parasternal RV outflow view (*left*), and pulsed Doppler PA flow recorded from a parasternal approach (*right*) for transpulmonic stroke volume calculation.

quantitated as the rate of change in pressure over time (*dP/dt*) by measuring the time interval between the mitral regurgitant jet velocity at 1 and at 3 m/s (Fig. 6–15). At each velocity the corresponding pressure gradient is $4v^2$ per the Bernoulli equation. Then,

$$dP/dt = [4(3)^2] - [4(1)^2]/\text{time interval}$$
$$= 32 \text{ mm Hg/time interval} \qquad (6\text{--}12)$$

A normal *dP/dt* is greater than 1000 mm Hg/s; a lower value reflects impaired LV contractility. Of course, the calculation of *dP/dt* can be performed only when a recordable mitral regurgitant jet is present and assumes a constant (and parallel) intercept angle between the mitral regurgitant jet and the ultrasound beam during the measurement period.

Myocardial Performance Index

The ratio of total LV isovolumic time to ejection time has been proposed as a global measure of systolic and diastolic function which can be applied to either the LV or RV. The myocardial performance (or Tei) index (MPI) is calculated as the sum of the duration of the iso-volumic relaxation (IVRT) and contraction (IVCT) times, divided by the systolic ejection period (SEP):

$$\text{MPI} = (\text{IVRT} + \text{IVCT/SEP}) \qquad (6\text{--}13)$$

The normal MPI is about 0.4 with higher values, typically ranging from 0.6 to > 1.0, indicating ventricular dysfunction either due to systolic dysfunction (with a prolonged IVCT) and/or diastolic dysfunction (prolonged IVRT). Although the MPI is not affected by abnormal ventricular geometry or changes in heart rate, it is affected by preload and afterload. MPI can be calculated using time intervals measured from conventional Doppler or, preferably, from tissue Doppler recordings. This index is widely used in pediatric heart disease but is less useful in adult populations (see Suggested Readings 13 to 15).

Limitations and Technical Considerations

The major limitation of Doppler evaluation of LV systolic function in adults is accurate diameter measurement for CSA calculations. While Doppler velocity curves can be recorded consistently with little interobserver measurement variability (2% to 5%), the variability of 2D diameter measurements is significantly greater (8% to 12%). For Doppler velocity data, the major source of measurement variability is data recording, given the critical importance of obtaining a parallel intercept angle between the ultrasound beam and the flow of interest. For 2D diameters, the major source of variability is measuring the 2D

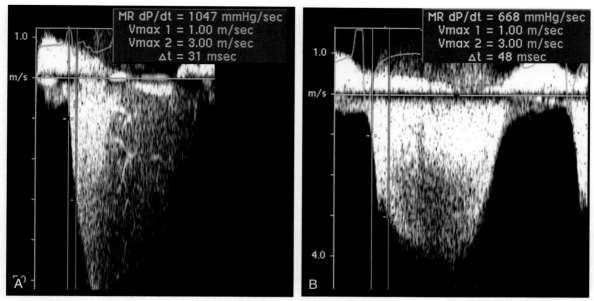

Figure 6–15 LV *dP/dt* is calculated from the MR-jet based on the interval between 1 and 3 m/s on the velocity curve with the scale expanded to optimize the accuracy of the measurement. Examples of normal ventricular systolic function (*dP/dt* > 1000 mm Hg/s) (**A**) and the slow rate of rise in MR velocity in a patient with dilated cardiomyopathy (**B**), corresponding to a *dP/dt* of 668 mm Hg/s, as shown by the parallel vertical lines.

images, particularly when image quality is suboptimal or when lateral resolution limits accurate border recognition. Despite these potential limitations, Doppler measurement of stroke volume has been well validated in a variety of clinical and research settings.

Measurement of *dP/dt* is limited by the need for enough mitral regurgitation to generate a Doppler signal with a well-defined velocity curve. Changes during ejection in the intercept angle between the ultrasound beam and the regurgitant jet will result in an erroneous measurement, since the assumption that cos θ = 1 in the Doppler equation will not be valid.

ECHO APPROACH TO RIGHT VENTRICULAR SYSTOLIC FUNCTION

Imaging of the Right Ventricle

Qualitative Evaluation

The RV is evaluated qualitatively by TTE 2D imaging (Fig. 6–16) from several different windows:

- ❑ Parasternal long- and short-axis
- ❑ RV inflow
- ❑ Apical four-chamber
- ❑ Subcostal four-chamber

On TEE imaging, similar views are obtained including the high TEE four-chamber view, a TEE short-axis view obtained by rotating the image plane to about 90° and the transgastric RV inflow view.

In each view on either TTE or TEE imaging, evaluation of the RV includes:

- ❑ Area of the chamber (relative to the LV chamber)
- ❑ Shape of the RV cavity
- ❑ Wall thickness
- ❑ Motion of the RV free wall
- ❑ Ventricular septal curvature and motion

The normal shape of the RV is complex in three dimensions, with the inflow segment located medial to the LV, the body and apex located anterior to the LV, and the RV outflow tract located superior to the LV and aortic valve. There is no simple geometric shape that approximates the RV chamber; rather, it is "wrapped around" the LV in a U-shaped fashion. Since echocardiographic long- and short-axis views are oriented with respect to the LV, the RV may appear abnormal in some individuals due to the position of the RV relative to the image plane. This occurs most often in parasternal views, where the RV may be imaged in an oblique orientation. Both subcostal and apical four-chamber windows tend to offer more consistent views of the RV, with the RV appearing somewhat triangular in shape with a broad base and narrow apex. The RV apex is slightly closer to the base than the LV apex (by about one third of the LV length) in normal individuals. On TEE imaging, RV size is best evaluated in the four-chamber view.

With RV dilation the RV outflow tract may be enlarged in the parasternal and TEE long-axis view. On apical, subcostal views and TEE transgastric views, the RV chamber will be larger and the RV apex is either closer to or encompasses the LV apex. The degree of RV dilation is best evaluated in the apical or subcostal four-chamber view in relation to

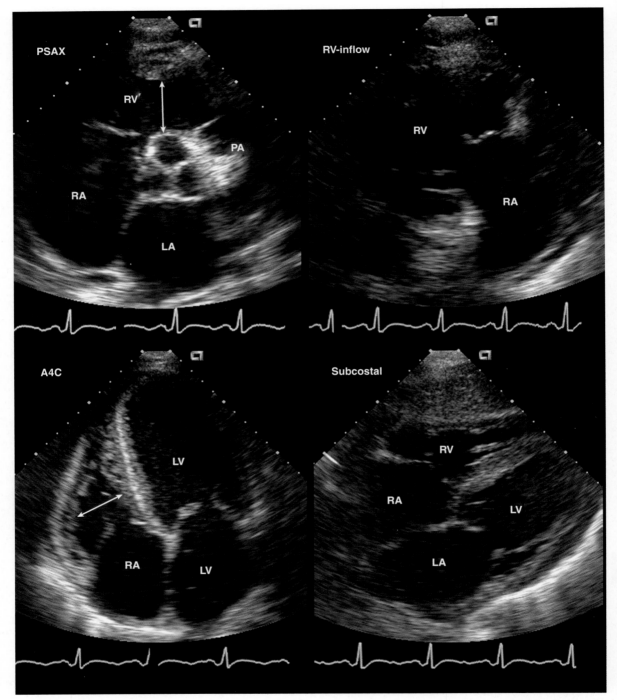

Figure 6–16 Evaluation of RV size and systolic function is based on multiple image planes including parasternal short-axis (PSAX) (**A**), RV inflow (**B**), apical four-chamber (A4C) with optimization of the RV (**C**), and subcostal (SC) four-chamber (**D**) views. Measurements of RV outflow diameter and mid-chamber dimension at end-diastole are shown.

the size of the LV, taking into consideration any abnormalities in LV size. RV size is described as:

❏ Normal (smaller than LV with RV apex more basal than LV apex)

❏ Mildly dilated (enlarged but a 2D area < LV area)
❏ Moderately dilated (RV = LV area)
❏ Severely dilated (RV > LV area)

RV dilation is the normal response of the ventricle to volume overload, and its presence mandates a careful search for etiology, such as an atrial septal defect, tricuspid regurgitation, or pulmonic regurgitation. Pressure overload of the RV also leads to dilation, so that evaluation of pulmonary pressures is mandatory when the RV is abnormal.

RV systolic function is evaluated qualitatively as:

❏ Normal
❏ Mildly reduced
❏ Moderately reduced
❏ Severely reduced

When ventricular systolic function is normal, the relative function of the two ventricles can be compared. When LV systolic function is depressed, the severity of LV dysfunction is used as an index of RV function; for example, a normal RV appears hyperdynamic when compared to an LV with reduced systolic function. If both ventricles have a similar qualitative pattern of contraction, the degree of RV dysfunction is similar to the degree of LV dysfunction.

RV hypertrophy is manifested as an RV free wall thickness >0.5 cm. RV wall thickness is best measured by 2D or 2D-guided M-mode in a subcostal four-chamber view at the tricuspid chordal level at the peak of the R wave on ECG. Epicardial fat and myocardial trabeculations are excluded from this measurement. The presence of RV hypertrophy suggests RV pressure overload and prompts a search for evidence of elevated pulmonary pressures or pulmonic valve stenosis. Increased thickness of the RV free wall also may be seen in some infiltrative cardiomyopathies or in hypertrophic cardiomyopathy.

Quantitative Evaluation

Quantitative evaluation of RV systolic function by 2D/M-mode echo is difficult. Standard geometric formulas for volume calculations have only limited applicability given the shape of the RV, and while 3D reconstructions have been shown to be accurate, the need for tedious endocardial border tracing and extensive data analysis has restricted its use to the research setting. However, simple linear RV dimension measurements can be made from TTE or TEE 2D images at end-diastole including:

❏ Four-chamber view basal diameter
❏ Four-chamber view mid-ventricular diameter
❏ Four-chamber view base to apex length
❏ Short-axis view RV outflow tract diameter
❏ Short-axis view pulmonic valve annulus diameter

RV systolic function can be evaluated based on the motion of the tricuspid annulus toward the apex in systole. A reduction in annular motion to less than 1.5 cm (normal 1.5–2.0 cm) indicates a significant reduction in systolic function. Other approaches to quantitative evaluation of RV systolic function include fractional area change from diastole to systole, and tissue Doppler imaging of tricuspid annulus motion.

Technical Considerations

Evaluation of RV systolic function on TTE imaging may be limited by poor ultrasound tissue penetration in some individuals. With careful patient positioning and a search from multiple windows the RV usually can be visualized, but endocardial definition may be suboptimal. If clinically indicated, TEE echo offers superior images of the RV both in the high esophageal four-chamber view and from a transgastric approach.

Patterns of Ventricular Septal Motion

The interventricular septum functions as part of the LV in the normal heart. During diastole the LV is circular in a short-axis view, with the normal septal curvature convex toward the RV and concave toward the LV. With the onset of systole, the septal myocardium thickens, and the septal endocardium moves toward the center of the LV such that at end-systole the short-axis image shows a circular LV chamber.

A number of cardiac disorders alter the pattern of ventricular septal motion, the most prominent being RV pressure and volume overload. The basic principle underlying the pattern of septal motion with RV dilation or hypertrophy is that the septum moves toward the center of mass of the entire heart. Normally, the center of cardiac mass coincides with the center of the LV. When RV and LV masses are equal, septal motion will be "flat" (on M-mode) or minimal (on 2D echo). When RV mass exceeds LV mass, the septum moves "paradoxically" anterior in systole (on M-mode) and flattens or reverses its curvature in diastole (on 2D echo) (Fig. 6–17).

On 2D echocardiography, pressure overload of the RV (increased mass due to increased wall thickness with a nondilated chamber) results in a leftward shift of septal motion throughout the cardiac cycle with the maximum reversed curvature at end-systole. With predominant RV volume overload, the maximum reversed curvature is seen in mid-diastole with normalization of curvature in systole. With increased RV mass due to volume overload, the additional factor of increased RV filling and emptying accentuates the diastolic reverse motion of the septum (due to rapid RV diastolic filling), resulting in a D shape of the LV chamber in early diastole, with the reversed curvature of the septum persisting throughout diastole. Anterior motion with systole may appear less prominent than with isolated pressure overload as the septum moves from its abnormal diastolic

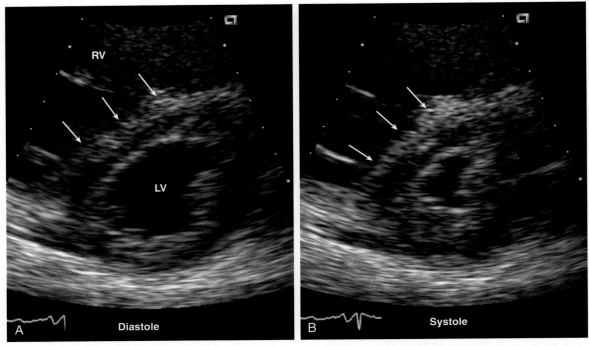

Figure 6–17 Example of abnormal septal motion in a patient with RV pressure overload due to primary pulmonary hypertension. The diastolic image (**A**) in a parasternal short-axis view shows a markedly dilated RV with flattening of the normal septal contour (*arrows*). The systolic image (**B**) shows persistent flattening of the septal contour, consistent with RV pressure overall.

position back toward the center of the heart, resulting in a more convex curve relative to the RV chamber. Often, the observation of abnormal septal motion during the examination is the first clue of RV pressure and/or volume overload.

Other abnormalities that affect the pattern of ventricular septal motion are summarized in Figure 6–18. Conduction defects affect the pattern of motion by altering the sequence of RV and LV contraction. Valvular disease can affect the timing of RV versus LV diastolic filling, particularly in early diastole. Pericardial tamponade or constriction results in a fixed total cardiac volume so that respiratory changes in RV filling result in respiratory shifts in the pattern of septal motion.

An abnormal pattern of septal motion may be appreciated on 2D imaging; however, M-mode echo offers more detailed time resolution for studying the pattern of motion. Abnormal septal motion rarely is diagnostic in and of itself, but it may raise a diagnostic possibility that had not been considered previously or may support a suspected diagnosis. For example, a pattern of paradoxical septal motion in association with RV and right atrial (RA) enlargement suggests the possibility of an atrial septal defect. This possibility then can be specifically excluded (or confirmed) during the echocardiographic examination. Another example is the patient with a pericardial effusion; in this

situation a changing pattern of septal motion with respiration supports a diagnosis of tamponade physiology.

Pulmonary Artery Pressure and Resistance Estimates

Clinically, one of the most important quantitative parameters of RV systolic function is an estimate of pulmonary artery pressure (PAP). Pulmonary hypertension often occurs in response to chronic left-sided heart diseases, such as mitral stenosis, mitral regurgitation, cardiomyopathy, and ischemic cardiac disease. Knowledge of the degree of pulmonary pressure elevation is critical in patient management (Table 6–5).

Tricuspid Regurgitant Jet

The most reliable method for estimating pulmonary systolic pressure noninvasively is based on measurement of the velocity in the tricuspid regurgitant jet. This velocity V_{TR} reflects the RV to RA pressure difference ΔP, as stated in the Bernoulli equation (Fig. 6–19):

$$\Delta P_{RV-RA} = 4(V_{TR})^2 \qquad (6\text{–}14)$$

When added to an estimate of right atrial pressure (RAP), RV systolic pressure (RVP) is obtained:

$$RVP = \Delta P_{RV-RA} + RAP \qquad (6\text{–}15)$$

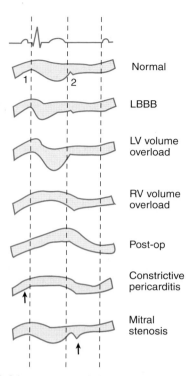

Figure 6–18 Schematic diagram of different patterns of septal motion on M-mode echocardiography. The normal pattern is characterized by systolic brief anterior motion (1) followed by posterior motion and myocardial thickening. In diastole, a small diastolic dip (2) following mitral valve opening may be seen. Left bundle branch block (LBBB) is characterized by systolic rapid downward septal motion. LV volume overload results in exaggerated septal (and posterior wall) motion. RV volume overload results in paradoxical anterior motion of the septum in systole. A similar pattern is seen in patients after cardiac surgery (Post-op). Constrictive pericarditis is characterized by anterior motion of the septum with atrial filling (before the QRS), while mitral stenosis typically shows a prominent early diastolic dip.

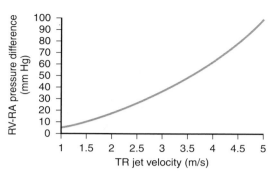

Figure 6–19 Relationship between the velocity in the tricuspid regurgitant (TR) jet and the RV-RA pressure difference as calculated with the simplified Bernoulli relationship.

In the absence of pulmonic stenosis (which is rare in adults), RV systolic pressure equals pulmonary artery systolic pressure, so that

$$PAP_{systolic} = 4(V_{TR})^2 + RAP \qquad (6\text{–}16)$$

as diagrammed in Figure 6–20.

This method has been shown to be highly accurate compared with invasive measurements of pulmonary pressure over a wide range of values (Table 6–6). Of course, the reliability of this approach is dependent on obtaining a parallel intercept angle between the tricuspid regurgitant jet and the ultrasound beam. Most often the apical or RV inflow view yields the highest velocity signal given careful angulation of the ultrasound beam in three dimensions (Fig. 6–21). Occasionally, the highest velocity tricuspid regurgitant jet is recorded from a subcostal approach. Although this

TABLE 6–5 Doppler Echo Methods for Pulmonary Artery Pressure Estimation		
Method	**Advantages**	**Potential Limitations**
TR jet: $PA_{systolic} = 4(V_{TR})^2 + RAP$	Accurate Measurable in a high percentage of patients overall (90%)	Nonparallel intercept angle between jet and ultrasound beam Misidentification of jet signal RAP estimate needed Presence of pulmonic stenosis Inadequate signal in some patients with chronic lung disease
PA flow: Time to peak velocity	Readily measured in nearly all patients, including patients with chronic lung disease Estimates *mean* PAP	Skewed flow profile in PA Measurement variability
PR ED velocity: $PA_{diastolic} = 4(V_{PR})^2 + RAP$	Reflects pulmonary diastolic pressure Adequate signal in 85% of patients Can be recorded continuously with a transthoracic transducer	Nonparallel intercept angle between jet and ultrasound beam RAP estimate needed

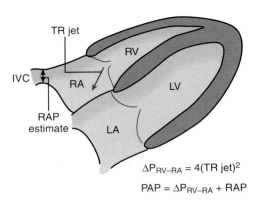

$$\Delta P_{RV-RA} = 4(TR\ jet)^2$$

$$PAP = \Delta P_{RV-RA} + RAP$$

Figure 6–20 Pulmonary artery pressure (PAP) can be calculated noninvasively based on the velocity in the TR-jet and the respiratory variation in inferior vena cava (IVC) size as an estimate of RA pressure (RAP).

method requires the presence of tricuspid regurgitation, this rarely is a limitation, since about 90% of normal individuals and patients have some degree of tricuspid regurgitation.

The same concept can be applied to the pulmonic regurgitant velocity curve. The end-diastolic pulmonic regurgitant velocity reflects the pulmonary artery to right ventricular end-diastolic pressure gradient per the Bernoulli equation. When added to an estimate of RA pressure, this provides a noninvasive estimate of diastolic pulmonary pressure (Fig. 6–22).

RA pressure is best estimated from evaluation of the inferior vena cava during respiration (Fig. 6–23). From a subcostal window, this segment of the inferior vena cava is imaged during quiet respiration. If the inferior vena cava diameter is normal (<7 cm) and

TABLE 6–6 Selected Studies Validating Noninvasive Pulmonary Artery Pressure Measurement

First Author and Year	Method	n	r	Regression Equation	SEE
Pulmonary Artery Pressure					
Kitabatake 1983	Time to peak flow (RVOT)	33	−0.88	Log(mean PAP) = 0.0068 (AcT) + 2.1 mm Hg	—
Stevenson 1989	TR jet Time to peak flow (PA) IVRT PR	50	0.96 0.63 0.97 0.96		6.9 mm Hg 16.4 mm Hg 5.4 mm Hg 4.5 mm Hg
Yock 1984	TR jet	62	0.95	DOP RV-RA ΔP = 1.03 ΔP + 0.71 mm Hg	7 mm Hg
Berger 1985	TR jet	69	0.97	Systolic PAP = 1.23 (DOP ΔP) − 0.09 mm Hg	4.9 mm Hg
Currie 1985	TR jet	127	0.96	DOP RV-RA ΔP = 0.88 ΔP + 2.2 mm Hg	7 mm Hg
Lee 1989	PR	29	0.94	Diastolic PAP (echo) = 0.95 (cath) − 1.0 mm Hg	Mean difference: 3.3 ± 2.2 mm Hg
Chandraratna 2002	PR	50	0.91	DOP = 0.82 Inv + 0.96	3.3 mm Hg
Pulmonary Vascular Resistance					
Gurudevan 2007	Systolic velocity tricuspid annulus (tS_m)	50	−0.71	PVR = 3698 − 1227 × ln (tS_m) dyne s cm^{-5}	tS_m > 10 has a sensitivity of 80% and specificity of 100% for PVR > 1000 dyne s cm^{-5}.
Abbas 2003	V_{TR}/VTI_{RVOT}	44	0.93	PVR = (V_{TR}/VTI_{RVOT}) × 10 + 0.16	SD 0.0 ± 0.41 Wood units
Farzaneh-Far 2008	V_{TR}/VTI_{RVOT}	22	0.70	(V_{TR}/VTI_{RVOT}) > 0.12 predicts PVR > 1.5 Wood units.	Sensitivity 100% Specificity 86%

AcT, acceleration time; DOP, Doppler; IVRT, isovolumic relaxation time; PAP, pulmonary artery pressure; PR, pulmonic regurgitation; PVR, pulmonary vascular resistance.

Data sources: Kitabatake et al: Circulation 68:302–309, 1983; Stevenson et al: J Am Soc Echocardiogr 2:157–171, 1989; Yock and Popp: Circulation 70:657–662, 1984; Berger et al: J Am Coll Cardiol 6:359–365, 1985; Currie et al: J Am Coll Cardiol 6:750–756, 1985; Lee et al: Am J Cardiol 64:1366–1370, 1989; Chandraratna et al: J Am Soc Echo 15:1381–1386, 2002; Gurudevan SV: J Am Soc Echocardiogr 20:1167–1171, 2007; Abbas et al: J Am Coll Cardiol 41:1021–1027, 2003; Farzaneh-Far et al: Am J Cardiol 101:259–262, 2008.

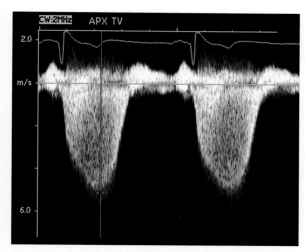

Figure 6–21 Tricuspid regurgitant jet in a patient with severe pulmonary hypertension. The maximum jet velocity of 5 m/s corresponds to a 100 mm Hg pressure difference between the RV and RA in systole.

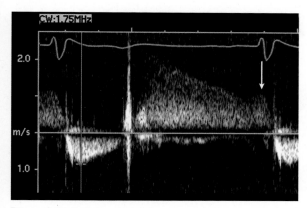

Figure 6–22 Pulmonic regurgitation recorded from a parasternal approach with continuous-wave Doppler shows an end-diastolic velocity of about 1 m/s, indicating low diastolic pulmonary pressures.

the segment adjacent to the RA collapses by at least 50% with respiration, then RA pressure is equal to normal intrathoracic pressures (i.e., 5–10 mm Hg). Failure to collapse with respiration and/or dilation of the inferior vena cava and hepatic veins is associated with higher RA pressures (Table 6–7). When no response is noted with normal respiration, the patient is asked to "sniff." This generates a sudden decrease in intrathoracic pressure, normally resulting in a decrease in inferior vena cava diameter.

Pulmonary Artery Velocity Curve

Another approach to estimating pulmonary pressure is based on the shape of the pulmonary artery Doppler velocity curve. Comparison of the normal LV and RV ejection curves reveals that LV ejection shows very rapid acceleration with a short time from flow onset to maximum velocity, whereas RV ejection shows a slower acceleration, a longer time from onset of flow to peak flow, and a more "rounded" velocity curve. As pulmonary vascular resistance (PVR) increases, the shape of the RV ejection curve more closely approximates the LV ejection curve, suggesting that the shapes of these velocity curves are related to the downstream resistance or impedance.

The time to peak velocity estimates of pulmonary pressure are not as reliable as tricuspid regurgitant jet estimates for two reasons. First, this method depends on measurement of a relatively short time interval, so measurement error is high and reproducibility is low. Second, the spatial flow velocity profile in the pulmonary artery is skewed, with higher acceleration and velocity along the inner edge of the curvature. Even when the sample volume appears positioned in the center of the vessel in a 2D image plane, it may be near the inner wall in the elevational plane, since this curvature is 3D. Thus, the shape of the pulmonary artery velocity curve is most helpful when it is normal. An apparent short time to peak velocity can be due to measurement variability or to the nonuniform spatial flow velocity distribution in the vessel.

Pulmonary Vascular Resistance

Pulmonary pressure is not an ideal measure of the vascular properties of the pulmonary bed, because pressure is affected by volume flow rate (increased pressures with higher flow rates and vice versa) and by the LA pressure. Pulmonary vascular resistance is calculated as the pressure drop across the pulmonary bed (mean systolic pulmonary pressure minus mean LA pressure) divided by stroke volume. Pulmonary vascular resistance is expressed in dimensionless Wood units where normal is <1 Wood unit, or an conversion factor is used for units of dynes s cm^{-5}, where normal is <160 dynes s cm^{-5}.

Noninvasive calculation of pulmonary resistance is problematic because of difficulty in measuring mean LA pressure and because of the measurement variability in noninvasive pulmonary pressure and right heart cardiac output calculations. One proposed approach is based on the tissue Doppler systolic motion of the tricuspid annulus, based on the concept that the RV is very responsive to an increased afterload so that an increase in pulmonary resistance will result in a decrease in tricuspid annular motion. The other approach is to estimate the pressure drop across the pulmonary bed using the peak tricuspid regurgitant jet velocity (V_{TR} in m/s) (ignoring LA pressure) and to estimate stroke volume using the VTI of flow in the RV outflow tract (VTI_{RVOT} in cm). This ratio is multiplied by 10 to approximate PVR in Wood units:

$$PVR \cong 10(V_{TR})/VTI_{RVOT} \qquad (6-17)$$

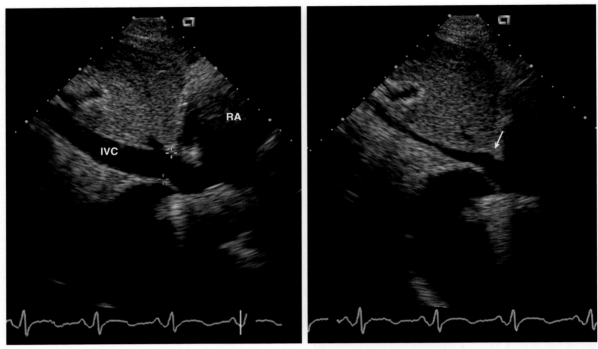

Figure 6–23 Subcostal view of the junction between the inferior vena cava (IVC) and the RA during normal expiration (*top*) and inspiration (*bottom*).

TABLE 6–7   Estimation of Right Atrial Pressure

IVC Diameter (1–2 cm from RA junction)	Change with Respiration or "Sniff"	Estimated RA Pressure
Small (<1.2 cm)	Spontaneous collapse	Intravascular volume depletion
Normal (<1.7 cm)	Decrease by ≥ 50%	0–5 mm Hg
Dilated (> 1.7 cm)	Decrease by ≥50%	5–10 mm Hg
Dilated (>1.7 cm)	Decrease by <50%	10–15 mm Hg
Dilated (>1.7 cm)	No change	15–20 mm Hg
Dilated with dilated hepatic veins	No change	>20 mm Hg

Adapted from Kircher BH, Himelmann RB, Schiller NG: Am J Cardiol 66:493, 1990; and from Lang RM, Bierig M, Devereux RB et al: J Am Soc Echocardiogr 18:1440, 2005.

This approach may be helpful in identification of patients with a normal PVR, despite a high pulmonary systolic pressure, and, conversely, those with a high PVR but low pressures due to a low cardiac output.

This approach is reasonably accurate in the absence of primary pulmonary hypertension. When pulmonary diastolic pressures are elevated, this approach may significantly underestimate PVR measured in Wood units; however, this approach still is useful for identifying patients with an elevated PVR and for tracking relative changes over time. Doppler-based PVR estimates also may be inaccurate with severe pulmonary artery or outflow tract dilation, severe elevation of RA pressure, or severe pulmonic regurgitation.

Limitations and Technical Considerations

Determination of PA systolic pressure derived from the continuous-wave Doppler tricuspid regurgitant (TR) jet velocity is only as accurate as the primary data. Underestimation of TR jet velocity due to a nonparallel intercept angle between the jet and the ultrasound beam results in underestimation of pulmonary pressure. Overestimation of pulmonary pressure can occur if the mitral regurgitant jet is mistaken for tricuspid regurgitation. Although both signals occur in systole and are directed away from the LV apex, the duration of tricuspid regurgitation is slightly longer than mitral regurgitation (when RV and LV systolic function are normal) due to a slightly longer RV systolic ejection period. The shapes of the velocity curves tend to differ as well, with TR having a slower upstroke and a peak later in systole, although the shapes of both velocity curves are affected by changes in ventricular function or atrial pressure. Note that the velocity of mitral regurgitation always is high, since it reflects the systolic LV (approximately 100 mm Hg) to LA (approximately 10 mm Hg) pressure difference. With normal pulmonary pressures, TR jet velocity is 2 to 2.5 m/s. With severe pulmonary hypertension, pulmonary pressure may approach systemic pressures, with a corresponding TR jet velocity in the range of 5 m/s.

It is important to keep separate the concepts of regurgitant *volume flow rate* (which relates to regurgitant severity) and regurgitant jet *velocity*, which reflects the instantaneous pressure gradient across the valve.

The TR jet can be used to estimate pulmonary pressure when RV and pulmonary artery systolic pressures are equal, specifically in the absence of pulmonic stenosis. *When pulmonic stenosis is present*, pulmonary pressures can be estimated by subtracting the RV to pulmonary artery pressure difference derived from the pulmonic stenotic jet velocity (V_{PS}) from the estimated RV systolic pressure:

$$PAP = [4(V_{TR})^2 + RAP] - [4(V_{PS})^2] \qquad (6\text{--}18)$$

The estimate of RA pressure from the appearance of the inferior vena cava also can affect the accuracy of Doppler echo pulmonary pressure estimates. The importance of this source of error is greatest at intermediate tricuspid regurgitant jet velocities: A TR jet velocity of 2.5 m/s with an RA pressure of 5 mm Hg indicates a pulmonary pressure of only 30 mm Hg (normal to mildly elevated), but if RA pressure is 20 mm Hg, then pulmonary pressure is 45 mm Hg (moderate pulmonary hypertension). At the extreme (i.e., a TR jet of 5 m/s), pulmonary hypertension clearly is severe regardless of the RA pressure estimate.

If images of the inferior vena cava are suboptimal, or if the degree of change with respiration is equivocal, it is appropriate to report the range of possible pulmonary pressures or to indicate that the RV to RA pressure gradient is added to a clinical estimate of RA pressure. Evaluation of respiratory variation in inferior vena cava diameter can be confounded by respiratory motion in the position of the inferior vena cava such that the center of the vessel moves in and out of the image plane. Of course, evaluation of inferior vena cava size and respiratory variation is not helpful in patients supported by positive-pressure ventilation, since intrathoracic pressures are abnormal.

Even when pulmonary pressure is normal, the time to peak velocity in the pulmonary artery can appear short when the Doppler sample volume is positioned along the inner curve of the pulmonary artery. Conversely, impaired RV systolic function may result in an apparently normal time to peak velocity even in the presence of pulmonary hypertension.

ALTERNATE APPROACHES

Left Ventricular Systolic Function

Cardiac magnetic resonance (CMR) imaging provides precise and accurate measures of LV volumes, mass, EF, and cardiac output. Other approaches include contrast angiography in the cardiac catheterization laboratory (Fig. 6–24) and radionuclide ventriculography (Fig. 6–25). The choice of imaging technique in an individual patient will depend on what other clinical questions are present (e.g., possible valvular disease) as well as availability and cost.

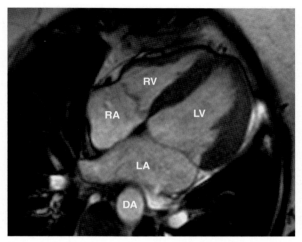

Figure 6–24 Cardiac magnetic resonance image of the heart in a four-chamber image plane. These images can be viewed in real time to provide qualitative evaluation of RV and LV global and regional function. Ventricular volumes and ejection fraction are calculated from traced borders.

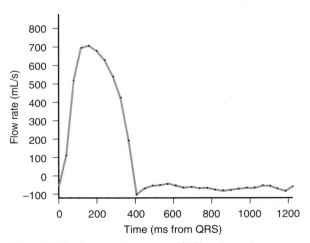

Figure 6–25 Cardiac magnetic resonance (CMR) can be used to measure volume flow rate in the aorta based on the velocity and cross-sectional area of flow. This CMR volume flow curve shows a typical systolic ejection curve, with little flow in diastole.

Cardiac output can be measured by the thermodilution technique via a right-sided heart catheter both in the catheterization laboratory and in the coronary care unit. Thermodilution outputs offer the advantages that measurements can be repeated frequently by the nurse caring for the patient and pulmonary pressures can be monitored continuously as well. Disadvantages of this approach are that it is invasive (risks, discomfort) and it provides only a volumetric flow rate, without direct visualization of ventricular function. Stroke volume can be maintained despite a low EF due to compensatory LV dilation. For example, the same stroke volume of 60 mL may result from an EF of 20% with an LV EDV of 300 mL or from a normal EF (60%) with a smaller LV EDV (100 mL).

Right Ventricular Systolic Function

Cardiac magnetic resonance imaging provides accurate measurement of RV volumes and EF and is increasingly utilized when these measurements are needed for clinical decision making, particularly in adults with congenital heart disease. RV contrast angiography can be performed at catheterization, but there is wide variability in the appearance of the normal RV. Radionuclide ventriculography can be used to derive an RV ejection fraction.

The alternative to noninvasive Doppler echo estimate of pulmonary pressures is direct measurement in the coronary care unit or cardiac catheterization laboratory with a pulmonary artery (Swan-Ganz) catheter. This approach has the advantages of precision, a high degree of accuracy (assuming appropriate transducer calibration and balancing), and the ability to continuously record measurements over a period of several days. In addition, pulmonary vascular resistance can be measured based on invasive measurement of cardiac output and pulmonary pressures. Disadvantages are its costs and potential complications of line placement.

SUGGESTED READING

Physiology of Left Ventricular Systolic Function

1. Sengupta PP, Korinek J, Belohlavek M, et al: Left ventricular structure and function: Basic science for cardiac imaging. J Am Coll Cardiol 48:1988–2001, 2006.
   Detailed discussion of the structure and function of the LV myocardium with illustrations of the helical architecture of the muscle bundles. The relationship between myocardial contraction and relaxation and the events of the cardiac cycle is reviewed and illustrated.

2. Thomas JD, Popovic ZB: Assessment of left ventricular function by cardiac ultrasound. J Am Coll Cardiol 48:2012–2025, 2006.
   Review of basic principles of ventricular function including cardiac hemodynamics (conservation of mass, energy and momentum), cardiac mechanics (global and regional function), and measures of diastolic function (relaxation, compliance, pressure differences, and shear strain and torsion).

Two-dimensional Echocardiographic Measures of Ventricular Function

3. Lang RM, Bierig M, Devereux RB, et al: Chamber Quantification Writing Group; American Society of Echocardiography's Guidelines and Standards Committee; European Association of Echocardiography. Recommendations for chamber quantitation: A report from the American Society of Echocardiography's Guidelines and Standards Committee and the Chamber Quantification Group, developed in conjunction with the European Association of Echocardiography, a branch of the European Society of Cardiology. J Am Soc Echocardiogr 18:1440–1463, 2005.
   Detailed discussion of methods for quantitation of LV and RV systolic function by 2D echocardiography and measurement of atrial size and aortic root dimensions. Technical details of image acquisition, diagrams illustrating quantitative methods, and tables of normal values are included.

4. Aurigemma GP, Gaasch WH: Quantitative evaluation of left ventricular structure, wall stress and systolic function. In Otto CM (ed): The Practice of Clinical Echocardiography, 3rd ed. Philadelphia: Elsevier/Saunders, 2007, pp 187–211.
   Advanced-level discussion of ventricular geometry, wall stress, and systolic function. This chapter provides a detailed and critical discussion of these approaches including LV ejection fraction, mass, and circumferential and meridional stress. 137 references.

5. Picard MH, Popp RL, Weyman AE: Assessment of left ventricular function by echocardiography: A technique in evolution. J Am Soc Echocardiogr 21:14–21, 2008.
   Historical review of echocardiographic evaluation of ventricular function starting with M-mode measures and progression to 2D echocardiographic measurements of volume and ejection fraction. Emerging approaches including 3D echocardiography and tissue Doppler are briefly discussed. 51 references.

6. Oxorn DC: Monitoring ventricular function in the operating room. Impact on clinical outcome. In Otto CM (ed): The Practice of Clinical Echocardiography, 3rd ed. Philadelphia: Saunders-Elsevier, 2007, pp 31–62.
   LV volumes and ejection fraction can be measured by TEE imaging using standard four-chamber and two-chamber views. Systolic function also can be assessed by calculation of stroke volume in the pulmonary artery or LV outflow tract.

Other Imaging Measures of Systolic Function

7. Sheehan FH: Ventricular shape and function. In Otto CM (ed): The Practice of Clinical Echocardiography, 3rd ed. Philadelphia: Elsevier/Saunders, 2007, pp 212–236.
   The 3D shapes of the left and right ventricles are altered in different disease states. Using 3D echocardiography to evaluate ventricular shape and to assess myocardial function in three

dimensions may have clinical utility in patients with cardiomyopathies, ischemic disease, and congenital heart disease.

8. Simonson JS, Schiller NB: Descent of the base of the left ventricle: An echocardiographic index of left ventricular function. J Am Soc Echocardiogr 2: 25–35, 1989.

The motion of the mitral annulus toward the ventricular apex in systole (lengthwise ventricular shortening) provides a simple method for quantitation of LV systolic function. Average motion in normal individuals is 12 ± 2 mm, with motion <8 mm sensitive (98%) and specific (82%) for diagnosis of an ejection fraction of less than 50%.

9. Soliman OI, Kirschbaum SW, van Dalen BM, et al: Accuracy and reproducibility of quantitation of left ventricular function by real-time three-dimensional echocardiography versus cardiac magnetic resonance. Am J Cardiol 102:778–783, 2008.

In a series of 24 patients, real-time 3D echocardiography (RT3DE) was used to calculate LV volumes using semi-automated border tracing from endocardial speckle tracking. RT3DE LV volumes correlated well with CMR measurements, with a mean difference of only 7 mL for EDV and 4 mL for ESV. Interobserver variability was 7.6% for EF measurement by RT3DE.

Doppler Evaluation of Systolic Function

10. Goldman JH, Schiller NB, Lim DC, et al: Usefulness of stroke distance by echocardiography as a surrogate marker of cardiac output that is independent of gender and size in a normal population. Am J Cardiol 15:499–502, 2001.

The velocity-time integral of antegrade flow in the LV outflow tract provides a simplified estimate of forward cardiac output. This approach is similar to calculation of stroke volume except that measurement of outflow tract diameter is eliminated. Thus, this measure represents "stroke distance" and is effectively indexed for body size. The normal range for stroke distance is 18 to 22 cm.

11. Chandraratna PA, Brar R, Vijayasekaran S, et al: Continuous recording of pulmonary artery diastolic pressure and cardiac output using a novel ultrasound transducer. J Am Soc Echo 15:1381–1386, 2002.

A small steerable transthoracic transducer that attaches to the chest wall was used to continuously measure cardiac output and pulmonary artery diastolic pressure in 50 patients in the intensive care unit. Adequate signals were

obtained in 86% for calculation of cardiac output based on pulmonary artery diameter, flow and heart rates, and pulmonary diastolic pressure based on the end-diastolic velocity of the pulmonic regurgitant jet and estimated right atrial pressure. Correlation of Doppler and invasive data was excellent for cardiac output (r = 0.90) and pulmonary artery diastolic pressure (r = 0.92).

12. Chung N, Nishimura RA, Holmes DR Jr, et al: Measurement of left ventricular dP/dt by simultaneous Doppler echocardiography and cardiac catheterization. J Am Soc Echocardiogr 5:147–152, 1992.

Doppler measurement of LV dP/dt from the mitral regurgitant velocity curve was most accurate using the time interval from 1 to 3 m/s on the velocity curve.

13. Tei C, Nishimura RA, Seward JB, et al: Noninvasive Doppler-derived myocardial performance index: Correlation with simultaneous measurements of cardiac catheterization measurements. J Am Soc Echocardiogr 10:169–178, 1997.

The use of the ratio of isovolumic contraction plus isovolumic relaxation, divided by the systolic ejection period is proposed as a combined measure of systolic and diastolic ventricular function. In this series of 34 adults with ischemic heart disease or a dilated cardiomyopathy, the Doppler myocardial performance index correlated with invasive measures of both systolic (+dP/dt) and diastolic function (−dP/dt and tau).

14. Su HM, Lin TH, Voon WC, et al: Correlation of Tei index obtained from tissue Doppler echocardiography with invasive measurements of left ventricular performance. Echocardiography 24:252–257, 2007.

Measurement of the myocardial performance index from mitral annular tissue velocity recordings has the advantages that all the time intervals can be measured on the same cardiac cycle. The myocardial performance index is calculated as (b − a)/b, where a is the time interval from the end to onset of the mitral annular diastolic velocity (which includes isovolumic contraction and relaxation, as well as the systolic ejection period) and b is the duration of the s-wave (which is equivalent to the systolic ejection period). When compared to invasive data, the myocardial performance index correlated with LV ejection fraction and the time constant of diastolic relaxation on multivariate analysis in 34 patients undergoing cardiac catheterization for suspected coronary artery disease.

15. Mishra RK, Kizer JR, Palmieri V, et al: Utility of the myocardial performance index in a population with high

prevalences of obesity, diabetes, and hypertension: The strong heart study. Echocardiography 24:340–347, 2007.

In 1862 Native Americans without coronary disease, valve disease, or a low ejection, but with a high prevalence of diabetes (48%), hypertension (44%), and obesity (54%), the value of the myocardial performance index as a predictor of clinical events was examined. Although there was a weak correlation with serum C-reactive protein and several hemodynamic variable, this index was not predictive of cardiovascular events at a mean follow-up of 7 years.

Right Ventricular Systolic Function

16. Forfia PR, Wiegers SE: Echocardiographic findings in acute and chronic pulmonary disease. In Otto CM (ed): The Practice of Clinical Echocardiography, 3rd ed. Philadelphia: Elsevier/Saunders, 2007, pp 848–876.

This chapter provides a concise review of RV anatomy and physiology followed by a detailed discussion of the approach to echocardiographic imaging and Doppler assessment. The response of the right heart to pressure and volume overload is presented followed by a discussion of cardiac changes in both acute and chronic pulmonary disease. 200 references.

17. Redington A, Sheehan F: The right ventricle:anatomy, physiology and clinical imaging. Heart 94:1510–1515, 2008.

This review summarizes the anatomy and physiology of the RV, emphasizing differences from the LV. Approaches to clinical imaging and determination of RV volumes and function are discussed.

Noninvasive Pulmonary Pressures

18. Currie PJ, Seward JB, Chart K-L, et al: Continuous-wave Doppler determination of right ventricular pressure: A simultaneous Doppler-catheterization study in 127 patients. J Am Coll Cardiol 6:750–756, 1985.

Validation of the use of tricuspid regurgitant jet velocity to estimate RV systolic pressure in a large series of patients. An adequate tricuspid regurgitant jet velocity signal was obtained in 111 of 127 (87%) of patients. The average coefficient of variation for measurement of maximum velocity was 2% (range 0 to 18%).

19. Ulett KB, Marwick TH: Incorporation of pulmonary vascular resistance measurement into standard echocardiography: Implications for assessment of

pulmonary hypertension. Echocardiography 24:1020–1022, 2007.

In 578 consecutive patients undergoing echocardiography with a measurable tricuspid regurgitant jet velocity (V_{TR}), pulmonary artery systolic pressure (PASP) was calculated as:

PASP = $4(V_{TR})2$ + right atrial pressure

Pulmonary vascular resistance (PVR) in Wood units was calculated from the maximum tricuspid regurgitant velocity and the velocity-time integral of RV outflow (VTI_{RVOT}) as:

PVR = 10 (V_{TR})/ VTI_{RVOT}

Calculation of PVR showed that 33% of patients with a PASP > 35 mm Hg had a normal PVR (<2 Wood units).

20. Farzaneh-Far R, Na B, Whooley MA, et al: Usefulness of noninvasive estimate of pulmonary vascular resistance to predict mortality, heart failure, and adverse cardiovascular events in patients with stable coronary artery disease (from the Heart and Soul Study). Am J Cardiol 101:762–766, 2008.

The ratio of tricuspid regurgitant velocity (V_{TR}) to the velocity-time integral of antegrade flow in the RV outflow tract (VTI_{RVOT}) correlates well with invasive measurement of PVR:

PVR $\cong$ (VT_R/ VTI_{RVOT})

In 795 ambulatory patients with coronary artery disease, Doppler VT_R/ VTI_{RVOT} predicted mortality and adverse cardiovascular events over a 4.3-year follow-up interval.

7 Ventricular Diastolic Filling and Function

V entricular emptying and filling are complex interdependent processes, but the cardiac cycle often is conceptually divided into systole and diastole to allow clinical measurements of disease severity. *Diastolic* ventricular dysfunction plays a key role in the clinical manifestations of disease in patients with a wide range of cardiac disorders. For example, many patients with clinical heart failure have normal systolic function with predominant diastolic dysfunction. Diastolic dysfunction may be an early sign of cardiac diseases (as in hypertension), often antedating clinical or echocardiographic evidence of systolic dysfunction. In addition, the degree of diastolic dysfunction may explain differences in clinical symptoms between patients with similar degrees of systolic dysfunction.

Echocardiographic techniques allow evaluation of right and left ventricular (RV and LV) diastolic filling patterns, the velocity of myocardial motion, and right and left atrial (RA and LA) filling patterns. The relationship between these noninvasive measures and ventricular diastolic function and the utility of these measures in patient evaluation are discussed in this chapter.

157

BASIC PRINCIPLES

Phases of Diastole

Although several different definitions of diastole have been proposed, the most widely accepted clinical definition is the interval from aortic valve closure (end-systole) to mitral valve closure (end-diastole) (Fig. 7–1). The isovolumic contraction period, from mitral valve closure to aortic valve opening, typically is considered to be part of systole.

Diastole can be divided into four phases:

❑ Isovolumic relaxation
❑ The early rapid diastolic filling phase
❑ Diastasis
❑ Late diastolic filling due to atrial contraction

During the isovolumic relaxation interval, LV pressure falls rapidly following aortic valve closure. At the point where LV pressure falls below LA pressure, the mitral valve opens, ending the isovolumic relaxation period. With mitral valve opening, blood flows from the LA to the LV, with the rate and time

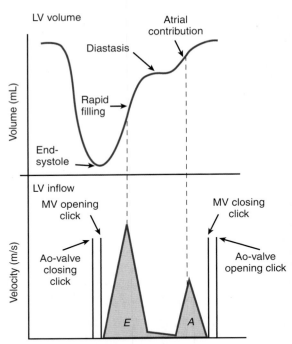

Figure 7–2 The relationship between LV volume and the diastolic LV Doppler filling pattern is shown. Early rapid filling coincides with the E velocity, followed by diastasis, with little or no flow from LA to LV, and atrial contraction, which coincides with the late diastolic A velocity. The Doppler velocity curve, in effect, is the first derivative of the LV volume curve.

course of flow being determined by several factors, including the pressure difference along the flow path, ventricular relaxation, and the relative compliances of the two chambers. Maximal opening of the mitral leaflets typically occurs rapidly, within 100 ± 10 ms of valve opening, in normal individuals.

As the ventricle fills, pressures in the atrium and ventricle equalize, resulting in a period of *diastasis*, during which there is little movement of blood between the chambers and the mitral leaflets remain in a semi-open position. The duration of diastasis is dependent on heart rate, being longer at slow heart rates and entirely absent at faster heart rates. With atrial contraction, LA pressure again exceeds LV pressure, resulting in mitral leaflet opening and a second pulse of LV filling. In normal individuals the atrial contribution to ventricular filling typically is small, comprising only about 20% of total ventricular filling (Fig. 7–2).

The phases of diastole for the RV are analogous to those described for the LV, with the difference that the total duration of diastole is slightly shorter in normal individuals due to a slightly longer RV systolic ejection period.

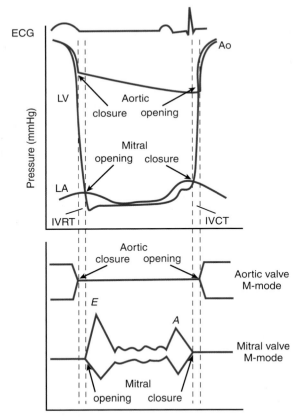

Figure 7–1 The relationship between LV, LA, and Ao pressures and M-mode tracings of the aortic and mitral valves is shown. The isovolumic relaxation time (IVRT) is the interval from Ao valve closure to MV opening. During this interval LV pressure declines rapidly. A rapid rise in LV pressure occurs during the isovolumic contraction time (IVCT), the interval between MV closure and Ao valve opening.

Parameters of Diastolic Function

There are several physiologic parameters that can be used to describe different aspects of diastolic function, but there is no single measure of overall diastolic function. The most clinically relevant parameters of diastolic function are:

- ❏ ventricular relaxation,
- ❏ myocardial or chamber compliance, and
- ❏ filling pressures.

Additional parameters of interest include elastic recoil of the ventricle and the effect of pericardial constraint, but the importance of these factors in normal diastolic ventricular function remains controversial.

Ventricular Relaxation

LV relaxation, occurring during isovolumic relaxation and the early diastolic filling period, is an active process involving utilization of energy by the myocardium. Factors affecting isovolumic relaxation include internal loading forces (cardiac fiber length), external loading conditions (wall stress, arterial impedance), inactivation of myocardial contraction (metabolic, neurohumoral, and pharmacologic), and nonuniformity in the spatial and temporal patterns of these factors. Abnormal relaxation results in prolongation of the isovolumic relaxation time (IVRT), a slower rate of decline in ventricular pressure, and a consequent reduction in the early peak filling rate (due to a smaller pressure difference between the atrium and the ventricle when the atrioventricular valve opens). Measures of LV relaxation include the IVRT, the maximum rate of pressure decline $(-dP/dt)$, and the time constant of relaxation (tau or τ). There are several different mathematical approaches to calculation of τ, but basically it reflects the rate of pressure decline from the point of maximum $-dP/dt$ to mitral valve opening. While peak rapid filling rate is affected by ventricular relaxation, it is only an indirect measure of this physiologic parameter, since several other factors also affect peak filling (Fig. 7–3).

Ventricular Compliance

Compliance is the ratio of change in volume to change in pressure (dV/dP). Stiffness is the inverse of compliance: the ratio of change in pressure to change in volume (dP/dV). Conceptually, compliance can be divided into myocardial (the characteristics of the isolated myocardium) and chamber (the characteristics of the entire ventricle) components. Chamber compliance is influenced by ventricular size and shape, as well as by the characteristics of the myocardium. Extrinsic factors also may affect measurement of compliance, including the pericardium, RV volume, and pleural pressure. Evaluation of ventricular compliance is based on diastolic passive pressure-volume curves showing the degree to which pressure and volume change in relation to each other over the physiologic range (Fig. 7–4).

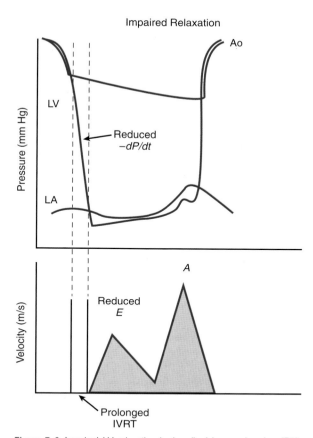

Figure 7–3 Impaired LV relaxation is described by a reduced $-dP/dt$, and a prolonged time constant of relaxation. The Doppler velocity curve shows a prolonged isovolumic relaxation time (IVRT), reduced *E* velocity (corresponding to a low LA-LV gradient at MV opening), and an increased *A* velocity.

Ventricular Diastolic Pressures

Clinically, evaluation of diastolic pressures alone often is used in patient management. Diastolic "filling" pressures include LV end-diastolic pressure (LV EDP) and mean left atrial pressure (LAP). LV EDP reflects ventricular pressure after filling is complete, while LAP reflects the average pressure in the LA during diastole. Clinically, LAP is estimated by the pulmonary capillary wedge pressure (PCWP) either at a single time point in the cardiac catheterization laboratory or at many time points with an indwelling right heart (Swan-Ganz) catheter in the intensive care unit.

Ventricular Diastolic Filling (Volume) Curves

Another clinically available measure related to diastolic function is the time course of ventricular filling: the ventricular diastolic filling curve. Experimentally, filling curves can be measured on a beat-to-beat basis from implanted sonocrystal-derived ventricular dimensions or from impedance catheter data. Clinically, filling curves can be generated for an individual cardiac

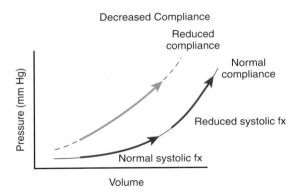

Decreased Compliance

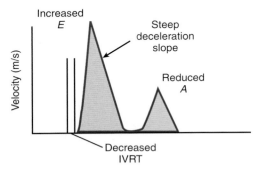

Figure 7–4 Reduced diastolic compliance is described by a steeper passive pressure-volume relationship of the LV. As LV volume increases in diastole, pressure rises rapidly, resulting in an initial high LA-LV pressure gradient with a rapid decrease in the filling gradient during diastole. The Doppler velocity curve shows a decreased IVRT, steep deceleration slope, and reduced *A* velocity. Note that even with normal compliance, reduced systolic function (fx) results in a rightward shift along the normal pressure-volume relationship, resulting in a pattern of diastolic filling similar to decreased compliance.

cycle from frame-by-frame measurements of ventricular volumes using angiographic, computed tomographic, magnetic resonance, or echocardiographic images or from high-temporal-resolution radionuclide studies. Doppler echocardiography offers the ability to measure LV diastolic filling, noninvasively, on a beat-to-beat basis.

Unfortunately, while ventricular *diastolic function* is one of the major factors affecting the pattern of *diastolic filling*, these two concepts are not identical. Several physiologic parameters other than diastolic function affect diastolic filling. Given no change in diastolic function (i.e., relaxation, compliance, etc.), the peak *early diastolic filling rate* will be affected by:

- ❏ Changes in preload that affect the initial diastolic pressure difference (or opening pressure) between the atrium and the ventricle (e.g., increased with volume loading, decreased with volume depletion)
- ❏ A change in transmitral volume flow rate (e.g., increased with coexisting mitral regurgitation)

- ❏ A change in atrial pressure (e.g., elevated LV EDP or a *v* wave due to mitral regurgitation)

Late diastolic filling is affected by:

- ❏ Cardiac rhythm
- ❏ Atrial contractile function
- ❏ Ventricular end-diastolic pressure
- ❏ Heart rate
- ❏ The timing of atrial contraction (PR interval)
- ❏ Ventricular diastolic function

The importance of considering how these factors impact the Doppler pattern of diastolic filling is discussed in more detail in the following sections. In addition, it is obvious that the utility of ventricular diastolic filling patterns for assessing diastolic function is valid only in the absence of obstruction at the atrioventricular valve level (i.e., mitral stenosis). In patients with rhythms other than normal sinus rhythm (e.g., atrial fibrillation), evaluation of diastolic function with Doppler is more challenging due to the absence of atrial contraction and the varying length of the diastolic filling period.

Atrial Pressures and Filling Curves

Another component in the evaluation of ventricular diastolic function is measurement of atrial filling patterns and pressures. The atrium serves as a "conduit" for flow from the venous circulation to the ventricle, especially in early diastole when the atrial is not contracting. In addition, elevations in ventricular diastolic pressures will be reflected in elevated pressures in the atrium (Fig. 7–5).

Right atrial pressures normally are quite low (0 to 5 mm Hg), with only small increases in pressure following atrial (*a* wave) and ventricular (*v* wave) contraction.

Right atrial filling is characterized by a:

- ❏ Small reversal of flow following atrial contraction (*a* wave)
- ❏ Systolic phase (which is effectively "diastole" for the atrium) when blood flows from the superior and inferior vena cava into the atrium
- ❏ Small reversal of flow at end-systole (*v* wave)
- ❏ Diastolic filling phase when the atrium serves as a conduit for flow from the systemic venous return to the RV

These filling phases are reflected in the patterns of jugular venous pulsation familiar to the clinician: the *a* wave following atrial contraction, the *x* descent corresponding to atrial filling during ventricular systole, the *v* wave at end systole, and the *y* descent corresponding to atrial filling during ventricular diastole. Disease processes affect the jugular venous pulsations and the Doppler pattern of RA filling in similar ways.

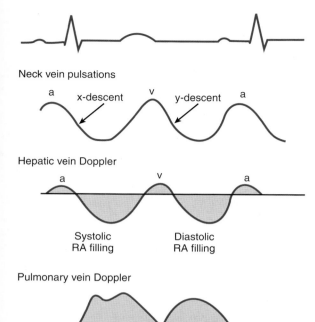

Figure 7–5 Schematic diagram of RA (hepatic vein) and LA (pulmonary vein) filling patterns and the close correspondence with the pattern of jugular venous pulsations. Pulmonary and hepatic vein patterns appear "opposite" in direction, because the direction of flow in the hepatic vein using a transthoracic subcostal view is away from the transducer (into the RA), while the direction of flow from a transthoracic apical view of the pulmonary vein is toward the transducer (into the LA).

LA filling from the pulmonary veins also is characterized by a:

☐ Small reversal of flow following atrial contraction (*a* wave)
☐ Systolic filling phase
☐ Blunting of flow or brief reversal at end-systole (*v* wave)
☐ Diastolic filling phase

In normal individuals the systolic and diastolic filling phases are approximately equal in volume. Normal LA pressure is low (5 to 10 mm Hg), corresponding to the normal LV end-diastolic pressure, with slight increases in pressure following atrial (*a* wave) and ventricular (*v* wave) contraction.

Normal Respiratory Changes

There is normal respiratory variation in RV and LV diastolic filling. With inspiration, negative intrapleural pressure results in an increase in systemic venous return into the thorax and, thus, into the RA. This increased RA volume and pressure results in a transient increase in RV diastolic filling volumes and velocities, with a normal magnitude of increase of up to 20% compared with end-expiratory values.

LA filling does *not* increase with inspiration, since pulmonary venous return is entirely intrathoracic and thus not affected significantly by respiratory changes in intrathoracic pressure. In fact, LA and, consequently, LV diastolic filling is slightly higher at end-expiration than during inspiration. The mechanism of the observation remains controversial. Some postulate a delay in transit of the increased RV filling to the left side of the heart. Others suggest a decrease in LA filling during inspiration due to an increased volume (or "pooling") in the pulmonary venous bed. Less likely, in normal individuals, is impaired LV diastolic filling due to an increase in RV diastolic volume within a fixed-volume pericardium. This last mechanism may become important in patients with pericardial disease (constriction, tamponade) and may partly account for the exaggerated respiratory changes in RV and LV diastolic filling seen in these conditions.

Causes of Diastolic Dysfunction

While diastolic dysfunction can be seen with a wide range of cardiac disorders, there are four basic mechanisms of disease (Table 7–1) that lead to diastolic dysfunction:

☐ Primary myocardial disease
☐ Secondary LV hypertrophy
☐ Coronary artery disease
☐ Extrinsic constraint

ECHOCARDIOGRAPHIC IMAGING

Evaluation of ventricular chamber dimensions and wall thickness is an integral part of the echocardiographic evaluation of diastolic function. Heart failure

TABLE 7–1	Causes of Diastolic Dysfunction
Cause	**Examples**
Primary myocardial disease	Dilated cardiomyopathy Restrictive cardiomyopathy Hypertrophic cardiomyopathy
Secondary hypertrophy	Hypertension Aortic stenosis Congenital heart disease
Coronary artery disease	Ischemia Infarction
Extrinsic constraint	Pericardial tamponade Pericardial constriction

due to diastolic dysfunction typically is evident on two-dimensional (2D) imaging with a thick-walled small ventricle (concentric remodeling) and atrial enlargement due to chronic elevation of filling pressures. Heart failure due primarily to systolic ventricular dysfunction usually is associated with a dilated ventricle (eccentric remodeling) and reduced ejection fraction. However, diastolic dysfunction usually accompanies systolic dysfunction, and measures of diastolic function are important for patient management and prognosis. In addition, there is a continuum of disease presentations from predominant systolic to isolated diastolic dysfunction, and the balance of systolic versus diastolic dysfunction may shift during the disease course. Other findings on echocardiographic imaging that raise the question of diastolic dysfunction include pericardial thickening (as in constrictive pericarditis), the pattern of ventricular septal motion with respiration (especially with tamponade physiology), and dilation of the inferior vena cava and hepatic veins (consistent with elevated RA pressures).

DOPPLER EVALUATION OF LEFT VENTRICULAR FILLING

Description of Left Ventricular Filling by Doppler Echo

Doppler recordings of LV diastolic filling velocities correspond closely with ventricular filling parameters measured by other techniques. The normal Doppler ventricular inflow pattern is characterized by a brief time interval between aortic valve closure and the onset of ventricular filling (the isovolumic relaxation time, IVRT). Immediately following mitral valve opening, there is rapid acceleration of blood flow from the LA to the ventricle with an early peak filling velocity of 0.6 to 0.8 m/s occurring 90 to 110 ms after the onset of flow in young, healthy individuals (Table 7–2). This early maximum filling velocity (E velocity) occurs simultaneously with the maximum pressure gradient between the atrium and ventricle. After this maximum velocity, flow decelerates rapidly (i.e., with a steep slope) in normal individuals with a normal deceleration slope of 4.3 to 6.7 m/s^2. Deceleration time, defined as the time interval from the E peak to where a line following the deceleration slope intersects with the zero baseline, ranges from 140 to 200 ms. Early diastolic filling is followed by a variable period of minimal flow (diastasis), depending on the total duration of diastole. With atrial contraction, LA pressure again exceeds ventricular pressure, resulting in a second velocity peak (late diastolic or atrial velocity), which typically ranges from 0.19 to 0.35 m/s in young, normal individuals (Fig. 7–6).

TABLE 7–2	Selected Normal Parameters of Diastolic Function	
Parameter	**Normal Value**	
Velocities		
E/A ratio	1.32 ± 0.42	
Deceleration slope	5.0 ± 1.4 m/s^2	
Intervals		
IVRT	63 ± 11 ms	
Deceleration time	150 – 200 ms	
$A_{dur} - a_{dur}$	<20 ms	
Derived Measures		
τ	33 ± 6 ms	
$-dP/dt$	2048 ± 335 mm Hg/s	
Filling Rates		
Peak filling rate	288 ± 66 mL/s	
Peak filling rate normalized to LVEDV	2.9 ± 1.0 s^{-1}	
Atrial filling rate	229 ± 83 mL/s	
Ratio of early to atrial VTI	1.71 ± 0.43	
Myocardial Doppler Velocities		
E'	10.3 ± 2.0 cm/s	
A'	5.8 ± 1.6 cm/s	
Ratio of E'/A'	2.1 ± 0.9	
Ratio of E/E'	<8	

IVRT, isovolumic relaxation time; VTI, velocity-time integral.
Data sources: Tebbe et al: Clin Cardiol 3:19, 1980; Shapiro and McKenna: Br Heart J 51:637, 1984; Pearson et al: Am Heart J 113:1417, 1987; Snider R et al: Am J Cardiol 56:921, 1985; Garcia-Fernandez et al: Eur Heart J 20:496, 1999.

Quantitative Ventricular Filling Velocity and Time Interval Measurements

Quantitative measurements that can be made from the Doppler velocity curve include (Fig. 7–7):

1. *Maximum velocities:* The E velocity, the A velocity, and their ratio (E/A ratio).
2. *Velocity-time integrals (VTIs):* Total, early diastolic, atrial contribution, first third or half of diastole, and their ratios.
3. *Time intervals:* The IVRT, the total duration of diastole, the deceleration time, and the atrial filling period.
4. *Measures of acceleration and deceleration:* The time from onset of flow to the E velocity, the maximum rate of rise in velocity, and the slope of early diastolic deceleration.

Volumetric Flow Rates

In order to convert the Doppler ventricular inflow *velocity* curve to a *volume* curve, the cross-sectional area (CSA) of flow must be taken into account. As described in

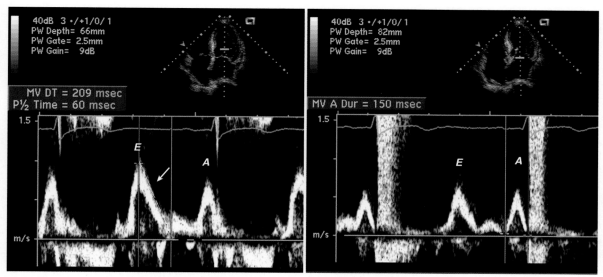

Figure 7–6 Normal pattern of LV diastolic filling recorded with pulsed Doppler in an A4C view at the mitral leaflet tips (*left*) and at the mitral annulus level (*right*). The recording at the mitral tips level is used to measure *E* velocity, *A* velocity, and the deceleration time (DT). The annular flow signal is used for measurement of atrial flow duration. If transmitral stroke volume is calculated, the annular flow signal is used for the velocity-time integral (VTI).

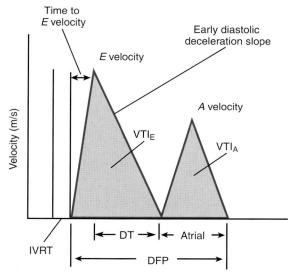

Figure 7–7 Schematic diagram of quantitative measurements that can be made from the Doppler LV filling curve. DFP, diastolic filling period; DT, deceleration time; IVRT, isovolumic relaxation time; VTI, velocity-time integral.

Chapter 6, volumetric flow rates can be calculated as the product of velocity and CSA in regions where flow is laminar with a spatially symmetric flow pattern. Thus the instantaneous volume flow rate across the mitral valve can be calculated as instantaneous velocity times the flow CSA. Similarly, transmitral stroke volume (SV) can be determined from the integral of the flow velocity curve (VTI) over the diastolic filling period:

$$SV_{transmitral} = VTI \times CSA$$

The standard approach to determining the CSA of flow across the mitral valve is to calculate mitral annular area. Motion of the mitral leaflets is a passive process,

with the degree of motion reflecting flow across the valve (in the absence of mitral stenosis). Although there is some tapering of the flow area from the annulus to the leaflet tips, the more rigid mitral annulus is a preferable site for flow measurement rather than the flexible, mobile leaflets. Even though the shape of the mitral annulus is complex in three dimensions, in clinical practice assuming either a circular or elliptical geometry is a reasonable approximation, based on a diameter measurement in the apical four-chamber and/or parasternal long axis (Fig. 7–8).

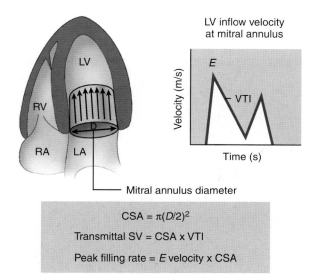

Figure 7–8 Calculation of volumetric flow rates across the mitral annulus. Mitral annular diameter can be measured from both A4C and parasternal long-axis views to calculate an elliptical cross-sectional area (CSA). If a circular CSA is used as an approximation, the parasternal long-axis annular diameter is used in the calculations.

Combining Doppler LV inflow velocity data with the CSA of the mitral annulus, additional filling parameters that can be calculated include:

1. *Peak filling rates:* Peak rapid filling rate, atrial peak filling rate, and their ratio
2. *Stroke volume*
3. *Fractional filling rates:* For example, first third filling fraction or the ratio of early to late filling

For each of these parameters, the filling rate is calculated by multiplying the appropriate velocity or VTI by CSA. For example, peak rapid filling rate (PRFR) is:

$$\text{PRFR (mL/s)} = E \text{ velocity (cm/s)} \times \text{CSA (cm}^2)$$

Of course, volume flow measurements are accurate only when velocities and diameters are measured at the same anatomic location, for example, at the annulus level.

Doppler Data Recording

LV inflow can be recorded in nearly all patients from an apical approach in either a four-chamber or long view on transthoracic (TTE) imaging. This window allows parallel alignment between the ultrasound beam and the direction of LV filling. On transesophageal (TEE) echocardiography, LV inflow can be recorded from a high esophageal position, taking care to align the Doppler beam parallel to the inflow stream (Fig. 7–9). In some patients, a transgastric apical view also may allow recording of LV inflow, although caution is needed to avoid foreshortening of the ventricle and a nonparallel intercept angle (with resultant underestimation of velocities) from this window.

Inflow velocities should be recorded using pulsed Doppler with the 2- to 3-mm sample volume positioned either at the mitral leaflet tips (for evaluation

of diastolic function) or at the mitral annulus level (for measurement of volume flow rates and the duration of atrial filling) (see Fig 7–6). For diastolic function evaluation, with the beam aligned parallel to the flow stream, the 2- to 3-mm sample volume is moved slowly along the length of the ultrasound beam to identify the site of maximal velocity, usually at the mitral leaflet tip level. The velocity range is adjusted to maximize the display of the velocity of interest and avoid signal aliasing. The sweep speed of the spectral display is maximized (100 cm/s) and wall filters are reduced (as allowed by signal quality) so that the velocities approach the baseline, allowing accurate time interval measurements. Flows are recorded at end-expiration during normal breathing.

Standard clinical measurements of LV inflow include:

- ❑ Early diastolic filling velocity (E)
- ❑ Atrial filling velocity (A)
- ❑ Deceleration time (DT) all at the leaflet tips
- ❑ Atrial filling duration (A_{dur}), measured at the mitral annulus

MYOCARDIAL TISSUE DOPPLER IMAGING

As the LV fills in diastole, the chamber lengthens from base to apex, expanding in both radial and circumferential directions. The velocity of longitudinal myocardial lengthening in diastole (and shortening in systole) can be measured using pulsed Doppler with the velocity scale, gain, and wall filters adjusted to display the velocity of the movement of the myocardium, rather than the intracavity blood flow velocities. Tissue Doppler myocardial velocities are less dependent on preload than transmitral flow velocities and thus are useful measures in evaluation of diastolic function.

Compared to transmitral blood flow velocity, the myocardial velocity curve is similar, but inverted and lower in velocity (Fig. 7–10). When myocardial tissue velocities are recorded near the mitral annulus from an apical approach, there is a brief early diastolic velocity peak away from the transducer, corresponding to early diastolic relaxation, with a normal velocity between 0.10 and 0.14 cm/s. This early diastolic velocity is abbreviated as E' (E-prime) in this book; other common abbreviations are E_a (for annular) or E_m for myocardial. Following atrial contraction, a second velocity peak away from the apex is seen (A'), with a normal ratio of $E'/A' > 1.0$. A reduced E'/A' indicates impaired relaxation. The pattern of E'/A' also helps distinguish normal LV filling from the pseudo-normalized pattern seen in patients with moderate to severe diastolic dysfunction.

Myocardial tissue Doppler signals are recorded using pulsed Doppler in an apical four-chamber view with a small sample volume (2–3 mm in length)

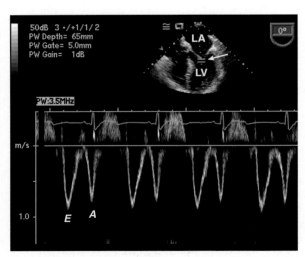

50dB 3 •/+1/1/2
PW Depth= 65mm
PW Gate= 5.0mm
PW Gain= 1dB
0°
LA
LV
PW:3.5MHZ
m/s
1.0
E A

Figure 7–9 TEE recording of LV filling. Flow is directed away from the transducer from this approach.

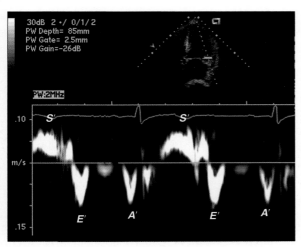

Figure 7–10 Myocardial tissue Doppler recording in a young normal patient with the early myocardial velocity (E') greater than the atrial velocity (A'). The systolic velocity toward the transducer is termed S'. Note that the velocity scale has a maximum of only 0.15 m/s, compared with 1.0 m/s for LV inflow in Figure 7–6 in the same patient.

positioned in the myocardium within the basal ventricular wall, within 1 cm of the mitral annulus. For evaluation of diastolic function, signals are recorded from the basal septum, because this location is more reproducible than lateral wall recordings and septal values have been used in validation studies. The velocity scale is decreased to show a range of only about 0.2 m/s, gain is turned to very low levels, and wall filters are reduced to obtain a well-defined signal with clear E' and A' peaks. Some instruments have a tissue Doppler setting that automatically makes these adjustments to the pulsed Doppler modality. Recordings are made at end-expiration during normal quiet respiration. Standard clinical measurements from the myocardial tissue Doppler include:

- ❏ Early diastolic filling velocity (E')
- ❏ Filling velocity after atrial contraction (A')
- ❏ Ratio of early to atrial diastolic myocardial velocity (E'/A')
- ❏ Ratio of transmitral blood flow velocity to tissue Doppler velocity (E/E')

The rationale for the ratio of blood flow to tissue velocity is that the transmitral E velocity reflects both the LA-to-LV opening pressure gradient and the amount of blood entering the ventricle in diastole. In contrast, the tissue Doppler velocity reflects only the amount of blood entering the ventricle (the volume increase in ventricular size), so that this ratio normalizes the E velocity for volume flow rate, thus providing a measure of filling pressure. However, although a very high E/E' ratio (>15) is specific for an elevated filling pressure, this ratio is not very sensitive and many patients with elevated filling pressures have a ratio between 8 and 15.

ISOVOLUMIC RELAXATION TIME

The IVRT is simply the time interval between aortic valve closure and mitral valve opening. A normal IVRT is approximately 80 to 100 ms, but the normal range varies with age and heart rate. Impaired relaxation is associated with a prolonged IVRT, whereas decreased compliance and elevated filling pressures are associated with a shortened IVRT. Thus, this measurement is useful in determining the severity of diastolic dysfunction, particularly in serial studies of patients on medical therapy or with disease progression.

The IVRT is measured from an apical four-chamber view angulated anteriorly to show the outflow tract and aortic valve. Using pulsed Doppler, a 3- to 5-mm sample volume is positioned midway between the aortic and mitral valves to obtain a clear signal showing both aortic outflow and mitral inflow, optimally with a defined aortic valve closing click. After adjusting gain and decreasing the wall filters, the IVRT is measured as the time interval in milliseconds from the middle of the aortic closure click to the onset of mitral flow (Fig. 7–11).

LEFT ATRIAL FILLING

Doppler Assessment

LA filling is evaluated by Doppler recordings of pulmonary vein flow either from a TEE or a TTE approach. Again, the Doppler pattern of velocities parallels the normal filling curves, with inflow into the LA occurring in two phases, systolic and diastolic. In addition, there is flow deceleration following ventricular contraction and a small reversal of flow after atrial contraction (Fig. 7–12). On TEE recordings the systolic inflow pattern is biphasic in some patients,

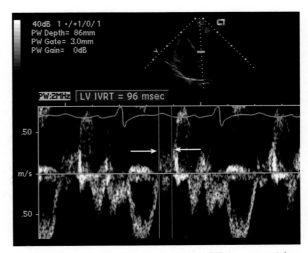

Figure 7–11 The isovolumic relaxation time (IVRT) is measured from aortic valve closure and the onset of mitral flow (*arrows*) and measures 96 ms in this example.

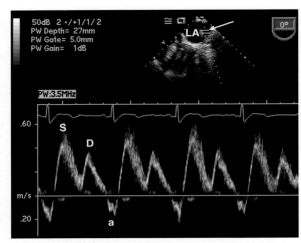

Figure 7–12 Normal pattern of LA inflow recorded in the left superior pulmonary vein from a TEE approach.

with an early systolic peak related to atrial relaxation and a second late systolic peak related to displacement of the mitral annulus toward the LV apex. Respiratory variation in flow may be seen in left heart filling patterns (atrial and ventricular) but is less prominent than the variation seen in right heart filling *and* is directionally opposite: left heart filling diminishes slightly with inspiration. Both the pulmonary veins and the LA are intrathoracic in their entirety, so negative intrathoracic pressure does not result in a pressure gradient between them. Instead, atrial filling may diminish during inspiration as blood "pools" briefly in the expanded pulmonary veins, which then empty during expiration.

Doppler Data Recording

From a TEE approach, LA inflow patterns can be easily recorded in each of the four pulmonary veins in the transverse plane. Careful positioning and angulation are needed to ensure that the pulsed Doppler sample volume is located in the pulmonary vein itself rather than in the adjacent LA. A sample volume size of 5 mm typically is used with wall filters lowered to show the low-velocity components associated with atrial and ventricular contraction. The flow pattern varies somewhat with distance from the pulmonary vein orifice. A distance about 1 cm from the orifice provides optimal signal strength with the most consistent inflow pattern.

The left superior pulmonary vein is most easily visualized adjacent to the LA appendage, directed somewhat anteriorly. The left inferior pulmonary vein can be visualized by advancing the transducer a short distance to see the inflow pattern from this horizontally directed vein. The right pulmonary veins can be imaged by turning the transducer medially to identify the superior right pulmonary vein (again anteriorly directed) and advancing the probe slightly

to image the horizontally positioned right inferior pulmonary vein.

From a TTE approach, recording pulmonary venous flow patterns is more challenging. Most echocardiographers use the apical four-chamber view, which allows a parallel alignment between the right superior pulmonary vein flow stream and the ultrasound beam. Signal strength may be a limiting factor at this depth of interrogation (typically about 14 cm), so careful attention to sample volume position, wall filters, and gain settings is needed to optimize the velocity data. Sample volume positioning may be facilitated by the use of color flow imaging to identify the flow stream from the pulmonary vein into the LA. Again, the sample volume should be positioned *in* the pulmonary vein 1 to 2 cm from the orifice. Of note, the biphasic pattern of systolic inflow and atrial reversal may be more difficult to demonstrate on TTE compared with TEE imaging due to a lower signal-to-noise ratio (Fig. 7–13). In addition, the flow pattern in the left upper pulmonary vein (on TEE imaging) shows a more laminar flow pattern than the right upper pulmonary vein (on TEE or TTE imaging). Alternate transthoracic windows that may allow recording of pulmonary vein flow in some individuals include subcostal and parasternal short-axis views at the aortic valve level or suprasternal notch views of the LA and pulmonary veins. However, intercept angle tends to be suboptimal from these windows.

Standard clinical measures of *pulmonary venous inflow* include:

- Peak systolic velocity (PV_S)
- Peak diastolic velocity (PV_D)
- Peak atrial reversal velocity (PV_a)
- Duration of pulmonary vein atrial reversal (a_{dur})

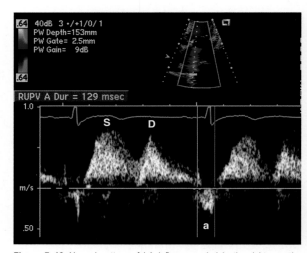

Figure 7–13 Normal pattern of LA inflow recorded in the right superior pulmonary vein from a transthoracic apical four-chamber view using color flow imaging to aid in positioning the sample volume approximately 1 to 2 cm into the vein. Note the systolic (S) and diastolic (D) filling phases with a slight flow reversal following atrial contraction (a).

COLOR DOPPLER M-MODE PROPAGATION VELOCITY

Color Doppler M-mode recordings of LV inflow from an apical approach can be used to measure the propagation velocity as blood moves from the annulus to the apex. The flow propagation velocity is decreased with restrictive ventricular filling and increased with constrictive pericarditis.

Color M-mode propagation velocity is recorded from an apical four-chamber view using color flow imaging to place a color M-mode cursor parallel to mitral inflow in the center of the flow stream (Fig. 7–14).

Using a narrow sector, minimum depth needed to include the annulus and apex, and an aliasing velocity of 0.5 to 0.7 m/s, the color M-mode signal is recorded at a fast sweep speed (100–200 mm/s). With normal diastolic function, the blood flows quickly from the annulus toward the apex resulting in a near vertical M-mode color pattern. The slope of the line along the edge of the color Doppler M-mode in early diastole is termed the propagation velocity, with a normal value >50 cm/s. With decreased relaxation, the movement of blood from the annulus to apex is slower so that the slope of color M-mode is prolonged. Accurate recording and measurement of the propagation velocity requires considerable expertise and is not used in all laboratories.

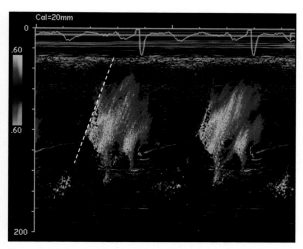

Figure 7–14 Color Doppler M-mode propagation velocity (*dashed line*) recorded with the color Doppler M-mode cursor positioned in the center of the mitral annulus in an apical four-chamber view. The slope of the Doppler flow as it moves from the annulus (*bottom of scale*) to the apex (*top of scale*) reflects the rate of LV relaxation.

MITRAL REGURGITANT JET (–dp/dt)

The rate of decline in velocity of the mitral regurgitant jet at end-systole reflects the rate of decrease in LV pressure in early diastole (Fig. 7–15). This allows measurement of negative dP/dt from the end-systolic segment of the mitral regurgitant jet, analogous to measurement of positive dP/dt from the initial segment of the jet (see Chapter 6). Unfortunately, the mitral regurgitant jet velocity is also affected by LA pressure, which may be elevated with mitral regurgitation independent of abnormalities in diastolic function. In addition, reproducibility of this measurement is suboptimal due to poor signal strength in some patients and measurement of a short time interval so that it has not been widely accepted as a standard method for evaluation of diastolic dysfunction.

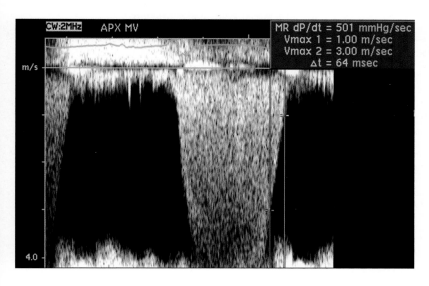

Figure 7–15 Measurement of –dP/dt from the deceleration curve of the mitral regurgitation jet signal.

FACTORS THAT AFFECT DOPPLER EVALUATION OF LEFT VENTRICULAR DIASTOLIC FUNCTION

Normal Variation

Evaluation of LV diastolic function is confounded by the normal variation in ventricular filling related to:

- ❑ Respiration
- ❑ Heart rate
- ❑ Age
- ❑ PR interval

There is normal slight variation (<20%) in LV inflow velocities with respiration. At higher heart rates, diastole is shorter—particularly the period of diastasis—so that the A velocity more closely succeeds the E velocity. When overlap of these two velocity curves occurs, the A velocity, in effect, is "added" to the E velocity curve, resulting in a higher A velocity and lower E/A ratio (Fig. 7–16). Similarly, a longer PR interval results in an A velocity earlier in diastole that may become superimposed on the E velocity curve. At very high heart rates (short diastolic filling periods), the E and A velocity curves become merged into a single E/A velocity. Evaluation of a patient with heart block or an atrial arrhythmia often demonstrates this

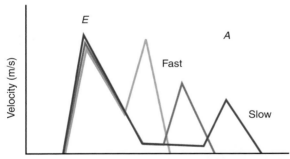

LV Inflow
Effect of Heart Rate

Figure 7–16 Schematic diagram showing the overlap or "summation" of A velocity with E velocity that occurs with higher heart rates.

Figure 7–17 LV filling in a patient with an atrial arrhythmia showing the effect of a shorter diastolic interval on the E/A pattern.

nicely, with the location of the A velocity relative to the E velocity affecting its magnitude accordingly (Fig. 7–17).

In children and young adults, the majority of ventricular filling occurs in early diastole, with a prominent E velocity and only a small contribution to ventricular filling due to atrial contraction (20% of total LV volume). With age the E velocity diminishes, and the atrial contribution becomes more prominent, with equalization of E and A velocities at approximately age 60 years and reversal of the E/A ratio after that age in normal individuals (Table 7–3). Early diastolic deceleration time also is progressively prolonged, and there is a slight increase in IVRT with age (Fig. 7–18). Presumably the mechanism of the changes in LV filling patterns with age is a gradual reduction in the rate of early diastolic relaxation. Keeping in mind that E velocity and E/A ratio usually decrease with age, the finding of a "normal" LV filling pattern in an older patient should raise the question of abnormal ventricular compliance.

LA filling is affected by many of the same variables that affect LV diastolic filling. Higher heart rates result in merging of the systolic and diastolic phases of LA filling, while lower heart rates result in clearer separation between them. Changes in LA inflow with aging have been described, including a reduction in the diastolic filling phase, a compensatory increase in the systolic filling phase, and a more prominent atrial reversal in subjects older than age 50 years.

Nondiastolic Physiologic Factors

Several physiologic variables, other than LV diastolic function, that also affect the pattern of LV diastolic filling include:

- ❑ Preload
- ❑ Volume flow rate
- ❑ LV systolic function
- ❑ Atrial contractile function

LAP, *preload*, dramatically affects the pattern of LV filling (Fig. 7–19). Increased preload results in an increase in the E velocity, a shortened IVRT, and

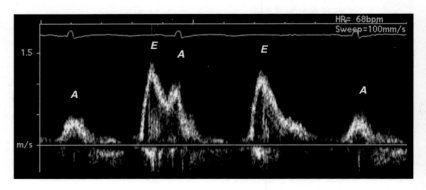

TABLE 7–3 Effect of Aging on Parameters of Left Ventricular Diastolic Filling in Normal Subjects			
Parameter	Age >21–49 yr* Mean (95% CI)	Age >50 yr* Mean (95% CI)	Age >70 yr[†] Mean (95% CI)
E velocity (m/s)	0.72 (0.44–1.00)	0.62 (0.34–0.90)	0.44 (0.25–0.76)
A velocity (m/s)	0.40 (0.20–0.60)	0.59 (0.31–0.87)	59 (0.38–0.84)
E/A ratio	1.9 (0.7–3.1)	1.1 (0.5–1.7)	0.8 (0.5–1.2)
Deceleration time (ms)	179 (139–219)	210 (138–282)	140 (90–230)
IVRT (ms)	76 (54–98)	90 (56–124)	

*Data from Cohen GI, Pietrolungo JF, Thomas JD, Klein AL: A practical guide to assessment of ventricular diastolic function using Doppler echocardiography. J Am Coll Cardiol 27:1753–1760, 1996. Normal reference values were derived from 61 subjects aged 21 to 49 years and 56 subjects older than 50 years.

[†]Data from Sagie A, Benjamin EJ, Galdersisi M et al; Reference values for Doppler indexes of left ventricular diastolic filling in the elderly. J Am Soc Echocardiogr 6:570–576, 1993. Reference values were derived from 114 healthy elderly subjects in the Framingham Heart Study.

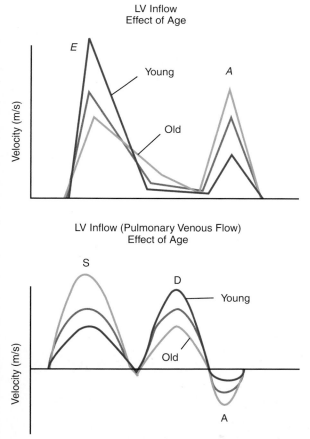

Figure 7–18 Schematic diagram showing the changes in LV (*top*) and LA inflow and pulmonary venous flow (*bottom*) patterns that occur with age. The typical pattern seen in younger (age 50 years) subjects (*red*) is compared with middle-aged (*blue*) and older (age 70 years) subjects (*yellow*).

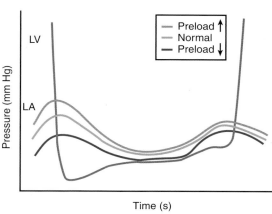

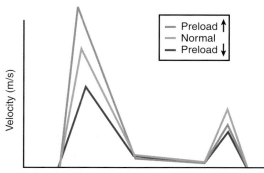

Figure 7–19 Effect of preload on LV filling pattern. With increased preload, an increased pressure gradient from the LA to the LV at the time of MV opening results in a higher *E* velocity. The *A* velocity remains the same or is reduced if a high end-diastolic pressure results in a smaller LA-to-LV pressure gradient following atrial contraction. The opposite changes occur with decreased preload.

steeper deceleration slope of early diastolic filling. As the LV fills rapidly in early diastole, LV diastolic pressure rises, so atrial contraction results in only a small pressure gradient between the LA and the LV and a small *A* velocity. Examples of elevated preload include volume infusion or an elevated LA pressure due to elevation of LV diastolic pressure.

Mitral regurgitation also results in an increase in *E* velocity both via the mechanism of an elevated LA pressure and because of the increased volume flow rate across the mitral valve. Again, the *A* velocity tends to be reduced (Fig. 7–20).

Figure 7–20 LV inflow in a patient with severe mitral regurgitation showing a high *E* velocity due to increased volume flow across the mitral valve and an increased LA pressure.

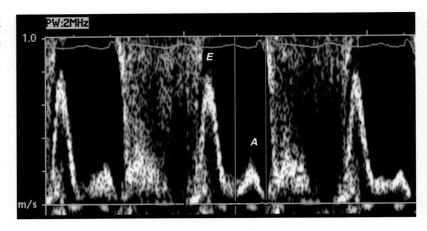

Situations with a reduced LA pressure have a reduced *E* velocity due to a smaller gradient between the LA and LV at mitral valve opening. Thus, hypovolemia or use of a venodilator (such as nitroglycerin) results in a decrease in the *E* velocity, with a much smaller effect on *A* velocity. Preload is transiently decreased during the strain phase of the Valsalva maneuver. Thus, if the *E/A* ratio appears normal but preload is elevated, with Valsalva maneuver the decrease in *E* velocity results in normalization or reversal of the *E/A* ratio. This response to the Valsalva maneuver may be used to separate a normal from a pseudo-normal pattern of diastolic filling, and to distinguish reversible from irreversible severe diastolic dysfunction.

LV systolic function affects the pattern of diastolic filling in that, for a given diastolic pressure-volume curve, an increased end-systolic volume results in a shift to a steeper portion of the pressure-volume curve. Diastolic filling then occurs with a greater increase in pressure for a given increase in volume. Thus, this shift along the diastolic pressure volume curve results in an increased *E* velocity and reduced *A* velocity, similar to the pattern seen with decreased compliance (see Fig. 7–4).

Atrial contractile function, though not always recognized clinically, can affect the pattern of LV diastolic filling. This is obvious in the case of atrial fibrillation, when no atrial contribution to ventricular filling is seen (Fig. 7–21), or with atrial flutter, when small "flutter" waves in the inflow velocity pattern may be noted, but is less obvious in sinus rhythm with ineffective atrial contraction, which may result in a small *A* velocity.

Pulmonary venous flow patterns also are affected by physiologic factors other than diastolic function, with the *systolic filling phase* most affected by:

❑ LA size
❑ LA pressure
❑ LA compliance
❑ Atrial contractile function

The velocity and duration of the *atrial reversal* is affected by:

❑ LA contraction
❑ LA compliance
❑ Cardiac rhythm

Figure 7–21 LV inflow in a patient with atrial fibrillation shows a single velocity peak and no *A* velocity.

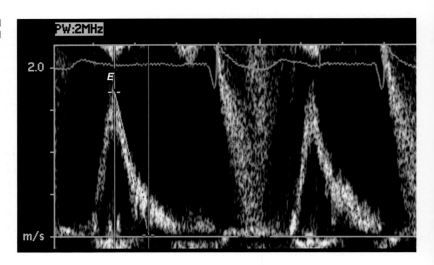

Despite the potential influence of all these factors on the pattern of LV diastolic filling, the Doppler velocity data still can provide useful information on diastolic dysfunction if carefully interpreted.

CLINICAL CLASSIFICATION OF DIASTOLIC FUNCTION

In the clinical setting, evaluation of diastolic ventricular function is complicated by the coexistence of more than one of the factors that affect diastolic filling. For example, patients with reduced compliance often have an elevated preload. Thus, an elderly patient with reduced compliance may have a pattern of LV filling similar to a younger patient with normal diastolic function (a pattern referred to as *pseudo-normalization*). Conversely, a patient with impaired relaxation may have coexisting mitral regurgitation, resulting in an increased *E/A* ratio due to the increased transmitral volume flow rate instead of the expected decrease in *E/A* ratio due to impaired relaxation. As these examples illustrate, sorting out the relative contribution of diastolic dysfunction from other physiologic parameters can be difficult in an individual patient. Furthermore, the factors that affect diastolic filling are not independent. A change in one physiologic parameter (such as LA pressure) may affect other parameters (such as atrial compliance and LV contractility). The interdependence of these physiologic parameters complicates not only our ability to evaluate individual patients but also our understanding of the physiology of diastolic filling. From a practical point of view, the combination of transmitral flow patterns, myocardial tissue velocity and the pattern of pulmonary venous inflow, allow a clinically useful classification of the type and severity of diastolic dysfunction. The simplified classification system in Table 7–4 is based on the Canadian Consensus Guidelines with modifications to reflect the recent literature.

The recent American Society of Echocardiography guidelines also provide a clinical framework for evaluation of diastolic dysfunction (see Suggested Reading 8).

The clinical indications and optimal examination for diastolic dysfunction continue to evolve, so that each laboratory needs to develop a protocol for when and how to evaluate diastolic function. My recommendation is that detailed evaluation of diastolic dysfunction be performed in patients referred for evaluation of heart failure symptoms, including dyspnea, and in those with evidence for any of the conditions listed in Table 7–1 based on clinical or echocardiographic criteria (Fig. 7–22).

Estimates of Diastolic Filling Pressures

In clinical practice, it is difficult to separate the effects of changes in ventricular relaxation and compliance from changes due to elevated filling pressures, because each of these factors affects both of the others. Nevertheless, these parameters are conceptually different. In addition, the elusive goal of accurate noninvasive assessment of LA pressure or of LV end-diastolic pressure would be of great clinical utility. Doppler data are not accurate or precise enough to replace invasive pressure measurements in critically ill patients when treatment is being titrated based on hemodynamic parameters. On the other hand, several Doppler parameters are useful for identification of patients with elevated filling pressure, even when an exact numerical value cannot be provided (Table 7–5).

Doppler parameters that indicate an elevated LV filling pressure include:

❒ A ratio of transmitral E velocity to the myocardial tissue E' velocity (E/ E') > 15
❒ A pulmonary vein atrial reversal velocity (PV_a) > 0.35 m/s

---

TABLE 7–4   Classification of Diastolic Dysfunction

	Normal	Mild	Moderate	Severe*
Pathophysiology		↓ Relaxation	↓ Relaxation ↑ LV EDP	↓ Compliance ↑↑ LV EDP
E/A ratio	1–2	<0.8	0.8–2.0[†]	≥2.0
DT (ms)	150–200	>200	150–200	<140
E' velocity (cm/s)	≥10	<8	<8	<5
E/E' ratio	≤8	<8	9–14	≥15
IVRT (ms)	50–100	≥100	60–100	≤60
PV_s/PV_D	≅1	S > D	S < D	S << D
PV_a (m/s)	<0.35	<0.35[‡]	≥0.35	≥0.35
$a_{dur} - A_{dur}$ (ms)	<20	<20[‡]	≥30	≥30 ms

*An additional grade of irreversible severe dysfunction is characterized by the absence of a decrease in E velocity with the strain phase of the Valsalva maneuver.
[†]*E/A* with Valsalva is <1.0.
[‡]Pulmonary atrial reversal duration and velocity may be increased if filling pressures are elevated.
Modified from Canadian Consensus Guidelines (Rakowki et al: J Am Soc Echocardiogr 9:736–760); 1996; Yamada et al: J Am Soc Echocardiogr, 15:1238–1244, 2002; Redfield: JAMA; 289.194–202, 2003; Lester et al: J Am Coll Cardiol 51:679–689, 2008. See also Suggested Reading 8.

Figure 7–22 Suggested algorithm for evaluation of diastolic dysfunction on routine clinical studies. When LV size, wall thickness, and ejection fraction (EF) are normal, further evaluation of diastolic function is needed only if there is LA enlargement or an abnormal *E/A* ratio for age. In patients with ventricular hypertrophy or dilation with a normal EF, diastolic function should be fully evaluated, particularly if there is a clinical concern that diastolic dysfunction may account for symptoms. When EF is reduced, the first step is to evaluate for elevated filling pressures. If simple criteria for elevated filling pressures are not present, a more complete evaluation of diastolic function is appropriate. See Table 7–4 for classification of diastolic dysfunction. DT, deceleration time; IVRT, isovolumic relaxtion time; PV, pulmonary vein.

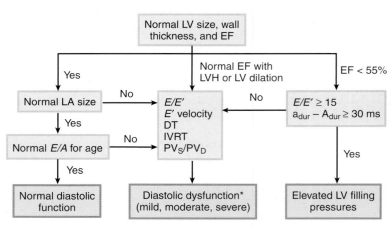

*See table for classification of diastolic dysfunction

- A pulmonary atrial reversal duration (a_{dur}) at least 20 ms greater than transmitral atrial flow duration (A_{dur})
- A pulmonary venous systolic flow less than diastolic flow (S < D)
- A ratio of the early to atrial transmitral velocity (*E/A* ratio) > 2
- An *E* velocity DT < 140 ms

In clinical practice, several of these variables are considered in examination of patients with suspected diastolic dysfunction with the confounding factors of diastolic relaxation and compliance affecting the data in each patient. In patients with a low LV ejection fraction, an *E/E'* ratio greater than 15 is a reasonably accurate indicator of elevated filing pressures. When LV systolic function is normal, a very low (≤8) or very high (>15) *E/E'* ratio is diagnostic, but the additional parameters listed above should be considered when the *E/E'* ratio is between 8 and 15. The diagnosis of elevated filling pressures is most secure when multiple parameters are congruent. Additional findings, such as LA enlargement and pulmonary hypertension improve diagnostic reliability.

Mild Diastolic Dysfunction

Mild diastolic dysfunction is characterized by impaired ventricular relaxation with a classic pattern of impaired early diastolic filling and an increased atrial contribution to total LV filling (Fig. 7–23). *Impaired relaxation is* associated with:

- A reduced *E* velocity
- A lengthened IVRT
- A prolonged early diastolic DT
- An *E'* velocity <8 cm/s

If LV relaxation is impaired but filling pressures are not elevated, the *E/E'* ratio is <8 and the pulmonary venous pattern is normal with:

- A systolic greater than diastolic phase
- A normal atrial reversal duration and velocity

If impaired relaxation is accompanied by elevated filling pressures, the LV inflow pattern continues to show an *E/A* ratio less than 1 with a prolonged DT. However, the ratio of early diastolic blood flow to tissue velocity (*E/E'*) now is elevated, the IVRT is in the normal range, and the pulmonary venous atrial reversal is prolonged in duration and increased in velocity. This pattern is consistent with mild-to-moderate diastolic dysfunction.

Moderate Diastolic Dysfunction

More severe diastolic dysfunction is characterized by abnormal compliance, often in addition to impaired relaxation. Abnormal ventricular compliance results in rapid early diastolic filling following mitral valve opening with a short IVRT and acceleration time. As the ventricle fills, LV diastolic pressure rises rapidly due to a stiff ventricle with decreased compliance, so a high *E* velocity is followed by a steep deceleration slope (Fig. 7–24). The atrial contribution to filling is relatively small, since filling is now occurring on the steep portion of the pressure-volume relationship. In addition, LV EDP typically is elevated, so there is only a small LA to LV pressure gradient following atrial contraction. With moderate diastolic dysfunction, this results in a pattern of ventricular filling often called "pseudo-normal" because the *E/A* ratio looks similar to normal.

Moderate diastolic dysfunction, with a normal *E/A* ratio (pseudo-normal), is distinguished from normal ventricular filling by:

- A short early diastolic DT
- A reduced *E'* velocity, an *E'/E_a* < 1, and an *E/E'* ratio of 9–14
- A decreased IVRT
- A pulmonary venous diastolic greater than systolic velocity

TABLE 7-5 Selected Studies Validating Doppler Measures of Left Ventricular Filling Pressures

Echo Parameter	Reference Standard	r	Breakpoints	Sensitivity (%)	Specificity (%)	First Author and Year
Transmitral Flow						
E/A	PAWP	0.72	$E/A > 1.1$ predicts PAWP > 12 mm Hg			Appleton 1993
E/A	LV EDP		$E/A > 2.0$ associated with LV EDP > 20 mm Hg	100	100	Channer 1986
DT	PAWP	−0.90	$DT \leq 120$ ms predicts PAWP ≥ 20 mm Hg	100	99	Giannuzzi 1994
DT	LV EDP	−0.74	$DT < 140$ ms predicts LV EDP ≥ 20 mm Hg	90	99	Cecconi 1996
DT	LAP	0.73	$DT < 180$ ms predicts LAP ≥ 20 mm Hg	100	100	Nishimura 1996
ΔA velocity with Valsalva	LV EDP	0.85	↓A wave by 21 ± 15 cm/s with LV EDP < 15 mm Hg ↑A wave by 18 ± 13 cm/s with LV EDP > 25 mm Hg			Schwammenthal 2000
Pulmonary Vein Flow						
a_{dur}	LV EDP		$a_{dur} > 0.35$ m/s predicts LV EDP > 15 mm Hg			Nishimura 1990
a_{dur}	LV EDP		$a_{dur} > A_{dur}$ predicts LV EDP > 15 mm Hg	85	79	Rossvold 1993
a_{dur}	LV EDP		$a_{dur} > A_{dur} + 20$ ms predicts LV EDP > 12 mm Hg	71	95	Appleton 1993
A_{dur}/a_{dur}	LV EDP	−0.70	$A_{dur}/a_{dur} \leq 0.9$ predicts LV EDP ≥ 20 mm Hg	90	90	Cecconi 1996
$PV_s/(PV_s + PV_D)$	LAP	−0.88	$PV_s/(PV_s + PV_D) < 55\%$ indicates LAP ≥ 15 mm Hg	91	87	Kuecherer 1990
PV_s/PV_D	LAP	0.94				Hoit 1992
$PV_D DT$	LAP	−0.92	DT of $PV_D < 175$ ms predicts LAP > 17 mm Hg	100	94	Kinnaird 2001
Tissue Doppler						
E/E'	PAWP	0.87	$PCWP = 1.24\ (E/E') + 1.9$ mm Hg			Nagueh 1997
E/E'	Mean LVDP	0.64	$E/E' < 8$ predicts normal LV EDP $E/E' > 15$ predicts mean LV EDP > 15 mm Hg		86	Ommen 2000
E/E'	LV EDP (pre-a wave)	0.74	$E/E' \geq 9$ predicts elevated LV EDP (>12 mm Hg)	81	80	Kim 2000

A_{dur}, time duration of transmitral A velocity; a_{dur}, time duration of pulmonary venous a velocity; DT, deceleration time (of E-wave); E, early diastolic transmitral flow velocity; E', early diastolic myocardial Doppler tissue velocity; E/A, ratio of early to late diastolic filling velocity; LAP, left atrial pressure; LV EDP, LV end-diastolic pressure; LVDP, LV diastolic pressure; PAWP, pulmonary artery wedge pressure; PV_D, diastolic pulmonary vein velocity; PV_s, systolic pulmonary vein velocity; $PV_D DT$, deceleration time of PV_D.

Data sources: Spirito et al: J Am Coll Cardiol 7:518–526, 1986; Appleton et al: J Am Coll Cardiol 22:1972–1982, 1993; Channer et al: Lancet, 1:1005–1007, 1986; Giannuzzi et al: J Am Coll Cardiol 23: 1630–1637, 1994; Cecconi et al: J Am Soc Echocardiogr 9:241–250, 1996; Nishimura et al: J Am Coll Cardiol 28:1226–1233, 1996; Schwammenthal et al: Am J Cardiol 86:169–174, 2000; Nishimura et al: Circulation 8:1488–1497, 1990; Rossvold et al: J Am Coll Cardiol 21: 1687, 1993; Kuecherer et al: Circulation 82:1127–1139, 1990; Hoit et al: Circulation 86:651–659, 1992; Kinnaird et al: J Am Coll Cardiol 37:2025–2030, 2001; Naugeh et al: J Am Coll Cardiol 15:1527–1533, 1997; Ommen et al: Circulation 102:1788–1794, 2000; Kim and Sohn: J Am Soc Echocardiogr 13:980–985, 2000.

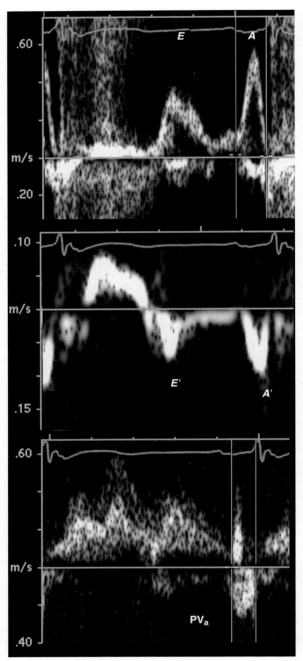

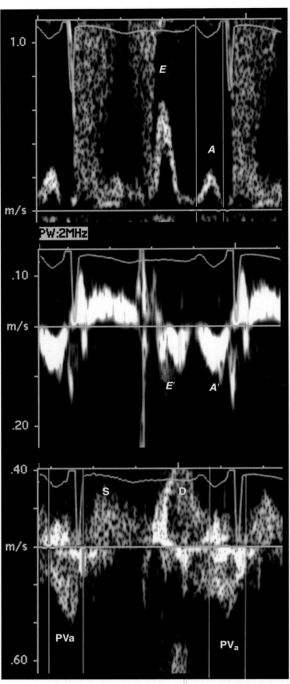

Figure 7–23 Mild diastolic dysfunction in a patient with LV hypertrophy and decreased relaxation. The mitral inflow at the leaflet tips (*top*) shows an *E/A* < 1 and a prolonged deceleration time. The myocardial tissue Doppler (*center*) confirms impaired relaxation with an *E′/A′* < 1, indicating the mitral flow pattern is not related to loading conditions. The pulmonary venous inflow (*bottom*) shows relatively slightly greater systolic compared with diastolic flow and a normal atrial reversal velocity and duration (PV$_a$), consistent with normal LV filling pressures. In addition, the *E/E′* ratio is only 4.

Figure 7–24 Moderate diastolic dysfunction a patient with impaired compliance and an elevated LV end-diastolic pressure. The mitral inflow at the leaflet tips (*top*) shows an *E/A* > 1 and a short deceleration time. The myocardial tissue Doppler (*center*) shows about equal *E′* and *A′* velocities, with an *E′* < 0.8 m/s, consistent with decreased compliance. The *E/E′* ratio is just over 8. The pulmonary venous inflow (*bottom*) shows a relatively larger diastolic than systolic component and an increased atrial reversal (PV$_a$) velocity (~0.40 m/s) and duration, consistent with elevated LV filling pressures.

In addition, the pulmonary venous flow pattern shows a prominent diastolic phase with an increased velocity and duration of atrial flow reversal, confirming the diagnosis of moderate diastolic dysfunction. Although the E/A ratio at rest is typically 1 to 2, with the strain phase of the Valsalva maneuver (decreased preload), the E velocity decreased more than the A velocity with an E/A ratio < 1.

Severe Diastolic Dysfunction

With severe diastolic dysfunction, the progressive reduction in compliance and elevation of filling pressures results in a further increase in the E velocity and decrease in the DT. The myocardial tissue velocities decrease to less than 5 cm/s and the ratio of E to E' increases to 15 or greater. The IVRT becomes very short, and the pulmonary venous inflow pattern is dominated by diastolic flow. Atrial reversal is prominent as well, with an increased velocity and duration of atrial flow, since a high LV diastolic pressure reduces late diastolic LV filling so that atrial contraction results in reversal of flow in the pulmonary veins (Fig. 7-25).

In summary, severe diastolic dysfunction with *reduced compliance* is associated with:

- ❏ Increased E velocity and E/A ratio
- ❏ Decreased DT
- ❏ A low E' velocity with an E/E' ratio ≥ 15
- ❏ Short IVRT
- ❏ Pulmonary venous diastolic greater than systolic flow
- ❏ Increased velocity and prolonged duration of pulmonary vein atrial reversal

Some classifications of diastolic dysfunction include another category of severe irreversible diastolic dysfunction characterized by the lack of a decrease in E velocity with Valsalva maneuver, along with even more severe abnormalities in the other parameters of diastolic function.

CLINICAL UTILITY

Myocardial Disease

Although systolic dysfunction with a low ejection fraction is the primary feature of a dilated cardiomyopathy, diastolic dysfunction often is also present (see Chapter 9). In addition, noninvasive estimates of filling pressures may be helpful in clinical management. When systolic dysfunction is present, the elevated end-systolic volume results in a shift along the pressure-volume curve to a steeper segment. This means that for a given diastolic pressure-volume relationship, compliance is reduced at higher LV volumes. Thus, the expected pattern of diastolic filling in dilated cardiomyopathy is that of reduced compliance: a high E velocity, rapid deceleration slope, low A velocity, and an E/A ratio > 1.

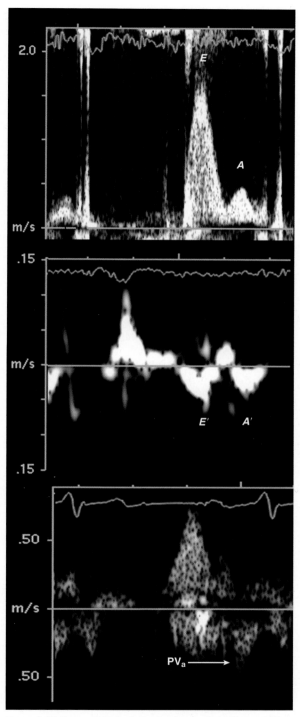

Figure 7–25 Severe diastolic dysfunction in a patient with heart failure and a low ejection fraction. The transmitral inflow shows a very high E/A ratio of 4 and a steep deceleration time (*top*). The myocardial tissue Doppler (*center*) shows a very low E' velocity of 0.5 m/s and a very high E/E' ratio of 32. The pulmonary venous inflow pattern is suboptimal, but diastolic flow is seen with no systolic component and the atrial reversal (PV_a) velocity is at the upper limits of normal (∼0.35 m/s), with a duration slightly longer than the mitral A duration, also supporting the diagnosis of elevated LV filling pressures.

In cardiac amyloidosis, a specific example of restrictive cardiomyopathy, the patterns of LV diastolic filling and the change in these patterns during the disease course are particularly instructive. With amyloid infiltration of the myocardium, the first change is impaired relaxation, resulting in the classic pattern of mild diastolic dysfunction with a reduced E velocity and increased A velocity (see Fig. 7–23) As the disease progresses, compliance also becomes abnormal, with moderate diastolic dysfunction resulting in a shift from E/A < 1 to an E/A > 1, with all the other findings of reduced compliance. This "pseudo-normalized" pattern can be distinguished from normal (if the patient is seen at only one point in the disease course) by the pattern of pulmonary venous inflow, which shows a diastolic component greater than the systolic component with an enhanced atrial reversal. The myocardial tissue Doppler signal will show an E'/A' < 1 (see Fig. 7–25). To some extent, this description oversimplifies the changes seen in amyloid heart disease, since concurrent changes in LV systolic function, the degree of mitral regurgitation, and LA filling pressures also occur, all of which affect the pattern of LV diastolic filling. However, it does serve as a useful framework for understanding the complex changes that occur with diastolic dysfunction.

Patients with hypertrophic cardiomyopathy often have a pattern of LV diastolic filling consistent with impaired relaxation. Some studies have suggested that Doppler evaluation of LV diastolic filling can be used to assess the effects of medical therapy (e.g., beta blockers or calcium channel blockers), and that subclinical disease can be detected by abnormalities in diastolic function using tissue Doppler or strain rate imaging. However, evaluation of diastolic dysfunction in patients with hypertrophic cardiomyopathy is problematic due to the numerous confounding factors in these patients. Many of the parameters validated in other patient groups are not accurate in patients with hypertrophic cardiomyopathy, including only a modest correlation between E/E' and LV filling pressures (see Suggested Readings 25 and 26).

Left Ventricular Hypertrophy

The "classic" pattern of mild LV diastolic dysfunction is seen with LV hypertrophy due to hypertension or to valvular aortic stenosis. The predominant abnormality is impaired relaxation, resulting in a pattern of reduced early diastolic filling and an enhanced atrial contribution to filling. The Doppler velocity curve typically shows a prolonged IVRT, reduced acceleration to a reduced E velocity, prolonged early diastolic deceleration slope, an increased A velocity, and an E/A ratio < 1. When LV systolic dysfunction supervenes, the elevated LV EDP and elevated LAP may result in "pseudo-normalization" of this pattern with an enhanced E velocity (related to a higher mitral valve opening gradient) and reduced A velocity (due to the elevated LV EDP). Coexisting mitral regurgitation also can lead to a "paradoxical" higher E velocity despite impaired ventricular relaxation.

Ischemic Cardiac Disease

In patients with coronary artery disease and no prior myocardial infarction, induction of ischemia results in diastolic dysfunction prior to systolic dysfunction (see Chapter 8). Diastolic filling curves with ischemia induced by balloon inflation during percutaneous transluminal angioplasty show rapid onset of a reduced E velocity, with resolution of these changes as ischemia is relieved. In acute myocardial infarction, a pattern of delayed relaxation is seen acutely. At follow-up, different patterns of LV filling may be observed: (1) with successful reperfusion and little myocardial damage, LV diastolic filling returns to normal; (2) with myocardial infarction but preserved LV systolic function, the pattern of impaired relaxation often persists; and (3) with a large infarction and significant LV systolic dysfunction, there is a "pseudo-normalized" pattern with a high E velocity and low A velocity due to a combination of reduced compliance, a high LV EDP, and a shift along the diastolic pressure-volume curve (increased end-systolic volume). Thus, an apparent "normal" pattern of LV filling late after myocardial infarction may be due to normal LV diastolic and systolic function or to impaired diastolic and systolic function. As with cardiomyopathy patients, pseudo-normal can be distinguished from normal based on a high E/A ratio, short IVRT, steep deceleration slope, and the pattern of myocardial tissue Doppler and pulmonary venous flow.

Pericardial Disease

With both pericardial tamponade and pericardial constriction, cardiac filling is impaired by pericardial "extrinsic constraint," and there is marked reciprocal respiratory variation in the LV and RV filling velocities. In the case of tamponade physiology, filling is impaired in both early and late diastole. With constrictive pericarditis, early diastolic filling tends to be normal, with marked impairment of filling late in diastole when the heart has expanded to the maximum allowed by the fibrotic pericardial encasement (see Chapter 10).

RIGHT VENTRICULAR DIASTOLIC FUNCTION

Right Ventricular Filling

The pattern of RV diastolic filling is similar to LV diastolic filling except that maximal velocities are lower (because the tricuspid annulus is larger) and the diastolic

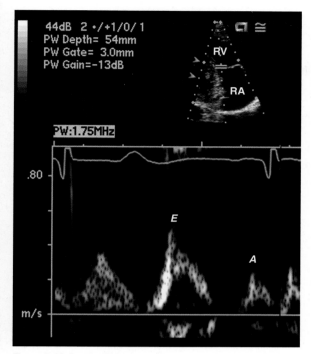

Figure 7-26 Doppler RV inflow shows an E velocity and A velocity similar to LV inflow.

filling period is slightly shorter (Fig. 7–26). Although few studies have addressed RV diastolic filling, the same measurements described for LV diastolic filling are applicable.

Doppler Data Recording

On TTE, RV inflow can be recorded from the parasternal RV inflow view or from the apical four-chamber view. Pulsed Doppler is used with the same technical considerations as apply to recording LV inflow velocities. Evaluation of respiratory variation on inflow velocities is complicated by the respiratory motion of the heart, so care is needed to ensure a parallel intercept angle between the ultrasound beam and inflow stream throughout the respiratory cycle. This can be accomplished in most patients by using a window where 2D echo shows little respiratory variation in the image plane itself or in the Doppler beam orientation relative to the 2D image.

Physiologic Factors That Affect Right Ventricular Filling

RV filling appears to be affected by all the same physiologic parameters that affect LV filling, although less attention has been directed toward RV inflow patterns. Again, the major differences between RV and LV filling are (1) timing, (2) reciprocal respiratory variation (as described earlier), and (3) absolute velocities,

which are lower for RV inflow because the tricuspid annulus is larger than the mitral annulus.

Right Atrial Filling

Doppler velocity curves of RA filling can be recorded in the superior vena cava (from a suprasternal notch approach) or the central hepatic vein (from a subcostal approach), since these central veins empty directly into the RA without intervening venous valves. The pattern of RA filling recorded by Doppler parallels the jugular venous pressure curves seen clinically (Fig. 7–27). However, the Doppler data represent a more reliable approach, since evaluation of jugular venous patterns is difficult in some patients due to body habitus and interpretation is subjective (with no recorded data).

Again, RA filling patterns show respiratory variation in normal individuals with augmentation of RA inflow during inspiration, as is seen in the RV inflow pattern. A plausible explanation for these observations is that the negative intrathoracic pressure with voluntary inspiration (but not with mechanical ventilation) results in an extrathoracic-to-intrathoracic pressure gradient from the great veins into the RA, leading to increased blood flow into the right side of the heart. RA pressure can be estimated by echocardiographic evaluation (from the subcostal window) of the inferior vena cava as it enters the RA as discussed in Chapter 6.

RA filling is most often evaluated from the subcostal window. After the long-axis view of the inferior vena cava is obtained, the transducer is rotated and

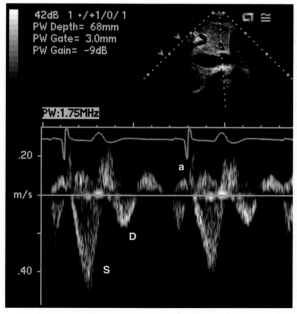

Figure 7-27 Normal pattern of RA inflow recorded in the central hepatic vein from a subcostal approach. Systolic (S) and diastolic (D) antegrade filling with slight flow reversal following atrial (A) contraction is seen.

angulated to visualize the central hepatic vein, which tends to be directed toward the transducer in this view, allowing a parallel intercept angle between the pulsed Doppler beam and hepatic vein flow. Hepatic vein flow is assumed to be representative of inferior vena caval flow, since both enter into the RA without intervening venous valves. Direct study of inferior vena caval flow is limited by a nearly perpendicular intercept angle.

RA inflow also can be recorded in the superior vena cava from the suprasternal notch window. From the standard aortic arch view, the transducer is angulated toward the patient's right to visualize the superior vena cava adjacent and slightly anterior to the ascending aorta. The pulsed Doppler sample volume is positioned in the superior vena cava, with adjustment of transducer angle and sample volume depth to obtain a well-defined velocity curve. As for

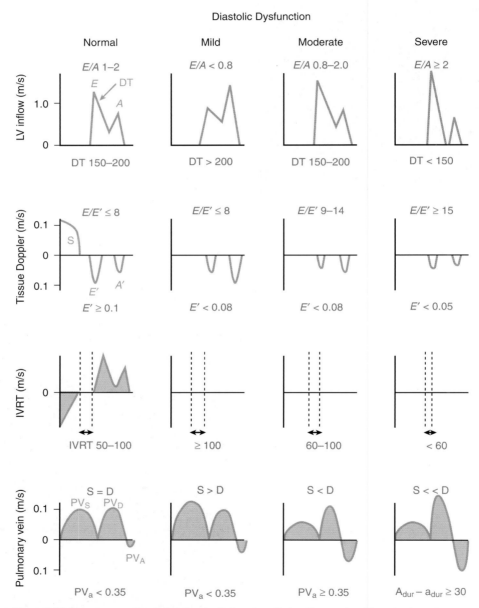

Figure 7–28 Diagram comparing typical Doppler findings in patients with normal, mild, moderate, and severe diastolic dysfunction. The top row shows LV inflow with early (E) and atrial (A) phases of diastolic filling, the second row shows tissue Doppler recorded at the septal side of the mitral annulus with the myocardial early (E′) and atrial (A′) velocities and the expected ratio of E/E′, the third row shows the isovolumic relaxation time (IVRT), and the bottom row shows the pulmonary venous inflow pattern with systolic (S) and diastolic (D) antegrade flow and the pulmonary vein atrial (PVₐ) reversal of flow.

other inflow patterns, wall filters are minimized (as allowed by signal-to-noise ratio) to demonstrate the low-velocity flows associated with atrial filling.

From both the superior vena cava and hepatic vein recordings it is important to distinguish respiratory variation in the Doppler curves due to (1) respiratory variation in the angle between the ultrasound beam and blood flow direction from (2) true variations in atrial filling volumes. The hepatic vein is small, so several positions often need to be tried to find one that maintains the sample volume in the hepatic vein throughout the respiratory cycle.

The physiologic factors that affect LA filling also affect RA filling, although (as for ventricular filling) less attention has been focused on physiologic parameters affecting the right side of the heart. Respiratory variation in RA filling typically is much more prominent than the respiratory variation seen in LA filling. When a non-sinus cardiac rhythm is present, the lack of atrial contraction results in an absent atrial reversal; systolic forward flow (the filling phase following atrial emptying) may be blunted or reversed.

ALTERNATE APPROACHES

Despite the numerous potential shortcomings of Doppler echocardiographic evaluation of diastolic filling, it has great promise as a repeatable, noninvasive, widely available method for evaluation of diastolic function (Fig. 7–28). Techniques used in the research laboratory (time constant of relaxation, pressure-volume curves, etc.) rarely are applicable to clinical patient management. The other available clinical modalities for evaluation of diastolic function include:

❑ Direct intracardiac pressure measurements
❑ Radionuclide high-resolution time-activity curves
❑ Cardiac magnetic resonance tissue tracking methods

The role of tissue Doppler or speckle tracking strain rate and strain measurements for clinical evaluation of diastolic dysfunction is in evolution.

SUGGESTED READING

Reviews

1. Desai MY, Klein AL: Assessment of diastolic function by echocardiography. In Otto CM (ed): The Practice of Clinical Echocardiography, 3rd ed. Philadelphia: Elsevier/Saunders, 2007, pp 237–261.
   Comprehensive book chapter that includes a review of the physiology of diastole, a detailed discussion of echocardiographic methods, and examples of clinical utility. 146 references.

2. Lester SJ, Tajik AJ, Nishimura RA, et al: Unlocking the mysteries of diastolic function: Deciphering the rosetta stone 10 years later. J Am Coll Cardiol 51:679–689, 2008.
   Detailed review of measures of diastolic dysfunction including practical tips for data recording. The classification of diastolic dysfunction severity and implications for therapy are discussed.

3. Maurer MS, Spevack D, Burkhoff D, et al: Diastolic dysfunction: Can it be diagnosed by Doppler echocardiography? J Am Coll Cardiol 44:1543–1549, 2004.
   This viewpoint emphasizes the difference between Doppler measures of diastolic filling and the intrinsic diastolic properties of the ventricle, defined by pressure-volume analysis. These points highlight some of the limitations of echocardiographic evaluation of diastolic dysfunction. The text and illustrations also provide a concise review of the physiology of diastole.

4. Oh JK, Hatle L, Tajik AJ, et al: Diastolic heart failure can be diagnosed by comprehensive two-dimensional and Doppler echocardiography. J Am Coll Cardiol 47:500–506, 2006.
   This viewpoint provides a rebuttal to Suggested Reading 3 and a brief review of the concept and diagnosis of diastolic heart failure. The authors argue that careful use of a combination of echocardiographic parameters does allow accurate diagnosis of diastolic dysfunction.

Consensus Guidelines

5. Rakowski H, Appleton C, Chan KL, et al: Canadian Consensus Recommendations for the Measurement and Reporting of Diastolic Dysfunction by Echocardiography. J Am Soc Echocardgr 9:736–760, 1996.
   Consensus document that first reviews the physiologic basis for Doppler measures of diastolic dysfunction and then summarizes recommended measurements and proposes classification on a scale from mild to severe dysfunction as summarized in Table 7–4. The use of Doppler myocardial velocity data (E' and A') is not addressed in this document but has been added to the figures and tables in this chapter.

6. Paulus WJ, Tschöpe C, Sanderson JE, et al: How to diagnose diastolic heart failure: A consensus statement on the diagnosis of heart failure with normal left ventricular ejection fraction by the Heart Failure and Echocardiography Associations of the European Society of Cardiology. Eur Heart J 28:2539–2550, 2007.
   This consensus statement recommends the term heart failure with normal ejection fraction (HFNEF) as a synonym for diastolic heart failure. The recommended diagnostic criteria for HRNEF are:
   1. Signs or symptoms of heart failure
   2. Normal LV systolic function (EF > 50% and LV end-diastolic volume index < 97 mL/m²)
   3. Evidence of diastolic dysfunction.
   Diastolic dysfunction is defined by invasive pressure measurements (LV EDP > 16 or pulmonary capillary wedge pressure [PCWP] > 12 mm Hg) or a Doppler E/E' > 15. When E/E' is between 8 and 15, additional diagnostic data include serum biomarkers, other Doppler diastolic function parameters (E/A, DT, PVₐ duration), LA volume index, LV mass index, and the presence of atrial fibrillation

7. Hatle L: How to diagnose diastolic heart failure: A consensus statement. Eur Heart J 28:2421–2423, 2007.
   This editorial, accompanying the consensus statement in Suggested Reading 6, provides a useful perspective. A specific concern is the reliance of the guidelines on the E/E' ratio, because a ratio over 15 is specific, but not sensitive, for an elevated diastolic pressure. Most patients with diastolic dysfunction and normal systolic function have an E/E' ratio between 8 and 15, emphasizing the need to

consider multiple parameters in evaluation for diastolic heart failure.

8. Nagueh SF, Appleton CP, Gillebert TG, et al: Recommendations for the evaluation of left ventricular diastolic function by echocardiography. J Am Soc Echocardiogr 22:107–133, 2009.

This consensus statement from the American Society of Echocardiography and the European Society of Echocardiography reviews the physiology of diastole, provides a detailed discussion of parameters of diastolic function (including validation), includes tables of normal values, proposes algorithms for clinical diagnosis of diastolic function, and classifies diastolic dysfunction (grades I, II, and III) based on LV filling and tissue Doppler parameters. A key resource for every echocardiography laboratory.

Prevalence of Diastolic Dysfunction

9. Yamada H, Goh PP, Sun JP, et al: Prevalence of left ventricular diastolic dysfunction by Doppler echocardiography: Clinical application of the Canadian Consensus guidelines. J Am Soc Echocardiogr 15:1238–1244, 2002.

In a series of 520 consecutive patients, diastolic dysfunction was present in 56% and was classified as mild in 19%, mild-to-moderate in 2%, moderate in 22%, and severe in 12% using the Canadian Consensus classification. In the 99 patients with clinical evidence of heart failure, diastolic dysfunction was the primary etiology in 38%, with most patients having underlying hypertensive or coronary heart disease.

10. Redfield MM, Jacobsen SJ, Burnett Jr JC, et al: Burden of systolic and diastolic ventricular dysfunction in the community: Appreciating the scope of the heart failure epidemic. JAMA 1289:194–202, 2003.

In a cross-sectional survey of 2042 adults over age 45, the prevalence of heart failure was 2.2%. However, 44% of these patients had an ejection fraction > 50%, suggesting diastolic dysfunction as the cause of clinical symptoms. The approach to classification of diastolic dysfunction based on mitral inflow, response to Valsalva maneuver, Doppler tissue imaging, and pulmonary venous flow is summarized.

Validation of Doppler Parameters

11. Nishimura RA, Schwartz RS, Tajik AJ, et al: Noninvasive measurement of rate of left ventricular relaxation by Doppler echocardiography: Validation with simultaneous cardiac catheterization. Circulation 88:146–155, 1993.

The time constant of LV relaxation (τ) can be calculated from the Doppler mitral regurgitant velocity signal using a semilogarithmic method with a zero asymptote, after conversion of velocities to pressures, using the Bernoulli equation. However, this approach requires knowledge of LAP and has only limited accuracy for detection of changes in τ in an individual patient.

12. Chen C, Rodriguez L, Lethor JP, et al: Continuous wave Doppler echocardiography for non-invasive assessment of left ventricular dP/dt and relaxation time constant from mitral regurgitant spectra in patients. J Am Coll Cardiol 23:970–976, 1994.

In 12 patients with mitral regurgitation, Doppler-derived measures correlated well with invasive data for maximum +dP/dt (r = 0.91), maximum −dP/dt (r = 0.89), and τ (r = 0.93).

13. Berk MR, Xie G, Kwan OL, et al: Reduction of left ventricular preload by lower body negative pressure alters Doppler transmitral filling patterns. J Am Coll Cardiol 16:1387–1392, 1990.

To avoid confounding effects of pharmacologic intervention, preload was reduced by lower body negative pressure. Decreased preload resulted in a reduced E velocity, no change in A velocity, a reduced E/A ratio, and a reduction in mean acceleration and deceleration with a corresponding prolongation of the pressure half-time.

14. Thomas JD, Choong CYP, Flachskampf FA, et al: Analysis of the early transmitral Doppler velocity curve: Effect of primary physiologic changes and compensatory preload adjustment. J Am Coll Cardiol 16:644–655, 1990.

Elegant description of early diastolic filling with mathematical explanations (for the mathematically inclined) and clear diagrams showing the effects of changes in each parameter (for the rest of us).

15. Pozzoli M, Capamolla S, Pinna G, et al: Doppler echocardiography reliably predicts pulmonary artery wedge pressure in patients with chronic heart failure with and without mitral regurgitation. J Am Coll Cardiol 27: 883–893, 1996.

Simultaneous right heart catheterization and Doppler studies were performed in 231 patients with chronic heart failure. Pulmonary wedge pressure correlated most closely with the deceleration rate of early mitral filling and the systolic fraction of pulmonary venous flow. Regression equations for noninvasive calculation of pulmonary wedge pressure are proposed.

16. Hofmann T, Keck A, van Ingen G, et al: Simultaneous measurement of pulmonary venous flow by intravascular catheter Doppler velocimetry and transesophageal Doppler echocardiography: Relation to left atrial pressure and left atrial and ventricular function. J Am Coll Cardiol 26:239–249, 1995.

In 32 patients undergoing open heart surgery, simultaneous measurement of LAP, pulmonary venous flow velocity by Doppler catheter, and TEE recording of pulmonary venous flow demonstrate close agreement between Doppler catheter and velocity data. LAP correlated with the ratio of systolic to diastolic peak velocity, the systolic VTI, the time to maximal flow velocity, and the ratio of systolic to diastolic flow duration.

17. Nishimura RA, Appleton CP, Redfield MM, et al: Noninvasive Doppler echocardiographic evaluation of left ventricular filling pressures in patients with cardiomyopathies: A simultaneous Doppler echocardiographic and cardiac catheterization study. J Am Coll Cardiol 28:1226–1233, 1996.

In patients with systolic LV dysfunction, LAP correlated directly with the E/A ratio, and inversely with the early diastolic DT. In contrast, correlation was poor in patients with hypertrophic cardiomyopathy due to multiple other factors affecting diastolic filling in these patients.

18. Takatsuji H, Mikami T, Urasawa K, et al: A new approach for evaluation of LV diastolic function: Spatial and temporal analysis of left ventricular filling flow propagation by color M-mode Doppler echocardiography. J Am Coll Cardiol 27:365–371, 1996.

Propagation velocity on a color M-mode of LV filling from an apical approach was defined as the distance/time ratio between the mitral orifice and the point where velocity decreased to 70% of its initial value. Compared to micromanometer pressure data, propagation velocity correlated with the time constant of relaxation (τ) and with peak −dP/dt in a series of 40 patients.

19. Ommen SR, Nishimura RA, Appleton CP, et al: Clinical utility of Doppler echocardiography and tissue Doppler imaging in the estimation of left ventricular filling pressures: A comparative simultaneous Doppler-catheterization study. Circulation 102:1788–1794, 2000.

Simultaneous catheter pressures and Doppler data were recorded in 100 consecutive patients undergoing cardiac catheterization. Isolated parameters of LV filling correlated with mean LV diastolic pressure only in patients with an ejection fraction < 50%. The best Doppler predictor of mean LV diastolic pressure was the ratio of the early mitral inflow velocity (E) to the early diastolic velocity of the mitral annulus (E').

A stepwise approach to evaluation of diastolic function, using multiple parameters, is recommended.

20. Schwammenthal E, Popescu BA, Popescu AC, et al: Nonivasive assessment of left ventricular end-diastolic pressure by the response of the transmitral *a*-wave velocity to a standardized Valsalva maneuver. Am J Cardiol 86:169–174, 2000.

Recording LV inflow during the Valsalva maneuver allows unmasking of elevated filling pressures when the E/A ratio is < 1.0. The change in the A velocity during Valsalva correlates closely (r = 0.87) with LV EDP, regardless of resting E/A ratio, with an increase in A velocity ≥ 9 cm/s during Valsalva indicating an LV EDP > 25 mm Hg.

21. Talreja DR, Nishimura RA, Oh JK: Estimation of left ventricular filling pressure with exercise by Doppler echocardiography in patients with normal systolic function: A simultaneous echocardiographic–cardiac catheterization study. J Am Soc Echocardiogr 20:477–479, 2007.

In 12 patients with dyspnea but a normal ejection fraction (>50%), exercise stress testing was performed with simultaneous Swan Ganz catheter and Doppler echocardiography. The sensitivity of a Doppler E/E′ ≤ 15 was 89% for predicting a normal (≤20 mm Hg) exercise pulmonary wedge pressure; the specificity of an E/E′ > 15 was 100% in identifying patients with a pulmonary wedge pressure over 20 mm Hg. Although this is a small study, it suggests that exercise measures of diastolic function may be useful in patients with unexplained exertional dyspnea.

Clinical Outcomes

22. Liang HY, Cauduro SA, Pellikka PA, et al: Comparison of usefulness of echocardiographic Doppler variables to left ventricular end-diastolic pressure in predicting future heart failure events. Am J Cardiol 97:866–871, 2006.

The value of measures of diastolic function in prediction of clinical outcome were evaluated in 289 patients with echocardiographic and catheterization data within 30 days of each other. The mean age was 64 ± 13 years, 37% were women, 39% had an ejection fraction < 50%, and 46% had significant (>70% stenosis) coronary artery disease. Multivariate predictors of heart failure events (n = 24 at a mean follow-up of 11 ± 10 months), adjusted for age, sex, ejection fraction, and previous heart failure, were invasively measured LV EDP ≥20 mm Hg (HR 1.09, confidence interval [CI] 1.03–1.16), Doppler E/E′ ratio ≥15 (HR 1.09, CI 1.03–1.15), and LA volume indexed to body surface area ≥ 23 m/m² (HR 1.05, CI 1.01–1.09). The best Doppler correlate of LV EDP was the E/E′ ratio (r = 0.31).

23. Persson H, Lonn E, Edner M, et al: Diastolic dysfunction in heart failure with preserved systolic function: need for objective evidence: Results from the CHARM Echocardiographic Substudy–CHARMES. J Am Coll Cardiol 49:687–694, 2007.

In 312 patients with heart failure symptoms and a mean ejection fraction of 50 ± 10%, diastolic dysfunction was present in 67% based on LV and LA filling patterns, compared with age-adjusted normal values. Mild dysfunction (present in 22%) was defined as impaired relaxation, moderate as a pseudonormal pattern (present in 37%), and severe as a restrictive pattern of diastolic filling (present in 7%). On multivariate analysis, the only independent predictors of outcome at a mean of 19 months were moderate (hazard ratio 3.5, 95% CI 1.2–11.2) and severe diastolic dysfunction (hazard ratio 5.7, CI 1.4–24.0).

24. Nishimura RA, Jaber W: Understanding "diastolic heart failure": The tip of the iceberg. J Am Coll Cardiol 49: 695–697, 2007.

This editorial accompanies Suggested Reading 23, suggesting that evaluation of diastolic function only with Doppler LV and LA filling patterns is overly simplistic and may miss patients with diastolic dysfunction. The different potential pathophysiologic explanations for heart failure symptoms with normal systolic function are discussed, including increased intrinsic muscle stiffness, increased ventricular and vascular stiffness resulting in increased sensitivity to changes in preload, and LV remodeling resulting in volume-dependent elevation of filling pressures.

25. Geske JB, Sorajja P, Nishimura RA, et al: Evaluation of left ventricular filling pressures by Doppler echocardiography in patients with hypertrophic cardiomyopathy: Correlation with direct left atrial pressure measurement at cardiac catheterization. Circulation 116:2702–2708, 2007.

Echocardiographic and catheter measurements of LAP were compared in 100 symptomatic hypertrophic cardiomyopathy patients, with simultaneous measurements in 42 patients. The correlation between the E/E′ ratio (using septal tissue velocities) was only fair (r = 0.44). The specificity of E/E′ for an elevated filling pressure was low (75%) in patients with hypertrophic cardiomyopathy; LAP was <15 mm Hg in 17 of 68 patients with an E/E′ > 15. However, a E/E′ > 15 identified 51 of the 61 patients with a mean LAP > 15 mm Hg (sensitivity 84%).

26. Rakowski H, Carasso S: Quantifying diastolic function in hypertrophic cardiomyopathy: The ongoing search for the Holy Grail. Circulation 116:2662–2665, 2007.

Editorial accompanying Suggested Reading 25 provides a perspective on the challenges of assessing diastolic function in patients with hypertrophic cardiomyopathy.

Ischemic Cardiac Disease

G iven the high prevalence of coronary artery disease, evaluation of patients with suspected or documented ischemic disease is one of the most common indications for echocardiography. Echocardiographic evaluation typically focuses on the functional outcome of coronary artery disease—specifically systolic wall thickening and endocardial motion—rather than on direct imaging of the coronary arteries. Although the proximal left main and right coronary arteries often can be identified, even on transthoracic (TTE) images, ultrasound imaging currently does not provide the detailed knowledge of distal vessel anatomy or the location and severity of coronary artery narrowing that is needed for patient management. Coronary angiography remains the procedure of choice for direct assessment of coronary artery anatomy.

However, echocardiography offers detailed functional assessment of segmental and global left ventricular (LV) systolic function both at rest and after interventions to induce ischemia. In many cases this functional assessment provides critical data for patient management. For example, stress echocardiography is a reliable approach for the initial diagnosis of coronary artery disease, especially in patients with a nondiagnostic stress electrocardiogram (ECG). Another example is the use of echocardiography in the emergency department for early diagnosis of acute myocardial infarction in patients with equivocal ECGs. In addition, the central role of echocardiography in evaluation for complications of acute myocardial infarction has long been recognized. Finally, echocardiography often provides important prognostic data in patients with coronary artery disease.

BASIC PRINCIPLES

Coronary Artery Anatomy

While coronary anatomy varies to some degree from patient to patient, the overall pattern of coronary artery branching is relatively uniform (Fig. 8–1). The left main coronary artery arises from the superior aspect of the left coronary sinus of Valsalva and divides into (1) the left anterior descending (LAD) artery, which extends via the interventricular groove down the anterior wall to (and sometimes around) the LV

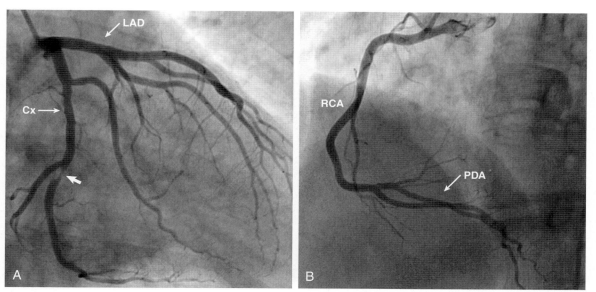

Figure 8–1 Normal left coronary artery in a right anterior oblique projection showing the left anterior descending (LAD) and circumflex (Cx) coronary arteries (**A**). Normal right coronary artery (RCA) anatomy with the posterior descending artery (PDA) seen in a right anterior oblique projection (**B**).

apex, and (2) the circumflex (Cx) artery, which continues laterally in the atrioventricular groove. The right coronary artery (RCA) arises from the superior aspect of the right coronary sinus of Valsalva and extends inferomedially following the atrioventricular groove. Approximately 80% of patients have a *right-dominant* coronary circulation; the right coronary artery gives rise to the posterior descending artery (PDA), which lies in the inferior interventricular groove. In about 20% of patients the coronary circulation is *left dominant;* the circumflex artery gives rise to the posterior descending artery.

Segmental wall motion abnormalities seen by echocardiography correspond closely with the coronary artery blood supply to the myocardium (Fig. 8–2). The left anterior descending artery supplies the anterior portion of the interventricular septum via septal perforating branches and the anterior wall via diagonal branches. The posterior descending artery supplies the inferior aspect of the ventricular septum and the inferior free wall. The lateral wall is supplied by obtuse marginal branches of the circumflex artery. The posterior LV wall may be supplied by extension branches from the right coronary artery or by obtuse marginal branches of the circumflex arteries. There is marked individual variability in the blood supply to the LV apex. In some cases, the left anterior descending artery extends around the apex to supply the apical segment of the inferior wall. In other cases, the posterior descending artery extends around the apex to supply the apical segment of the anterior wall. More commonly, the blood supply to the apex arises from both the left anterior descending and the posterior descending coronary arteries.

A standardized nomenclature for tomographic imaging of the heart allows consistency of terms, correlations between different imaging techniques, and a known relationship of each segment to coronary anatomy. The standardized terminology for tomographic planes is short axis, vertical long axis (equivalent to echocardiographic two-chamber plane), and horizontal long axis (equivalent to echocardiographic four-chamber plane). From base to apex the LV is divided into three segments—basal, mid-cavity, and apical—to correspond to proximal, middle, and apical lesions of the coronary arteries (Fig. 8–3). In a short-axis view, both at the basal (mitral valve) and mid-cavity (or papillary muscle) levels, the ventricle is divided clockwise, beginning with the interventricular groove, into six segments: the anterior wall, the anterolateral wall, the posterior (or inferolateral) wall, the inferior wall, the inferior septal, and the anterior septal walls. The apical region is divided into four segments because of the normal tapering of the ventricle toward the apex: anterior, lateral, inferior, and septal, with an additional segment for the tip of the apex. This results in a total of 17 myocardial segments. The location of wall motion abnormalities can be reported descriptively, using a series of drawings showing different echocardiographic views or using more quantitative display formats.

The segmental wall motion abnormalities seen with ischemia or infarction correspond to the coronary anatomy as follows:

1. Left anterior descending artery disease results in wall motion abnormalities of the anterior septum,

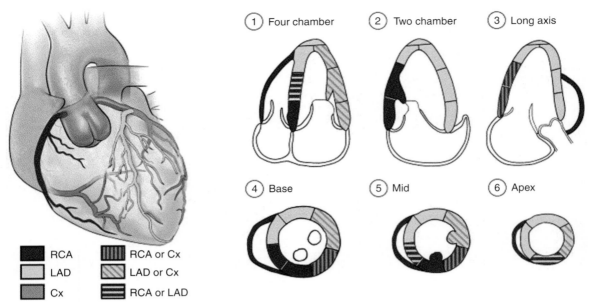

Figure 8–2 Typical distributions of the right coronary artery (RCA) and the left anterior descending artery (LAD) and circumflex (Cx) coronary arteries. The coronary anatomy is shown on the left with the corresponding wall segments in standard echocardiographic views on the right. The arterial distribution varies between patients. Some segments have variable coronary perfusion as indicated by the hatched regions. *(From Lang RM, Bierig M, Devereux RB et al: Recommendations for chamber quantification: a report from the American Society of Echocardiography's Guidelines and Standards Committee and the Chamber Quantification Writing Group, developed in conjunction with the European Association of Echocardiography, a branch of the European Society of Cardiology. J Am Soc Echocardiogr 18:1440–1463, 2005.)*

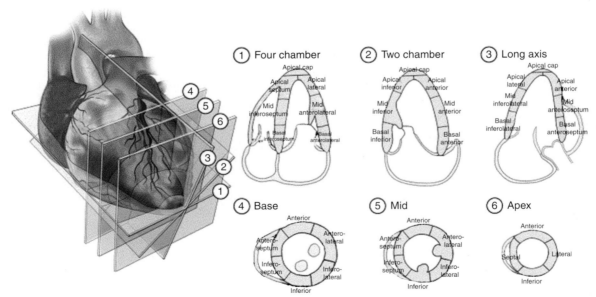

Figure 8–3 Segmental analysis of LV walls based on schematic views, in a PSAX and PLAX orientation, at three different levels. The apex segments are usually visualized from apical four-chamber, apical two-chamber, and apical three-chamber views. The apical cap can only be appreciated on some contrast studies. A 16-segment model can be used, without the apical cap, as described in an ASE 1989 document. A 17-segment model, including the apical cap, has been suggested by the American Heart Association Writing Group on Myocardial Segmentation and Registration for Cardiac Imaging. *(From Lang RM, Bierig M, Devereux RB, et al: Recommendations for chamber quantification: a report from the American Society of Echocardiography's Guidelines and Standards Committee and the Chamber Quantification Writing Group, developed in conjunction with the European Association of Echocardiography, a branch of the European Society of Cardiology. J Am Soc Echocardiogr 18:1440–1463, 2005.)*

anterior free wall, at the base and mid-cavity level and of the septal and anterior apical segments and the LV apex. Depending on the degree to which diagonal branches supply the lateral wall, the anterolateral wall also may be affected. If the left anterior descending artery extends around the apex, the affected area includes apical segments of the inferior and inferolateral walls. The location of the lesion along the length of the coronary artery affects the pattern of wall motion. A lesion in the distal third of the vessel affects only the apex, a lesion in the midsegment of the vessel affects the mid-cavity and apical segments, while a proximal lesion affects the entire wall including the basal segments.

2. Circumflex artery disease affects wall motion of the anterolateral and posterolateral LV walls. Again the extent of segmental wall motion is related to the exact coronary anatomy in an individual patient. Echocardiography is particularly helpful in patients with circumflex disease, because this myocardial region often is "silent" electrocardiographically and is not well seen on a single-plane right anterior oblique LV angiogram.

3. Posterior descending artery disease results in abnormal wall motion in the inferior septum, inferior free wall, and inferolateral (posterior) LV segments. If the posterior descending artery is a short vessel, the apex will not be affected, while extensive wall motion abnormalities of the apex may be seen if the posterior descending artery extends to supply the ventricular apex.

Other patterns of abnormal wall motion are seen with lesions of the branches of the three major coronary arteries. For example, isolated disease in a diagonal branch of the left anterior descending artery results in a discrete wall motion abnormality in the portion of the anterolateral wall supplied by that vessel. Proximal right coronary artery disease can result in ischemia or infarction of the right ventricular (RV) free wall.

Collateral vessels and previous bypass surgery also affect the pattern of wall motion. If a myocardial segment has a balanced oxygen demand-to-supply ratio, wall motion will be normal whether blood flow is supplied antegrade by the native vessel, by collateral vessels, or by a bypass graft.

Evaluation of Left Ventricular Wall Motion

Transthoracic Imaging

Regional systolic function for each segment of the LV can be assessed on TTE imaging by combining data from multiple image planes (Fig. 8–4). Standard views for evaluation of wall motion are:

- ❑ Short-axis (base, mid-LV, and apex) view
- ❑ Four-chamber view
- ❑ Two-chamber view
- ❑ Long-axis view

In the parasternal long-axis view, the basal and midventricular segments of the anterior septum and posterior LV walls are seen. In the parasternal short-axis view, circumferential images of the LV at the base and midventricular levels are obtained. Note that if the transducer is angulated toward the apex from a fixed parasternal position, progressively more apical segments of the posterior wall are imaged while the *same* segment of the septum is included in the ultrasound image plane. A more parallel alignment between image planes may be obtained by moving the transducer apically to obtain short-axis mid-cavity and (sometimes) apical views of the LV (Fig. 8–5). In either case, evaluation of wall motion from other windows is helpful for avoiding misdiagnosis related to an oblique image plane. Of note, the apical segments rarely are adequately visualized from the parasternal window or on transesophageal (TEE) images.

From the apical window, evaluation of LV wall motion is performed in four-chamber, two-chamber, and long-axis views. Detailed evaluation of the extent of abnormal myocardium is possible by slow rotation of the image plane between the standard views. In the four-chamber view, the inferior septum and anterolateral wall are seen. Anterior angulation to include the aortic valve allows visualization of portions of the anterior septum. In the two-chamber view, the anterior and inferior free walls are seen. Endocardial and epicardial definition of the anterior wall may be difficult due to attenuation by adjacent overlying lung tissue. This problem can be alleviated by careful patient positioning and imaging during held respiration. In the apical long-axis view, the anterior septum and inferolateral (posterior) wall are seen (analogous to the parasternal long-axis view).

Note that while these three apical image planes are oriented approximately 60° to each other, there is some individual variation in their exact relationship. In addition, variation in coronary anatomy between individuals results in variable patterns of abnormal wall motion. Care is needed in positioning the transducer at the apex to avoid foreshortening of the ventricle from this approach. Integration of data from parasternal and apical approaches, taking into account image quality in each view, allows assessment of each myocardial segment in at least two views.

Finally, evaluation from a subcostal approach may be helpful. In the subcostal four-chamber view, the inferior septum and anterolateral wall are imaged. In the subcostal short-axis view, the inferior and inferolateral (posterior) walls are nearest the transducer and the anterior and anterolateral walls most distal (Fig. 8–6).

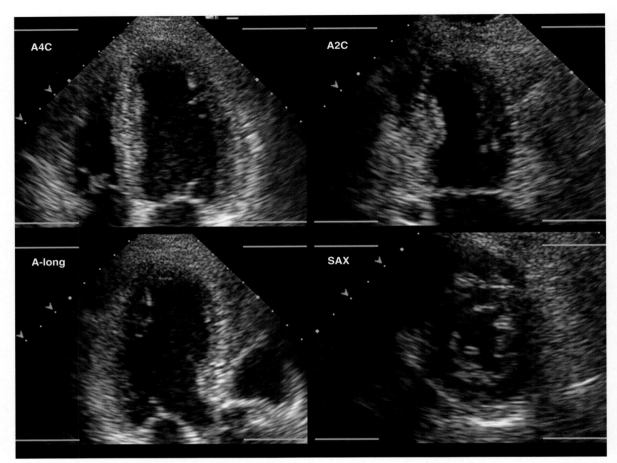

Figure 8–4 Example of the standard image planes used for stress echocardiography: apical four-chamber (A4C), apical two-chamber (A2C), apical long-axis (A-long), and parasternal short-axis (PSAX). Images are acquired in a digital cine-loop format at each stress stage and then re-sorted to show the baseline and peak stress images side-by-side for each view. Images are gated to show only systole so that endocardial motion and wall thickening appear to occur in the same time frame, even though there is a substantial difference in HR between baseline and peak stress. Image depth is adjusted to show only the LV.

Real-time volumetric imaging from an apical approach avoids many of these limitations. Simultaneous apical views at set angles of rotation or multiple parallel short-axis views can be generated from the three-dimensional (3D) volume set allowing rapid evaluation of wall motion in multiple myocardial segments on the same cardiac cycles. A limitation of apical volumetric scans is that the endocardium is imaged using the lateral, rather than axial, resolution of the ultrasound beam, which may limit identification of endocardial borders for quantitative analysis (see Fig. 4-1).

Transesophageal Imaging

When TTE images are inadequate, or in certain monitoring situations (e.g., intraoperative monitoring of LV function), regional LV function can be evaluated from a TEE approach (Fig. 8–7). From the high left atrial (LA) position a four-chamber view of the LV is obtained (in the 0° plane of the TEE probe) showing the inferior septum and lateral wall. Rotating the image plane to approximately 60° provides a two-chamber view with visualization of the anterior and inferior walls, while further rotation to about 120° results in a long-axis view with imaging of the anterior septum and inferolateral (posterior) wall. Again, the exact degree of rotation to obtain these views varies slightly from patient to patient. In addition, transducer position and angulation may require adjustment as the image plane is rotated using anatomic landmarks to ensure optimal images with inclusion of the apical segments. Even with optimal technique these views may be foreshortened; that is, the apparent apex represents an oblique plane through the anterolateral wall, while the true LV apex is not seen.

From the transgastric position, the transverse image plane provides short-axis views of the LV at the base (mitral valve) and mid-cavity (papillary muscle) level.

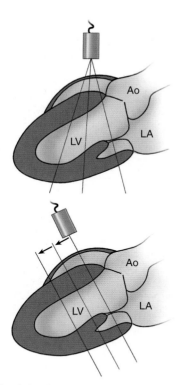

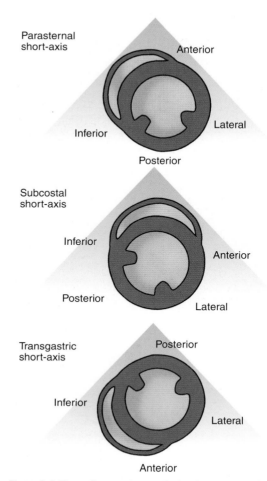

Figure 8–5 Angulation of the transducer from a fixed parasternal position results in short-axis views that intersect similar segments of the septum but progressively more apical segments of the posterior wall. By moving the transducer apically, more parallel image planes can be obtained.

Rotation of the image plane at this position provides a two-chamber view, although the apex may be fore-shortened. Further advancement of the probe may allow acquisition of an "apical" four-chamber view (in the 0° plane) by flexing the probe tip. However, the ventricle may be foreshortened and the true apex missed if the LV apex does not lie on the diaphragm without intervening lung tissue in a position accessible from the transgastric approach.

TEE imaging of LV wall motion is indicated:

❏ For intraoperative assessment of global and segmental LV function
❏ In critically ill patients when TTE views are inadequate

TEE imaging also may be used with stress protocols, although this is not a routine approach.

Sequence of Events in Ischemia

Irreversible myocardial damage (e.g., infarction) results in wall motion abnormalities that are present at rest. With an acute infarction, wall thickness is normal, but systolic wall thickening and endocardial motion are reduced or absent. An old myocardial infarction is characterized by thinning and increased echogenicity of the affected segments due to scarring

Figure 8–6 The wall segments seen in the short-axis view from TTE parasternal and subcostal, and TEE transgastric approach are shown. Correct identification of wall segments is facilitated by noting the position of the septum and the papillary muscles.

and fibrosis, in addition to abnormal motion and absent wall thickening.

In contrast, ischemia is a reversible imbalance in the myocardial oxygen demand-to-supply ratio. Even with substantial coronary artery narrowing, blood flow is adequate for myocardial oxygen demands at rest. However, when the narrowing exceeds approximately 70% of the luminal cross-sectional area, blood flow becomes inadequate to meet increased myocardial oxygen demands with exercise, pharmacologic interventions, or mental stress, resulting in ischemia. When oxygen demand returns to baseline, blood flow again is adequate, ischemia resolves, and wall motion returns to normal. Thus, wall motion *at rest* is normal in patients with coronary artery disease if there has been no prior myocardial infarction.

The sequence of changes as a region of myocardium becomes ischemic is as follows (Fig. 8–8). The first detectable changes associated with heterogeneity of

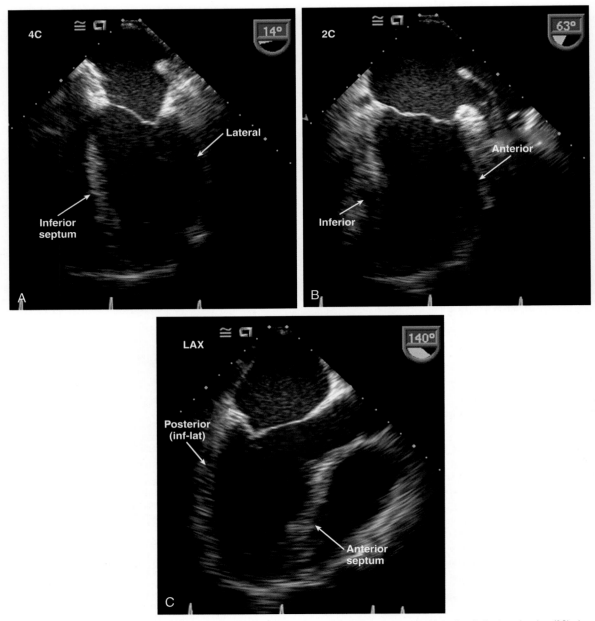

Figure 8–7 In the standard high TEE views, the four-chamber (4C) view shows the inferior septum and lateral wall, the two-chamber (2C) view shows the anterior and inferior walls, and the long-axis view (LAX) shows the anterior septum and posterior or inferolateral (inf-lat) wall. The apical segments are best visualized by decreasing transducer frequency and adjusting probe angulation, but apical abnormalities may be difficult to appreciate. Subcostal short-axis and two-chamber views also are helpful for evaluation of wall motion.

flow to the LV are biochemical followed by a significant perfusion defect (detectable by radionuclide and magnetic resonance techniques). Next, regional myocardial dysfunction, characterized by both abnormal diastolic function and impaired systolic wall thickening, occurs in rapid succession (within a few cardiac cycles). Ischemic ST-segment depression on ECG and clinical angina are relatively late manifestations of ischemia and are not seen consistently. Echocardiography, by detecting abnormal regional wall motion, provides a useful noninvasive method for evaluating ischemia that is more sensitive than ECG given this sequence of events. Echocardiography differs from radionuclide techniques in that the functional consequences of ischemia, rather than the pattern of myocardial perfusion, are assessed.

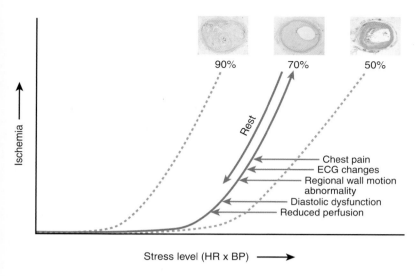

90%   70%   50%

Ischemia →

Rest

Chest pain
ECG changes
Regional wall motion
abnormality
Diastolic dysfunction
Reduced perfusion

Stress level (HR x BP) →

Figure 8–8 Schematic diagram of the sequence of events in myocardial ischemia. The level of stress is shown on the horizontal axis, often estimated by the heart rate × blood pressure product, with the degree of ischemia shown on the vertical axis. With a 70% coronary artery narrowing (*blue*), ischemia begins when the stress level results in inadequate coronary blood flow to that region of myocardium. As ischemia increases, the sequence of events is shown. With rest (*downward blue arrow*), these events reverse unless the duration of ischemia is long enough to cause infarction. The onset and slope of the ischemic response is earlier and steeper with more severe coronary stenosis (as shown for a 90% lesion), and later and less steep with milder coronary disease (as shown for a 50% stenosis).

Evaluation of Global and Regional Ventricular Function

Global LV systolic function can be evaluated either qualitatively or quantitatively in patients with coronary artery disease using the approaches described in Chapter 6. Since the pattern of LV dysfunction typically is *not* uniform, it is important that qualitative evaluation be based on multiple tomographic views. If quantitative methods are applied, approaches that incorporate endocardial borders from at least two tomographic planes are most appropriate. In patients with coronary artery disease, LV ejection fraction measurement provides essential clinical data because it is a crucial variable in clinical decision making and for predicting long-term outcome.

Segmental (or regional) LV systolic function most often is evaluated using a semiquantitative scoring system. The endocardial motion for each defined myocardial segment is graded as normal, hyperdynamic, hypokinetic, akinetic, dyskinetic, or aneurysmal (Table 8–1). Some clinicians prefer to subclassify the degree of hypokinesis as mild, moderate, or severe, but such a subclassification often has significant interobserver and intraobserver variability. Ischemia results both in a decrease in the total amplitude and velocity of endocardial motion and wall thickening and in a delay in the onset of contraction and relaxation. Some centers use a numerical scoring system for wall motion from 1 (normal) to 4 (dyskinetic) for each segment. An overall wall motion score index can be derived by dividing the sum of scores for each segment by the number of segments evaluated:

$$\text{Wall motion score} = \frac{\text{Sum of individual segment scores}}{\text{Number of segments visualized}}$$

Several more sophisticated approaches to quantitation of wall motion have been proposed based on the

TABLE 8–1	**Qualitative Scale for Assessment of Segmental Wall Motion**
Wall Motion Grade	**Definition**
Hyperdynamic	Increased amplitude and velocity of endocardial inward motion and wall thickening in systole
Normal	Normal endocardial inward motion and wall thickening in systole
Hypokinesis	Reduced amplitude and velocity of endocardial motion and wall thickening in systole, delay in the onset of contraction and relaxation.
Akinesis	Absence of inward endocardial motion or wall thickening in systole
Dyskinesis	Outward motion or "bulging" of the segment in systole, usually associated with thin, scarred myocardium
Aneurysmal	Diastolic contour abnormality and dyskinesis

total amplitude of endocardial motion, the extent of wall thickening, the velocity of myocardial motion, or the timing of the onset of contraction. Quantitative evaluation of regional function by echocardiography requires:

❏ Identification and tracing of the endocardium at end-diastole and end-systole
❏ Evaluation of wall motion for all segments of the myocardium

❒ Knowledge of the degree of variability of normal wall motion

❒ Correction for the effects of LV translation, rotation, and torsion

❒ High temporal resolution for analysis of the onset and velocity of myocardial thickening

Approaches that incorporate 3D reconstruction of the LV may improve data acquisition times and may diminish the effects of cardiac motion that potentially result in imaging different regions of myocardium in systole versus diastole for a given tomographic plane. Although wall thickening or the timing and velocity of motion may be more sensitive methods for evaluation of regional ventricular function, most current approaches continue to rely on endocardial motion. Other promising approaches include (1) contrast echocardiography to improve endocardial definition or evaluate myocardial perfusion and (2) tissue Doppler or speckle-tracking strain and strain rate imaging (see Suggested Reading and Chapter 4).

MYOCARDIAL ISCHEMIA

Since echocardiographic wall motion at rest is normal in a patient with significant coronary artery disease and no prior myocardial infarction, imaging *during ischemia* is needed for diagnosis. Inducing ischemia during echocardiographic imaging is referred to as *stress echocardiography*. Ischemia can be induced by increasing myocardial oxygen demand either with exercise or by pharmacologic interventions (Table 8–2).

Basic Principles of Stress Echocardiography

Stress echocardiography is based on the concept that an increased cardiac workload is needed to elicit signs of physiologic dysfunction in many types of cardiac disease. For example, in patients with coronary artery disease, resting myocardial blood flow is adequate so that myocardial function, seen on echocardiography as wall thickening and endocardial motion, is normal at rest. However, when cardiac workload is increased, the increased oxygen demands of the myocardium cannot be balanced by an increase in flow in the coronary artery, resulting in ischemia with impairment of myocardial thickening and endocardial motion (Fig. 8–9). An increase in cardiac workload typically is achieved by having the patient exercise, either on a supine bicycle or an upright treadmill or by infusion of a pharmacologic agent, such as dobutamine, that increases heart rate (HR). In addition to echocardiographic imaging, key elements in interpretation of stress test results include the:

❒ Duration of exercise

❒ Maximum workload—approximated by heart rate × blood pressure (HR × BP) product

❒ Symptoms

❒ BP response

❒ Arrhythmias

❒ ST-segment changes on ECG

The basic principles of image acquisition for stress echocardiography are to use standard image planes, ensure that all myocardial segments are visualized in at least one (and preferably two) views, use comparable

TABLE 8–2 Stress Echocardiography

Type of Stress	Advantages	Disadvantages
Treadmill exercise	Widely available High workload	Imaging post-ETT only
Upright bicycle	Imaging during exercise	Imaging may be technically difficult. Lower workload
Supine bicycle	Imaging during exercise	Lower workload Supine position affects exercise physiology
Dobutamine + atropine	Continuous imaging Does not require physically active patient	Potential adverse effects of dobutamine Lower level of stress achieved
Vasodilator	Continuous imaging Does not require physically active patient	Potential adverse effects of vasodilator agent Induction of relative flow inequality rather than ischemia per se
Atrial pacing	Continuous imaging Does not require physically active patient	Requires permanent pacer Does not simulate exercise

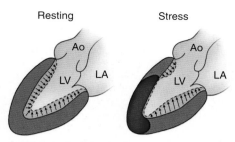

Resting   Stress

Figure 8–9 Diagram illustrating the concept of stress echocardiography in a patient with a 70% stenosis in the proximal third of the left anterior descending coronary artery (LAD). At rest (*left*), endocardial motion and wall thickening are normal. After stress (*right*), either exercise or pharmacologic, the middle and apical segments of the anterior wall become ischemic, showing reduced endocardial wall motion and wall thickening. If the LAD extends around the apex, the apical segment of the posterior wall also will be affected, as shown here. The normal segment of the posterior wall shows compensatory hyperkinesis.

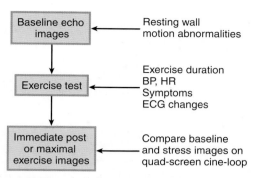

Figure 8–10 Flow chart of an exercise echocardiography protocol. HR, heart rate.

views at rest and stress, and record images in a digital cine-loop format with side-by-side display of rest and stress images. The cine-loop format is essential because otherwise the change in heart rate between rest and stress makes interpretation of wall motion difficult.

For evaluation of regional ventricular function, optimal endocardial definition is essential. When endocardial definition remains suboptimal despite careful patient positioning, use of harmonic imaging and other imaging adjustments, contrast echocardiography, or a non-echocardiographic imaging approach should be considered.

The sensitivity of stress echocardiography for detection of coronary disease depends on acquiring stress images at the maximal cardiac workload. With pharmacologic stress testing, this is rarely an issue, because the stress level can be maintained until image acquisition is complete. However, with exercise stress, the workload declines rapidly on cessation of exercise, so that images must be acquired as quickly as possible after exercise. Both the time from stopping exercise and the heart rate at the time of image acquisition compared to maximum heart rate are recorded as indicators of workload. 3D echocardiographic acquisition systems that allow simultaneous real-time imaging in multiple image planes offer the promise of faster acquisition times at peak stress, with the potential for improved diagnostic sensitivity.

Exercise Echocardiography

Exercise echocardiography typically is performed using standard exercise test protocols. Supine or upright bicycle exercise protocols have the advantage that echocardiographic imaging can be performed during exercise at each progressive level of exertion, including maximal exercise. Treadmill exercise protocols have the advantage that a higher total workload can be achieved but the disadvantage that imaging

can only be performed after exercise. Wall motion abnormalities that resolve very rapidly after exercise may be missed.

Resting images are acquired in digital cine-loop format for standard views of the LV. Standard exercise protocols are used with monitoring of the 12-lead ECG, BP, and symptoms by a qualified medical professional during and following the exercise protocol. The risks of exercise echocardiography are the risks of the exercise test itself. Either during maximal exercise (supine or sitting bicycle) or immediately after exercise (treadmill), digital cine-loop image acquisition is repeated. Typically, four or more sequential cycles are recorded digitally, and the examiner subsequently chooses the best image for comparison with the baseline views (Fig. 8–10). This allows elimination of poor-quality images due to respiratory motion. Next, the rest and exercise cine-loop digital images are displayed side by side so that endocardial motion and wall thickening for each myocardial region can be compared.

Interpretation of an exercise stress echocardiogram includes incorporation of data on the maximum workload achieved (exercise duration), the heart rate and BP response to exercise, the presence of arrhythmias, and clinical symptoms, as well as evaluation of the echocardiographic images. A systematic approach, comparing each segment in turn, is needed for detection of subtle abnormalities (Fig. 8–11).

Dobutamine Stress Echocardiography

Evaluation for Ischemia

Pharmacologic stress testing with intravenous dobutamine is based on the increased heart rate and contractility induced by this potent beta-agonist. Dobutamine is started at a low dose (5 µg/kg/min) and increased incrementally every 3 minutes with a calibrated intravenous infusion pump to (10, 20, 30, and 40 µg/kg/min) until the maximum dose or an endpoint has been reached. Atropine is used as needed, in divided doses of 0.25 to 0.5 mg (maximum

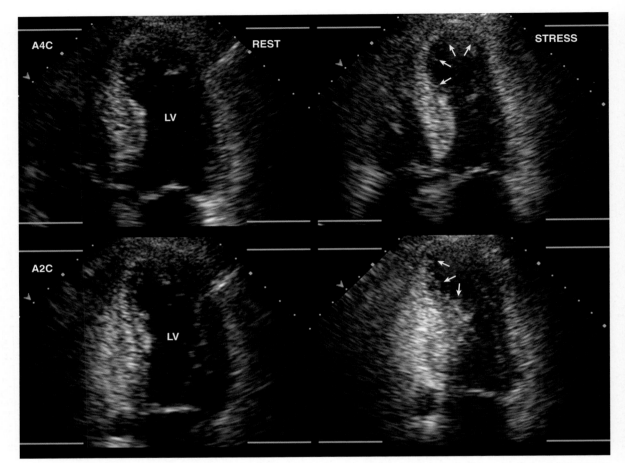

Figure 8–11 Frames from an abnormal exercise echo study showing the development of apical akinesis (*arrows*) with exercise. End-systolic images are shown at rest on the left and immediately after exercise on the right in the four-chamber view (*top*) and two-chamber view (*bottom*). Regional function was normal at rest with normal endocardial motion and wall thickening in all segments. With stress, the apical inferior septum and inferior wall become akinetic, consistent with inducible ischemia in the distal LAD coronary artery territory.

total 2.0 mg), to achieve the target goal of 85% of the patient's maximum predicted heart rate. In order to minimize the likelihood of significant adverse effects and to optimize the quality of the data obtained, a dobutamine stress echocardiography examination requires a well-defined study protocol performed in the appropriate clinical setting.

Patient monitoring during dobutamine stress echocardiography includes:

❑ Periodic BP measurement (usually every 2 to 3 minutes)
❑ Continuous ECG monitoring
❑ Careful observation for clinical symptoms or signs

Appropriate equipment, medications, and trained personnel should be immediately available in the event of an adverse effect, including a cardiac defibrillator, emergency cardiac medications, intravenous esmolol (a beta-blocker that counteracts the effects of dobutamine), and a qualified physician.

After an intravenous line for administration of the dobutamine has been placed, the patient is positioned in a left lateral decubitus position on an echo-stretcher with an apical cutout to allow optimal image acquisition throughout the study protocol. Initially the intravenous line is filled only with saline solution while resting data are obtained. Data collection at baseline, at each dosage level, and during recovery includes heart rate, BP, symptoms, a 12-lead ECG, and echocardiographic images (Fig. 8–12). Standard views include parasternal short-axis images at the base and mid-cavity levels and apical four-chamber, two-chamber, and long-axis images with digital image acquisition in each view. Some centers also record Doppler LV filling and ejection velocities at each stage of the stress protocol.

Endpoints for stopping the test are:

❑ reaching the maximum protocol dose,
❑ patient discomfort,
❑ a definite wall motion abnormality involving two or more adjacent segments,

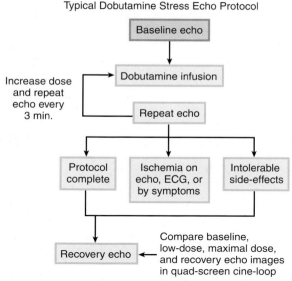

Typical Dobutamine Stress Echo Protocol

Baseline echo

Dobutamine infusion

Repeat echo

Increase dose and repeat echo every 3 min.

Protocol complete

Ischemia on echo, ECG, or by symptoms

Intolerable side-effects

Recovery echo

Compare baseline, low-dose, maximal dose, and recovery echo images in quad-screen cine-loop

Figure 8–12 Flow chart of dobutamine stress echo protocol.

each myocardial segment, wall motion is compared on these images in a systematic fashion. Since wall thickening and endocardial motion normally increase with dobutamine, an abnormal test is defined as the observation of hypokinesis or akinesis in a region that had normal wall motion at rest (Figs. 8–13 and 8–14).

Evaluation for Myocardial Viability

In addition to detection of ischemic myocardium, dobutamine stress echocardiography has been proposed as a method to evaluate for myocardial viability in regions that are "stunned" or "hibernating." For example, after treatment of myocardial infarction with thrombolytic therapy, the extent of residual viable myocardium in the area at risk may be unclear early after the event because of myocardial "stunning." Alternatively, a patient with chronic coronary artery disease may have hypokinesis or akinesis at baseline due to "hibernating" myocardium, which may recover with revascularization. In both these settings, echocardiographic imaging during low-dose (5 to 10 µg/kg/min) dobutamine infusion has been reported to show improved wall thickening and endocardial motion in viable segments of the myocardium. Of course, at higher dobutamine doses, worsening of regional function may occur due to induction of ischemia. This pattern of initial improvement at low dose, with subsequent worsening of myocardial function at higher dobutamine doses, is referred to as a *biphasic response.*

Other Stress Modalities

Vasodilators (dipyridamole or adenosine) have been proposed for echocardiographic stress testing by some investigators based on the differential pattern of coronary blood flow induced by these agents: increased blood flow in normal coronary arteries with a *relative* decrease in blood flow in diseased vessels. Overall success with this approach has been higher with nuclear perfusion imaging because the difference in blood flow between regions supplied by normal versus abnormal coronary arteries can be seen on the radionuclide images. Results with echocardiographic imaging have been less consistent, since actual ischemia (not just a relative difference in blood flow) is needed to discern a wall motion abnormality. In patients with a permanent pacer, atrial pacing to achieve the target heart rate is another option.

Limitations/Technical Aspects

Stress echocardiography has a high sensitivity and specificity for diagnosis of significant coronary artery disease (Tables 8–3 and 8–4). In addition, it allows reliable definition of the anatomic location and extent of ischemic myocardium. However, stress

- ☐ ST-segment elevation on ECG,
- ☐ reaching 85% of maximum predicted heart rate for age,
- ☐ a systolic BP >200 or <100 mm Hg *or* a diastolic BP >120 mm Hg, or
- ☐ significant ventricular arrhythmias.

Although serious complications are uncommon when appropriate precautions are observed, reported adverse effects include anxiety, tremulousness, palpitations, arrhythmias, paresthesias, and chest pain. About 10% of patients have premature atrial or ventricular beats and up to 4% of patients experience nonsustained supraventricular or ventricular tachycardia. Because the purpose of the test is to induce ischemia, some patients will have either echocardiographic changes or ECG evidence of ischemia and may experience angina. However, the frequency of angina may be less than with standard ECG stress testing, because the protocol can be stopped as soon as wall motion abnormalities are seen (which often is before angina occurs). Hypotension occurs in up to 10% of patients because of peripheral β2-receptor–mediated vasodilation but, unlike hypotension with exercise testing, is *not* a predictor of severe coronary disease or a worse prognosis. Overall, the risk of myocardial infarction or ventricular fibrillation is about 1 in 2000 studies. Contraindications to dobutamine stress echocardiography include unstable angina, uncontrolled hypertension, or sensitivity to dobutamine.

The echocardiographic images are interpreted after reformatting the digital images so that each quadrant of the screen shows a single view at rest (upper left), low-dose (upper right), maximal dose (lower left), and recovery phase (lower right). For

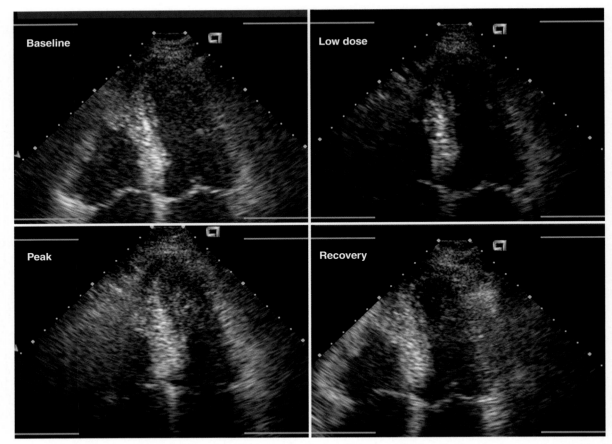

Figure 8–13 Normal dobutamine stress echocardiography showing the standard display format for the apical four-chamber view at end-systole at baseline (*upper left*), low-dose (5 μg/kg/min) dobutamine (*upper right*), high-dose (40 μg/kg/min) dobutamine (*lower left*), and recovery images (*lower right*). Note the marked decrease in end-systole cavity area from baseline to peak dose images. This format is also used for the apical two-chamber, long-axis, and parasternal short-axis views.

echocardiography does have potential technical and physiologic limitations:

- ❏ Endocardial definition
- ❏ Cardiac and respiratory motion
- ❏ Inadequate stress or workload
- ❏ Abnormal resting LV function

Assessment of endocardial wall motion and wall thickening requires adequate delineation of the endocardium for each myocardial segment. Careful attention to patient positioning, transducer orientation, and image processing parameters can improve image quality, but definition of certain segments, particularly the anterior wall, may be difficult in some individuals due to adjacent lung tissue. Some centers use contrast agents that opacify the LV after intravenous administration to enhance detection of regional wall motion abnormalities when endocardial definition is suboptimal even with harmonic imaging (Fig. 8–15).

Exercise and postexercise imaging can be limited by respiratory interference due to a rapid respiratory rate. Digital acquisition in cine-loop format of several cycles, followed by selection of the best images, is necessary for correct interpretation. The possible effects of cardiac translation and rotation, both between systole and diastole and between baseline and stress, should be considered in comparisons of wall motion. The interpretation of a stress echocardiographic study includes a description of image quality as an indicator of the reliability of these results. Suboptimal images should be interpreted with caution.

Potential physiologic limitations are related to the fact that abnormal wall motion occurs only *during* ischemia. First, if the "stress" used does *not* induce ischemia, no wall motion abnormality will be seen even if significant coronary disease is present. For example, a patient with limited exercise duration due to hip pain may not achieve a level of exertion that results in ischemia. Similarly, a pharmacologic "stress" that does not induce ischemia will not induce a wall motion abnormality. Second, the duration of ischemia is important. If ischemia has resolved by the time imaging is performed, the wall motion abnormality will not be detected. This is of particular concern with treadmill exercise, since

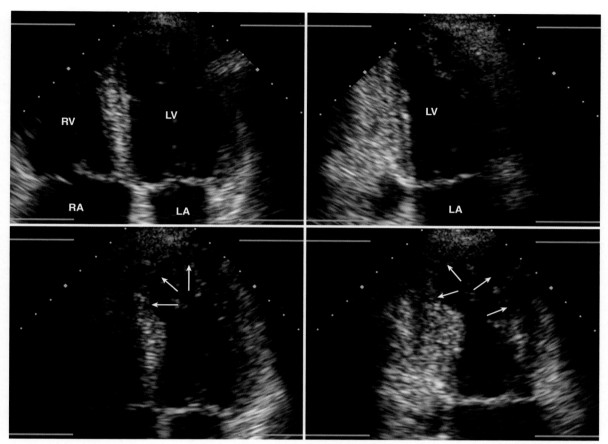

Figure 8–14 Example of an abnormal dobutamine stress echocardiographic study with baseline images (*top*) at end-systole in an apical four-chamber view (*left*) and apical two-chamber view (*right*), and the peak dose (40 µg/kg/min dobutamine plus 0.5 mg atropine) end-systole images on the *bottom*. The apical segments of the septum, anterior, and inferior walls became akinetic at peak dobutamine dose (*arrows*), indicating significant coronary artery disease in the left anterior descending coronary artery distribution.

TABLE 8–3   Selected Studies on the Diagnostic Accuracy of Exercise Echocardiography Compared with Coronary Angiography*

First Author and Year	N	CAD Present (%)	Sensitivity (%)	Specificity (%)
Limacher 1984	73	—	91	88
Armstrong 1987	123	82	87	86
Ryan 1988	64	47	78	100
Sawada 1989	57 (women)	49	86	86
Crouse 1991	228	77	97	64
Marwick 1992	179	64	84	86
Quinones 1992	112	77	74	88

*In all studies, significant coronary artery disease (CAD) was defined as a 50% stenosis in an epicardial vessel.
CAD, coronary artery disease.
Data sources: Limacher et al: Circulation 67:1211–1218, 1984; Armstrong et al: J Am Coll Cardiol 10:531–538, 1987; Ryan et al: J Am Coll Cardiol 11:993–999, 1988; Sawada et al: J Am Coll Cardiol 14:1440–1447, 1989; Crouse et al: J Am Coll Cardiol 67:1213–1218, 1991; Marwick et al: J Am Coll Cardiol 19:74–81, 1992; Quinones et al: Circulation 85:1026–1031, 1992.

echocardiographic imaging is performed after exertion, although this possible limitation may be offset by the higher maximum workload achieved prior to the recovery period compared with bicycle exercise protocols.

Stress echocardiography in patients with abnormal global or regional function at rest is more difficult to interpret than in subjects with normal resting LV systolic function. The presence of a segmental motion

First Author and Year	Source of Subjects	N	CAD Present (%)	Stenosis Considered Significant (%)	Sensitivity (%)	Specificity (%)
Berthe 1986	Post-acute MI	30	100	50	85	88
Cohen 1991	Chest pain	70	27	70	86	95
Sawada 1991	Coronary angio	103	44	50	89	85
Mazeika 1992	Coronary angio	50	26	70	78	93
Martin 1992	Coronary angio	40	35	50	76	60
Segar 1992	Coronary angio	85	—	50	95	82
Marcovitz 1992	Coronary angio	141	21	50	96	66
Marwick 1993	Coronary angio	217	65	50	72	83

TABLE 8–4   Selected Studies on Diagnostic Accuracy of Dobutamine Stress Echocardiography Compared with Coronary Angiography

MI, myocardial infarction.
Data sources: Berthe et al: Am J Cardiol 58:1167–1172, 1986; Cohen et al: Am J Cardiol 67:1311–1318, 1991; Sawada et al: Circulation 83:1602–1614, 1991; Mazeika et al: J Am Coll Cardiol 19:1203–1211, 1992; Martin et al: Ann Intern Med 116:190–196, 1992; Segar et al: J Am Coll Cardiol 19:1197–1202, 1992; Marcovitz et al: Am J Cardiol 69:1269–1273, 1992; Marwick et al: J Am Coll Cardiol 22:159–167, 1993.

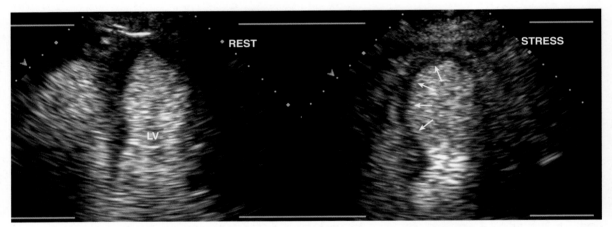

Figure 8–15 This patient had suboptimal endocardial definition even with harmonic imaging and careful patient positioning. After intravenous injection of a left heart contrast agent, opacification of the LV chamber is seen with clear definition of the endocardial border, at rest and with stress in the apical four-chamber view, demonstrating inducible ischemia in the mid and apical inferior septum.

abnormality at rest implies that coronary artery disease, with prior myocardial infarction, is present. With stress imaging, new wall motion abnormalities in regions remote from the site of resting abnormal wall motion indicate additional areas of ischemia. Evaluation of areas adjacent to the resting wall motion abnormality may be problematic due to a potential tethering effect by the abnormal region. In patients with global systolic dysfunction at rest—which may be due to end-stage ischemic disease, cardiomyopathy, or chronic valvular disease—stress echocardiography is less specific for the diagnosis of coronary disease.

Alternate Approaches

In patients with suspected or known coronary artery disease, the choice of stress and imaging modality depend on patient factors and on the specific clinical question. Optimally, the method of stress is chosen to allow an adequate workload in that patient—with pharmacologic testing used in those who cannot exercise to a maximal workload due to orthopedic, neurologic, pulmonary, or other conditions. The choice of imaging modality is chosen based on image quality in each patient and the type of information needed.

Exercise Electrocardiography

Exercise ECG remains a standard test for evaluation of patients with suspected or known coronary artery disease. Even though it has a lower sensitivity and specificity for diagnosis of coronary disease compared with imaging techniques, it continues to provide important prognostic data at a low cost in many patients. Imaging techniques most often are needed in subgroups with high false-positive (e.g., women with chest pain) or false-negative rates and in patients with an abnormal resting ECG that obscures exercise-induced ischemic changes.

Direct Visualization of Coronary Anatomy

The origins of the right and left coronary arteries often can be identified on TTE imaging (Fig. 8–16). On TEE imaging the proximal left coronary can be followed to its bifurcation into left anterior descending and circumflex arteries (Figs. 8–17 and 8–18), and often these branches can be imaged for a portion

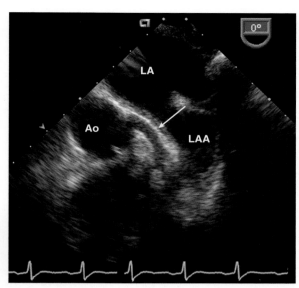

Figure 8–18 In the same patient as Figure 8–17, slight withdrawal of the probe with angulation toward the apex shows the left main coronary artery continuing into the left anterior descending coronary artery (*arrow*). The circumflex coronary artery extends out of the image plane. LAA, left atrial appendage.

of their length, as can the right coronary artery (see Suggested Reading 34). However, clinical decision making usually requires detailed knowledge of the entire extent of the coronary anatomy. Ultrasound imaging is a suboptimal method for evaluation of the relatively small coronary vessels that move with the epicardial surface of the heart.

Coronary angiography remains the standard of reference for evaluation of coronary artery disease. Cardiac catheterization with injection of contrast directly in the coronary vessels allows detailed assessment of both proximal and distal coronary anatomy and can be performed at the time of percutaneous revascularization. Noninvasive computed tomographic coronary angiography provides high-resolution images of the coronary arteries, allowing diagnosis of coronary anomalies and detailed assessment of atherosclerotic plaques (Fig. 8–19). Disadvantages of coronary angiography are use of a contrast agent and radiation exposure.

Radionuclide Techniques/Positron Emission Tomography

Radionuclide perfusion imaging techniques with thallium or sestamibi immediately after exercise and at rest after redistribution are well-validated methods for evaluation of coronary artery disease patients (Fig. 8–20). These techniques also can be performed using a vasodilator to induce heterogeneity in blood flow or with dobutamine to induce ischemia. Compared with stress echocardiography, radionuclide techniques have the advantage that image quality is less

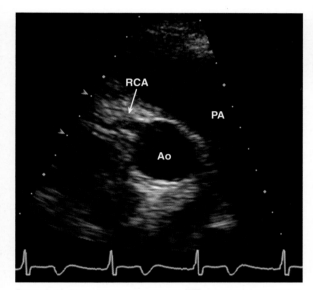

Figure 8–16 Right coronary artery seen on a TTE parasternal short-axis view.

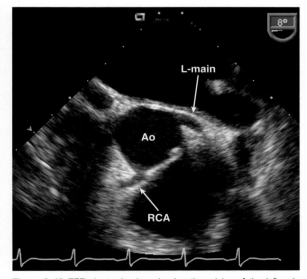

Figure 8–17 TEE short-axis view showing the origins of the left-main (L-main) and right coronary artery (RCA).

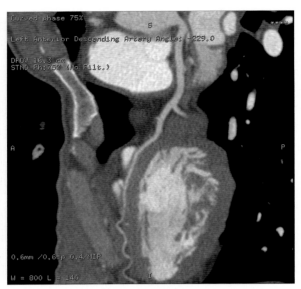

Figure 8–19 Example of computed tomographic coronary angiography showing the degree of detail in definition of coronary anatomy from the left-main to the distal left anterior descending coronary artery.

dependent on each patient's body habitus, although attenuation due to breast tissue may be a problem in women. Disadvantages of the use of radionuclide techniques include a higher cost, it is less easily performed at the bedside, and it uses ionizing radiation (albeit a low dose). Technical factors are important with both techniques, and data quality at a particular institution depends in part on experience. Positron emission tomography provides optimal stress images in larger patients.

Cardiac Magnetic Resonance Imaging

CMR imaging allows identification of coronary anomalies. In addition, viable myocardium can reliably be distinguished from infarcted tissue. Wall motion at rest and stress also can be evaluated using CMR cine images with a pharmacologic stress test.

Clinical Utility

The utility of stress echocardiography in patients with known or suspected coronary artery disease includes:

❑ Detection of coronary artery disease
❑ Assessment of the area of myocardium at risk
❑ Risk stratification after myocardial infarction
❑ Evaluation after revascularization
❑ Detection of myocardial viability

Stress echocardiography is particularly useful for detection of coronary artery disease in specific patient groups including:

❑ Women with chest pain symptoms and/or cardiac risk factors

❑ Patients after heart transplantation
❑ Patients being considered for renal transplantation
❑ Patients undergoing vascular surgery

Stress echocardiography also can be used to evaluate changes in cardiac hemodynamics including valve gradients and areas, regurgitant severity, and pulmonary pressures. As discussed in Chapters 11 and 17, echocardiography is used in patients with valvular or congenital heart disease for evaluation of changes with stress in:

❑ Aortic valve area in calcific aortic stenosis
❑ Mitral regurgitant severity in myxomatous mitral valve disease
❑ Pulmonary pressures in mitral stenosis or regurgitation
❑ Aortic coarctation pressure gradients
❑ Dynamic outflow obstruction in hypertrophic cardiomyopathy

Diagnosis of Coronary Artery Disease

The accuracy of stress echocardiography for diagnosis of significant coronary artery disease is highly dependent on image quality, specifically endocardial definition, with most investigators reporting success rates for obtaining diagnostic images after treadmill exercise of 85% to 100% of patients. The success rate for image acquisition and the quality of the images obtained tend to be greater with supine exercise (in which the patient can be positioned optimally) and with pharmacologic stress (which has the added advantage of little increase in respiratory interference).

Compared with coronary angiography, with significant disease defined as 50% narrowing of an epicardial coronary artery, exercise echocardiography has an overall sensitivity of 74% to 97% and a specificity of 64% to 100% for diagnosing the presence of coronary artery disease (see Table 8–4). Sensitivity is highest for multivessel disease (>90%) and lowest for single-vessel disease (60% to 80%) in these studies. In comparison, exercise ECG had a much lower sensitivity at 51% to 63% and specificity at 62% to 74%, while exercise thallium-201 perfusion imaging tends to have an accuracy similar to echocardiography, with a sensitivity of 61% to 94% and a specificity of 81%.

Extent and Location of Ischemic Areas

When image quality is adequate, stress echocardiography also allows accurate evaluation of the location and extent of the area of ischemic myocardium. By integrating data from multiple views, a reasonable estimate of the location of significant coronary lesions can be made. Echocardiographic estimates of which and how many coronary arteries are affected correlate well with angiographic findings.

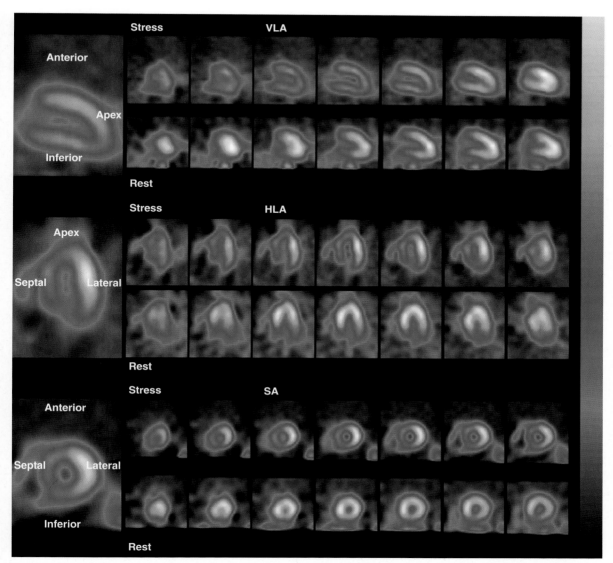

Figure 8–20 Exercise stress dual-isotope radionuclide study; resting images were acquired with thallium-201 and exercise images with Tc-Sestamibi. Three views are shown. *Top,* The vertical long-axis (VLA) images from the septum to lateral wall are shown with the stress images on the top and the rest images on the bottom. *Middle,* Horizontal long-axis (HLA) images are shown from posterior to anterior. *Bottom,* Short-axis (SA) images from apex to base are displayed. On the exercise images there is an inferior wall perfusion defect starting in the apical slice on the short-axis view and extending to the mid-cavity and basal slices. On the rest images there is complete redistribution consistent with ischemia without previous infarction in the inferior wall. *(Courtesy of James H. Caldwell, Jr., MD.)*

Prognostic Implications

The relationship between stress echocardiographic results and clinical outcome has been evaluated in several studies and in a recent meta-analysis (Tables 8–5 and 8–6 and Suggested Reading 4). In patients with known or suspected coronary artery disease, a normal stress echocardiogram has a 98% negative predictive value for myocardial infarction or cardiovascular death over the next 3 years. Interpretation of a stress test depends on the pre-test likelihood of disease, including clinical risk factors such as age, gender, diabetes, smoking, hypertension, and hypercholesterolemia. In addition, indicators of a higher likelihood of an adverse outcome with exercise echocardiography, as with all exercise stress tests, include exercise capacity, exercise-induced angina, and the BP response to exercise. However, echocardiographic images provide additional prognostic information, with the key predictors of clinical outcome including resting wall motion abnormalities, ejection fraction, and the extent of ischemia. Similarly, with dobutamine stress, echocardiography provides incremental value with resting wall motion and evidence of inducible ischemia predicting cardiovascular events.

TABLE 8–5   Selected Studies on the Prognostic Value of Exercise Stress Echocardiography

First Author and Year	N	Female	Study Group	Outcomes (Event Rate)	Median Follow-up (yr)	Multivariate Predictors of Outcome*
Arruda-Olson 2002	5798	43%	CAD	Cardiac death/ MI (4.4%)	3.2	Exercise workload (METs) Exercise WMSI
Marwick 2001	5375	37%	CAD	All deaths (12%)	5.5	Duke treadmill score Resting wall motion (scar) Exercise wall motion (ischemia)
Elhendy 2002	4347	49%	CAD	Cardiac death/ MI (3.1%)	3.0	Resting EF Exercise wall motion (ischemia)
Bergeron 2004	3260	55%	Chest pain and/or dyspnea	Cardiac death/ MI (3.3%)	3.1	Previous MI Ejection fraction Rest to exercise ΔWMSI
Arruda 2001a	2632	44%	CAD ≥ age 65 yr	Cardiac death/ MI (5.6%)	2.9	Exercise workload Exercise ΔEF Rest to exercise ΔESV
Arruda 2001b	718	18%	Previous CABG	Cardiac death/ MI (10.6%)	2.9	Exercise workload Exercise ΔEF
Elhendy 2001	563	40%	Diabetes and CAD	Cardiac death/ MI (8.9%)	3.0	Exercise workload Resting EF Extent of ischemia
Elhendy 2003	483	42%	CAD and LVH on ECG	Cardiac death/ MI (12.4%)	3.0	Exercise workload Resting WMSI Rest to exercise ΔEF
Olmos 1998	225	24%	CAD	Cardiac death/ MI (28%)	3.7	Exercise WMSI Inducible ischemia

Δ, change in; CABG, Coronary artery bypass graft; CAD, suspected or known coronary artery disease; EF, ejection fraction; ESV, end-systolic volume; LVH, left ventricular hypertrophy; METs, metabolic equivalents; MI, myocardial infarction; WMSI, wall motion score index.
*In addition to clinical factors including male gender, age, diabetes, hypertension, smoking, and previous CABG.
Data sources: Arruda et al: Am J Cardiol 87:1069–1073, 2001b; Arruda et al: J Am Coll Cardiol 37:1036–1041, 2001a; Arruda-Olson et al: J Am Coll Cardiol 39:625–631, 2002; Bergeron et al: J Am Coll Cardiol 43:2242–2246, 2004; Elhendy et al: J Am Coll Cardiol 20:1623–1629, 2002; Elhendy et al: J Am Coll Cardiol 37:1551–1557, 2001; Elhendy et al: J Am Coll Cardiol 41:129–135, 2003; Marwick et al: Circulation 103:2566–2571, 2001; Olmos et al: Circulation 98:2679–2686, 1998.

MYOCARDIAL INFARCTION

Basic Principles

Myocardial infarction is irreversible injury to the myocardium due to prolonged ischemia, usually secondary to acute thrombotic occlusion of an epicardial coronary artery at the site of an atherosclerotic plaque. Initially the affected myocardium becomes akinetic, with normal wall thickness. Over time (4–6 weeks), the involved myocardial segments show thinning of the wall and increased echogenicity. An ST-elevation myocardial infarction results in a definite area of akinesis and wall thinning. A non-ST elevation myocardial infarction may result in a lesser degree of wall thinning and in hypokinesis rather than akinesis.

Echocardiographic Imaging

The myocardial segments affected and the echocardiographic views for assessment of myocardial infarction are the same as described for myocardial ischemia. An occlusion of the left anterior descending artery results in akinesis of the anterior septum, anterior free wall, and apex (Fig. 8–21). Imaging in parasternal long-and short-axis views and in apical views demonstrates these segmental wall motion abnormalities.

TABLE 8–6   Selected Studies on the Prognostic Value of Pharmacologic Stress Echocardiography

First Author and Year	N	Female	Study Group	Outcomes (Event Rate)	Median Follow-up (yr)	Multivariate Predictors of Outcome*
Biagini 2005a	3381	33%	CAD	Cardiac death, MI (30%)	7 ± 3.4	Resting WMA Ischemia
Marwick 2001	3156	43%	CAD	Cardiac death (8%)	3.8 ± 1.9	Resting WMA Ischemia
Chaowalit 2006	2349	43%	Diabetes	Death, MI, late coronary revascularization (57%)	5.4 ± 2.2	Extent of ischemia Ventricular function Failure to reach target heart rate
Biagini 2005b	1434	33%	CAD ≥ 65 yr	Cardiac death/ MI (40%)	6.5	Resting WMI Ischemia
Chuah 1998	860	44%	CAD	Cardiac death/ MI (10%)	2 ± 0.8	Stress WMA Rest to exercise ΔESV
Poldermans 1997	316	16%	Before vascular surgery	Perioperative and late cardiac events (10%)	1.6 ± 0.9	Previous infarction Inducible ischemia

CAD, known or suspected coronary artery disease; ΔESV, change in end-systolic volume; MI, myocardial infarction; WMA, wall motion abnormality.

*In addition to clinical factors including male gender, age, diabetes, smoking, history of heart failure, and previous coronary artery bypass graft.

Data sources: Biagini et al: J Am Coll Cardiol 45:93–97, 2005a; Marwick et al: J Am Coll Cardiol 37:754–760, 2001; Chaowalit et al: J Am Coll Cardiol 47:1029–1036, 2006; Biagini et al: Gerontol A Biol Sci Med Sci 60:1333–1338, 2005b; Chuah et al: Circulation 97:1474–1480, 1998; Poldermans et al: Circulation 95:53–58, 1997.

In the acute setting (Fig. 8–22) the unaffected walls may be hyperkinetic. Overall LV systolic function typically is moderately depressed with an average ejection fraction of 41% ± 11% after an un-reperfused anterior myocardial infarction due to a proximal left anterior descending artery occlusion.

Occlusion of the posterior descending artery results in an inferior myocardial infarction with akinesis of the inferior septum, the inferior free wall, and (to a variable extent) the inferolateral (posterior) wall. Parasternal and apical views again are used. The subcostal approach may be particularly helpful in patients with poor image quality from parasternal and apical windows. Typically, overall LV systolic function is only mildly depressed, with an average post-infarction ejection fraction of 53% ± 10% after an un-reperfused inferior infarction. With inferior infarction the echocardiographer also should evaluate for possible concurrent RV infarction.

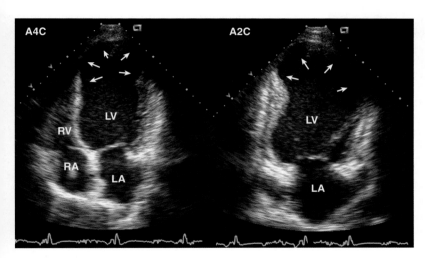

Figure 8–21 Old anterior-apical myocardial infarction with a diastolic contour abnormality, thinning and akinesis of the distal septum, anterior wall, and apical third of the left ventricle seen in the apical four-chamber (A4C) and apical two-chamber (A2C) views.

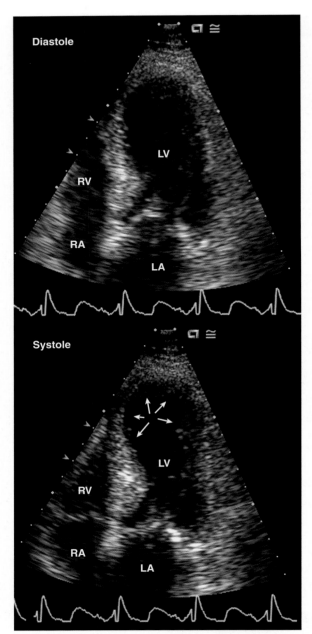

Figure 8–22 Acute anterior myocardial infarction seen in an apical four-chamber view in diastole (*top*) and systole (*bottom*). The apical septum is akinetic (*arrows*), although the myocardium is not yet thinned and scarred.

Occlusion of the circumflex artery, resulting in a lateral myocardial infarction, is less common and often is electrocardiographically "silent." Akinesis of the anterolateral and posterolateral walls is seen, with a mild to moderately depressed ejection fraction depending on the extent of myocardium supplied by the circumflex artery in that individual.

Note that these "classic" patterns of wall motion abnormalities will vary with individual variation in coronary anatomy and the location of the occlusion along the length of the coronary artery. Also, these patterns will be altered by the use of reperfusion therapy.

In acute myocardial infarction, diastolic function, as well as systolic function, is abnormal. Acutely, diastolic relaxation is impaired with normalization over the subsequent 1 to 2 weeks when reperfusion is successful. With late or ineffective reperfusion resulting in a large infarction, an initial pattern of impaired relaxation is followed by pseudo-normalization of diastolic filling with a high E velocity reflecting an increased LV end-diastolic pressure. In patients with moderate to severely reduced systolic function, the E/A ratio correlates positively with LV end-diastolic and LA pressures (i.e., a higher E/A ratio indicates a higher LV end-diastolic pressure) due to the overriding effect of LA pressure on the early diastolic filling velocity. It is most helpful to interpret patterns of LV diastolic filling in a coronary disease patient over time with side-by-side comparisons of the echocardiographic findings and integration with other clinical data (see Chapter 7).

Limitations/Alternate Approaches

As for other applications of echocardiography, image quality can be a limiting factor in patients with poor ultrasound tissue penetration. However, with optimal patient positioning, an experienced sonographer, and a state-of-the-art instrument, diagnostic images can be obtained in nearly all patients.

The standard approach to the diagnosis of acute myocardial infarction includes two of the following three findings:

- ❑ A typical clinical presentation
- ❑ Diagnostic ECG changes
- ❑ A consistent pattern of elevation in serum cardiac enzyme levels

When typical findings of acute myocardial infarction are present, the diagnosis rarely is in doubt. Unfortunately, many patients have an atypical clinical presentation, and ECG changes may be nondiagnostic.

Radionuclide imaging for acute myocardial infarction is based on the principle of detection of areas of hypoperfusion. The finding of a normal radionuclide perfusion pattern in patients presenting with chest pain has a high specificity for the absence of acute myocardial infarction. Sensitivity for acute infarction is lower, since an old infarction cannot be distinguished from an acute infarction with this approach.

Coronary angiography remains the standard of reference for identification of an occluded coronary artery. Concurrent left ventriculography can identify wall motion abnormalities. The current standard of care for acute myocardial infarction often includes percutaneous coronary revascularization, so many of these patients go directly to the catheterization laboratory at the time of presentation.

Clinical Utility

Diagnosis in the Emergency Department

In a patient presenting to the emergency department with chest pain and a nondiagnostic ECG, echocardiographic assessment of global and segmental wall motion can be helpful in clinical decision making. The presence of a segmental wall motion abnormality indicates that coronary artery disease is present—which may be acute infarction, ischemia, or an old infarction. Associated hyperkinesis of uninvolved segments suggests an acute event. Many emergency departments now use small portable ("hand-held") ultrasound devices for this indication.

Since ischemic myocardium also is akinetic in a patient with chest pain, echocardiography cannot distinguish acute infarction from ongoing ischemia. Normal wall motion implies that there was no ischemia *at the time* the images were acquired. Thus, normal wall motion *between* episodes of chest pain does not exclude a diagnosis of unstable angina. In patients presenting with chest pain, a nondiagnostic ECG, and normal cardiac enzymes, some clinical centers now use exercise echocardiography to allow triage to further inpatient versus outpatient evaluation.

Evaluation of Interventional Therapy

In a patient with a definite myocardial infarction by clinical and ECG criteria, echocardiography allows assessment of the location and extent of "myocardium at risk." Once reperfusion therapy has been initiated, echocardiography can be used to assess its effects. However, there often is a several-day time lag between successful reperfusion and normalization of wall motion ("stunned" myocardium), so evaluation is most meaningful before hospital discharge or at outpatient follow-up. Prolonged persistence of wall motion abnormalities that can be reversed by reperfusion also can occur—termed *hibernating myocardium*. Echocardiographic imaging cannot distinguish between these conditions, since it shows the regional myocardial function at the time imaging is performed. In patients with post-infarction chest pain, echocardiography may help separate those with recurrent ischemia, and new wall motion abnormalities, from those with post-infarction pericarditis or noncardiac chest pain. At long-term follow-up after myocardial infarction, echocardiography allows assessment of global ventricular function and long-term ventricular dilation due to infarct expansion.

Mechanical Complications of Myocardial Infarction

Echocardiography is the procedure of choice for initial evaluation of the post–myocardial infarction patient with a new systolic murmur with a differential diagnosis of:

- ❐ Mitral regurgitation
- ❐ Ventricular septal defect
- ❐ Ventricular rupture with pseudoaneurysm formation

Most commonly, the etiology of the murmur is *mitral regurgitation* due to papillary muscle dysfunction, abnormal wall motion of the segment underlying a papillary muscle, or papillary muscle rupture. The presence and severity of mitral regurgitation are evaluated using Doppler techniques (see Chapter 12), and the etiology is inferred from two-dimensional (2D) imaging. Partial or complete rupture of the papillary muscle is a catastrophic complication that can be recognized as a flail leaflet with an attached mass (the papillary muscle head) that prolapses into the LA in systole (Fig. 8–23). TEE imaging is indicated when this diagnosis is suspected unless the diagnosis is clear on TTE images.

Another cause of a new systolic murmur after myocardial infarction is a *ventricular septal defect* due to necrosis and rupture of a focal area of the interventricular septum (Fig. 8–24). Identification of the rupture site may be difficult with 2D imaging, especially since this complication tends to occur with *small* infarcts so that the wall motion abnormality may be subtle. Evaluation with Doppler ultrasound establishes the diagnosis, with a high-velocity left-to-right systolic jet recorded with continuous-wave Doppler ultrasound and systolic turbulence on the RV side of the septum recorded with conventional pulsed Doppler or color flow imaging.

When *ventricular rupture* occurs in the free wall of the LV (instead of in the septum), mortality is extremely high due to extravasation of blood into the pericardial space and acute pericardial tamponade. However, some patients have a temporary respite due to containment of the rupture by pericardial adhesions or by thrombosis at the rupture site. In these patients, echocardiography may establish the diagnosis, prompting emergency surgery (Fig. 8–25). Echocardiographic clues of ventricular rupture (in the appropriate clinical setting) include a diffuse or localized pericardial effusion and a discrete segmental wall motion abnormality. Occasionally, the site of rupture can be visualized on 2D imaging, and rarely, flow from the ventricle into the pericardial space can be demonstrated with Doppler techniques.

A chronic, contained ventricular rupture is called a *pseudoaneurysm* (Figs. 8–26 and 8–27). An LV pseudoaneurysm has a wall composed of pericardium (no myocardial fibers). Characteristic features are:

- ❐ An abrupt transition from normal myocardium to the aneurysm
- ❐ An acute angle between the normal myocardium and aneurysm
- ❐ A narrow "neck" at the site of rupture
- ❐ A ratio of the "neck" diameter to the maximum diameter < 0.5
- ❐ Partial filling of the aneurysm with thrombus

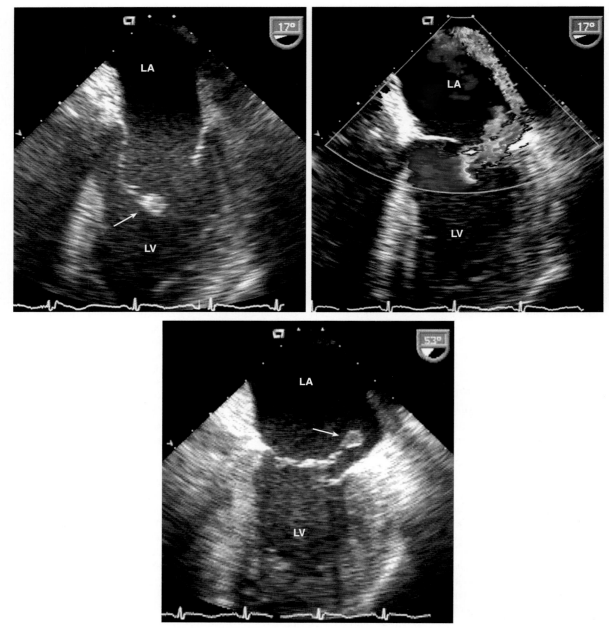

Figure 8–23 On a TEE image in the four-chamber (*top, left*) view, papillary muscle rupture is seen in diastole with an abrupt discontinuity in the anterolateral papillary muscle. In systole the papillary muscle head (*arrow*) prolapses into the LA as seen in the two-chamber view (*bottom*) in association with an eccentric jet of severe mitral regurgitation (*top, right*) with a wide vena contracta. The patient underwent emergency mitral valve repair.

Often, flow in and out of the pseudoaneurysm is seen, and clinically, a corresponding apical murmur may be appreciated on auscultation. While long-term survival has been described occasionally in patients with a pseudoaneurysm, correct echocardiographic diagnosis is essential. Surgical repair usually is recommended given a high likelihood of spontaneous rupture.

Other complications of acute myocardial infarction include:

❐ Pericardial effusion
❐ RV infarction
❐ LV aneurysm
❐ LV thrombus

A *pericardial effusion* also can be seen after myocardial infarction as a nonspecific response to transmural infarction. This effusion may be asymptomatic or may be associated with clinical symptoms (chest pain) and signs (ECG changes) of acute pericarditis. While usually

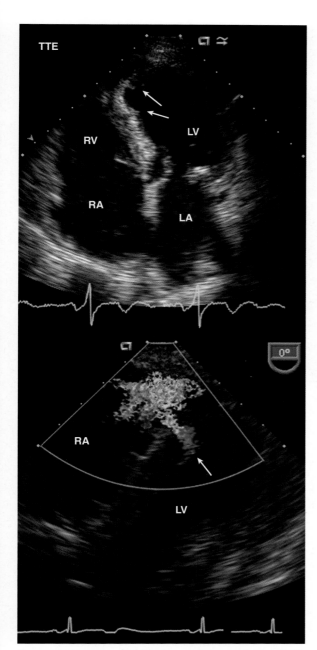

Figure 8–24 Post–myocardial infarction ventricular septal defect (VSD). The TTE apical four-chamber view shows a localized area of dyskinesis in the septum (*arrows*). The zoomed color Doppler image shows left-to-right flow across the VSD (*arrow*). *(From Schwaelger RG, Otto CM: Echocardiography Review Guide. Elsevier/Saunders, 2008, p 124, Fig. 8–19.)*

benign, an effusion may be complicated by tamponade physiology.

RV infarction may accompany an inferior infarction of the LV. Echocardiographic findings include RV hypokinesis or akinesis with variable degrees of RV dilation. With ECG leads placed on the right chest (in a mirror image pattern to the normal positions),

ST-segment elevation may be seen, but this finding is not as sensitive or specific as echocardiography.

Longer term complications of acute myocardial infarction include aneurysm formation, LV thrombi, and the sequelae of the irreversible decrease in LV systolic function. An *LV aneurysm* is defined echocardiographically as a dyskinetic region with a diastolic contour abnormality (Fig. 8–28). Apical aneurysms are most common, but inferior-basal aneurysms also may be seen. Note that a "true" LV aneurysm, unlike a "false" or pseudoaneurysm, is lined by (thinned) myocardium. There is a smooth transition from normal myocardium to the thinned area with an obtuse angle between the aneurysm and body of the LV. The ratio of the diameter of the junction between the aneurysm and the remainder of the LV to the maximum aneurysm diameter is > 0.5.

LV thrombi form in regions of stasis of blood flow, such as in an apical aneurysm or overlying an area of akinesis in other regions of the LV. Evidence of severely reduced overall ventricular function, an aneurysm, an akinetic area, and the appearance of a spontaneous contrast effect in the LV all increase the likelihood of LV thrombus formation. Only rarely (as in hypereosinophilic syndrome) do ventricular thrombi occur in the absence of an underlying wall motion abnormality.

A thrombus is identified as an area of increased echogenicity within the ventricular chamber, distinct from the endocardium (see Fig. 15–17). Often, the thrombus protrudes into the chamber with a convex contour, but laminated thrombus with a concave contour following the endocardial curve also can be seen. Care is needed to distinguish a thrombus from prominent apical trabeculation with a false tendon or "web" traversing the apex of the LV chamber (see Fig. 15–1.)

Diagnosis of apical thrombi is enhanced by using a 5-MHz transducer (improved near-field resolution), sliding the transducer laterally from the apical window and then angulating medially and superiorly to obtain a short-axis view of the apex. These procedures allow clear definition of the apical endocardium in most individuals. However, if images are suboptimal, appropriate interpretation should indicate that a thrombus "cannot be excluded," especially if the patient is at high risk of LV thrombus formation. Note that TEE imaging is less helpful for this diagnosis, because the apex often is not fully visualized and is in the far field of the image plane.

END-STAGE ISCHEMIC CARDIAC DISEASE

Differentiation from Other Causes of Left Ventricular Systolic Dysfunction

The diagnosis of coronary artery disease is clear in patients with definite segmental wall motion abnormalities that correspond to the distribution of coronary

Figure 8-25 LV rupture with pseudoaneurysm formation seen in an apical two-chamber (A2C) view. Color Doppler shows flow (*arrow*) from the LV into the contained pericardial space. *(From Schwaelger RG, Otto CM: Echocardiography Review Guide. Elsevier/Saunders, 2008, Fig. 8–16.)*

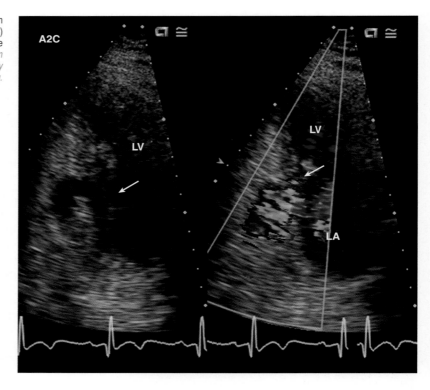

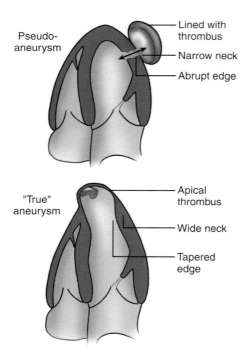

Figure 8-26 Schematic diagram of a pseudoaneurysm versus a true aneurysm.

blood flow. In end-stage ischemic disease, repeated transmural and subendocardial infarctions result in a diffuse pattern of abnormal wall thickening and endocardial motion. Thus, when global systolic dysfunction is present, it may be difficult to differentiate between end-stage ischemic disease and systolic dysfunction due to long-standing valvular disease or a dilated cardiomyopathy (Fig. 8–29).

Echocardiographic Approach

Several features of the echocardiographic examination help in this differentiation. The segmental pattern of LV wall motion is examined carefully in each tomographic plane. While patients with a dilated cardiomyopathy may have a somewhat asymmetric pattern of wall motion with relative preservation at the ventricular base, definite areas of akinesis or wall thinning suggest ischemic disease. The degree of reduction in overall ventricular function (ejection fraction) is important in patient management but does not assist in determining the etiology of disease.

RV size and systolic function are normal in patients with ischemic disease unless there has been a previous RV infarction. Dilated cardiomyopathy occasionally affects the two ventricles in differing degrees but most often results in a symmetric pattern of RV and LV dilation and reduced systolic function. Mitral valve regurgitation typically accompanies both dilated cardiomyopathy and end-stage ischemic

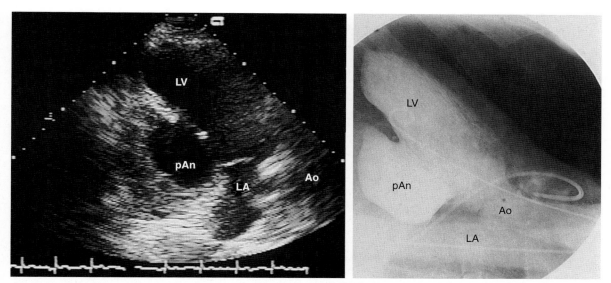

Figure 8–27 Apical long-axis view showing a chronic basal aneurysm filled with thrombus with a narrow neck (*left*) consistent with a pseudoaneurysm (pAn). Angiography (oriented to match the apical long-axis view) shows a similar appearance (*right*).

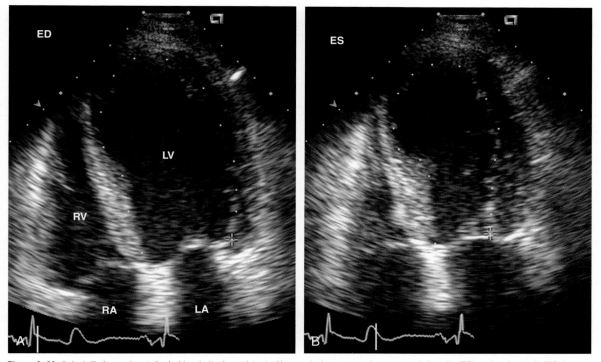

Figure 8–28 Apical dilation and systolic dyskinesis (*top*) consistent with an apical aneurysm shown on end-diastolic (ED) and end-systolic (ES) images in an apical four-chamber view. There is no obvious thrombus but evaluation with a higher frequency transducer and oblique views is needed.

disease due to one of several mechanisms, including mitral annular dilation, reduced papillary muscle systolic function, or malalignment of the papillary muscles. LV dilation and systolic dysfunction *due to* chronic mitral regurgitation, in contrast to mitral regurgitation due to ventricular dilation and dysfunction, usually are associated with anatomic abnormalities of the mitral leaflets themselves (e.g., myxomatous or rheumatic disease).

Pulmonary artery pressures are elevated to variable degrees in patients with LV dysfunction of any etiology, due to chronic elevation in LV end-diastolic pressure.

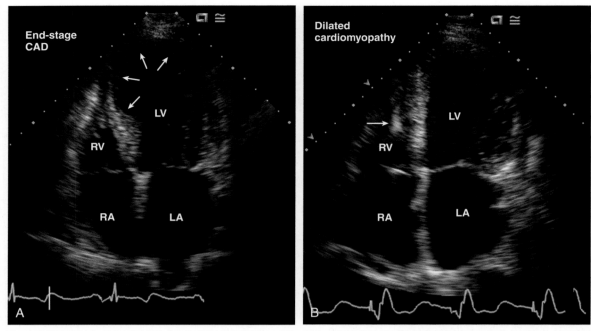

Figure 8–29 End-stage ischemic heart disease (**A**) and a dilated cardiomyopathy (**B**) often appear similar on 2D echocardiography. The patient with ischemic disease has apical dilation and dyskinesis (*arrows*) and a relatively normal right heart. The patient with a dilated cardiomyopathy has more diffuse and severe (note scales) four-chamber enlargement and biventricular dysfunction. The lead for an automated implanted defibrillator is seen in the RV (*arrow*).

Pulmonary pressures can be estimated from the tricuspid regurgitant jet velocity or from the pulmonary artery systolic velocity curve as described in Chapter 6. Mild degrees of tricuspid valve regurgitation are common in ischemic disease, but moderate or severe regurgitation usually is a response to chronic pulmonary hypertension or chronic RV dilation and systolic dysfunction.

Note that aortic regurgitation is *not* a consequence of LV dilation or systolic dysfunction. LV dilation typically does not result in an increase in the diameter of the aortic annulus or adjacent outflow tract. The finding of moderate or severe aortic regurgitation implies primary valvular disease or aortic root dilation.

LV thrombi may be present with severe LV dysfunction of any etiology. The observation of reduced systolic function should prompt a search for apical thrombi, but this finding does not help in the differential diagnosis.

Limitations/Alternate Approaches

If a diagnosis of end-stage ischemic disease versus a primary cardiomyopathy would alter patient management, coronary angiography may be needed for a definitive diagnosis, to document the exact site and severity of coronary lesions, and to assess the distal vessel anatomy. Other useful approaches include computed tomographic coronary angiography or CMR imaging for visualization of coronary anatomy and identification of myocardial scar.

SUGGESTED READING

General

1. Pellikka PA, Nagueh DF, Elhendy AA, et al: American Society of Echocardiography: Recommendations for performance, interpretation and application of stress echocardiography. J Am Soc Echocardiogr 20:1021–1041, 2007.
   These guidelines from the American Society of Echocardiography summarize the optimal methods of performing pharmacologic and stress echocardiography. Details include the imaging technique, required equipment, personnel, and analysis techniques. Contraindications, accuracy, and prognostic implications also are summarized with inclusion of clinical outcome data and issues in specific patient groups.
2. Cerqueira MD, Weissman NJ, Dilsizian V, et al: Standardized myocardial segmentation and nomenclature for tomographic imaging of the heart. American Heart Association Writing Group on Myocardial Segmentation and Registration for Cardiac Imaging. Circulation 105:538–542, 2002.
   Standards for defining cardiac image orientation and myocardial segments that can be used by all imaging modalities to enhance correlation between different approaches. The standard reference for cardiac displays is defined as the long axis of the LV. The names used for image planes are short axis (90° to long axis), vertical long axis (apical two-chamber plane), and horizontal long axis (four-chamber plane). Myocardial segments are defined at the basal

and midventricular level as (clockwise from the anterior septal insertion) as anterior, anterolateral, inferolateral, inferior, inferoseptal, and anteroseptal. There are four apical segments (anterior, septal, inferior, and lateral).

Exercise Echocardiography

3. Freeman RV: Exercise echocardiography. In Otto CM (ed): The Practice of Clinical Echocardiography, 3rd ed. Philadelphia: Elsevier/Saunders, 2007, pp 326–352.

    The clinical application of exercise echocardiography is discussed in detail, including necessary equipment and personnel, interpretation of stress images, a comparison of treadmill versus bicycle exercise testing, and the relative advantages and disadvantages of exercise echocardiography compared to other diagnostic approaches. Topics include the utility of exercise echocardiography for detection of coronary artery disease, and evaluation after revascularization or acute myocardial infarction. 208 references.

4. Metz LD, Beattie M, Hom R, et al: The prognostic value of normal exercise myocardial perfusion imaging and exercise echocardiography: A meta-analysis. J Am Coll Cardiol 49:227–237, 2007.

    This meta-analysis includes prospective cohort studies of patients with known or suspected coronary artery disease, published between 1990 and 2005, which include outcome data on myocardial infarction and cardiac death with at least 3 months' follow-up. Both a normal myocardial perfusion imaging study and a normal exercise echocardiogram had a high negative predictive value ($\cong$98%) for these outcomes over about 3 years of follow-up. Annualized event rates were 0.45% per year for a normal myocardial perfusion imaging study and 0.54% per year for a normal stress echocardiogram. Prognostic value was similar in men and women.

5. Shoyeb A, Weinstein H, Roistacher N, et al: Preoperative exercise echocardiography and perioperative cardiovascular outcomes in elderly patients undergoing cancer surgery. Am J Geriatr Cardiol 15:338–344, 2006.

    The prognostic value of exercise echocardiography was evaluated in 221 consecutive patients over age 75 years undergoing intermediate or high-risk cancer surgery. The exercise echocardiographic study showed a resting wall motion abnormality or inducible ischemia in 22.6%. Perioperative adverse cardiac events occurred in 11.8% including atrial fibrillation (8.1%), congestive heart failure (3.6%), acute coronary syndrome (0.9%), and cardiac arrest (0.5%). Perioperative events were more likely in those

with an abnormal stress echocardiogram (22% vs 8.8%, p < 0.025).

6. Shaw LJ, Vasey C, Sawada S, et al: Impact of gender on risk stratification by exercise and dobutamine stress echocardiography: Long-term mortality in 4,234 women and 6,898 men. Eur Heart J 26:447–456, 2005.

    In 11,132 patients undergoing stress echocardiography (exercise or dobutamine), risk factors for cardiac death (3% at 5 years) were LV systolic function and the extent of inducible ischemia. Dobutamine stress echocardiography in women predicted a 5-year survival of 95% for those with no inducible ischemia, 89% for ischemia in the distribution of a single coronary artery, and 86.6% for findings consistent with two- or three-vessel coronary disease.

7. Shaw LJ, Marwick TH, Berman DS, et al: Incremental cost-effectiveness of exercise echocardiography vs. SPECT imaging for the evaluation of stable chest pain. Eur Heart J 27:2448–2458, 2006.

    The cost-effectiveness of exercise echocardiography (n = 4884) was compared to nuclear single-photon emitted computed tomography (SPECT) imaging (n = 4637) in intermediate-risk patients with chest pain. The model considered a test cost-effective for a cost under $5000 per year of life saved. Exercise echo was cost-effective when the annual risk of myocardial infarction or death was less than 2%, whereas nuclear perfusion imaging was cost-effective in patients with established coronary disease and an annual risk of 2% or higher.

Dobutamine Stress Echocardiography

8. Marwick TH: Stress echocardiography with non-exercise techniques: Principles, protocols, interpretation, and clinical applications. In Otto CM (ed): The Practice of Clinical Echocardiography, 3rd ed. Philadelphia: Elsevier/Saunders, 2007, pp 353–392.

    Concise summary of the principles, technical aspects, and clinical utility of pharmacologic stress echocardiography. Comprehensive tables summarize clinical studies evaluating the sensitivity and specificity of dobutamine stress, vasodilator stress, and atrial pacing stress echocardiography. 281 references.

9. Mertes H, Sawada SG, Ryan T, et al: Symptoms, adverse effects, and complications associated with dobutamine stress echocardiography: Experience in 1118 patients. Circulation 88:15–19, 1993.

    Complications of dobutamine stress echocardiography that required termination of the test protocol included noncardiac symptoms

(nausea, anxiety, headache, tremor, urgency) in 3%, and angina pectoris in 19.3% (which was relieved by sublingual nitroglycerin or a short-acting beta-blocker in all cases). Arrhythmias included premature ventricular contractions in 15%, premature atrial contractions in 8%, and nonsustained ventricular tachycardia in 40 (3.5%) patients. There were no deaths, myocardial infarctions, or episodes of sustained ventricular tachycardia.

10. Geleijnse ML, Fioretti PM, Roelandt JR: Methodology, feasibility, safety and diagnostic accuracy of dobutamine stress echocardiography. J Am Coll Cardiol 30:595–606, 1997.

    This review summarizes the data from 2246 patients having dobutamine stress echocardiography at 28 different centers. The risk of ventricular fibrillation or myocardial infarction was 1/2000, and there were no reported deaths. Dobutamine stress echocardiography was nondiagnostic in about 5% due to poor image quality and in 10% due to submaximal stress. In the remainder the overall sensitivity was 80% with a specificity of 84% for detection of coronary artery disease. Sensitivity was higher for three-vessel (92%) compared with two-vessel (86%) or one-vessel (74%) disease and was lowest for circumflex artery disease.

11. Chaowalit N, McCully RB, Callahan MJ, et al: Outcomes after normal dobutamine stress echocardiography and predictors of adverse events: Long-term follow-up of 3014 patients. Eur Heart J 27:3039–3044, 2006.

    In 3014 patients with a normal dobutamine stress echocardiogram, cardiac events, defined as myocardial infarction and coronary revascularization, occurred in 231 (7.7%) at a median follow-up of 6.3 years. A normal dobutamine stress echocardiogram was defined as normal wall motion at rest and with stress. The probability of freedom from cardiac events was 98% at 1 year, 93% at 5 years, and 89% at 10 years. Overall mortality was 31% with a survival of 95% at 1 year, 78% at 5 years, and 56% at 10 years. Independent predictors of mortality and cardiac events were age, diabetes, and failure to achieve 85% of maximum predicted HR.

12. Moir S, Shaw L, Haluska B, et al: Left ventricular opacification for the diagnosis of coronary artery disease with stress echocardiography: An angiographic study of incremental benefit and cost-effectiveness. Am Heart J 154:510–518, 2007.

    Routine use of echocardiographic contrast for dobutamine stress echocardiography improved identification of wall motion abnormalities with an increased sensitivity for detection of coronary disease (80% to 91%, p = 0.03) with no

change in specificity (72% to 77%, p = NS).
However, cost-effectiveness analysis based on
cardiac outcomes showed that this improvement
in sensitivity was not cost-effective, with an
increase in cost of $1069 per additional correct
diagnosis.

13. Poldermans D, Arnese M, Fioretti PM,
    et al: Sustained prognostic value of
    dobutamine stress echocardiography
    for late cardiac events after major non-
    cardiac vascular surgery. Circulation
    95:53–58, 1997.
    The risk of cardiac events after major noncar-
    diac vascular surgery (mean follow-up
    19 ± 11 months) is increased in those with
    extensive (risk 6.5 times higher) or limited
    inducible ischemia (risk 2.9 times higher) on
    preoperative dobutamine stress echocardiography
    compared with those with no wall motion
    abnormalities. Risk also is increased (3.8
    times) in those with a resting wall motion
    abnormality on echocardiography. See accom-
    panying editorial by Bach and Eagle on
    pp 8–10 in the same issue.

14. Sicari R, Pasanisi E, Venneri L, et al,
    for the Echo Persantine International
    Cooperative (EPIC) Study Group and
    the Echo Dobutamine International
    Cooperative (EDIC) Study Group.
    Stress echo results predict mortality:
    A large-scale multicenter prospective
    international study. J Am Coll Cardiol
    41:589–595, 2003.
    In 7333 patients undergoing pharmacologic
    stress echocardiography, followed for a mean of
    2.6 years, there was evidence for ischemia in
    35%. Cardiac events (sudden death and fatal
    myocardial infarction) occurred in 2.1% of the
    study group with a Kaplan-Meier survival of
    92% for those with a normal stress test, com-
    pared to 71% for those with ischemia.

Chest Pain in the Emergency Department

15. Weeks S, Fleischmann KE: The role of
    echocardiographic evaluation in patients
    presenting with acute chest pain in the
    emergency room. In Otto CM (ed): The
    Practice of Clinical Echocardiography,
    3rd ed. Philadelphia: Elsevier/Saunders,
    2007, pp 285–298.
    Review of the potential utility of echocardiog-
    raphy for triage, risk stratification, and detec-
    tion of other causes of chest pain in patients
    with suspected myocardial infarction. The
    concept of a chest pain center and cost-effec-
    tiveness of various approaches are discussed.

16. Tong KL, Kaul S, Wang XQ, et al:
    Myocardial contrast echocardiography
    versus Thrombolysis In Myocardial
    Infarction score in patients presenting to

the emergency department with chest pain
and a nondiagnostic electrocardiogram.
J Am Coll Cardiol 46:920–927, 2005.
In 957 patients presenting to the emergency
department with chest pain and a nondiagnostic
ECG, contrast echocardiography was performed
to evaluation regional function and myocardial
perfusion. Echocardiography was superior to
the Thrombolysis in Myocardial Infarction
score is identifying high-risk patients. Only 2 of
523 patients with a normal echocardiogram
had an acute cardiac event.

17. Hernandez AF, Velazquez EJ, Solo-
    mon SD, et al; VALIANT Registry.
    Left ventricular assessment in myocar-
    dial infarction: The VALIANT registry.
    Arch Intern Med 165:2162–2169,
    2005.
    In the Valsartan in Acute Myocardial Infarc-
    tion (VALIANT) registry, evaluation of LV
    function by echocardiography or ventriculogra-
    phy was performed in 77.4% of the 1423
    patients with heart failure and in 54% of the
    3968 patients without heart failure. The use of
    imaging was associated with a shorter time to
    hospital discharge, increased use of appropriate
    medical therapy, and lower in-hospital mor-
    tality in both those with and those without
    heart failure.

18. Conti A, Sammicheli L, Gallini C, et al:
    Assessment of patients with low-risk
    chest pain in the emergency depart-
    ment: Head-to-head comparison of
    exercise stress echocardiography and
    exercise myocardial SPECT. Am Heart
    J 149:894–901, 2005.
    In 503 consecutive patients with chest pain and a
    nondiagnostic ECG and negative cardiac enzymes
    after 6 hours of observation, exercise echocardi-
    ography and exercise nuclear SPECT imaging
    were performed. The stress test was abnormal in
    20% by echocardiography and 24% by nuclear
    imaging. Echocardiography, compared to nuclear
    stress, was more sensitive (93% vs 88%) and
    specific (95% vs 90%) for diagnosis of coronary
    disease and had a higher overall positive predictive
    value (81% vs 67%).

19. Nucifora G, Badano LP, Sarraf-Zade-
    gan N, et al: Comparison of early
    dobutamine stress echocardiography
    and exercise electrocardiographic test-
    ing for management of patients pre-
    senting to the emergency department
    with chest pain. Am J Cardiol
    100:1068–1073, 2007.
    Dobutamine and exercise stress echocardiogra-
    phy for evaluation of low-risk patients present-
    ing to the emergency department with chest pain
    was evaluated by randomization of 199 con-
    secutive patients to dobutamine versus exercise
    stress. Most patients (84%) were discharged
    after a normal stress test. At two-month follow-
    up, cardiac events occurred in 11% of the

exercise patients compared with 0% of the
dobutamine stress patients, suggesting this is an
appropriate approach to triage in low-risk
patients with chest pain.

Myocardial Viability

20. Schinkel AF, Bax JJ, Poldermans D,
    et al: Hibernating myocardium: diag-
    nosis and patient outcomes. Curr Probl
    Cardiol 32:375–410, 2007.
    This review discussion approaches to evaluation
    of hibernating myocardium including dobuta-
    mine echocardiography, thallium-201 and
    technetium-99m nuclear imaging, positron
    emission tomography, and CMR imaging.

21. Dwivedi G, Janardhanan R, Hayat SA,
    et al: Prognostic value of myocardial
    viability detected by myocardial con-
    trast echocardiography early after acute
    myocardial infarction. Am Coll Cardiol
    50:327–334, 2007.
    Residual myocardial viability, as assessed by
    contrast echocardiographic myocardial perfusion,
    was a predictor of survival and recurrent myo-
    cardial infarction in 95 patients evaluated an
    average of 1 week after myocardial infarction.

Complications of Acute Myocardial Infarction

22. Gerber IL, Foster E: Echocardiography
    in the coronary care unit: management
    of acute myocardial infarction, detec-
    tion of complications, and prognostic
    implications. In Otto CM (ed): The
    Practice of Clinical Echocardiography,
    3rd ed. Philadelphia: Elsevier/Saunders,
    2007, pp 299–325.
    This chapter summarizes the pathophysiologic
    correlates of the echocardiographic findings in
    acute myocardial infarction, the role of echo-
    cardiography in patient management, and the
    utility of echocardiography for detecting com-
    plications of acute myocardial infarction. Post-
    myocardial complications and risk stratification
    are reviewed. 219 references.

23. Vargas-Barrón J, Molina-Carrión M,
    Romero-Cárdenas A, et al: Risk factors,
    echocardiographic patterns, and out-
    comes in patients with acute ventricular
    septal rupture during myocardial
    infarction. Am J Cardiol 95:1153–1158,
    2005.
    This paper describes the transthoracic and
    transesophageal echocardiography findings in
    17 patients with a post–myocardial infarction
    ventricular septal defect. Myocardial infarction
    location was inferior in 3 and anterior in 14,
    most had persistent ST elevation on ECG, the
    defect was complex in 9, and RV involvement
    was common.

24. Oliva PB, Hammill SC, Edwards WD: Cardiac rupture, a clinically predictable complication of acute myocardial infarction: Report of 70 cases with clinicopathologic correlations. J Am Coll Cardiol 22:720–726, 1993.

Cardiac rupture should be suspected after myocardial infarction in the setting of pericarditis, repetitive emesis, restlessness and agitation, or if there is a deviation from the expected pattern of T-wave evolution on ECG. Prompt echocardiography can establish the diagnosis of cardiac rupture, allowing rapid intervention.

25. Amigoni M, Meris A, Thune JJ, et al: Mitral regurgitation in myocardial infarction complicated by heart failure, left ventricular dysfunction, or both: Prognostic significance and relation to ventricular size and function. Eur Heart J 28:326–333, 2007.

In 496 patients with heart failure or systolic dysfunction after myocardial infarction, echocardiography 5 days after infarction showed that mitral regurgitant severity was associated with large LV volumes, increased ventricular sphericity, and reduced ejection fraction. Moderate to severe mitral regurgitation at baseline and progressive mitral regurgitation on follow-up studies were associated with an increased risk of cardiovascular death and recurrent heart failure.

26. Assali AR, Teplitsky I, Ben-Dor I, et al: Prognostic importance of right ventricular infarction in an acute myocardial infarction cohort referred for contemporary percutaneous reperfusion therapy. Am Heart J 153:231–237, 2007.

RV infarction is seen in 28% of patients with an inferior myocardial infarction and is associated with increased hospital and long-term mortality. Complete revascularization of the right coronary was associated with improved RV function.

27. Galiuto L, Barchetta S, Paladini S, et al: Functional and structural correlates of persistent ST elevation after acute myocardial infarction successfully treated by percutaneous coronary intervention. Heart 93:1376–1380, 2007.

In 33 patients with persistent ST elevation after myocardial infarction, LV aneurysm was present in 27%, compared with 8% of 49 patients without persistent ST elevation, even though the degree of LV dilation was similar in both groups.

28. Yeo TC, Malouf JF, Oh JK, et al: Clinical profile and outcome in 52 patients with cardiac pseudoaneurysm. Ann Intern Med 128:299–305, 1998.

LV pseudoaneurysms are rare, with only 52 cases diagnosed on echocardiography over a 16-year period at three Mayo Clinic sites. Clinical presentation was no cardiac symptoms (echocardiography requested for other reasons) in

48%, heart failure (15%), chest pain (13%), syncope or arrhythmia (10%), systemic embolism (6%), acute myocardial infarction (6%), or cardiac tamponade (2%). Pseudoaneurysm developed after cardiac surgery (58%) or after myocardial infarction (42%). Most pseudoaneurysms were located in the inferior or posterolateral wall (82%) after myocardial infarction or adjacent to the valve annulus after cardiac surgery.

29. Gueret P, Khalife K, Jobic Y, et al: Echocardiographic assessment of the incidence of mechanical complications during the early phase of myocardial infarction in the reperfusion era: A French multicentre prospective registry. Arch Cardiovasc Dis 101:41–47, 2008.

The prevalence of post-myocardial complications was assessed in a contemporary series of 908 patients. Mitral regurgitation was the most common complication, present in 28%, and was due to LV remodeling (43%) or papillary muscle dysfunction (57%). Pericardial effusion occurred in only 6.6% and was more common after anterior infarction. Other complications were unusual: LV thrombus in 2.4%, early infarct expansion in 4%, septal rupture in 0.6%, and free wall rupture in 0.8%. Mechanical complications were more likely in the absence of early revascularization and with older age.

Clinical Outcome after Myocardial Infarction

30. Khumri TM, Nayyar S, Idupulapati M, et al: Usefulness of myocardial contrast echocardiography in predicting late mortality in patients with anterior wall acute myocardial infarction. Am J Cardiol 98:1150–1155, 2006.

Myocardial contrast echocardiography was performed 2 days after admission in 167 anterior myocardial infarction patients with LV dysfunction. The only multivariate predictors of long-term survival (mean follow-up 39 months) were age and perfusion score index (odds ratio 4.5 for each 1.0 increase in score index, confidence interval 1.3–15.4).

31. Mollema SA, Liem SS, Suffoletto MS, et al: Left ventricular dyssynchrony acutely after myocardial infarction predicts left ventricular remodeling. J Am Coll Cardiol 50:1532–1540, 2007.

Echocardiographic evaluation—including 2D quantitation of ventricular volumes and function, Doppler measures of diastolic function, evaluation of mitral regurgitation, and speckle-tracking radial strain dyssynchrony analysis—was performed in 178 consecutive patients with acute myocardial infarction treated with primary percutaneous coronary revascularization.

Multivariate analysis identified dyssynchrony as the strongest predictor of ventricular remodeling at 6 months (present in 20%). A cutoff value of 130 ms for dyssynchrony had a sensitivity of 92% and specificity of 95% for prediction of ventricular remodeling after acute myocardial infarction.

32. Witt N, Samad BA, Frick M, et al: Detection of left ventricular dysfunction by Doppler tissue imaging in patients with complete recovery of visual wall motion abnormalities 6 months after a first ST-elevation myocardial infarction. Clin Physiol Funct Imaging 27:305–308, 2007.

In 68 patients with no prior coronary disease and an ST-elevation myocardial infarction, complete recovery of wall motion was seen in 28% at 6 months. However, even with complete recovery as assessed by 2D imaging, mitral annular tissue Doppler systolic and diastolic velocities remained reduced compared with normal controls, possibly reflecting residual subendothelial damage.

33. Tani T, Tanabe K, Kureha F, et al: Transthoracic Doppler echocardiographic assessment of left anterior descending coronary artery and intramyocardial artery predicts left ventricular remodeling and wall-motion recovery after acute myocardial infarction. J Am Soc Echocardiogr 20: 813–819, 2007.

In 24 patients with an acute anterior myocardial infarction, coronary flow velocity was recorded in the left anterior descending and intramyocardial coronary arteries by TTE 2 days after successful percutaneous revascularization. Acutely, there were no differences in LV wall motion score or ejection fraction, comparing the group with a rapid (<600 ms) to the group with normal (>600 ms) coronary diastolic deceleration time (DDT). However, at 6-month follow-up the wall motion score index was higher and ejection fraction was lower (38 ± 9 vs 55 ± 10%, p = 0.001) in those with a rapid DDT, suggesting that coronary DDT predicts recovery of function in the infarct region.

34. Watanabe N: Echocardiographic evaluation of coronary blood flow: Approaches and clinical applications. In Otto CM (ed): The Practice of Clinical Echocardiography, 3rd ed. Philadelphia: Elsevier/Saunders, 2007, pp 393–402.

This chapter describes the approach to echocardiographic and Doppler evaluation of coronary anatomy and blood flow. Clinical applications are summarized, including coronary flow reserve measurements, noninvasive diagnosis of coronary stenosis, and the role of coronary flow measurement in acute myocardial infarction.

Cardiomyopathies, Hypertensive and Pulmonary Heart Disease

C ardiomyopathy is defined as a primary disease of the myocardium, excluding myocardial dysfunction due to ischemia or chronic valvular disease. There are several possible approaches to classification of cardiomyopathies, such as etiology or anatomy, but a physiologic classification is most useful clinically. The three basic physiologic categories of cardiomyopathy are:

❑ Dilated
❑ Hypertrophic
❑ Restrictive

The disease process in an individual patient may correspond closely with one of these physiologic categories; however, overlap between these categories (particularly between dilated and restrictive) can occur. Echocardiographic evaluation focuses on confirming the diagnosis and type of cardiomyopathy present and on defining the physiologic consequences of the disease process in that individual.

While hypertensive and pulmonary heart disease are not primary diseases of heart muscle, they are included in this chapter because their clinical and echocardiographic presentation may mimic a cardiomyopathy. In addition, evaluation of the patient after cardiac transplant is included. End-stage coronary disease resulting in left ventricular (LV) systolic dysfunction, sometimes referred to as "ischemic cardiomyopathy," is discussed in Chapter 8.

DILATED CARDIOMYOPATHY

Basic Principles

Dilated cardiomyopathy is characterized by four-chamber enlargement with impaired systolic function of both ventricles. There are many causes as summarized in Table 9–1. The physiology of dilated cardiomyopathy is characterized predominantly by:

❐ Impaired LV contractility
❐ Reduced cardiac output
❐ Elevated LV end-diastolic pressure

Clinically, patients most often present with heart failure, with initial complaints ranging from symptoms of pulmonary or systemic venous congestion to symptoms of low forward cardiac output. Coexisting mitral regurgitation frequently is present secondary to LV and mitral annular dilation. In addition, pulmonary hypertension develops in most patients in response to the chronic elevation in left atrial (LA) pressure. Typically, LV diastolic dysfunction coexists with systolic dysfunction, although separating the hemodynamic effects of diastolic dysfunction from concurrent systolic dysfunction is challenging.

Echocardiographic Approach

Echocardiographic imaging from standard windows allows evaluation of the size and function of all four cardiac chambers with particular attention to the two ventricles (Figs. 9–1 and 9–2):

❐ LV systolic function
  ❐ Qualitative global and regional function
  ❐ Quantitative end-diastolic and end-systolic dimensions or volumes
  ❐ Ejection fraction
❐ Right ventricular (RV) systolic function
  ❐ Qualitative size and systolic function
  ❐ Pulmonary artery systolic pressure and estimated resistance

In addition to two-dimensional (2D) imaging, other signs of poor LV systolic function include:

❐ M-mode
  ❐ Increased mitral E-point to septal separation (EPSS)
  ❐ Reduced anteroposterior aortic root motion
  ❐ Delayed mitral valve closure

TABLE 9–1   Examples of Causes of Cardiomyopathies, Functional Classification

Dilated Cardiomyopathy

Genetic
Infectious
• Postviral (myocarditis)
• Chagas' disease
Toxins and drugs
• Alcohol
• Anthracycline medications
Metabolic
• Thiamine deficiency
• Hypo- or hyperthyroidism
• Pheochromocytoma
Nutritional
• Beriberi (thiamine deficiency)
Peripartum
Systemic inflammatory disease
Neuromuscular diseases
• Duchenne-Becker muscular dystrophy
Stress-induced
• Tako-tsubo

Hypertrophic Cardiomyopathy

Nonobstructive
Obstructive
Latent obstructive

Restrictive Cardiomyopathy

Infiltrative systemic diseases
• Amyloidosis
• Gaucher disease
Inflammatory (granulomatous)
• Sarcoidosis
Storage diseases
• Hemochromatosis
• Fabry's disease
Endomyocardial
• Hypereosinophilic syndrome
• Radiation-induced
Noninfiltrative
• Scleroderma

Other Cardiomyopathies

Arrhythmogenic RV dysplasia
Isolated LV noncompaction

❐ Doppler
  ❐ Reduced aortic ejection velocity
  ❐ Reduced rate of rise in ventricular pressure (dP/dt)
  ❐ Associated mitral regurgitation
  ❐ Diastolic dysfunction

The increase in EPSS is due to a combination of LV dilation and reduced mitral leaflet motion resulting

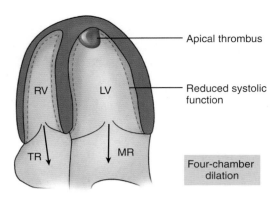

Figure 9–1 Schematic diagram of the key features of dilated cardio-myopathy in an apical four-chamber view. All four chambers are enlarged with reduced LV and RV systolic function. Dashed lines indicate the limited extent of endocardial motion between end-diastole and end-systole. An apical thrombus is present. Secondary mitral and tricuspid regurgitation are indicated by the *arrows*.

from low transmitral flow rates. Reduced anteroposter-ior aortic root motion reflects reduced LA filling and emptying (Fig. 9–3). A reduced aortic ejection velocity indicates a reduced stroke volume, although compensa-tory mechanisms (including LV dilation) often result in a normal stroke volume at rest. A slow rate of rise in velocity of the mitral regurgitant jet indicates a reduced rate of rise in LV pressure in early systole (dP/dt).

The cause of functional mitral valve regurgitation (with an anatomically normal valve) is related to malalignment of the papillary muscles, ventricular systolic dysfunction, and annular dilation. Regurgi-tant severity ranges from mild to severe, as assessed with Doppler techniques (see Chapter 12) (Fig. 9–4). Pulmonary artery (PA) pressures usually are elevated and can be estimated from the velocity of the tricus-pid regurgitant jet, as described in Chapter 6.

The echocardiographic appearance of a dilated cardiomyopathy is fairly uniform despite a wide range of disease processes. Exceptions include fulmi-nant myocarditis, in which there may be little ventric-ular dilation, despite severe systolic dysfunction. In Chagas' heart disease, an LV apical aneurysm is seen in about one half of patients, often with thrombus for-mation, although global hypokinesis is typical with advanced disease (Fig. 9–5). Tako-tsubo cardio-myopathy is an acute, transient, stress-induced car-diomyopathy characterized by "apical ballooning" with apical dilation and dyskinesis but preserved dimensions and function of the cardiac base (Fig. 9–6).

The pattern of LV diastolic filling can be evaluated with Doppler recordings of LV inflow. Early in the disease course, a reduced E velocity and increased A velocity consistent with impaired early diastolic relaxation may be observed. However, once LV func-tion has deteriorated significantly, the pattern changes to that of an increased E velocity and reduced A veloc-ity. In this situation, the high ratio of E to A velocity most likely indicates a high LA pressure (increased

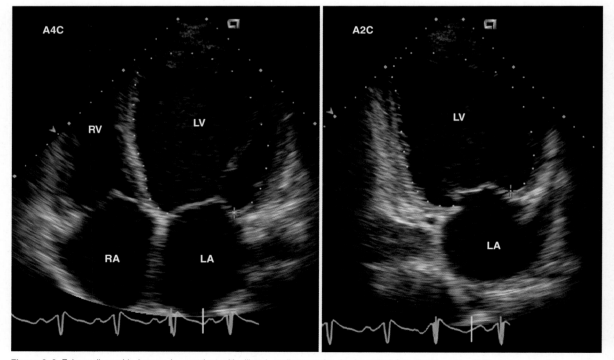

Figure 9–2 Echocardiographic images in a patient with dilated cardiomyopathy. In the apical four-chamber view (*left*), dilation of all four cardiac chambers is seen. In the apical two-chamber view (*right*), the LV and LA are seen. In real time, RV and LV systolic function were severely reduced.

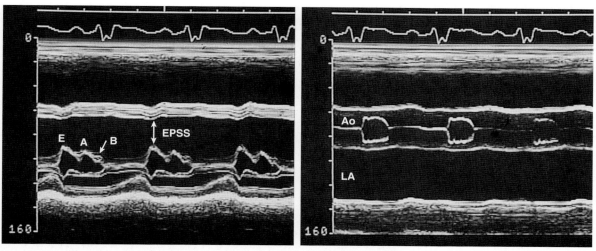

Figure 9–3 M-mode findings in dilated cardiomyopathy. There is increased mitral E-point septal separation (EPSS) and a "B-bump" (*left*) and decreased aortic root motion with early closure of the aortic valve (*right*).

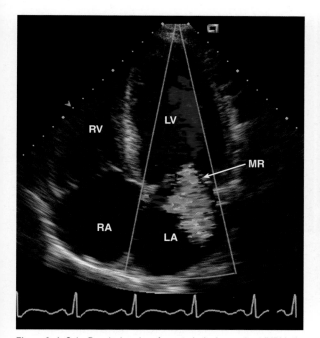

Figure 9–4 Color Doppler imaging of a central mitral regurgitant (MR) jet in an apical four-chamber view in a patient with dilated cardiomyopathy. The mitral valve leaflets are normal with functional MR due to ventricular dilation and abnormal alignment of the papillary muscles resulting in leaflet tethering.

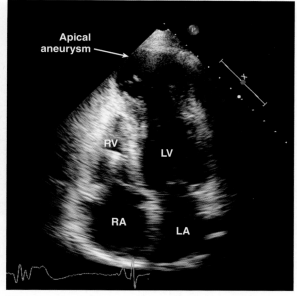

Figure 9–5 Large apical aneurysm in a 47-year-old woman with chronic Chagas cardiomyopathy complaining of palpitations and dizziness. The basal and medial segments of the LV walls had near normal or increased contractility. A pacemaker wire is seen in the RV. Coronary angiography was normal. Apical abnormalities are seen in 1% to 10% of asymptomatic subjects and in about half of patients with Chagas' disease. *(Courtesy of Dr. Harry Acquatella, Centro Medico, San Bernardino, Caracas, Venezuela.)*

gradient from LA to LV at mitral valve opening) and a high LV end-diastolic pressure (reduced *A* velocity) (Fig. 9–7). This pattern of mitral inflow, often termed *pseudo-normalization*, can be distinguished from a normal inflow pattern by the pulmonary venous inflow signal, which shows both an increased atrial reversal velocity and an increased diastolic to systolic flow

ratio, and by the Doppler tissue velocities at the mitral annulus, which shows a decreased *E′* velocity. The M-mode finding of a delayed rate of mitral valve closure, termed a *B-bump* or *AC-shoulder* also correlates with an elevated end-diastolic pressure (see Fig. 9–3).

When significant LV systolic dysfunction is present (ejection fraction <35%), a careful search for apical

Figure 9–6 This 28-year-old woman developed acute heart failure after emergency noncardiac surgery. In the apical four-chamber view the LV apex is dilated with systolic dyskinesis (*arrows*) with relatively preserved contraction at the myocardial base. The degree of annular apical motion from diastole to systole is indicated by the *double-headed arrow*. Coronary angiography was normal and ventricular systolic function returned to normal within 2 weeks.

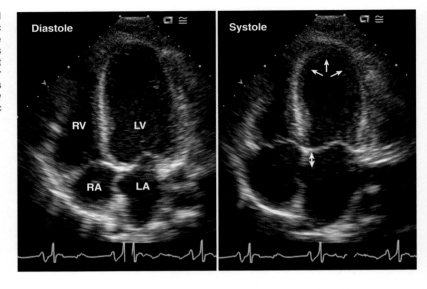

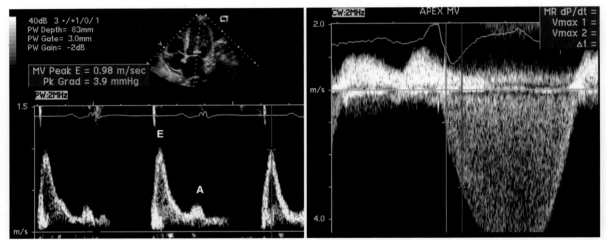

Figure 9–7 Doppler findings in dilated cardiomyopathy. LV diastolic inflow shows a high *E* velocity and low *A* velocity suggestive of "pseudo-normalization" due to an elevated end-diastolic pressure (*left*). The mitral regurgitation jet shows a slow rate of rise in velocity consistent with a reduced *dP/dt* (*right*).

LV thrombus is indicated, although prevalence is low with current medical therapy (Fig. 9–8). Details on the technical aspects of identifying an LV thrombus are given in Chapter 8.

Limitations/Technical Considerations

Echocardiography rarely can establish the etiology of a dilated cardiomyopathy, even though it is instrumental both in confirming the presence of ventricular dysfunction and in providing prognostic data. The accuracy of measures of ventricular volumes and ejection fraction depend on attention to data acquisition and analysis as discussed in Chapter 6. In addition to the technical aspects in evaluation of diastolic dysfunction, as discussed in Chapter 7, diastolic and systolic function are inseparable parts of cardiac performance. Isolating the effects of diastolic dysfunction from that of altered loading conditions related to systolic dysfunction can be problematic. Most patients have combined systolic and diastolic dysfunction, with both contributing to clinical symptoms and outcomes.

Clinical Utility

Echocardiographic evaluation is indicated at the initial presentation of a patient with symptoms consistent with heart failure. If echocardiography shows no significant impairment of LV systolic dysfunction, other possible diagnoses include:

- ❑ Coronary artery disease
- ❑ Valve disease
- ❑ Hypertensive heart disease
- ❑ Pericardial disease
- ❑ Pulmonary heart disease

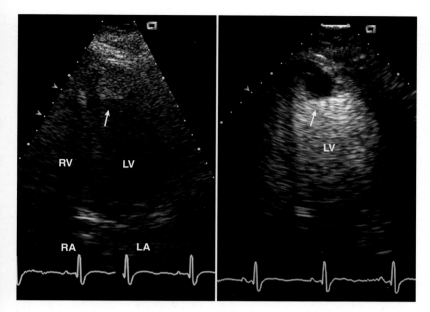

Figure 9–8 An apical LV thrombus (*arrow*) is poorly seen on 2D imaging (*left*) but appears as a definite filling defect using left-sided echo contrast (*right*).

Whenever the clinical presentation suggests heart failure, a comprehensive examination of systolic and diastolic function is needed, even when the core echocardiographic examination does not show obvious evidence of dysfunction. If the echocardiogram is consistent with the clinical diagnosis of dilated cardiomyopathy, detailed information on ventricular function, chamber sizes, associated valvular disease, and pulmonary pressure is obtained.

Periodic echocardiography is essential for optimal care of patients with dilated cardiomyopathy. The detailed assessment available by echocardiography aids in appropriate tailoring of medical therapy. In addition, repeat echocardiography may be helpful when a change in clinical status suggests an interval change in ventricular function. A severe decrease in ventricular systolic function may prompt consideration of cardiac transplantation in appropriate candidates.

The role of echocardiography in selection of patients for cardiac resynchronization therapy is in evolution. Myocardial dyssynchrony can be evaluated by tissue Doppler and speckle-tracking techniques as discussed in Chapter 4 and in Suggested Reading 1. After resynchronization with biventricular pacing, benefit can be measured by the reduction in LV size, improvement in systolic function and decrease in mitral regurgitant severity.

In the intensive care unit, echocardiographic evaluation can be helpful in patients with dilated cardiomyopathy to assess LV function, PA pressure, and the degree of coexisting mitral regurgitation, and to estimate LV filling pressure. Evaluation of an individual patient's response to afterload reduction therapy can be performed by repeat ejection fraction measurements or by sequential noninvasive measurements of PA pressure and cardiac output (Fig. 9–9).

Alternate Approaches

Evaluation of a patient with new-onset heart failure typically includes a careful clinical evaluation and laboratory data. In many patients with dilated cardiomyopathy an exact etiology cannot be identified, even when all diagnostic modalities are used. Coronary angiography may be appropriate to evaluate for an ischemic cause. If exact measurement of pulmonary vascular resistance is needed (e.g., in a heart transplant candidate), cardiac catheterization is indicated because noninvasive approaches provide only an estimate of pulmonary vascular resistance.

HYPERTROPHIC CARDIOMYOPATHY

Basic Principles

Hypertrophic cardiomyopathy is an autosomal dominant inherited disease of the myocardium (with variable penetrance) related to abnormalities in genes coding for contractile proteins. Characteristic anatomic features of this disease (Fig. 9–10) include:

- ❑ Asymmetric hypertrophy of the LV
- ❑ Normal ventricular systolic function
- ❑ Impaired diastolic LV function
- ❑ Subaortic dynamic obstruction

Other important clinical features of this disease are a high risk of sudden death (especially during exertion); symptoms of angina, exercise intolerance, and syncope, a high prevalence of atrial fibrillation, and a systolic murmur on cardiac auscultation.

The *pattern* of LV hypertrophy in patients with hypertrophic cardiomyopathy can be quite variable, ranging from "classic" septal hypertrophy to isolated

Figure 9–9 Calculation of stroke volume in a patient with dilated cardiomyopathy is based on measurement of LV outflow tract diameter from a parasternal long-axis view (*top*) for calculation of a circular cross-sectional area (CSA$_{LVOT}$). and the LV outflow tract velocity-time integral (VTI$_{LVOT}$) recorded just proximal to the Ao valve from an apical approach using a pulsed Doppler sample volume length of 5 to 10 mm (*bottom*). Stroke volume is calculated as VTI × CSA. Cardiac output is stroke volume times heart rate. Calculation of stroke volume in this patient is complicated by mechanical alternans related to severe systolic dysfunction with marked variation in the outflow velocity (*arrows*) on alternating beats despite normal sinus rhythm.

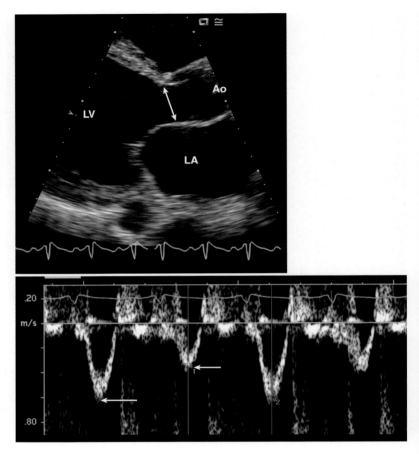

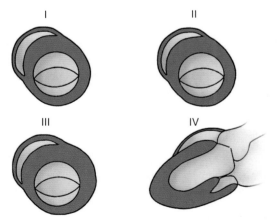

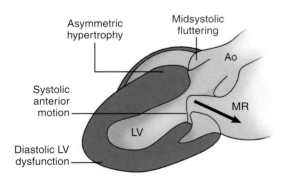

Figure 9–10 Schematic diagram of the typical features of hypertrophic cardiomyopathy in a long-axis view. There is midsystolic closure and coarse fluttering of the aortic valve leaflets, asymmetric septal hypertrophy with sparing of the basal posterior wall, normal LV systolic function with impaired diastolic function, dynamic outflow tract obstruction with systolic anterior motion of the mitral valve leaflets, and mitral regurgitation.

Figure 9–11 Schematic diagram of patterns of ventricular hypertrophy in hypertrophic cardiomyopathy in a basal short-axis view. Type I = hypertrophy confined to anterior septum; type II = anterior and posterior septum involved; type III = extensive hypertrophy sparing only the basal posterior wall; type IV = apical hypertrophy (in a long-axis schematic view).

apical hypertrophy (Fig. 9–11). In addition, the *degree* of myocardial thickening is quite variable, even within a family. In about 10% of cases, hypertrophy is confined to the anterior segment of the ventricular septum (type I) and about 20% have involvement of both the anterior and posterior segments of the

septum (type II) with sparing of the lateral, posterior, and inferior walls. The most common pattern of hypertrophy, seen in 52% of patients, involves the septum and anterolateral free wall (type III).

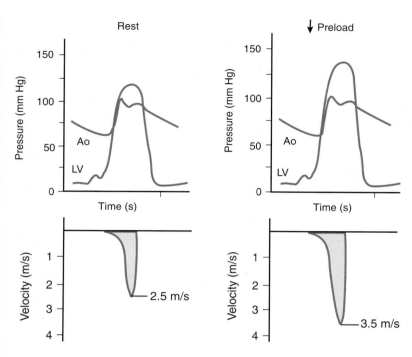

Figure 9–12 Schematic diagrams of the pressure gradient and velocity curve in dynamic outflow obstruction due to hypertrophic cardiomyopathy. At rest, a small gradient is present only in late systole between the LV and aorta (Ao). The continuous-wave Doppler curve (*bottom*) shows a late-peaking velocity of 2.5 m/s, with the origin of this velocity being the subaortic region. With alterations in loading conditions (decreased preload), the degree of obstruction increases dramatically. A late-peaking, high-velocity (3.5 m/s) Doppler curve now is obtained.

Involvement of other regions of the ventricle, including apical hypertrophic cardiomyopathy (type IV) accounts for about 18% of cases. The common feature of all these hypertrophy patterns is normal thickness (or "sparing") of the basal posterior LV wall. In the parasternal long- and short-axis views, this region is seen at the base (between the papillary muscle and mitral annulus) posterior to the mitral valve leaflets.

Hypertrophic cardiomyopathy is classified as nonobstructive (about one third of patients) if the outflow gradient at rest and with provocation is <30 mm Hg, obstructive if the gradient at rest is ≥30 mm Hg (>2.7 m/s), and inducible or latent if the resting gradient is <30 mm Hg but obstruction occurs with exercise (or other maneuvers). With dynamic obstruction there is an increase in flow velocity, and corresponding pressure gradient, proximal to the aortic valve, in association with systolic anterior motion of the mitral valve toward the hypertrophied ventricular septum. Obstruction is dynamic rather than fixed, both in the sense that it occurs only in mid to late systole and in the sense that the presence and severity of obstruction can be altered by loading conditions. These features contrast with the relatively fixed obstruction of aortic valve stenosis, which persists from the onset to the end of ejection and in which the severity of the stenosis is relatively insensitive to changes in loading conditions. Dynamic outflow obstruction in hypertrophic cardiomyopathy typically has a pattern of onset in mid-systole, with the maximum LV to aortic pressure gradient occurring in late systole (Fig. 9–12).

Obstruction can be diminished by maneuvers that increase ventricular volume—such as an increase in preload or a decrease in contractility—or by maneuvers that increase afterload. Conversely, the degree of obstruction is increased by:

- a reduction in preload,
- an increase in contractility, or
- a decrease in afterload.

Each of these physiologic changes results in a decrease in LV volume and an increase in the degree of dynamic obstruction, with a louder murmur and an increased Doppler velocity.

Dynamic outflow obstruction usually is associated with mitral regurgitation, since the systolic anterior motion of the leaflets disrupts normal coaptation. A posteriorly directed mitral regurgitant jet of mild to moderate severity originates at the mal-coapted segment of the leaflets (Fig. 9–13).

LV systolic function typically is normal in patients with hypertrophic cardiomyopathy. However, LV diastolic function is abnormal, with impaired relaxation and decreased compliance, accounting for many of the heart failure symptoms in patients with hypertrophic cardiomyopathy.

Echocardiographic Approach

Left Ventricular Asymmetric Hypertrophy

Evaluation of the pattern and extent of LV hypertrophy is made from multiple tomographic views. In the parasternal long-axis view, particular attention is focused on the posterobasal wall between the papillary muscle and the mitral annulus. Although

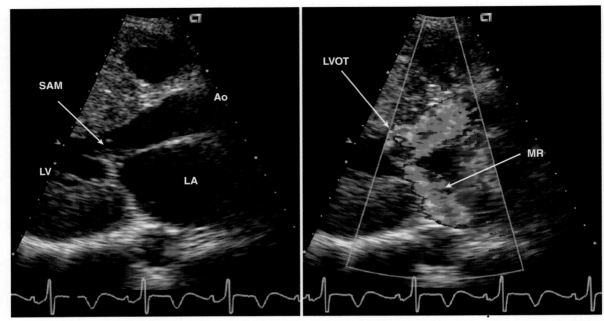

Figure 9–13 Parasternal long-axis 2D image (*left*) and color flow image (*right*) showing systolic anterior motion of the mitral leaflets (SAM) and mitral regurgitation (MR) in a patient with hypertrophic cardiomyopathy. The posteriorly directed MR jet originates from the malcoapted segment of the mitral leaflets in association with systolic anterior motion. Turbulence in the LV outflow tract (LVOT) is seen due to subaortic dynamic obstruction.

the wall in this region is not thickened in most patients with hypertrophic cardiomyopathy, it is thickened in patients with concentric hypertrophy due to other etiologies (e.g., hypertension, infiltrative cardiomyopathy). 2D-guided M-mode tracings are used for measurement of septal and posterior wall thickness, using both long- and short-axis views to ensure that the measurements are perpendicular to the LV wall and to avoid inclusion of RV trabeculation in the septal wall thickness. Careful measurements of diastolic septal thickness provide prognostic information (e.g., risk of sudden death) and are essential for decision making about septal reduction procedures.

The parasternal long-axis view also offers the best opportunity to define the exact relationship between the pattern of septal hypertrophy and the outflow tract (Fig. 9–14). This is important when a surgical approach, such as myotomy-myectomy, is being considered, since surgical visualization usually is retrograde across the aortic valve, allowing only limited direct inspection of the septal endocardium and little information on the extent of septal thickening or the degree of septal curvature. The extent and pattern of hypertrophy also is relevant if percutaneous catheter ablation is being considered. Parasternal short-axis views from base to apex allow assessment of the lateromedial extent of the hypertrophic process.

It is important to recognize that some degree of bulging of the septum into the LV outflow tract, often called a septal "knuckle," is seen in normal older individuals. This apparent septal prominence most likely

is due to increased tortuosity of the aorta resulting in a more acute angle between the basal septum and aortic root. There is no evidence that this septal contour pattern is inherited or associated with clinical events so that these patients should not be considered to have hypertrophic cardiomyopathy.

Apical views again allow visualization of the pattern and extent of hypertrophy. Diagnosis of apical hypertrophy can be difficult, since endocardial definition may be poor and the endocardial surface (which may be located up to one third the distance from the apical epicardium to the base) may be missed if image quality is suboptimal (Fig. 9–15). In some cases the epicardium may be mistaken for the apical endocardium. A careful examination, when the referring physician has alerted the echocardiographer to this possible diagnosis, avoids this potential pitfall. Color or pulsed Doppler examination is helpful in demonstrating the absence of blood flow in the "apical" region, which is occupied by the hypertrophied myocardium. If needed, echo contrast can be used to better define the endocardial border.

Qualitative and quantitative evaluation of LV systolic function is performed using standard approaches (see Chapter 6).

Left Ventricular Diastolic Function

LV diastolic function is evaluated using Doppler recordings of:

❏ LV inflow across the mitral valve
❏ LA inflow in the pulmonary vein

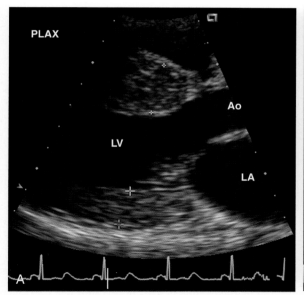

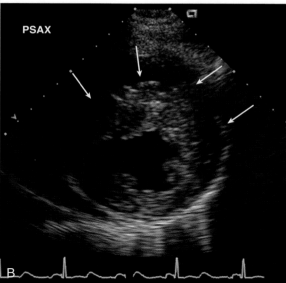

Figure 9–14 **A,** Two-dimensional images of hypertrophic cardiomyopathy in a parasternal long-axis view at end-diastole for measurement of septal and posterior wall thickness. The septal thickness is 2.1 cm, taking care to avoid the trabeculation on the RV side of the septum. **B,** The parasternal short-axis view shows hypertrophy involving the anterior septum and anterior free wall (*arrows*).

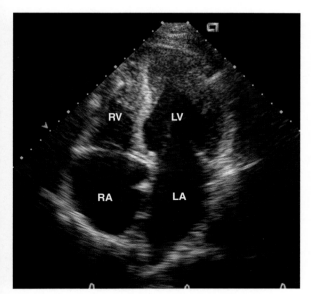

Figure 9–15 Apical hypertrophic cardiomyopathy with marked thickening of the apical segments in an apical four-chamber view.

❑ Mitral annular Doppler tissue velocity
❑ Isovolumic relaxation time (IVRT)

Parameters of diastolic function are evaluated as described in Chapter 7. Typical changes in patients with hypertrophic cardiomyopathy include a prolonged IVRT, reduced *E* velocity, enhanced *A* velocity, and increased duration and velocity of the pulmonary vein *a*-reversal. These findings are consistent with impaired diastolic relaxation and an elevated

LV end-diastolic pressure. However, there is marked patient variability depending on the severity of diastolic dysfunction in each patient. Sequential studies may show changes after medical or surgical therapies that are consistent with improved diastolic filling.

Dynamic Outflow Tract Obstruction

In a subset of patients with hypertrophic cardiomyopathy, subaortic obstruction is present, characterized by:

❑ Systolic anterior motion of the mitral leaflet
❑ Mid-systolic closure of the aortic valve
❑ Late-peaking high-velocity flow in the outflow tract
❑ Variability in the severity of obstruction with maneuvers:
  ❑ Post–premature ventricular contraction (PVC) beats
  ❑ Valsalva maneuver
  ❑ Exercise

IMAGING. In a patient with dynamic LV outflow tract obstruction, long-axis images show the classic finding of systolic anterior motion of the mitral valve with apposition of the mitral leaflet and septum in mid to late systole. M-mode recordings may be helpful in that with pathologic systolic anterior motion, the rate of anterior leaflet motion is more rapid than the anterior motion of the posterior wall in systole (Fig. 9–16). A "contact lesion" on the ventricular septum at the site of mitral leaflet impingement may be seen in some patients.

Short-axis views also show the systolic anterior motion of the mitral valve leaflets. Frame-by-frame

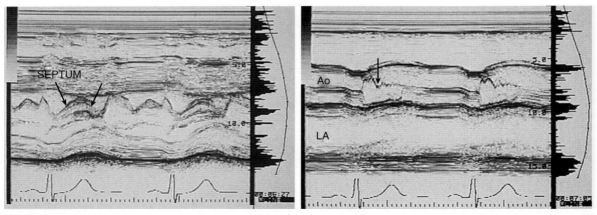

Figure 9–16 M-mode at the mitral valve level (*left*) in a patient with dynamic outflow obstruction due to hypertrophic cardiomyopathy showing the classic septal hypertrophy and systolic anterior motion of the mitral valve leaflets (*arrows*). An M-mode view at the aortic valve level (*right*) shows midsystolic closure of the valve (*arrow*) followed by coarse fluttering of the leaflets.

analysis shows the cross-sectional area of the outflow tract throughout systole.

Apical 2D views are helpful for demonstrating the abnormal mitral leaflet motion, especially the apical long-axis and the anteriorly angulated four-chamber views. Note that the degree of systolic anterior motion may not be uniform from medial to lateral across the mitral leaflets, so imaging in multiple planes with slight adjustments in transducer angulation may be needed to demonstrate the presence and extent of dynamic outflow obstruction.

The aortic valve shows normal leaflet opening in early systole, followed by mid-systolic abrupt partial closure with coarse fluttering of the aortic valve leaflets in late systole due to late systolic dynamic outflow obstruction. Again, these rapid leaflet movements are best documented on M-mode recordings. The aortic leaflets themselves may be sclerotic because of the long-term effect of a turbulent jet as a result of subaortic obstruction, and some degree of coexisting aortic regurgitation may be noted.

DOPPLER EVALUATION. Doppler studies provide a more direct evaluation of the presence, location, and degree of dynamic subaortic obstruction than do imaging techniques. With conventional pulsed or color flow imaging, the site of obstruction is identified based on the location of the post-stenotic turbulence. Both parasternal and apical long-axis views are useful for this examination.

Using pulsed Doppler from an apical approach, the sample volume is slowly moved from the apex progressively toward the base, recording the velocity curve at each step. Proximal to the outflow obstruction, velocities are normal. At the site of obstruction the velocity increases abruptly to a velocity reflecting the degree of obstruction (as stated in the Bernoulli equation). This approach, using stepwise evaluation with pulsed Doppler ultrasound, is advantageous in that intracavity gradients due to apical hypertrophy or apposition

of the papillary muscle with the septum will be recognized and not mistaken for subaortic dynamic obstruction.

Continuous-wave Doppler from an apical approach typically shows a late-peaking high-velocity systolic jet in patients with dynamic LV outflow tract obstruction (Fig. 9–17). The shape of this curve is distinctive, corresponding to the temporal course of the LV to aortic pressure gradient (see Fig. 9–12).

Latent Outflow Obstruction. Some patients with hypertrophic cardiomyopathy have dynamic outflow obstruction with exercise but not at rest. Traditionally, maneuvers to "provoke" outflow obstruction at rest were performed during the echocardiography examination. A spontaneous PVC results in an increased degree of obstruction on the post-PVC beat due to increased LV contractility. Alternatively, the strain phase of the Valsalva maneuver increases obstruction by decreasing preload (smaller LV cavity size) but is difficult to perform simultaneously with echocardiography due to changes in cardiac position and lung interference as the patient performs the maneuver. In the past, amyl nitrate inhalation was used to induce a brief decrease in preload (venodilation) and decrease in afterload (arterial dilation), both of which increase the degree of obstruction. However, these maneuvers are no longer recommended due to low reproducibility and limited clinical value.

The optimal approach to evaluation for inducible obstruction is a treadmill or bicycle exercise stress test. Continuous-wave Doppler outflow velocity recordings are made at rest and immediately after exercise to assess for inducible outflow obstruction, defined as an exercise outflow tract gradient ≥ 30 mm Hg (velocity ≥ 2.7 m/s). Pharmacologic stress testing with dobutamine is not recommended, because it is nonspecific (mid-cavity obstruction is seen even in normal individuals) and does not provide information on exercise capacity or the relationship of symptoms to exertion.

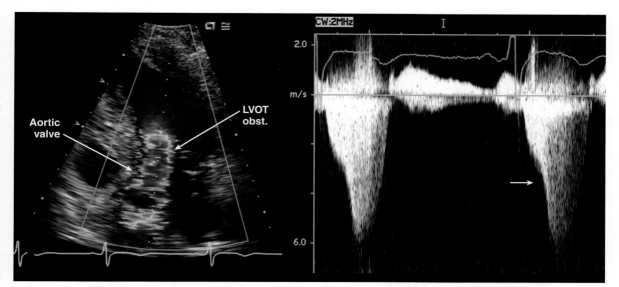

Figure 9–17 Resting LV outflow obstruction in this patient with hypertrophic cardiomyopathy was evaluated from the apical view (*left*) with color and pulsed Doppler to localize the level of obstruction. The pulsed Doppler sample volume was moved sequentially from the ventricular cavity toward the aortic valve to identify the site of increased velocity. Continuous-wave Doppler (*right*) shows the high-velocity late-peaking (*arrow*) jet typical of dynamic outflow obstruction.

Mitral Valve Abnormalities

The mitral valve is anatomically and functionally abnormal in the majority of patients with hypertrophic cardiomyopathy. Anatomically, the leaflets are larger than in normal individuals. Functionally, mitral regurgitation results from systolic anterior motion of the leaflets into the outflow tract leading to late systolic failure of coaptation and a consequent posteriorly directed regurgitant jet. Mitral regurgitant severity typically is moderate but ranges from mild to severe and varies dynamically with the severity of outflow obstruction. Evaluation of mitral valve anatomy and severity of regurgitation is detailed in Chapter 12.

Limitations/Technical Considerations

When a high-velocity outflow signal is detected with continuous-wave Doppler, other techniques are needed to determine the depth of origin of the signal because velocities are measured along the entire length of the ultrasound beam. In patients with hypertensive heart disease or hypovolemia, the combination of LV hypertrophy and hyperdynamic systolic function may result in a late-peaking high-velocity systolic waveform (Fig. 9–18) similar to that seen in hypertrophic cardiomyopathy. However, in these patients the site of obstruction is not subaortic; it is closer to the apex, at the midventricular level.

The distinction between hypertrophic cardiomyopathy and a hyperdynamic concentrically hypertrophied ventricle can be made by careful attention to the 2D images (sparing of the basal posterior wall in hypertrophic cardiomyopathy) and by evaluation of the depth of origin of the high-velocity jet using conventional pulsed, high pulse repetition frequency, and color Doppler techniques. The patient's clinical and family histories also are important for making this distinction. Genetic testing may be reasonable in some cases.

Distinguishing between the signal due to dynamic subaortic obstruction and mitral regurgitation can be challenging because both are common with hypertrophic cardiomyopathy and both are high-velocity systolic signals directed away from the apex. The two features that are helpful in this distinction are (1) the shape of the velocity curve (late peaking with subaortic obstruction versus a rapid early systolic rise in velocity with mitral regurgitation) and (2) the timing of flow (mitral regurgitation is longer in duration, starting earlier and ending later in the cardiac cycle).

Another difficult problem is separating the degree of outflow obstruction due to dynamic subaortic obstruction from that due to valvular aortic stenosis in the rare patient with both conditions. In the presence of serial stenoses, an accurate measure of the pressure drop across each narrowing may not be possible, since the simplified Bernoulli equation applies to a single stenosis. However, high pulse repetition frequency Doppler may allow examination of velocities at several levels, indicating the relative contribution of each site to the total degree of obstruction to ventricular outflow. Occasionally a patient with valvular aortic stenosis and a hypertrophied ventricle will demonstrate dynamic subaortic obstruction only after aortic valve replacement. Some of these patients have hypertrophic cardiomyopathy that is "unmasked" by the afterload reduction of valve replacement. Others have a hyperdynamic ventricle with a mid-cavity pressure gradient that may resolve as the degree of LV hypertrophy decreases postoperatively.

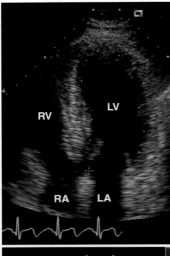

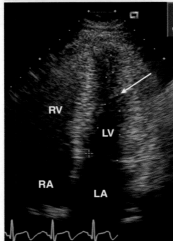

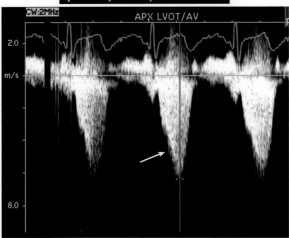

Figure 9–18 Example of a concentrically hypertrophied hyperdynamic LV in diastole (*top*) with mid-cavity obliteration at end-systole (*middle*) resulting in a late-peaking high-velocity outflow tract Doppler curve (*bottom*). This patient was anemic and febrile at the time of this examination. Hypertensive hyperdynamic mid-cavity obstruction must be distinguished from the dynamic subaortic obstruction seen in hypertrophic cardiomyopathy.

Clinical Utility

Diagnosis and Screening

Echocardiography is the procedure of choice for accurate diagnosis of hypertrophic cardiomyopathy. Since this is an inherited disorder, screening with echocardiography is indicated for all first-degree relatives of the affected individual. This diagnosis significantly impacts clinical management even in asymptomatic individuals, given the high risk of sudden death with exertion, and has important implications for genetic counseling. Doppler diastolic tissue velocities are reduced even in the absence of LV hypertrophy and may help identify genetically affected family members early in the disease course.

Evaluation of Medical Therapy

In patients with a definite diagnosis of hypertrophic cardiomyopathy, Doppler findings can be used to assess the impact of medical therapy. Specifically, the pattern of LV diastolic filling after institution of therapy to improve diastolic function (such as beta-blockers or calcium channel blockers) may show an improvement in early diastolic filling. The degree of dynamic outflow obstruction also may show improvement on medical therapy.

Selection of Patients for Automatic Implanted Defibrillators

Primary prevention of sudden cardiac death in patients with hypertrophic cardiomyopathy is based on placement of automatic implanted defibrillation in patients with a combination of risk factors for sudden death. Definite risk factors are sustained or frequent nonsustained ventricular tachycardia, recurrent unexplained syncope, a family history of sudden death, an abnormal blood pressure response to exercise, and extreme LV hypertrophy (septal diastolic wall thickness >30 mm). Other risk factors include high-risk genetic defects. Outflow obstruction is considered only a minor risk factor for sudden cardiac death.

Monitoring of Percutaneous Septal Ablation

Echocardiography plays a key role in patient selection for catheter septal ablation procedures and for monitoring the procedure in the catheterization laboratory. In the patient being considered for percutaneous or surgical treatment for hypertrophic cardiomyopathy, knowledge of the extent, distribution, and curvature of septal hypertrophy determines the location and size of the muscle segment to be removed or ablated. In the catheterization laboratory, baseline and part-procedure Doppler data are used in conjunction with invasive hemodynamics to assess the reduction in outflow obstruction (Fig. 9–19). In addition, contrast is injected during echocardiographic imaging with the catheter positioned in a

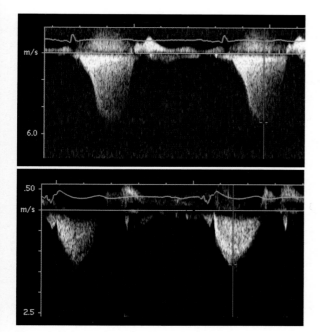

Figure 9–19 In a patient with obstructive hypertrophic cardiomyopathy undergoing a catheter septal ablation procedure, TTE in the catheterization laboratory demonstrates severe obstruction at baseline with a late-peaking outflow tract velocity of 5 m/s (*top*). After the septal ablation, the maximum velocity was 1.4 m/s (*bottom*).

septal coronary branch to show the specific location and extent of the area perfused by that vessel before delivery of the ablation agent (Fig. 9–20). After the procedure, sequential echocardiographic studies may show continued improvement in the extent of outflow obstruction due to healing and fibrosis of the infarcted septal myocardium.

Surgical Therapy

Intraoperative monitoring of myotomy-myectomy allows evaluation of the adequacy of the procedure in relieving outflow tract obstruction. Transesophageal echocardiographic (TEE) imaging often provides adequate images of the myectomy site; however, epicardial imaging can be helpful since the septum is located anteriorly relative to the esophagus. Doppler evaluation for residual obstruction following cardiopulmonary bypass should be performed under hemodynamic conditions as similar as possible to the baseline state, because the degree of obstruction is influenced by loading conditions. Color flow imaging is helpful in excluding residual obstruction, but when the subaortic flow pattern remains abnormal, quantitative Doppler velocity data are needed. Careful examination for a postoperative ventricular septal defect also should be performed.

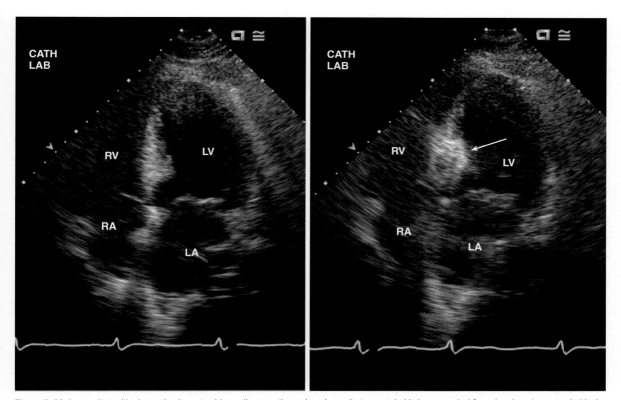

Figure 9–20 In a patient with obstructive hypertrophic cardiomyopathy undergoing catheter septal ablation, an apical four-chamber view recorded in the cardiac catheterization laboratory (Cath Lab) with the patient supine, the baseline image on the *left* shows septal hypertrophy. The image on the *right* shows contrast in the septum (*arrow*) defining the area perfused by the septal branch that will be injected with the ablation agent.

It may be difficult to obtain an accurate continuous-wave Doppler recording of the degree of outflow obstruction in the operating room, because the TEE approach rarely provides a transgastric apical view from which the beam can be aligned parallel to the jet. An epicardial apical position may not be obtainable with a median sternotomy, because the transducer often is too large to fit under the ribs at the apex. Placement of a sterile transducer on the ascending aorta with inferior angulation toward the outflow tract may allow a parallel intercept angle in some patients (see Chapter 18).

Alternate Approaches

Cardiac magnetic resonance (CMR) imaging provides accurate and detailed assessment of the pattern and degree of hypertrophy. Cine images demonstrate systolic anterior motion of the mitral valve and outflow obstruction. Patchy areas of late gadolinium enhancement in the myocardium are supportive of a diagnosis of hypertrophic cardiomyopathy.

In some patients cardiac catheterization may be helpful. First, evaluation of coronary anatomy may be indicated, since coexisting epicardial coronary artery disease may explain some symptoms in a patient with hypertrophic cardiomyopathy. Second, recordings of LV and aortic pressures at rest and after provocative maneuvers to increase or decrease dynamic outflow obstruction and with slow "pullback" across the outflow tract and aortic valve allow more detailed hemodynamic evaluation. This is particularly helpful in the patient with sequential stenoses in the subaortic region and at the aortic valve level. In the operating room, direct LV and aortic pressure measurements after myectomy may be helpful if residual obstruction is suspected.

RESTRICTIVE CARDIOMYOPATHY

Basic Principles

Restrictive cardiomyopathy is characterized by normal LV systolic function with impaired diastolic function due to stiff and thickened myocardium. Heart failure symptoms are due to the resultant elevation in LV end-diastolic pressure and the inability to increase cardiac output with exercise due to impaired diastolic filling. Note that heart failure—defined as the inability to maintain a normal cardiac output or maintenance of a normal cardiac output only with an elevated LV end-diastolic pressure—can occur with normal systolic function. In many patients with restrictive cardiomyopathy, right-sided failure predominates initially with peripheral edema and ascites.

As the disease progresses, an individual patient may progress from an anatomic/hemodynamic pattern consistent with restrictive cardiomyopathy to a pattern showing some features of dilated cardiomyopathy, ending with a picture indistinguishable from dilated cardiomyopathy.

Compared with dilated cardiomyopathy, restrictive cardiomyopathy is an uncommon diagnosis. Causes of restrictive cardiomyopathy include systemic diseases with accumulation of cells or protein in the myocardial interstitium, storage diseases with accumulation of material within myocardial cells, and processes that affect the endocardium. Some specific examples of the etiology of restrictive cardiomyopathy are shown in Table 9–1.

Echocardiographic Approach
Anatomic Features

Typical echocardiographic features (Figs. 9–21 and 9–22) in the untreated patient with restrictive cardiomyopathy include:

- ❐ Nondilated, thick-walled LV
- ❐ Normal LV systolic function
- ❐ Abnormal LV diastolic function
- ❐ RV free wall thickening
- ❐ Biatrial enlargement
- ❐ Moderate pulmonary hypertension
- ❐ Elevated right atrial pressure

Echocardiography usually cannot identify the cause of a restrictive cardiomyopathy, but there are some features that may support a specific diagnosis. The classic "speckled" myocardium of amyloidosis is nonspecific, particularly with harmonic imaging. However, amyloid frequently also affects the valves,

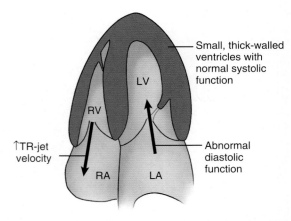

Figure 9–21 Schematic diagram of the typical features of restrictive cardiomyopathy, which include a thick-walled, small LV with impaired diastolic function, LA and RA enlargement, and signs of secondary pulmonary hypertension, including paradoxical septal motion and a high-velocity tricuspid regurgitant (TR) jet.

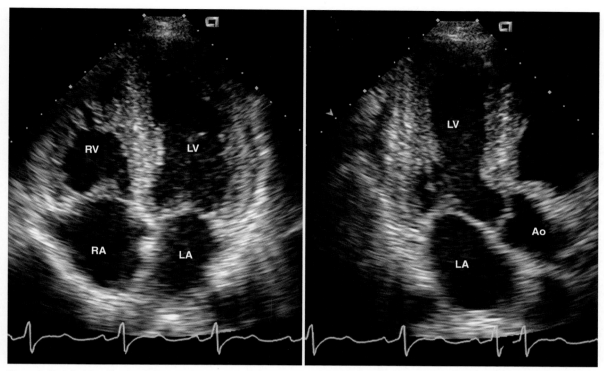

Figure 9–22 Apical four-chamber (*left*) and apical two-chamber (*right*) 2D echocardiographic images in a patient with a restrictive cardiomyopathy due to amyloidosis. There is biventricular hypertrophy, biatrial enlargement, and both systolic and diastolic dysfunction of the LV. Mild, diffuse valve thickening also is present.

with diffuse leaflet thickening; the conduction system; and the coronary microvasculature. Hemochromatosis results in conduction disease, as well as a dilated or restrictive cardiomyopathy. Fabry's disease is characterized by symmetric or asymmetric ventricular hypertrophy (which may appear similar to hypertrophic cardiomyopathy), conduction defects, and, late in the disease, aortic root dilation. A hyperechoic endocardium distinguishes Fabry's disease from other causes of ventricular hypertrophy (Fig. 9–23). Sarcoidosis often causes conduction defects and pericardial effusions are common. In hypereosinophilic syndrome, LV thrombus formation occurs in the absence of an underlying wall motion abnormality (particularly in the apex), resulting in gradual apical "obliteration" (as seen on angiography) or filling in of the apex with an echogenic mass (on echocardiography). Thrombus formation also occurs under the posterior mitral valve leaflet, leading to adherence of the posterior leaflet to the endocardium and significant mitral regurgitation. Heart disease related to radiation therapy results in a restrictive cardiomyopathy of both the LV and RV and in accelerated calcific valve disease and coronary atherosclerosis of the segments within the radiation field.

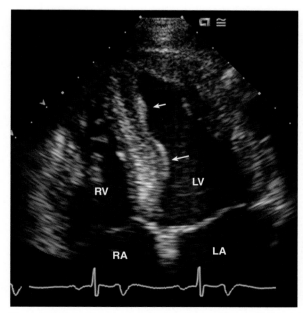

Figure 9–23 Apical four-chamber view in a 48-year-old man with Fabry's disease shows increased LV wall thickness with increased echodensity of the endocardium, particularly along the septum (*arrows*).

Diastolic Function

The pattern of LV diastolic filling parallels the abnormalities in LV diastolic function in this disease. However, interpretation is complicated both by the numerous confounding factors that affect LV diastolic filling (see Chapter 7) and by temporal changes in diastolic filling as the disease progresses in an individual patient.

Early in the disease course, impaired diastolic relaxation of the LV results in impaired early-diastolic filling. The Doppler LV inflow curve shows a reduced E velocity, increased A velocity, prolonged IVRT, and decreased early-diastolic deceleration slope. The mitral annular tissue Doppler signal shows a reduced E' and increased A' velocity (Fig. 9–24). The pulmonary vein flow curve shows a reduced diastolic filling phase and normal systolic filling phase, resulting in a decreased ratio of systolic to diastolic pulmonary venous flow.

RA filling patterns, recorded in the hepatic vein (or superior vena cava), correspond to physical examination of the neck vein pulsations seen in patients with restrictive cardiomyopathy. Using this analogy, the hepatic vein flow pattern typically shows a prominent reverse flow phase with atrial contraction (*a* wave) followed by a rapid filling curve in systole (*x* descent). The diastolic phase of RA filling is blunted, corresponding to a diminished *v* wave and *y* descent. These findings correspond to the pattern of RA pressure recordings at catheterization; the *x* descent represents the "dip," and the blunted systolic filling phase represents the "plateau" of the dip-and-plateau pattern.

As the disease progresses, LA pressure rises, resulting in an increased pressure gradient from the LA to LV at mitral valve opening. Along with reduced diastolic compliance of the LV, this increased mitral opening pressure leads to an increased E velocity and a rapid deceleration slope. The A velocity is reduced due to a combination of increased LV end-diastolic pressure and reduced atrial contractile function (Fig. 9–25). Thus the pattern of diastolic filling in established restrictive cardiomyopathy (which may coincide with the initial clinical presentation) is similar to the "big E, little A" pattern seen in normal young individuals. However, this "pseudo-normal" pattern of LV filling can be distinguished from normal by:

❏ The rapid early diastolic deceleration time
❏ A reduced E' velocity
❏ An increased PV_a velocity and duration
❏ The patient's age, clinical presentation other associated echocardiographic findings

With a pseudo-normal LV inflow pattern, the mitral annular velocity shows a marked reduction in the E' velocity with the ratio of the transmitral E velocity to the annular E' velocity corresponding to the elevation in LV end-diastolic pressure. In

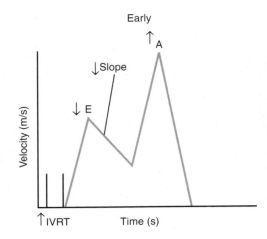

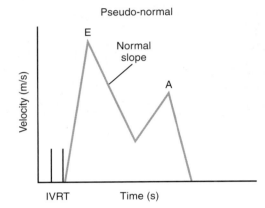

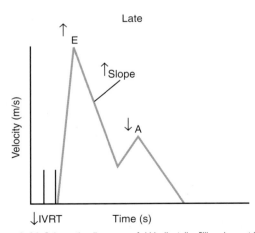

Figure 9–24 Schematic diagrams of LV diastolic filling in restrictive cardiomyopathy. Early in the disease course, ventricular relaxation abnormalities predominate, and the E velocity and early deceleration slope are reduced while the isovolumic relaxation time (IVRT) and A velocity are increased. Pseudo-normalization occurs as LV end-diastolic pressure rises, resulting in relatively normal E and A velocities. With advanced (late) disease, ventricular compliance decreases, resulting in a high E velocity, steep deceleration slope, short IVRT, and reduced A velocity.

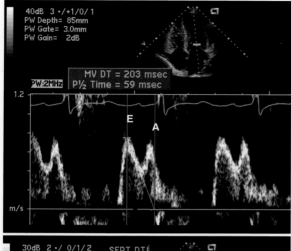

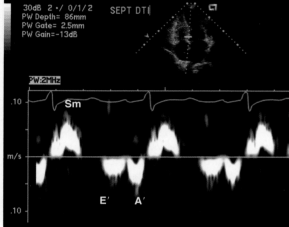

Figure 9–25 LV diastolic filling in a patient with a restrictive cardiomyopathy shows pseudo-normalization with an *E* velocity slightly greater than the *A* velocity (*top*). This pattern is distinguished from normal by the tissue Doppler myocardial velocity (*bottom*) showing reduced early motion (*E'*), compared with the motion after atrial contraction (*A'*). Same patient as Figure 9–22.

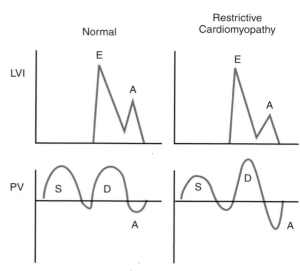

Figure 9–26 Schematic diagrams of LV inflow (LVI) and pulmonary vein (PV) Doppler flow patterns with normal diastolic function and in restrictive cardiomyopathy. Although the inflow patterns are similar superficially, the "pseudo-normal" pattern has a steeper deceleration slope and lower *A* velocity. The PV flow shows increased diastolic filling and a prominent *A* reversal compared with the normal pattern.

Limitations/Technical Considerations

Differentiation of restrictive cardiomyopathy from constrictive pericarditis is problematic. Both have a similar clinical presentation, and both are characterized by preserved LV systolic function with impaired diastolic filling. Features that distinguish these two conditions include the patterns of atrial and ventricular diastolic filling, the presence or absence of pericardial thickening, and the degree of associated pulmonary hypertension. However, no single feature is diagnostic of either condition (see Table 10–2).

Attention to technical details is necessary in recording Doppler atrial and ventricular filling patterns, particularly their relationship to the phase of respiration. Respiratory variation is assessed most reliably using a respirometer to mark the onsets of inspiration and expiration. Prior to recording Doppler signals, 2D and color flow imaging is used to convince the sonographer that there is no significant respiratory variation in the angle between the ultrasound beam and the direction of blood flow, since respiratory changes in intercept angle could result in apparent changes in velocity even under constant-flow conditions due to the erroneous assumption that cosine θ remains 1 in the Doppler equation. Once a constant intercept angle is ascertained, recordings of LV diastolic inflow are made with the sample volume positioned at the mitral leaflet tips.

Recording RA filling patterns is straightforward using a subcostal approach with the pulsed Doppler sample volume positioned in the central hepatic vein. This vein connects directly to the inferior vena cava

addition, pulmonary venous inflow in diastole is normal or increased as blood flows in a conduit from the pulmonary veins to LV. With atrial contraction, the increased resistance to LV filling results in an increase in the velocity and duration of the atrial flow reversal into the lower resistance pulmonary veins. Thus, pulmonary venous flow shows an increased diastolic phase, reduced systolic phase, and prominent *a*-wave flow reversal. This is in contrast to the normal pattern of nearly equal systolic and diastolic pulmonary venous inflow curves (Fig. 9–26) and a small *a* wave.

Late in the disease course, a restrictive pattern of LV filling is seen with an increased *E* velocity and reduced *A* velocity, steep early diastolic deceleration slope, and reduced IVRT.

and RA, with no intervening venous valve, and conveniently lies parallel to the direction of the ultrasound beam from the subcostal window.

LA filling is more technically challenging to record due to signal attenuation at the depth of the pulmonary veins from an apical approach. Other transthoracic acoustic windows rarely allow interrogation of pulmonary vein flow at a near-parallel intercept angle. A TEE approach is helpful if recordings of pulmonary vein flow are inadequate on transthoracic interrogation and are needed for patient management.

Tissue Doppler mitral annular velocity is recorded in the four-chamber apical view with a small sample volume (2 mm) positioned at the medial mitral annulus. Gain is reduced and wall filters are set at low (50–100 Hz) with the velocity scale expanded to optimally display the phasic waveform.

Clinical Utility

In a patient with symptoms of heart failure, a diagnosis of restrictive cardiomyopathy may not have been suspected on clinical grounds. In some cases, echocardiographic findings may provide the first clues pointing toward this diagnostic possibility. In a patient with known restrictive cardiomyopathy, echocardiography can be used to follow disease progression. A meticulous examination with careful attention to technical details and with integration of 2D, Doppler, and clinical data may allow differentiation of restrictive cardiomyopathy from constrictive pericarditis.

Alternate Approaches

Clinical history and laboratory tests are important in determining the cause of a restrictive cardiomyopathy. Diagnostic evaluation also may include cardiac catheterization with measurement of intracardiac pressures at rest and with volume loading. Endomyocardial biopsy can be diagnostic, although sensitivity is low because of nonhomogeneous myocardial involvement in many of these conditions. Biopsy of noncardiac tissue may be diagnostic for amyloidosis. Chest computed tomographic imaging can exclude pericardial calcification or thickening. CMR imaging can detect myocardial iron overload due to hemochromatosis, patchy late gadolinium enhancement with sarcoidosis, and can distinguish myocardial involvement due to restrictive cardiomyopathy from constrictive pericarditis.

OTHER CARDIOMYOPATHIES

Arrhythmogenic Right Ventricular Dysplasia

Arrhythmogenic RV dysplasia (ARVD) is a genetic form of cardiomyopathy that results in fibrofatty

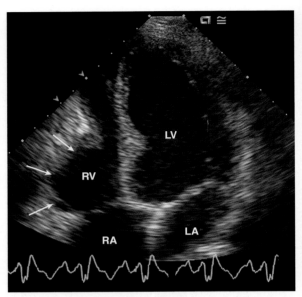

Figure 9–27 In this patient with arrhythmogenic RV dysplasia and a history of sudden death, the apical four-chamber view shows only mild RV dilation and systolic dysfunction, but there is an abnormal contour of the RV free wall (*arrows*).

replacement of the RV wall with clinical manifestations of RV systolic dysfunction, arrhythmias, and sudden death. Echocardiographic findings include RV dilation and systolic dysfunction in the presence of a relatively normal LV and normal PA pressures (Fig. 9–27). Prominent trabeculation of the RV, increased echogenicity of the moderator band, and small RV aneurysms also may be seen. However, echocardiographic findings are quite variable, and other imaging approaches, such as CMR, may be more accurate for this diagnosis.

Isolated Left Ventricular Noncompaction

Isolated LV noncompaction is a genetic cardiomyopathy characterized by thickened, prominently trabeculated myocardium with deep recesses that communicate with the ventricular chamber and by decreased coronary flow reserve (Fig. 9–28). A similar pattern of ventricular trabeculation may be seen with secondary cardiomyopathies due to neuromuscular diseases and other conditions. Features of noncompaction overlap with the clinical presentation of dilated, hypertrophic, and restrictive cardiomyopathy. Noncompaction presents clinically with heart failure, embolic events, and arrhythmias. Distinguishing echocardiographic features are hypokinesis and myocardial thickening localized to the apex, and midlateral and midinferior walls; a ratio of the thickness of the noncompacted to compacted myocardium at end-systole $\geq$ 2:1; and color Doppler showing flow extending into the trabecular recesses.

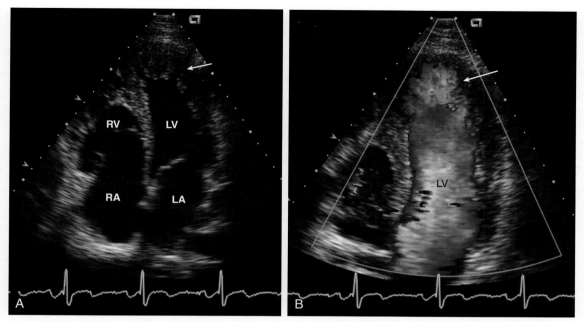

Figure 9–28 **A,** Noncompaction of the LV in an apical four-chamber view showing the thick wall with deep trabecular recesses (*arrow*). The color flow image (**B**) shows ventricular flow filling the trabeculated sections of the myocardium.

HYPERTENSIVE HEART DISEASE

Basic Principles

Hypertensive heart disease is an end-organ consequence of systemic hypertension. Chronic systemic pressure overload results in LV hypertrophy to maintain normal wall stress. Initially, diastolic function is impaired, while systolic function remains normal. With long-standing hypertension, systolic dysfunction and ventricular dilation can occur. Typical echocardiographic findings (Fig. 9–29) associated with chronic hypertension include:

- ❑ LV hypertrophy
- ❑ Diastolic dysfunction
- ❑ Aortic root dilation
- ❑ Aortic valve sclerosis
- ❑ Mitral annular calcification
- ❑ LA enlargement
- ❑ Atrial fibrillation

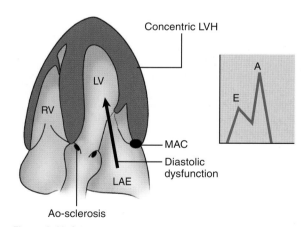

Figure 9–29 Schematic diagram of hypertensive heart disease in an anteriorly angulated apical four-chamber view. Note concentric LV hypertrophy, mitral annular calcification, LA enlargement, aortic valve sclerosis, aortic root dilation, and impaired early diastolic relaxation (*E* < *A*).

Echocardiographic Approach

Ventricular Hypertrophy

Standard imaging views demonstrate concentric LV hypertrophy with increased wall thickness and a nondilated chamber (Fig. 9–30). In contrast to hypertrophic cardiomyopathy, the pattern of hypertrophy is generally symmetric, including involvement of the basal posterior wall. 2D or 2D-guided M-mode recordings confirm an increased end-diastolic wall thickness

(>11 mm). LV mass can be estimated from M-mode data, assuming hypertrophy is symmetric, but preferably is calculated from 2D data (see Chapter 6).

Diastolic Function

LV diastolic function is characterized by impaired early diastolic relaxation (Fig. 9–31). This results in a prolonged IVRT, reduced *E* velocity, reduced *E/A* ratio, and prolonged deceleration slope. Interestingly, in

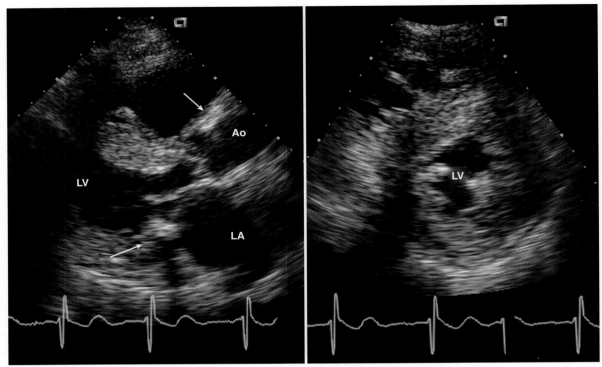

Figure 9–30 Parasternal long-axis (*left*) and short-axis (*right*) views with the typical echocardiographic findings in hypertensive heart disease with concentric LV hypertrophy, mitral annular calcification with shadowing (*large arrow*), aortic valve sclerosis, and increased echogenicity of the ascending aorta (*small arrow*).

individuals with physiologic hypertrophy or "athletes' heart," diastolic dysfunction is not seen even when increased wall thickness is present. In pathologic hypertrophy (due to hypertension), diastolic dysfunction often is the first evidence of end-organ damage, usually antedating clear evidence of anatomic hypertrophy.

Systolic Function

Typically, systolic function is preserved early in the disease course. Segmental wall motion abnormalities are not seen unless coexisting coronary artery disease is present. With a small, hypertrophied, normally functioning LV chamber, mid-cavity obliteration at end-systole may be seen with an associated Doppler velocity curve showing a brief, late-systolic high-velocity signal. The duration of this intracavity gradient is briefer than that seen with hypertrophic cardiomyopathy, the level of obstruction is midventricular rather than subaortic, and systolic anterior motion of the mitral leaflets is not seen. Mid-cavity obliteration is exacerbated by hypovolemia or increased contractility.

Other Echocardiographic Findings

Aortic root dilation often is present in hypertensive patients and is associated with increased tortuosity of

the ascending aorta, arch, and descending aorta. Increased irregular echogenicity of the aortic walls, representing atherosclerosis, also may be noted. In uncomplicated hypertension, the aortic annulus itself is not dilated. The aortic valve leaflets usually show sclerotic changes and associated mild aortic regurgitation. Mitral annular calcification frequently is present in patients with chronic hypertension and is one cause of mild to moderate mitral regurgitation in these patients. LA enlargement is due to a combination of a chronically elevated LV end-diastolic pressure and mitral regurgitation.

Limitations/Technical Considerations

LV mass determinations are dependent on optimal image quality with clear definition of endocardial and epicardial surfaces and on correct endocardial border tracing at end-diastole and end-systole. It remains controversial whether 2D or M-mode mass calculations are optimal, especially given cost considerations in large patient populations. Differentiation of hypertensive heart disease from hypertrophic or restrictive heart disease is based on the pattern of hypertrophy, associated echocardiographic findings, and integration of the echocardiographic and clinical data.

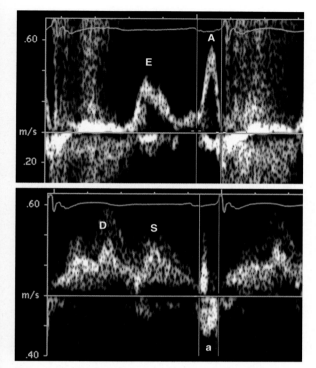

Figure 9–31 LV inflow (*top*) and pulmonary vein flow (bottom) in a patient with hypertension and concentric hypertrophy. Mild diastolic dysfunction is present with impaired relaxation as evidenced by the *E/A* ratio <1 and the prolonged deceleration time. However, LV end-diastolic pressure is normal with a low velocity and short duration of the pulmonary vein atrial reversal (*a*).

Clinical Utility

Diagnosis and Prognosis

LV mass, measured by echocardiography, is a strong predictor of clinical outcome in patients with hypertension. In subjects with borderline hypertension, increased LV mass identifies a subgroup of patients with a poor prognosis without medical therapy. In patients with definite hypertension, the degree of LV hypertrophy reflects the chronic elevation of systemic pressure, in theory serving as an index of the temporally averaged blood pressure over long periods of time. Thus, LV mass may be a more accurate method for assessing the severity of hypertension than occasional blood pressure recordings in the physician's office or even 24-hour recordings of blood pressure.

Choices of Medical Therapy

In theory, hypertension therapy could be tailored in each patient based on noninvasive Doppler echo evaluation of hemodynamics. Since blood pressure equals cardiac output times systemic vascular resistance, hypertension can be due to elevation of either

one or both of the components of this equation. To assess hemodynamics noninvasively in hypertensive patients, cardiac output can be measured using Doppler recordings of ascending aortic flow and 2D aortic diameter measurements (see Chapter 6). Systemic vascular resistance then is estimated from the cuff blood pressure and Doppler cardiac output. However, in clinical practice, hypertension therapy is based on established algorithms; hemodynamic evaluation is rarely performed.

Efficacy of Medical Therapy

Determination of LV mass may be useful in assessing the long-term effect of medical therapy. Again, rather than measuring blood pressure at rare intervals in the disease course, the chronic end-organ effects of hypertension on the LV are measured. It seems plausible that effective antihypertensive therapy should reverse end-organ changes; specifically, it should result in regression of LV hypertrophy.

Evaluation of Heart Failure Symptoms

In a patient with chronic hypertension, heart failure symptoms may be due to diastolic or systolic LV dysfunction, superimposed coronary artery disease, or superimposed valvular disease. Early in the disease course, pathologic hypertrophy is associated with impaired early-diastolic filling. Impaired LV filling leads to elevated LA pressure and pulmonary venous hypertension, resulting in dyspnea. Diagnosis of diastolic dysfunction with preserved systolic function can be made by echocardiography and has important clinical implications, since the therapy for heart failure symptoms is quite different for diastolic versus systolic dysfunction.

An extreme form of preserved systolic function with LV hypertrophy and heart failure symptoms has been observed in hypertensive patients and has been termed *hypertensive hypertrophic cardiomyopathy*. This condition is characterized by normal to hyperdynamic systolic function, concentric hypertrophy, diastolic dysfunction, and a midventricular late-systolic gradient due to cavity obliteration (see Fig. 9–18). Strictly speaking, this combination of findings is not a "cardiomyopathy" and is not an inherited disorder, but simply represents severe end-organ damage due to hypertension. However, awareness of this specific clinical picture results in consideration of this diagnosis in patients in whom hypertrophic or restrictive cardiomyopathy otherwise might be suspected.

With long-standing hypertension, impairment of LV contractility can occur, even in the absence of coexisting coronary artery disease. Physiologically, elevated afterload (as in valvular aortic stenosis) is the proximate cause of systolic dysfunction. However, systolic function may not improve even with aggressive antihypertensive therapy when systolic dysfunction is long-standing, suggesting that irreversible changes in ventricular contractility have occurred. End-stage hypertensive heart disease has an echocardiographic appearance similar to end-stage dilated cardiomyopathy.

Alternate Approaches

The need for routine echocardiographic evaluation of patients with hypertension is controversial. Medical management based on intermittent office blood pressure measurements remains standard practice at most medical centers. When needed, estimates of the chronicity of blood pressure elevation can be obtained by 24-hour blood pressure monitors or evaluation of other end-organ damage (e.g., renal function, retinal examination). While electrocardiographic estimates of LV hypertrophy are less accurate and precise than echocardiographic measurements, there is a substantial cost differential between these diagnostic tests.

EVALUATION OF THE PATIENT AFTER CARDIAC TRANSPLANT

Basic Principles

Echocardiographic evaluation of the patient after cardiac transplant typically is directed toward one of three goals: (1) assessment of cardiac anatomy and physiology prompted by a specific clinical problem, (2) the elusive goal of noninvasive diagnosis of early rejection of the transplanted heart, or (3) diagnosis of post-transplant coronary artery disease.

Common problems encountered in the patient after cardiac transplant include:

❐ Pericardial effusion, particularly early post-operatively
❐ RV systolic dysfunction due to inadequate myocardial preservation at the time of transplantation, persistently elevated pulmonary vascular resistance, or transplant rejection
❐ LV systolic dysfunction due to inadequate myocardial preservation, acute rejection early after transplantation, or superimposed coronary artery disease at a longer interval after transplantation

Primary valvular disease, of course, is uncommon due to screening of donor hearts before transplantation. However, mitral or tricuspid regurgitation secondary to ventricular dysfunction and annular dilation may be seen. Diastolic dysfunction is an early marker of rejection.

Echocardiographic Approach

Normal Findings after Cardiac Transplantation

Typically, RV and LV size, wall thickness, and systolic function are normal in the absence of perioperative complications or rejection. However, abnormal septal motion is the norm with anterior motion of the septum in systole with a slight decrease in the extent of systolic thickening of the septal myocardium. Valvular anatomy and function are normal, with small amounts of mitral, tricuspid, and pulmonic regurgitation present with a prevalence similar to that in normal individuals. The suture lines in the aorta and pulmonary artery may be difficult to appreciate depending on the distance of the suture lines from the valve planes and the type of surgical procedure. A small pericardial effusion is seen early in the postoperative period but rarely persists beyond a few weeks. PA pressures may show some degree of persistent elevation as calculated from the velocity in the tricuspid regurgitant jet and estimates of RA pressure.

If the surgical approach included anastomoses of the normal and donor atrium, a normal echocardiogram after cardiac transplantation will show biatrial enlargement (Fig. 9–32) with a variably prominent ridge between the donor and recipient portions of both RA and LA. The atrial suture line should not be mistaken for an abnormal atrial mass (Fig. 9–33). When transplantation is performed with anastomosis of the superior and inferior vena cava for the RA and a cuff of tissue with the pulmonary veins for the LA, there is little atrial enlargement and suture lines may not be evident.

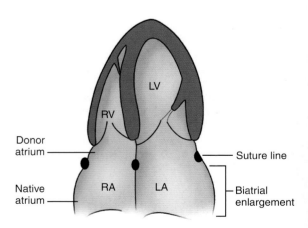

Figure 9–32 Schematic diagram of the post-transplant heart. Note the suture line between the donor and native atria resulting in an appearance of biatrial enlargement. RV and LV size and systolic function are normal. With the more recent surgical techniques, an atrial suture line is not present.

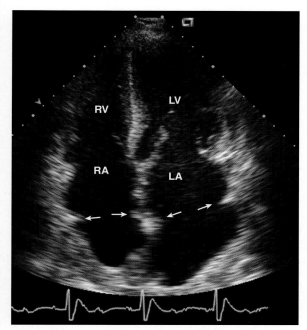

Figure 9–33 Apical four-chamber view in a post-transplant patient showing biatrial enlargement with a prominent suture line (*arrows*).

Evaluation of Abnormal Findings

The echocardiographic approach to the post-transplant patient with suspected cardiac dysfunction is similar to that in any patient, with the proviso that the expected findings after transplantation (such as the atrial suture line) are recognized. Pericardial effusions often are loculated due to postoperative pericardial adhesions, so careful examination in multiple tomographic planes from parasternal, apical, and subcostal windows is essential when this diagnosis is suspected.

Transplant Rejection

With acute severe rejection, echocardiography shows increased LV mass, decreased systolic function, and an increase in the echogenicity of the myocardium. However, with mild or early rejection, 2D echocardiographic changes are subtle and are not accurate or reproducible enough to allow adjustment of immunosuppressive medications in individual patients. Instead, proposed echocardiographic approaches to diagnosis of early rejection have focused on measures of diastolic function, specifically measures of early diastolic relaxation. The Doppler changes in acute rejection include:

- ❑ Decreased pressure half-time (increased early diastolic deceleration slope)
- ❑ Decreased IVRT
- ❑ Increased *E* velocity

Compared to the patient's own baseline study, a significant change (defined as >20% for *E* velocity and >15% for pressure half-time or IVRT) is consistent with rejection. Tissue Doppler measures are sensitive but not specific for detection of rejection. In addition, many post-transplant patients have resting tachycardia, with *E/A* fusion, due to cardiac denervation. Some transplant centers have found these measures clinically useful, but most centers continue to rely on endomyocardial biopsy.

Transplant Coronary Artery Disease

As survival after cardiac transplantation has improved, increasing numbers of patients are seen with post-transplant coronary artery disease. Transplant coronary disease differs from typical atherosclerosis in that both epicardial vessels and the microvasculature are diffusely involved with an accelerated form of intimal hyperplasia. Echocardiographic exercise stress testing has a high prevalence of false-negative results due to the diffuse disease process masking regional wall motion abnormalities. Dobutamine stress echocardiography is more accurate in this patient population and now is routine at many transplant centers. However, coronary angiography may be needed for a definitive diagnosis, often with concurrent intravascular ultrasound examination of the coronary arteries.

Limitations/Technical Considerations/ Alternate Approaches

The standard method for evaluation of transplant rejection remains transvenous endomyocardial biopsy. Some centers use echocardiographic (rather than fluoroscopic) guidance for this procedure. Since echocardiographic images are tomographic, any segment of the biopsy catheter going through the image plane will appear to be the "tip." Thus, it is crucial to identify the open forceps at the tip for correct identification of the biopsy site. A subcostal window often is most practical, since, with the patient supine, clear views of the RV and septum are obtained, and the sonographer is clear of the sterile field (usually the right internal jugular vein approach is used). In some cases, the apical view also may be helpful.

PULMONARY HEART DISEASE

Chronic versus Acute Pulmonary Disease

Chronic pulmonary hypertension, whether due to intrinsic lung disease, recurrent pulmonary emboli, or primary pulmonary hypertension, results in a group of clinical signs and symptoms termed *cor pulmonale*. The underlying pathophysiology of this clinical syndrome is chronic pressure overload of the RV as it ejects into a high-resistance pulmonary vascular bed. Initially, compensatory hypertrophy of the RV occurs with preserved

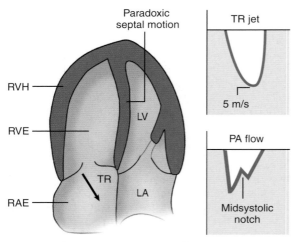

Figure 9–34 Schematic diagram of the key features of pulmonary heart disease. RV hypertrophy (RVH) and enlargement (RVE) are seen with paradoxic septal motion. Secondary tricuspid regurgitation (TR) and RA enlargement (RAE) are common. Elevated pulmonary pressures will be reflected in the high-velocity TR-jet velocity and mid-systolic notching in the pulmonary artery (PA) velocity curve.

systolic function. Over time, RV contractility deteriorates, and RV dilation, moderate to severe tricuspid regurgitation, and consequent RA enlargement are seen (Fig. 9–34).

Acute pulmonary embolism also can affect right-sided heart function due to the sudden onset of elevated pulmonary vascular resistance. Echocardiographic evaluation may be helpful in assessing PA pressures and RV function in patients with either chronic or acute pulmonary hypertension.

Echocardiographic Approach

Pulmonary Pressures

Standard approaches for noninvasive evaluation of PA pressure, as described in Chapter 6, are applicable to the patient with suspected or known pulmonary hypertension. The most reliable approach is to record the maximum tricuspid regurgitant jet velocity (V_{TR}) for calculation of the RV to RA systolic pressure difference (Fig. 9–35). Care is needed to interrogate the tricuspid regurgitant jet from multiple acoustic windows (apical, parasternal) with careful transducer angulation to obtain a parallel intercept angle between the ultrasound beam and jet. RA pressure (RAP) is estimated from the size and respiratory variation in the inferior vena cava. Then PA systolic pressure (PAP, in the absence of pulmonic stenosis) is calculated as

$$PAP = 4V_{TR}^2 + RAP$$

Diastolic PA pressure can be estimated from the velocity in the pulmonic regurgitant Doppler curve. Pulmonary vascular resistance (PVR) can be estimated from the ratio of the tricuspid regurgitant jet velocity to the velocity-time integral of RV outflow (VTI_{RVOT}), multiplied by 10 for conversion to Wood units (see Chapter 6):

$$PVR(Wood\ units) = 10(V_{TR}/VTI_{RVOT})$$

Indirect signs of pulmonary hypertension often are seen that indicate the presence, but not the exact severity, of pulmonary hypertension. For example, an M-mode recording through the pulmonic valve shows a reduced *a* wave and midsystolic closure of the valve.

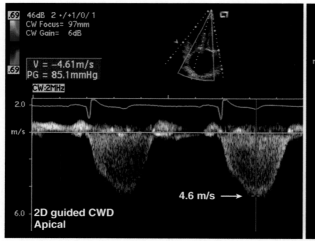
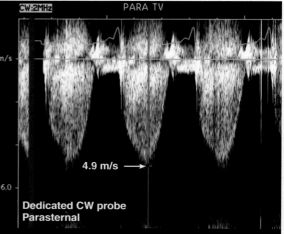

Figure 9–35 Tricuspid regurgitant jet in a patient with primary pulmonary hypertension. Using 2D and color-guided continuous-wave (CW) Doppler from the apex, a clear signal is obtained, although signal strength is low, with a maximum jet of only 4.6 m/s. The use of a dedicated CW probe (*right*) provides a stronger signal, and a higher jet velocity is obtained from a parasternal window. The maximum velocity of 4.9 m/s indicates an RV-to-RA pressure difference of 96 mm Hg. RA pressure was elevated at 10 mm Hg, so estimated PA systolic pressure is 106 mm Hg. Note the faint linear spread of the signal at peak of the curve (see third beat in *right panel*). This faint signal is due to the transit time effect, and care is needed to avoid including these signals in the velocity measurement.

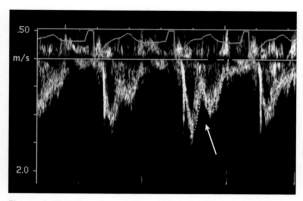

Figure 9–36 Pulmonary artery velocity curve showing mid-systolic notching (*arrow*) due to severe pulmonary hypertension.

This pattern has a reasonably high specificity (>90%) for detecting pulmonary hypertension but a low sensitivity (30% to 60%). This motion pattern is paralleled by the Doppler velocity curve, which shows an abrupt midsystolic deceleration of flow (Fig. 9–36). Signs of RV pressure overload, including abnormal ventricular septal motion, also may be valuable clues suggesting the presence of pulmonary hypertension.

Right Ventricular Pressure Overload

The response of the RV to chronic pressure overload is hypertrophy and dilation (Fig. 9–37). The increase in thickness of the RV free wall is best seen on the subcostal view. Ventricular septal motion is abnormal

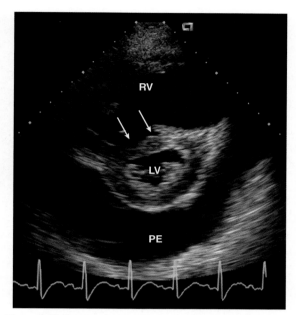

Figure 9–38 Parasternal short-axis view in a patient with pulmonary hypertension and a pericardial effusion (PE) shows severe RV enlargement with flattening of the ventricular septum (*arrows*) in diastole.

or "paradoxical" with anterior motion of the septum during systole both on M-mode and 2D imaging. A rational explanation for this pattern of septal motion is based on the concept that the septum moves toward the center of mass of the heart during systole. With RV hypertrophy, the center of mass is shifted anteriorly, so the septum moves toward the center of the RV instead of the normal pattern of motion toward the center of the LV. On 2D imaging the curvature of the septum is reversed in both systole and in early to mid-diastole. In contrast, RV volume overload is characterized by diastolic flattening of the septum in late diastole with a normal curvature in systole, due to increased volume flow into the RV (compared with the LV) in diastole but normal ventricular pressures in systole (Fig. 9–38).

With long-standing or acute pulmonary hypertension, RV systolic dysfunction can occur, with secondary dilation serving as a compensatory mechanism to maintain forward stroke volume. However, RV dilation leads to tricuspid regurgitation due to annular dilation and malalignment of the papillary muscles. This superimposed volume overload results in further RV dilation and more tricuspid regurgitation. RA dilation is due to both pressure (*v* wave) and volume (tricuspid regurgitation) overload of the RA.

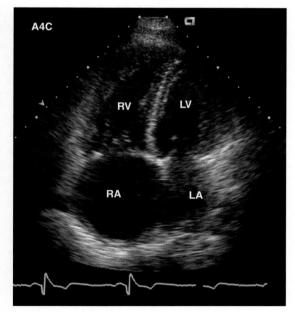

Figure 9–37 Apical four-chamber view at end-diastole in a patient with cor pulmonale. There is RV enlargement, RV hypertrophy, paradoxic septal motion, and reduced systolic function of the RV.

Secondary Tricuspid Regurgitation

Tricuspid regurgitation secondary to pulmonary hypertension and/or RV systolic dysfunction can be evaluated with color Doppler flow imaging from parasternal, apical, and subcostal views. Severe regurgitation results in systolic flow reversal in the inferior vena cava and hepatic veins. Careful attention to tricuspid valve anatomy is needed to ensure that other etiologies of tricuspid regurgitation (e.g., vegetation, rheumatic, carcinoid, Ebstein anomaly) are not present.

The intensity of the continuous-wave Doppler tricuspid regurgitant jet relates to the severity of regurgitation, but the velocity relates to the RV to RA pressure difference. With acute tricuspid regurgitation a rapid falloff in velocity in late systole may be seen consistent with an RA *v* wave.

Limitations/Technical Considerations

The major limitation of echocardiography in evaluation of cor pulmonale is poor ultrasound tissue penetration resulting in poor image quality and low Doppler signal strength. Hyperexpanded lungs obscure the standard acoustic windows in many patients with chronic lung disease. However, adequate image quality may be obtained with current instruments in nearly all patients.

Assessment of the severity of pulmonary hypertension depends on obtaining a parallel intercept angle between the ultrasound beam and tricuspid regurgitant jet. Underestimation of PA pressure should be considered in all patients, especially when Doppler signal strength is suboptimal or when the Doppler data and clinical setting are discrepant. The absence of a recordable tricuspid regurgitant jet does not indicate normal PA pressures. In this situation the report indicates that the data are inadequate and alternate diagnostic approaches should be considered. Overestimation of PA pressures from the tricuspid regurgitant signal can be avoided by measuring the outer edge of the dark spectral envelope, but avoiding the slight spectral broadening at peak velocity that results from the transit time effect (see Fig. 9–35).

Clinical Utility

In the patient with chronic lung disease and right heart failure, echocardiography allows confirmation of a clinical diagnosis of cor pulmonale, assessment of the degree of pulmonary hypertension, and evaluation of RV size and systolic dysfunction.

In patients with primary pulmonary hypertension, echocardiography is essential to exclude other causes of pulmonary hypertension, such as an atrial septal defect or mitral regurgitation. In addition, noninvasive measurement of pulmonary pressure now is routinely used for evaluating changes with medical therapy.

In the patient with an acute pulmonary embolus, imaging may show a residual thrombus originating from or in transit through (from a deep vein thrombosis) the right side of the heart. TEE imaging can demonstrate thrombus in the main, right, or left pulmonary artery. However, the sensitivity of echocardiography for diagnosis of pulmonary embolism based on demonstrating a thrombus is low because the thrombus is lodged more distally in the pulmonary vasculature in most cases. In addition, adequate visualization of the pulmonary artery bifurcation is not possible in all patients due to interposition of the air-filled trachea and bronchi. Indirect signs of pulmonary embolism include:

- ❏ Elevated PA pressures
- ❏ Evidence of acute RV pressure overload
- ❏ RV dilation and dysfunction
- ❏ Tricuspid regurgitation

Similar findings may be seen in patients with chronic recurrent pulmonary emboli. The possibility of pulmonary embolism should be strongly considered in patients with these findings even when a different working clinical diagnosis or "reason for echo" was entertained. Often patients in whom pulmonary embolism is subsequently diagnosed are initially referred for nonspecific indications including "chest pain," "dyspnea," or "heart failure."

Alternate Approaches

Cardiac catheterization allows direct measurement of RV and PA pressures and calculation of pulmonary vascular resistance. RV size and systolic function can be evaluated by angiography.

Clinically, the standard approach for diagnosis of pulmonary embolism is computed tomographic pulmonary angiography. When that procedure is not available, a radionuclide ventricular perfusion scan is appropriate. Pulmonary angiography with injection of contrast material directly into the main pulmonary artery is only rarely needed when other tests are inconclusive.

SUGGESTED READING

Dilated Cardiomyopathy

1. St John Sutton M: Doppler echocardiography in heart failure and cardiac resynchronization. In Otto CM (ed): The Practice of Clinical Echocardiography, 3rd ed. Philadelphia: Elsevier/Saunders Elsevier, 2007, pp 629–652.

Review of the echocardiographic approach to the patient with heart failure due to a dilated cardiomyopathy. This chapter addresses both systolic and diastolic dysfunction and right and left heart failure. The role of echocardiography in evaluation of ventricular assist devices is included along with a detailed discussion of resynchronization therapy.

2. Kirkpatrick JN, Vannan MA, Narula J, et al: Echocardiography in heart failure: Applications, utility and new horizons. J Am Coll Cardiol 50:381–396, 2007.

   This is a comprehensive review of the current echocardiographic approach to evaluation of patients with systolic and diastolic heart failure. There are excellent tables and references summarizing the numerous studies correlating echocardiographic data (including Doppler) with clinical outcomes in heart failure. Clear illustrations highlight newer echocardiographic approaches to diagnosis of heart failure including myocardial motion, strain and strain rate, tissue tracking, and three-dimensional (3D) echocardiography. 142 references.

3. Acquatella H: Echocardiography in Chagas heart disease. Circulation 115:1124–1131, 2007.

   Chagas' disease is endemic in Central and South America and is due to infection by the protozoa Trypanosoma cruzi. In the acute phase a pericardial effusion is common. Chronic disease develops over several decades. In the asymptomatic phase stress testing may be abnormal. As disease progresses apical aneurysms are common, but end-stage disease has an appearance similar to other causes of dilated cardiomyopathy.

4. Felker GM, Boehmer JP, Hruban RH, et al: Echocardiographic findings in fulminant and acute myocarditis. J Am Coll Cardiol 36:227–232, 2000.

   Myocarditis may present acutely after a viral prodrome (fulminant myocarditis) or may present with slowly progressive symptoms (acute myocarditis). On echocardiography there is severe LV systolic dysfunction with both fulminant and acute myocarditis. However, fulminant myocarditis is characterized by a relatively normal LV size and a high likelihood of recovery of systolic function within 6 months. With acute myocarditis the ventricle is more dilated and recovery is less likely.

5. Kurowski V, Kaiser A, von Hof K, et al: Apical and midventricular transient LV dysfunction syndrome (takotsubo cardiomyopathy): Frequency, mechanisms, and prognosis. Chest 132:809–816, 2007.

   Tako-tsubo cardiomyopathy typically occurs in postmenopausal women after a stressful event, and the electrocardiographic changes typically are greater than expected for the degree of cardiac enzyme elevation. In a registry of 3265 adults presenting with a troponin-positive acute coronary syndrome, only 1.2% met the criteria for tako-tsubo cardiomyopathy with transient LV dysfunction and normal coronary arteries.

   There was typical apical dilation and dyskinesis in 60% of patients, while the other 40% demonstrated a midventricular pattern of abnormal wall motion.

6. Kwan J, Shiota T, Agler DA, et al: Geometric differences of the mitral apparatus between ischemic and dilated cardiomyopathy with significant mitral regurgitation: Real-time three-dimensional echocardiographic study. Circulation 107:1135–1140, 2003.

   Real-time 3D echocardiography was used to study 26 patients with ischemic mitral regurgitation, 18 dilated cardiomyopathy patients with mitral regurgitation, and 8 control subjects. Asymmetric distortion of the angle between the annular plane and valve leaflets was seen with ischemic mitral regurgitation as compared with symmetric changes in patients with dilated cardiomyopathy.

Hypertrophic Cardiomyopathy

7. Woo A, Wigle ED, Rakowski H: Echocardiography in the evaluation and management of patients with hypertrophic cardiomyopathy. In Otto CM (ed): The Practice of Clinical Echocardiography, 3rd ed. Philadelphia: Elsevier/Saunders, 2007, pp 653–709.

   This chapter details the echocardiographic findings in hypertrophic cardiomyopathy and correlates the echocardiographic data with clinical, genetic, and pathophysiologic aspects of the disease process.

8. Nagueh SF, Mahmarian JJ: Noninvasive cardiac imaging in patients with hypertrophic cardiomyopathy. J Am Coll Cardiol 48:2410–2422, 2006.

   This is a detailed review of the echocardiographic evaluation of patients with hypertrophic cardiomyopathy including excellent illustrations of typical findings. The use of echocardiography in monitoring medical therapy, percutaneous and surgical interventions is discussed. Sections also address the role of nuclear and CMR imaging for hypertrophic cardiomyopathy.

9. Maron BJ, McKenna WJ, Danielson GK, et al: ACC/ESC clinical expert consensus document on hypertrophic cardiomyopathy: A report of the American College of Cardiology Task Force on Clinical Expert Consensus Documents and the European Society of Cardiology Committee for Practice Guidelines (Committee to Develop an Expert Consensus Document on Hypertrophic Cardiomyopathy). J Am Coll Cardiol 42:1687–1713, 2003.

   Consensus document with a detailed summary of the diagnosis, genetic aspects, natural history, medical and surgical therapy for hypertrophic cardiomyopathy. 273 references.

10. Nishimura RA, Holmes DR Jr: Clinical practice. Hypertrophic obstructive cardiomyopathy. N Engl J Med 350:1320–1327, 2004.

    This review provides a concise summary of the pathophysiology, clinical presentation, and management options for hypertrophic cardiomyopathy.

11. Maron MS, Olivotto I, Zenovich AG, et al: Hypertrophic cardiomyopathy is predominantly a disease of left ventricular outflow tract obstruction. Circulation 114:2232–2239, 2006.

    Resting or latent outflow obstruction was present in 70% of 320 consecutive patients with hypertrophic cardiomyopathy. An outflow gradient >50 mm Hg was present at rest in 37% of subjects. Exercise stress testing in the remaining 201 patients demonstrated inducible obstruction in 106 (33% of total). Only 95 patients (30% of total) had nonobstructive disease with a gradient <30 mm Hg at rest and with exercise. Other provocative maneuvers, such as Valsalva, underestimated the presence and degree of outflow obstruction.

12. Ho CY, Sweitzer NK, McDonough B, et al: Assessment of diastolic function with Doppler tissue imaging to predict genotype in preclinical hypertrophic cardiomyopathy. Circulation 105:2992–2997, 2002.

    A myocardial tissue Doppler velocity (E′ < 15 cm/s) in combination with an elevated ejection fraction (≥68%) is specific (100%) for detection of genetically affected individuals without other phenotypic evidence for hypertrophic cardiomyopathy. However, the low sensitivity (44%) of E′ and ejection fraction suggests that continued periodic evaluation of individuals with a family history but no overt findings for hypertrophic cardiomyopathy is warranted.

13. Nagueh SF, Ommen SR, Lakkis NM, et al: Comparison of ethanol septal reduction therapy with surgical myectomy for the treatment of hypertrophic obstructive cardiomyopathy. J Am Coll Cardiol 38:1701–1706, 2001.

    Outcomes with surgical myotomy-myectomy and with alcohol septal ablation were similar when patients from two institutions were compared. The used of contrast echocardiography to guide the percutaneous septal ablation seems to reduce the incidence of complete heart block requiring pacemaker implantation.

14. Firoozi S, Elliott PM, Sharma S, et al: Septal myotomy-myectomy and transcoronary septal alcohol ablation in hypertrophic obstructive

cardiomyopathy: A comparison of clinical, haemodynamic and exercise outcomes. Eur Heart J 23:1617–1624, 2002.

In a comparison of 20 patients treated with septal ablation and 24 patients undergoing surgical myectomy for symptoms refractory to medical therapy, although the reduction in outflow gradient was similar with both approaches (from about 85–90 mm Hg to 15–20 mm Hg), myectomy was associated with a greater improvement in exercise tolerance.

15. Ward RP, Weinert L, Spencer KT, et al: Quantitative diagnosis of apical cardiomyopathy using contrast echocardiography. J Am Soc Echocardiogr 15:316–322, 2002.

Contrast echocardiography improves the accuracy of the echocardiographic diagnosis of apical cardiomyopathy and should be considered in patients with unexplained symmetric precordial T-wave inversion or increased apical uptake on single-photon emission computed tomography, but a nondiagnostic transthoracic echo. A contrast-enhanced apical thickness >2.0 cm was seen in those with apical hypertrophic cardiomyopathy.

16. Geske JB, Sorajja P, Nishimura RA, et al: Evaluation of left ventricular filling pressures by Doppler echocardiography in patients with hypertrophic cardiomyopathy: Correlation with direct left atrial pressure measurement at cardiac catheterization. Circulation 116:2702–2708, 2007.

In 100 symptomatic hypertrophic cardiomyopathy patients, Doppler data were compared to directly measured LA pressures, with simultaneous measurements in 42 subjects. Although Doppler E/E' ratio statistically correlated with directly measured LA pressure, there was marked scatter in the data with wide 95% confidence limits of ±18 mm Hg. These findings suggest that noninvasive estimates of LV filling pressures are not accurate in hypertrophic cardiomyopathy patients, probably related to the multiple factors affecting diastolic function in these patients.

17. Abergel E, Chatellier G, Hagege AA, et al: Serial left ventricular adaptations in world-class professional cyclists: Implications for disease screening and follow-up. J Am Coll Cardiol 44:144–149, 2004.

This study compared 286 cyclists who had participated in the Tour de France race with 52 sedentary controls. Over 50% of high-level endurance athletes had LV dilation (diastolic dimension >60 mm), and about 12% had a reduced (<52%) ejection fraction. An increased ventricular wall thickness was uncommon, was always <15 mm, and rarely (<1%) occurred without LV dilation. The relatively normal wall thickness helps distinguish normal cardiac changes due to physical conditioning from hypertrophic cardiomyopathy.

Restrictive Cardiomyopathy

18. Naqvi TZ: Restrictive cardiomyopathy: diagnosis and prognostic implications. In Otto CM (ed): The Practice of Clinical Echocardiography, 3rd ed. Philadelphia: Elsevier/Saunders, 2007, pp 679–711.

Detailed discussion of the importance of echocardiography in the diagnosis, management, and evaluation of prognosis in patients with restrictive cardiomyopathies.

19. Bellavia D, Pellikka PA, Abraham TP, et al: Evidence of impaired left ventricular systolic function by Doppler myocardial imaging in patients with systemic amyloidosis and no evidence of cardiac involvement by standard two-dimensional and Doppler echocardiography. Am J Cardiol 101:1039–1045, 2008.

In 42 patients with systemic amyloidosis and no 2D or Doppler echocardiographic evidence of cardiac involvement, Doppler tissue parameters were reduced as compared with controls, suggesting early myocardial involvement.

20. Heidenreich PA, Hancock SL, Vagelos RH, et al: Diastolic dysfunction after mediastinal irradiation. Am Heart J 150:977–982, 2005.

Echocardiographic evidence of diastolic dysfunction was present in 14% of 294 patients with a history of radiation therapy a mean of 15 years previously for Hodgkin's lymphoma. Exercise-induced ischemia was present in 23% of those with diastolic dysfunction as compared with 11% of those with normal diastolic parameters. The presence of diastolic dysfunction predicted a poorer long-term survival on multivariate analysis with a hazard ratio of 1.66 (95% confidence interval [CI] 1.06–2.4) as compared with those with normal diastolic function.

21. Pieroni M, Chimenti C, De Cobelli F, et al: Fabry's disease cardiomyopathy echocardiographic detection of endomyocardial glycosphingolipid compartmentalization. J Am Coll Cardiol 47:1663–1671, 2006.

Fabry's disease is an X-linked inherited deficiency in alpha-galactosidase A activity that results in glycolipid accumulation and tissue deposition. Ventricular hypertrophy typically is the first sign of cardiac involvement and occasionally is the presenting feature in heterozygous females. In a comparison of patients with Fabry's disease, hypertrophic cardiomyopathy, hypertensive heart disease and normal adults (40 subjects in each group), the echocardiographic finding of a bright endocardium (or "binary appearance of the endocardial border") had a sensitivity of 94% and specificity of 100% for diagnosis of Fabry's disease. This echocardiographic finding is due to endomyocardial glycosphingolipid compartmentalization, as verified on histologic studies.

22. Shah R, Ananthasubramaniam K: Evaluation of cardiac involvement in hypereosinophilic syndrome: Complementary roles of transthoracic, transesophageal, and contrast echocardiography. Echocardiography 23:689–691, 2006.

23. Benezet-Mazuecos J, Marcos-Alberca P, Farré J, et al: Images in cardiovascular medicine. Early differential resolution of right and left ventricular obliteration in Löffler endocarditis after chemotherapy and anticoagulation. Circulation 114:e635–e637, 2006.

These two case reports have excellent echocardiographic images of hypereosinophilic syndrome and a brief literature review. Cardiac involvement is present in 30% to 40% of patients with the primary hypereosinophilic syndrome and is common in other causes of hypereosinophilia. The differential diagnosis of apical obliteration includes apical hypertrophic cardiomyopathy or ventricular thrombus due to apical infarction. These diagnoses can be distinguished by clinical features, echocardiography and other imaging approaches, including CMR imaging.

24. Mehta D, Lubitz SA, Frankel Z, et al: Cardiac involvement in patients with sarcoidosis: Diagnostic and prognostic value of outpatient testing. Chest 133:1426–1435, 2008.

In 62 patients with a diagnosis of sarcoidosis, cardiac involvement was present in 39%. In those with cardiac involvement as compared with those without it, cardiac symptoms were more common (46% vs 5%), the 24-hour electrocardiogram more often was abnormal (50% vs 3%) and transthoracic echocardiography showed more abnormalities (25% vs 5%). Echocardiographic features suggesting cardiac involvement included an LV ejection fraction <45%, wall motion abnormalities, significant diastolic dysfunction, and RV systolic dysfunction in the absence of pulmonary hypertension. However, cardiac positron emission tomography and CMR imaging were more sensitive for detection of cardiac sarcoidosis.

Other Cardiomyopathies

25. Yoerger DM, Marcus F, Sherrill D, et al: Echocardiographic findings in patients meeting task force criteria for

arrhythmogenic right ventricular dys-plasia: New insights from the multidis-ciplinary study of right ventricular dysplasia. J Am Coll Cardiol 45: 860–865, 2005.

Diagnosis of ARVD is challenging because of the normal variation in RV shape, size, and function. In a series of 29 patients with diag-nostic criteria for ARVD, compared to 29 control subjects, echocardiography showed a reduced RV fractional area change (27.2% ± 16% vs. 41.0% ± 7.1%, p = 0.0003). RV dimensions were increased with a dimen-sion of the RV outflow tract >30 mm, measured in the long-axis view, present in 89% of cases, but only 14% of controls. Other findings in ARVD included prominent trabec-ulation (54%), increased echogenicity of the moderate band (34%), and focal aneurysms (17%).

26. Frischknecht BS, Jost CH, Oechslin EN, et al: Validation of noncompaction criteria in dilated cardiomyopathy, and valvular and hypertensive heart disease. J Am Soc Echocardiogr 18:865–872, 2005.

Echocardiographic criteria for isolated ventric-ular noncompaction (IVNC) were evaluated in patients with noncompaction, dilated cardio-myopathy, hypertensive heart disease, and val-vular heart disease. In patients with IVNC, criteria were present as follows:

❑ *Thick ventricular wall with two-layered appearance (100%)*

❑ *Ratio 2:1 of noncompacted to compacted myocardium at end-systole (100%)*

❑ *Deep recesses with ventricular blood flow seen with color Doppler (95%)*

❑ *Hypokinesis of the affected segments (89%)*

❑ *Prominent trabecular meshwork at the apex or midventricular segments of the inferior and lateral walls (68%).*

Each of these findings was seen in some patients with other types of heart disease, but the combination of findings was very specific for the diagnosis of IVNC.

Hypertensive Heart Disease

27. Gottdiener JS: Hypertension: impact of echocardiographic data on the mecha-nism of hypertension, treatment options, prognosis and assessment of therapy. In Otto CM (ed): The Practice of Clinical Echocardiography, 3rd ed. Philadelphia: Elsevier/Saunders, 2007, pp 816–847.

This chapter reviews approaches to evaluation of LV mass in population-based studies with emphasis on technique reproducibility and cost. The clinical relevance of echocardiography in determining the prognosis and in tailoring medical therapy in the hypertensive patient is discussed.

28. Fox ER, Alnabhan N, Penman AD, et al: Echocardiographic left ventricular mass index predicts incident stroke in African Americans: Atherosclerosis Risk in Communities (ARIC) Study. Stroke 38:2686–2691, 2007.

In this population-based study of 1792 African Americans, an increased LV mass index, measured by echocardiography, was more prevalent in those with stroke (62% vs 39%). Echocardiographic LV mass index was an independent predictor of stroke risk, even after correction for traditional risk factors.

29. Pierdomenico SD, Lapenna D, Cuccur-ullo F: Regression of echocardiographic left ventricular hypertrophy after 2 years of therapy reduces cardiovascular risk in patients with essential hypertension. Am J Hypertens 21:464–470, 2008.

In 387 hypertensive patients with LV hyper-trophy by echocardiography, regression of hypertrophy after 2 years of medical therapy was associated with fewer cardiac and cere-brovascular events (RR 0.36, 95% CI 0.19–0.68, p = 0.002).

Evaluation after Heart Transplantation

29. Wu AH: End-stage heart failure: ven-tricular assist devices and the post-transplant patient. In Otto CM (ed): The Practice of Clinical Echocardiog-raphy, 3rd ed. Philadelphia: Elsevier/Saunders, 2007, pp. 735–752.

The structure and function of the normal transplanted heart are reviewed followed by a discussion of acute rejection and transplant vasculopathy. A detailed discussion of the echocardiographic evaluation of ventricular assist devices is included in this chapter. 71 references.

30. Sun JP, Niu J, Banbury MK, et al: Influence of different implantation techniques on long-term survival after orthotopic heart transplantation: an echocardiographic study. J Heart Lung Transplant 26:1243–1248, 2007.

Outcomes after heart transplantation were compared in groups defined by the type of sur-gical implantation (293 biatrial vs 322 bica-val). Preoperative characteristics and operative mortality were not different between groups. After transplantation the biatrial group had a greater degree of LA enlargement and a higher incidence of tricuspid regurgitation as compared with those with a bicaval anastomosis. In both groups, risk factors for mortality were LV ejection fraction, RV ejection fraction, and moderate to severe tricuspid regurgitation. Sur-vival at 10 years was 79.9% in the biatrial group and 87.3% in the bicaval group (p < 0.05).

Pulmonary Heart Disease

31. Forfia PR, Wiegers SE: Echocardio-graphic findings in acute and chronic respiratory disease. In Otto CM (ed): The Practice of Clinical Echocardiog-raphy, 3rd ed. Philadelphia: Elsevier/Saunders, 2007, pp 848–876.

This chapter provides a detailed review of echocardiographic imaging and Doppler evalu-ation of the RV and noninvasive measurement of pulmonary pressures. The pathophysiologic response of the RV to chronic pressure or vol-ume overload and the effect of pulmonary dis-ease on the right heart are discussed. 200 references.

32. Willens HJ, Chirinos JA, Gomez-Marin O, et al: Noninvasive differentiation of pulmonary arterial and venous hyper-tension using conventional and Doppler tissue imaging echocardiography. J Am Soc Echocardiogr 21:715–719, 2008.

Elevated PAPs due to primary pulmonary arterial hypertension can be distinguished from elevated PAPs due to pulmonary venous hypertension (with an elevated LA and pulmo-nary wedge pressure) by an LV diastolic filling pattern showing decreased compliance and ele-vated filling pressures. An E/E' ratio over 9.2 had a sensitivity of 95% and specificity of 96% for diagnosis of pulmonary venous hypertension.

33. Raymond RJ, Hinderliter AL, Willis PW, et al: Echocardiographic predic-tors of adverse outcomes in primary pulmonary hypertension. J Am Coll Cardiol 39:1214–1219, 2002.

In 81 patients with primary pulmonary hypertension, echocardiographic predictors of death or lung transplantation were pericardial effusion, indexed RA area, and paradoxical septal motion.

34. Cotton CL, Gandhi S, Vaitkus PT, et al: Role of echocardiography in detecting portopulmonary hypertension in liver transplant candidates. Liver Transpl 8:1051–1054, 2002.

In patients undergoing evaluation for orthotopic liver transplantation, echocardiographic esti-mates of pulmonary systolic pressure have a high negative predictive value (92%) for excluding significant portopulmonary hypertension. However, positive predictive value is low (38%) due to overestimation of PAPs by echocardiography, so that right heart catheterization is needed when the echocardio-graphic pulmonary pressure estimate is >50 mm Hg.

10 Pericardial Disease

PERICARDIAL ANATOMY AND PHYSIOLOGY

The pericardium consists of two serous surfaces surrounding a closed, complex, saclike potential space. The visceral pericardium is continuous with the epicardial surface of the heart. The parietal pericardium is a dense but thin fibrous structure that is apposed to the pleural surfaces laterally and blends with the central tendon of the diaphragm inferiorly. Around the right and left ventricles (RV and LV) and the ventricular apex, the pericardial space is a simple ellipsoid structure conforming to the shape of the ventricles. Around the systemic and pulmonary venous inflows and around the great vessels, the parietal and visceral pericardia meet to close the "ends" of the sac; these areas often are referred to as *pericardial reflections*. The pericardial space encloses the right atrium (RA) and RA appendage anteriorly and laterally, with pericardial reflections around the superior and inferior vena cavae near their junction with the RA. Superiorly, the pericardium extends a short distance along the great vessels; with a small "pocket" of pericardium surrounding the great arteries posteriorly—the *transverse sinus*. The pericardial space extends lateral to the left atrium (LA), and a blind pocket of the pericardium extends posterior to the LA, between the four pulmonary veins—the *oblique sinus*

(Fig. 10–1). The pericardial space normally contains a small amount (5–10 mL) of fluid that may be detectable by echocardiography.

Anatomically, the pericardium isolates the heart from the rest of the mediastinum and from the lungs and pleural space, serving as a barrier to infection and reducing friction with surrounding structures during contraction, rotation, and translation of the heart. In addition, the semi-rigid enclosure provided by the pericardium affects the pressure distribution to the cardiac chambers and mediates the interaction between RV and LV diastolic filling. The importance of the pericardium is most evident when affected by disease processes such as inflammation, thickening, or fluid accumulation.

PERICARDITIS

Basic Principles

Pericarditis is inflammation of the pericardium, and it can be due to a wide variety of causes, including bacterial or viral infection, trauma, uremia, and transmural myocardial infarction (Table 10–1). Clinically, the diagnosis of pericarditis is based on at least two of the four characteristic features:

❏ Typical chest pain
❏ Widespread ST elevation on electrocardiogram

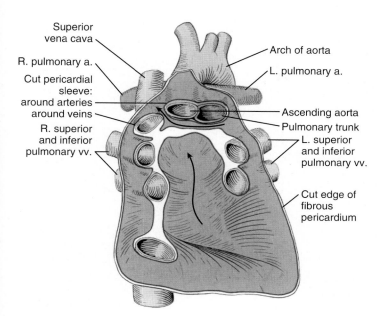

Superior
vena cava

R. pulmonary a.

Cut pericardial
sleeve:
around arteries
around veins

R. superior
and inferior
pulmonary vv.

Arch of aorta

L. pulmonary a.

Ascending aorta

Pulmonary trunk

L. superior
and inferior
pulmonary vv.

Cut edge of
fibrous
pericardium

Figure 10–1 The posterior wall of the pericardial sac after the heart has been removed by severing its continuity with the great arteries and veins and by cutting the two pericardial sleeves that surround the arteries and veins. The *horizontal arrow* is in the transverse sinus; the *vertical arrow* is in the oblique sinus of the pericardium. *(Reprinted with permission from Rosse C, Goddum-Rosse P: Hollinshead's Textbook of Anatomy, 5th ed. Philadelphia: Lippincott-Raven, 1997.)*

TABLE 10–1   Causes of Pericardial Disease (with Examples)

Idiopathic

Infections
- Viral
- Bacterial (*Staphylococcus*, *Pneumococcus*, tuberculosis)
- Parasitic (*Echinococcus*, amebiasis, toxoplasmosis)

Malignant
- Metastatic disease (e.g., lymphoma, melanoma)
- Direct extension (lung carcinoma, breast carcinoma)
- Primary cardiac malignancy

Inflammatory
- Post–myocardial infarction (Dressler's syndrome)
- Uremia
- Systemic inflammatory diseases (lupus, scleroderma)
- Post–cardiac surgery
- Radiation

Intracardiac-pericardial Communications
- Blunt or penetrating chest trauma
- Post-catheter procedures
- Post-infarction LV rupture
- Aortic dissection

❏ A pericardial rub on auscultation
❏ A new or increasing pericardial effusion

While it is probable that most patients with pericarditis have a pericardial effusion at some point in the disease course, a pericardial effusion is not a necessary criterion for diagnosis of pericarditis, nor does the presence of an effusion indicate a diagnosis of pericarditis. Interestingly, there is no correlation between the size of the pericardial effusion and the presence or absence of a pericardial "rub" on physical examination.

Echocardiographic Approach

In a patient with suspected pericarditis, the echocardiogram may show a pericardial effusion of any size, pericardial thickening with or without an effusion, or it may be entirely normal. A pericardial effusion is recognized as an echolucent space around the heart, as described in detail in the following sections (Fig. 10–2).

Pericardial thickening is evidenced by increased echogenicity of the pericardium on two-dimensional (2D) imaging and as multiple parallel reflections posterior to the LV on M-mode recordings (Fig. 10–3). However, since the pericardium typically is the most echogenic structure in the image, it can be difficult to distinguish normal from thickened pericardium and other imaging approaches, such as computed tomography (CT) or cardiac magnetic resonance (CMR), are more sensitive for this diagnosis.

A careful echocardiographic examination from several windows is needed when pericarditis is suspected, since effusion or thickening can be localized and may be seen in only certain tomographic views. If a pericardial effusion is present, the possibility of tamponade physiology should be considered. If pericardial thickening is present, examination for evidence of constrictive physiology should be considered.

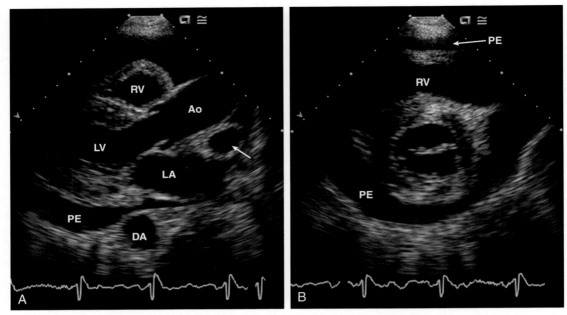

Figure 10–2 Parasternal long- (**A**) and short-axis (**B**) views of a moderate circumferential pericardial effusion (PE). In the long-axis view, the effusion tracks anterior to the descending aorta with a small amount of fluid posterior to the LA in the oblique sinus. Pericardial fluid in the transverse sinus (posterior to the Ao) delineates the right pulmonary artery (*arrow*), which is not usually seen in this view in adults. Pericardial fluid anterior to the RV is seen in both the long- and short-axis views.

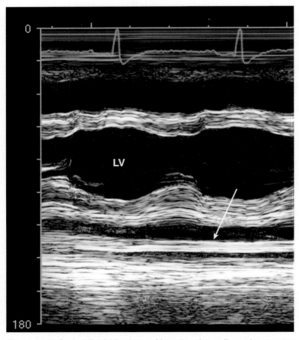

Figure 10–3 Pericardial thickening on M-mode echocardiography appears as multiple parallel dense echos (*arrow*) posterior to the LV epicardium. This patient also has a small pericardial effusion, seen on M-mode as an echo-free space between the flat pericardium and moving posterior wall.

Clinical Utility

Pericarditis is a clinical diagnosis that cannot be made independently by echocardiography. The goal of the echocardiographic examination is to evaluate for pericardial effusion or thickening and to evaluate for tamponade physiology.

PERICARDIAL EFFUSION

Basic Principles

A wide variety of disease processes can result in a pericardial effusion with a differential diagnosis similar to that for pericarditis (see Table 10–1). The physiologic consequences of fluid in the pericardial space depend both on the volume and rate of fluid accumulation. A slowly expanding pericardial effusion can become quite large (>1000 mL) with little increase in pericardial pressure, whereas rapid accumulation of even a small volume of fluid (50–100 mL) can lead to a marked increase in pericardial pressure (Fig. 10–4).

Tamponade physiology occurs when the pressure in the pericardium exceeds the pressure in the cardiac chambers, resulting in impaired cardiac filling. (Fig 10–5) As pericardial pressure increases, filling of each cardiac chamber is sequentially impaired, with lower pressure chambers (atria) affected before higher pressure chambers (ventricles). The compressive effect of the pericardial fluid is seen most clearly in the phase of the cardiac cycle when pressure is lowest in that chamber—

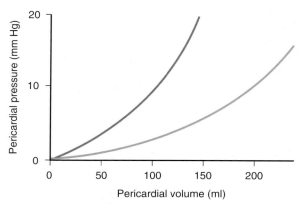

Figure 10–4 Schematic graph of pericardial pressure versus pericardial volume for an acute effusion (*blue line,* with a steep pressure-volume relationship) and for a chronic effusion (*yellow line,* where large volumes may lead to only mild pressure elevation).

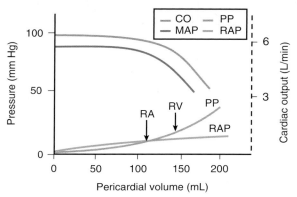

Figure 10–5 Schematic graph showing the relationship between pericardial pressure (PP), RA pressure, mean arterial pressure (MAP), and cardiac output (CO). Note that when PP exceeds RAP, MAP, and CO fall. When RV pressure is exceeded (*at the arrow*), CO and blood pressure fall further.

systole for the atrium, diastole for the ventricles. Filling pressures become elevated as a compensatory mechanism to maintain cardiac output. In fully developed tamponade, diastolic pressures in all four cardiac chambers are equal (and elevated) due to exposure of the entire heart to the elevated pericardial pressure.

Clinically, tamponade physiology is manifested as symptoms of low cardiac output, hypotension, and tachycardia. Jugular venous pressure is elevated and pulsus paradoxus (an inspiratory decline >10 mm Hg in systemic blood pressure) is present on physical examination. The clinical finding of pulsus paradoxus is closely related to the echo findings of reciprocal respiratory changes in RV and LV filling and emptying.

Diagnosis of Pericardial Effusion

Diffuse Effusion

A pericardial effusion is recognized on 2D echocardiography as an echolucent space adjacent to the cardiac structures. In the absence of prior pericardial disease or surgery, pericardial effusions usually are diffuse and

symmetric with clear separation between the parietal and visceral pericardium (Fig. 10–6). A relatively echogenic area anteriorly, in the absence of a posterior effusion, most likely represents a pericardial fat pad. M-mode recordings are helpful, especially with a small effusion, showing the flat posterior pericardial echo reflection and the moving epicardial echo with separation between the two in both systole and diastole.

In patients with recurrent or long-standing pericardial disease, fibrinous stranding within the fluid and on the epicardial surface of the heart may be seen. When a malignant effusion is suspected, it is difficult to distinguish this nonspecific finding from metastatic disease. Features suggesting the latter include a nodular appearance, evidence of extension into the myocardium, and the appropriate clinical setting (Fig. 10–7).

The size of the pericardial effusion is considered to be small when the separation between the heart and the parietal pericardium is <0.5 cm, moderate when it is 0.5 to 2 cm, and large when it is >2 cm. More quantitative measures of the size of the pericardial effusion rarely are needed in the clinical setting.

Loculated Effusion

After surgical or percutaneous procedures, or in patients with recurrent pericardial disease, pericardial fluid may be *loculated* (Fig. 10–8). In this situation the effusion is localized by adhesions to a small area of the pericardial space or consists of several separate areas of pericardial effusion, separated by adhesions. Recognition of a loculated effusion is especially important because hemodynamic compromise can occur with even a small, strategically located fluid collection. In addition, drainage of a loculated effusion may not be possible from a percutaneous approach.

Distinguishing from Pleural Fluid

In order to reliably exclude the possibility of a loculated pericardial effusion, echocardiographic evaluation requires a careful examination from multiple acoustic windows. The parasternal approach demonstrates the extent of the fluid collection at the base of the heart in both long- and short-axis views. Note that pericardial fluid may be seen posterior to the LA (in the oblique sinus), as well as posterior to the LV. Care should be taken that the coronary sinus or descending thoracic aorta is not mistaken for pericardial fluid. In fact, these structures can help in distinguishing pericardial from pleural fluid, since a left pleural effusion will extend posterolateral to the descending aorta, whereas a pericardial effusion will track anterior to the descending aorta (Fig. 10–9). When a large left pleural effusion is present, sometimes cardiac images can be obtained with the transducer on the patient's back (Fig. 10–10).

In the apical views the lateral, medial, and apical extent of the effusion can be appreciated. In the

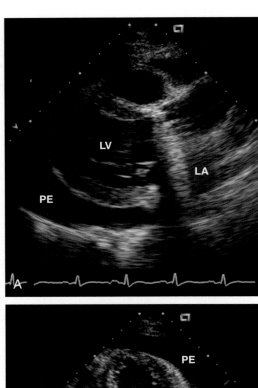

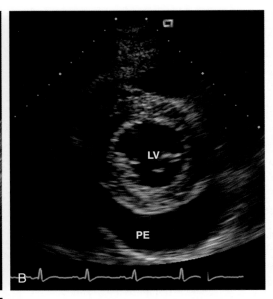

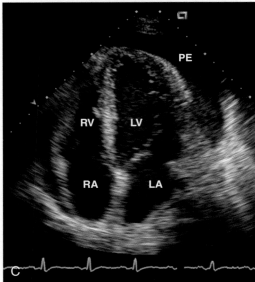

Figure 10–6 Pericardial effusion (PE) seen from a parasternal long-axis view (**A**), parasternal short-axis view (**B**), and apical four-chamber view (**C**) in a patient early after mechanical aortic valve replacement. Note the shadowing and reverberations from the valve in the long-axis view.

apical four-chamber view, an isolated echo-free space superior to the RA most likely represents pleural fluid. The subcostal view demonstrates fluid between the diaphragm and RV and is particularly helpful in echo-guided pericardiocentesis (Fig. 10–11). The sensitivity and specificity of echocardiography for detection of a pericardial effusion are very high.

Diagnosis of Pericardial Tamponade

When cardiac tamponade occurs with a diffuse moderate to large pericardial effusion, the associated physiologic changes are evident on echocardiographic and Doppler examination (Fig. 10–12), including:

- ❏ RA systolic collapse
- ❏ RV diastolic collapse
- ❏ Reciprocal respiratory changes in RV and LV volumes
- ❏ Reciprocal respiratory changes in RV and LV filling
- ❏ Reduced early-diastolic tissue Doppler velocity
- ❏ Inferior vena cava plethora

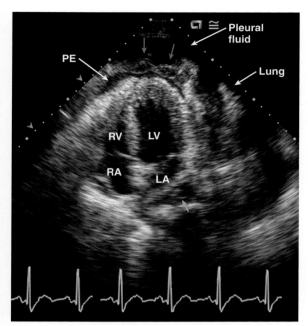

Figure 10–7 Apical four-chamber view in a patient with metastatic lymphoma shows a small pericardial effusion (PE) in the apical region with marked thickening and irregularity of the pericardium (*cyan arrows*), suggesting tumor involvement. Pleural fluid with compressed lung also is evident. The small fluid collection adjacent to the LA (*yellow arrow*) may be pericardial fluid in the oblique sinus of the pericardium.

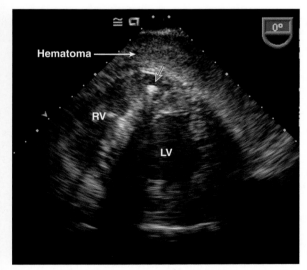

Figure 10–8 Transesophageal transgastric short-axis view in a patient with acute hypotension during an electrophysiology procedure shows a localized hematoma in the pericardial space with compression of the RV. The catheter in the RV (*cyan arrow*) casts a dark shadow that obscures part of the ventricular septum.

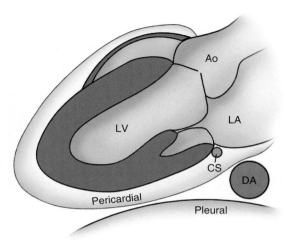

Figure 10–9 Schematic diagram of the relationship between a pericardial effusion and the descending aorta (DA) compared with a left pleural effusion. Pericardial fluid tracks posterior to the LA in the oblique sinus of the pericardium, anterior to the descending aorta. CS, coronary sinus.

Right Atrial Systolic Collapse

When intrapericardial pressure exceeds RA systolic pressure (lowest point of the atrial pressure curve), inversion or collapse of the RA free wall occurs. Since the RA free wall is a thin, flexible structure, brief RA wall inversion can occur in the absence of tamponade physiology. However, the longer the duration of RA inversion relative to the cycle length, the greater is the likelihood of cardiac tamponade. Inversion for greater than a third of systole has a sensitivity of 94% and a specificity of 100% for the diagnosis of tamponade. Careful frame-by-frame 2D-image analysis is needed for this evaluation (Fig. 10–13).

Right Ventricular Diastolic Collapse

RV diastolic collapse occurs when intrapericardial pressure exceeds RV diastolic pressure *and* when the RV free wall is normal in thickness and compliance. The presence of RV hypertrophy or infiltrative diseases of the myocardium may allow development of a pressure gradient between the pericardial space and RV chamber without inversion of the normal contour of the free wall. RV diastolic collapse is best appreciated in the parasternal long-axis view or from a subcostal window. If the timing of RV wall motion is not clear on 2D imaging, an M-mode recording through the RV free wall is helpful. The presence of RV diastolic collapse is somewhat less sensitive (60% to 90%) but more specific (85% to 100%) than brief RA systolic collapse for diagnosing tamponade physiology (Fig. 10–14).

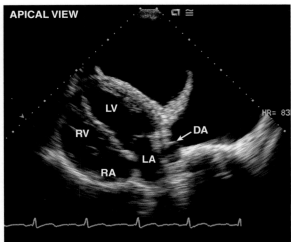

APICAL VIEW

HR= 83

LV

RV

DA

LA

RA

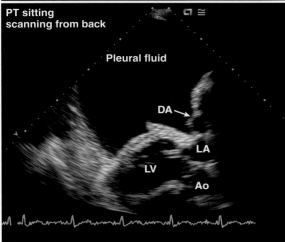

PT sitting
scanning from back

Pleural fluid

DA

LA

LV

Ao

Figure 10–10 In a view with the transducer moved laterally from the apical position (*top*) a large left pleural effusion is seen. This can be distinguished from pericardial fluid by the position of the descending aorta (DA), the presence of compressed lung, and identification of both layers of the pericardium adjacent to the myocardium. Images also were obtained with the transducer on the patient's back (*bottom*), demonstrating the relationship between the pleural fluid and the DA.

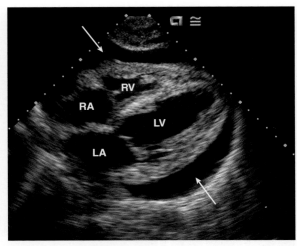

RV

RA

LV

LA

Figure 10–11 Subcostal four-chamber view showing a pericardial effusion (*arrows*) with a circumferential effusion around the right and left heart.

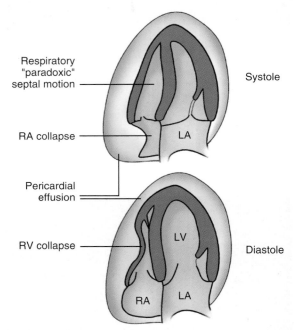

Respiratory "paradoxic" septal motion

Systole

LA

RA collapse

Pericardial effusion

RV collapse

LV

Diastole

RA   LA

Figure 10–12 Schematic diagram of 2D echo findings with tamponade physiology.

Reciprocal Changes in Ventricular Volumes

Reciprocal respiratory variation in RV and LV volumes may be seen on 2D imaging when tamponade is present. In the apical four-chamber view, an increase in RV volume with inspiration (shift in septal motion toward the LV in diastole and toward the RV in systole) and a decrease during expiration (normalization of septal motion) can be appreciated. This pattern of motion corresponds to the physical finding of pulsus paradoxus. The proposed explanation for this observation is that total pericardial volume (heart chambers plus pericardial fluid) is fixed in tamponade; thus, as intrathoracic pressure becomes more negative during inspiration, enhanced RV filling limits LV diastolic filling. This pattern reverses during expiration.

Respiratory Variation in Diastolic Filling

Doppler recordings of RV and LV diastolic filling in patients with tamponade physiology show a pattern that parallels the changes in ventricular volumes. With inspiration, the RV early-diastolic filling velocity is augmented, while LV diastolic filling diminishes (Figs. 10–15 and 10–16). In addition, the velocity time integral (VTI) in the pulmonary artery increases with inspiration, while the aortic velocity time integral decreases. In the acutely ill patient these changes

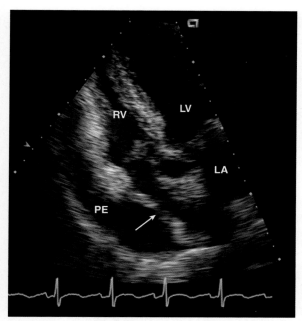

Figure 10–13 Apical four-chamber view showing systolic collapse on the RA free wall (*arrow*) in a patient with clinical tamponade physiology.

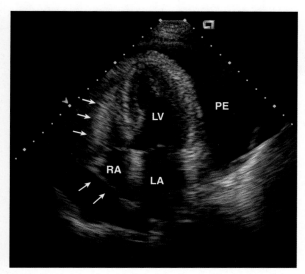

Figure 10–14 Apical four-chamber view with a large pericardial effusion (PE) and tamponade physiology resulting in the compression (or collapse) of the RV (*arrows*) and RA in diastole.

can be difficult to demonstrate, in part due to respiratory changes in the intercept angle between the Doppler beam and the flow of interest causing artifactual apparent velocity changes. Differentiating the normal respiratory variation in diastolic filling from the excessive variation (>25%) seen in tamponade may be subtle in borderline cases. Tamponade physiology is not an all-or-none phenomenon; a patient may exhibit varying degrees of hemodynamic

impairment as the degree of pericardial compression (pericardial pressure) increases.

Tissue Doppler Early-Diastolic Velocity

The early-diastolic mitral annular tissue Doppler velocity (E') is reduced when tamponade is present and returns to normal after pericardiocentesis, probably reflecting changes in cardiac output. However, respiratory variation is not seen, and the sensitivity and specificity of this finding have not been evaluated.

Plethora of the Inferior Vena Cava

Inferior vena cava plethora, a dilated inferior vena cava with <50% inspiratory reduction in diameter near the inferior vena cava–RA junction, also has been proposed as a sensitive (97%), albeit nonspecific (40%) indicator of tamponade physiology. This simple finding reflects the elevated RA pressure seen in tamponade.

Limitations and Alternate Approaches

Echocardiography is very sensitive for the diagnosis of pericardial effusion, even when loculated, if care is taken to examine the heart in multiple tomographic planes from multiple acoustic windows. Loculated effusions can be difficult to assess in certain locations, particularly if localized to the atrial region, since the effusion itself may be mistaken for a normal cardiac chamber. Transesophageal echocardiographic (TEE) imaging may better detect and define the extent of loculated effusions after cardiac surgery, especially when located posteriorly.

Pericardial adipose tissue is common, especially anterior to the RV, and may be mistaken for an effusion. Unlike pericardial fluid, adipose tissue exhibits a fine pattern of echogenicity that helps with identification of this normal finding. A pericardial cyst is an uncommon congenital fluid-filled sac, usually adjacent to the right heart. Pericardial cysts may be missed on echocardiography and are better evaluated by chest CT or CMR. However, when present they may be mistaken for a pericardial or pleural effusion.

The etiology of the pericardial effusion is not always evident on echocardiographic examination. Irregular pericardial or epicardial masses in a patient with a known malignancy certainly raise the possibility of a malignant effusion, but this appearance can be mimicked by fibrinous organization of a long-standing pericardial effusion. Masses adjacent to the cardiac structures (in the mediastinum) resulting in pericardial effusion can be missed by echocardiography. Wide-view tomographic imaging procedures, such as CT or magnetic resonance imaging (MRI), are helpful in these cases.

Figure 10–15 Doppler recording of LV inflow with superimposed respirometer tracing in a patient with tamponade showing increased tricuspid flow and decreased mitral (*arrows*) flow on the first beat after inspiration, reflecting the reciprocal respiratory changes in RV and LV diastolic filling.

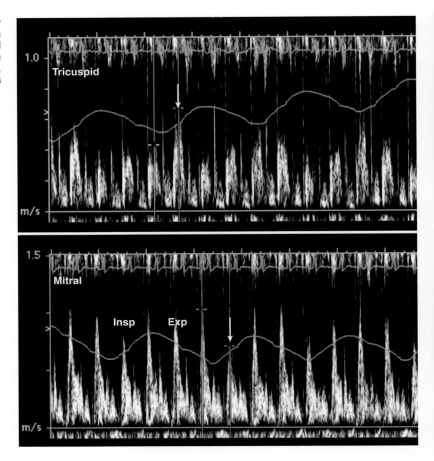

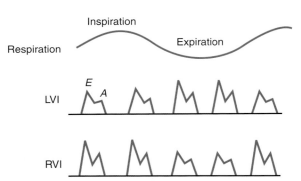

Figure 10–16 Schematic diagram of LV and RV diastolic inflow (RVI and LVI) Doppler curves with tamponade physiology showing enhanced RV (and reduced LV) diastolic filling with inspiration and a reversal of this pattern during expiration.

Obviously, whether a pericardial effusion is infected or inflammatory in etiology cannot be determined by echocardiography. Depending on the associated clinical findings in each case, diagnostic pericardiocentesis and/or pericardial biopsy may be indicated to establish the correct diagnosis.

With pericardial effusion due to aortic dissection or cardiac rupture (as a consequence of either myocardial infarction or a procedure) the entry site into the pericardium rarely can be detected, so a high level of suspicion is needed when these diagnoses are a possibility. The site of an LV rupture may be "contained" by pericardial adhesions, resulting in formation of a pseudoaneurysm. A *pseudoaneurysm* is defined as a saccular structure communicating with the ventricle with walls composed of pericardium. In contrast, the walls of a "true" aneurysm are composed of thinned, scarred myocardium (see Fig. 8–26).

Clinical Utility

Diagnosis of Pericardial Effusion

Echocardiography is the procedure of choice for diagnosis of pericardial effusion. When transthoracic images are inadequate, as occasionally occurs (especially in postoperative patients), TEE imaging or an alternate tomographic imaging procedure (MRI, CT) may be needed. Echocardiography can be helpful in establishing a diagnosis of pericardial tamponade but requires integration with other clinical data.

In evaluating a patient for cardiac tamponade, it is essential to remember that tamponade is a clinical and hemodynamic diagnosis. Furthermore, varying degrees of tamponade physiology may be seen. The most important finding on echocardiography in a patient with suspected pericardial tamponade is whether or not a pericardial effusion is present. The absence of a pericardial effusion *excludes* the diagnosis, again taking care that a loculated effusion is not missed. Only rarely does tamponade physiology result from other mediastinal contents under pressure (i.e., air due to barotrauma or a compressive mass). Conversely, in a patient with convincing clinical evidence for tamponade, the presence of a moderate to large pericardial effusion on echocardiography *confirms* the diagnosis; further evaluation with Doppler is not needed and may delay appropriate intervention.

In intermediate cases, either when the diagnosis has not been considered or when clinical evidence is equivocal, 2D findings of chamber collapse and inferior vena cava plethora and Doppler findings showing marked respiratory variation in RV and LV filling may be helpful, in conjunction with the clinical data. Another approach to making this diagnosis is right-sided heart catheterization showing a depressed cardiac output and equalization of RA, RV diastolic, and pulmonary artery wedge pressures.

Echo-Guided Pericardiocentesis

The success rate without complications of percutaneous needle pericardiocentesis can be enhanced by using echocardiographic guidance. With the patient in the position planned for the procedure, the optimal transcutaneous approach is identified based on the location of the effusion, the distance from the chest wall to the pericardium, and the absence of intervening structures. The transducer angle and pericardial depth are noted, and the transducer position is marked prior to prepping the site for the procedure. After the procedure, the residual amount of pericardial fluid is assessed using standard tomographic views (Fig. 10–17). If monitoring during the procedure is needed, an acoustic window that allows visualization of the effusion but does not compromise the sterile field is identified. (Alternatively, a sterile sleeve is used for the transducer.) Note that with *tomographic* imaging it is difficult to identify the *tip* of the needle, since any segment of the needle passing through the image plane may appear to be the tip. The source of error is minimized by scanning in both superior-inferior and lateral-medial directions during the procedure. Confirmation that the needle tip is

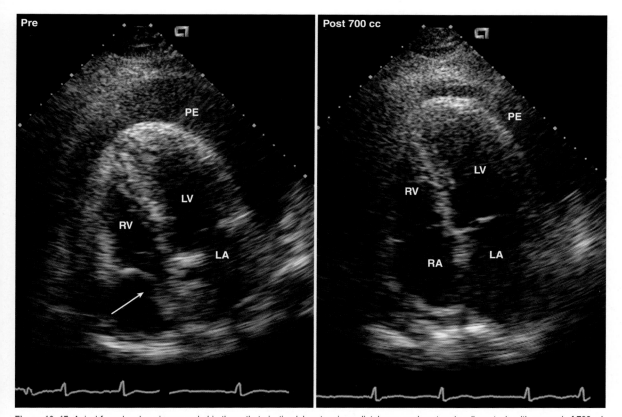

Figure 10–17 Apical four-chamber view recorded in the catheterization laboratory immediately pre- and post-pericardiocentesis with removal of 700 mL of fluid. On the pre-pericardiocentesis image (*left*) a large pericardial effusion (PE), small ventricular chambers, and RA collapse (*arrow*) are seen. The post-pericardiocentesis image (*right*) shows a reduction in size of the effusion, an increase in RV and LV volumes, and a normal contour of the RA wall.

in the pericardial space can be made by injecting a small amount of agitated sterile saline solution through the needle to achieve an echo-contrast effect.

PERICARDIAL CONSTRICTION

Basic Principles

In constrictive pericarditis the serous surfaces of the visceral and parietal pericardium are adherent, thickened, and fibrotic, with resultant loss of the pericardial space and impairment of diastolic ventricular filling. Pericardial constriction can occur after repeated episodes of pericarditis, after cardiac surgery, after radiation therapy, and from a variety of other causes. The diagnosis often is delayed because clinical symptoms are nonspecific—fatigue and malaise due to low cardiac output—and physical findings either are subtle (elevated jugular venous pressure, distant heart sounds) or occur only late in the disease course (ascites and peripheral edema).

The physiology of constrictive pericarditis is characterized by impaired diastolic cardiac filling due to the abnormal pericardium surrounding the cardiac structures, acting like a rigid "box" (Fig. 10–18). Early-diastolic filling is rapid, with an abrupt cessation of ventricular filling as diastolic pressure rises—when the "box" is full. Pressure tracings (Fig. 10–19) typically show:

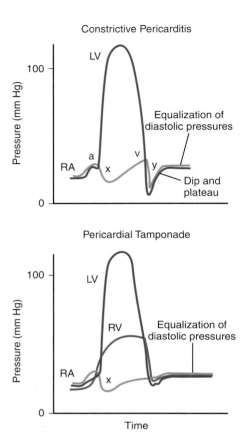

Figure 10–19 Typical pressure tracings in tamponade and constriction.

❑ A brief, rapid fall of LV pressure in early diastole followed by
❑ A high early-diastolic pressure plateau (*dip-plateau* or *square-root sign*),
❑ A rapid descent of RA pressure with the onset of ventricular filling (*y* descent),

❑ Only modest elevation of RV and pulmonary artery systolic pressures,
❑ An RV diastolic pressure plateau that is a third or more of systolic pressure, and
❑ Equalization of diastolic pressures in the RV and LV even after volume loading.

Figure 10–18 Schematic diagram of pericardial tamponade compared with pericardial constriction. With tamponade, diastolic filling is impaired in both early and late diastole due to the elevated pericardial pressures "compressing" the heart. With constriction, early-diastolic filling is rapid but ends abruptly when the volume limits of the rigid pericardial space are reached.

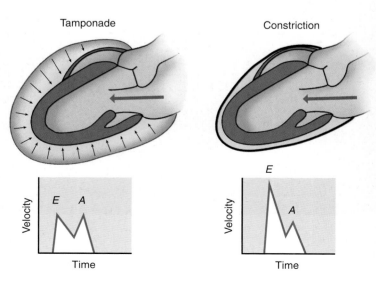

Pericardial Disease | Chapter 10   253

Echocardiographic Approach

Imaging

Typically, LV wall thickness, internal dimensions, and systolic function are normal in the patient with constrictive pericarditis. LA enlargement is seen due to chronic LA pressure elevation. Pericardial thickening may be evident on 2D imaging as increased echogenicity in the region of the pericardium (Fig. 10–20). Careful examination from several acoustic windows is needed because the spatial distribution of pericardial thickening may be asymmetric. From the parasternal approach, an M-mode recording shows multiple echo-densities, posterior to the LV epicardium, moving parallel with each other. These echo-densities persist even at a low-gain setting. High–time resolution M-mode recordings also may demonstrate abrupt posterior motion of the ventricular septum in early diastole, with flat motion in mid-diastole and abrupt anterior motion following atrial contraction (Fig. 10–21). This pattern of motion appears to be due to initial rapid RV diastolic filling, followed by equalization of filling of RV and LV as the "plateau" phase of the pressure curve is reached, and increased RV filling after atrial contraction. The LV posterior wall endocardium shows little posterior motion during diastole (<2 mm from early to late diastole) due to the impairment of diastolic filling resulting in a "flat" pattern of diastolic posterior wall motion. On subcostal views the inferior vena cava and hepatic veins are dilated, reflecting the elevated RA pressure.

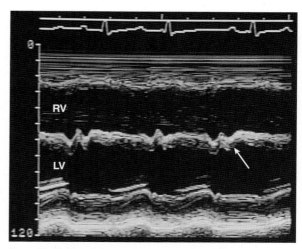

Figure 10–21 M-mode in constrictive pericarditis showing rapid anterior motion of the septum (arrow) with atrial contraction before the QRS on the ECG.

Doppler Examination

The Doppler findings in constrictive pericarditis reflect the abnormal hemodynamics in this condition (Fig. 10–22) including:

- Characteristic patterns of RA and LA filling
- Respiratory variation in LV and RV filling
- Respiratory variation in the isovolumic relaxation time (IVRT).

Pulsed Doppler recordings of hepatic vein flow (from a subcostal approach) measure RA filling and show a prominent a wave and a deep y descent (Fig. 10–23), and a marked increase in flow velocities with inspiration. Similarly, pulsed Doppler recordings of pulmonary vein flow (transthoracic apical four-chamber view or TEE approach) indicate LA filling and again show a prominent a wave, prominent y descent, a prominent diastolic filling phase, and blunting of the systolic phase of atrial filling.

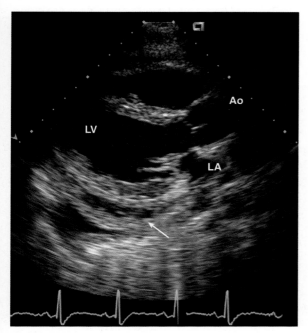

Figure 10–20 Constrictive pericarditis from a parasternal long-axis view with both thickened pericardium (arrow) and a small effusion.

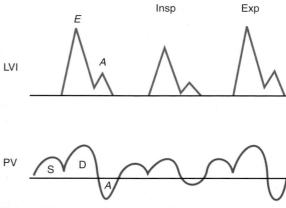

Figure 10–22 Schematic diagram of the Doppler flow patterns in constrictive pericarditis. LV inflow (LVI) shows reduced early diastolic filling with inspiration, while the pulmonary vein (PV) shows a prominent a wave and blunting of the systolic filling phase.

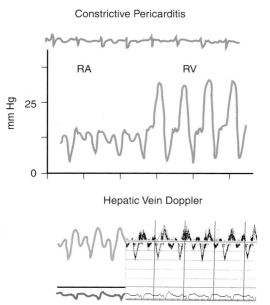

Figure 10–23 Pressure tracing and hepatic vein flow in a patient with constrictive pericarditis. Note the prominent *a* wave, flat diastolic segment, and prominent *y* descent, all consistent with the "square-root sign" or dip and plateau in the pressure tracings.

Both RV and LV diastolic filling show a high *E* velocity reflecting rapid early-diastolic filling due to the initial high atrial-to-ventricular pressure difference. As LV pressure rises, filling abruptly ceases, reflected in a short deceleration time of the *E*-velocity curve. Little ventricular filling occurs in late diastole due to the elevated LV diastolic pressure (the "plateau") and the constrictive effect of the thickened pericardium. Doppler recordings of ventricular inflow thus show a very small *A* velocity following atrial contraction.

Marked reciprocal respiratory variations in RV and LV diastolic inflow velocities are seen due to the differing effects of changes in intrapleural pressure on filling of the two ventricles (Fig. 10–24). With inspiration, intrapleural pressure becomes more negative, resulting in augmentation of RV diastolic filling and inflow velocity. In contrast, LV filling velocities *decrease* with inspiration and *increase* with expiration. Although similar directional changes in filling velocities occur in normal individuals, the respiratory changes are much greater (variation >25%) with constrictive pericarditis.

The IVRT—measured from the aortic closure to the mitral opening click on Doppler recordings—increases by a mean of 20% with inspiration in patients with constrictive pericarditis. Tissue Doppler findings in constrictive pericarditis include an increased early-diastolic velocity (*E′*), consistent with rapid early-diastolic filling.

Constrictive Pericarditis vs Restrictive Cardiomyopathy

Even though the hemodynamics of pericardial tamponade and pericardial constriction have some similarities, differentiating between these two diagnoses usually is straightforward based on the presence or absence of a pericardial effusion (Table 10–2). Differentiating constrictive pericarditis from a restrictive cardiomyopathy is more difficult. Both are characterized by clinical signs and symptoms of elevated venous pressure and low cardiac output, and both show a normal-sized LV chamber with normal systolic function on 2D echocardiography. Pericardial thickening may be difficult to appreciate, and other 2D and M-mode findings may not reliably differentiate between these two diagnoses. Doppler findings that favor constrictive pericarditis over restrictive cardiomyopathy include reciprocal respiratory changes in ventricular volumes and filling parameters with a 25% or greater difference in

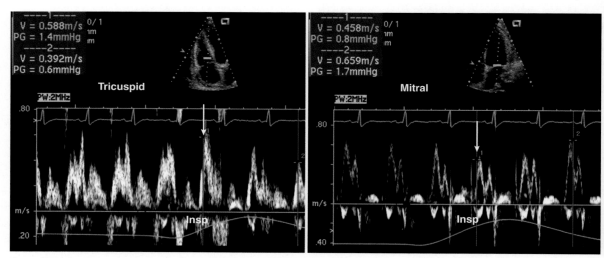

Figure 10–24 Respiratory variation in RV and LV diastolic filling in a patient with constrictive pericarditis. There in an increase in tricuspid and decrease in mitral flow velocities on the first beat after inspiration (*arrows*), with the decrease greater than 25% compared to the maximum velocities.

TABLE 10–2   Comparison of Pericardial Tamponade, Constriction, and Restrictive Cardiomyopathy

	Pericardial Tamponade	Constrictive Pericarditis	Restrictive Cardiomyopathy
Hemodynamics			
Right atrial pressure	↑	↑	↑
RV/LV filling pressures	↑, RV = LV	↑, RV = LV	↑, LV > RV
Pulmonary artery pressures	Normal	Mild elevation (35–40 mm Hg systolic)	Moderate-to-severe elevation (≥60 mm Hg systolic)
RV diastolic pressure plateau		>1/3 peak RV pressure	<1/3 peak RV pressure
Radionuclide Diastolic Filling			
		Rapid early filling, impaired late filling	Impaired early filling
2D Echo			
	Moderate-large PE IVC plethora	Pericardial thickening without effusion	LV hypertrophy Normal systolic function
Doppler Echo			
	Reciprocal respiratory changes in RV and LV filling	$E > a$ on LV inflow Prominent y descent in hepatic vein Pulmonary venous flow = prominent a wave, reduced systolic phase Respiratory variation in IVRT and in E velocity	(1) Early in disease $e < A$ on LV inflow (2) Late in disease $E > a$ (3) Constant IVRT (4) Absence of significant respiratory variation
Tissue Doppler			
	↓ E' without respiratory variation	↑ E'	↓ E' consistent with degree of diastolic dysfunction
Other Diagnostic Tests			
	Therapeutic/diagnostic pericardiocentesis	CT or MRI for pericardial thickening	Endomyocardial biopsy

CT, computed tomography; IVRT, isovolumic relaxation time; IVC, inferior vena cava; MRI, magnetic resonance imaging; PE, pericardial effusion.

maximum E velocity from expiration to inspiration, and normal or only mildly elevated pulmonary pressures. However, Doppler data are far from absolutely accurate due to overlap between groups in the Doppler findings and due to differing hemodynamics in patients with restrictive cardiomyopathy depending on disease stage (see Chapter 9).

Limitations and Alternate Approaches

When the diagnosis of constrictive pericarditis is in question, several alternate approaches may be helpful. Either chest CT or MRI scanning is more definitive for detection of pericardial thickening and calcification, especially when it is asymmetric (Fig. 10–25). Endomyocardial biopsy occasionally will confirm a diagnosis of restrictive cardiomyopathy due to an infiltrative process.

Right- and left-sided heart catheterization shows equalization of diastolic pressure in the four cardiac chambers when constrictive pericarditis is present.

Differentiation of constrictive pericarditis from restrictive cardiomyopathy is further complicated by the concurrent presence of both conditions in some patients—for example, in radiation-induced heart disease. Similarly, while constrictive pericarditis typically occurs in the absence of a pericardial effusion, some patients have an overlap condition with a clinical presentation consistent with effusive-constrictive pericarditis.

Clinical Utility

The diagnosis of pericardial constriction remains problematic, with no single diagnostic feature on echocardiographic or Doppler examination. However, the

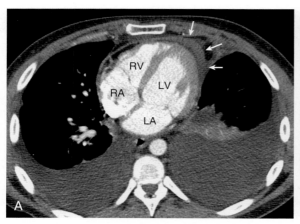 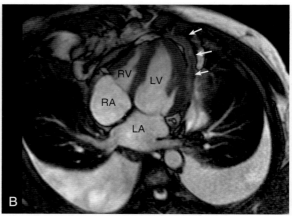

Figure 10–25 In a 32-year-old man with radiation therapy 15 years ago, chest CT (**A**) shows thickening of the pericardium (*arrows*) and bilateral pleural effusions. **B**, In the same patient, a similar CMR view shows pericardial thickening as a low signal band (*arrows*) at the apex and around the lateral LV wall, anterior to the RV (*arrow*).

conjunction of several findings in a patient in whom the level of clinical suspicion is high increases the likelihood of this diagnosis and may be definitive in some cases. Conversely, the echo and Doppler findings may provide the first clues for this diagnosis in a patient in whom it was not previously considered, for example, a patient presenting with ascites and no prior cardiac history.

SUGGESTED READING

General

1. Munt MI, Moss RR, Thompson CR: Pericardial disease. In Otto CM (ed) The Practice of Clinical Echocardiography, 3rd ed. Philadelphia: Elsevier/Saunders, 2007, pp 710–734.

   This comprehensive chapter provides additional information and illustrations about echocardiographic evaluation of pericardial disease. A detailed step-by-step protocol for echo-guided pericardiocentesis is provided. Case examples are included on the accompanying DVD. 128 references.

2. Goldstein J: Cardiac tamponade, constrictive pericarditis, and restrictive cardiomyopathy. Curr Probl Cardiol 29:503–567, 2004.

   This article reviews the physiology of the normal pericardium and the pathophysiology of cardiac tamponade, constrictive pericarditis, and restrictive cardiomyopathy. There are 21 figures illustrating the physiology of pericardial disease and findings on clinical imaging studies.

3. Maisch B, Seferovic P, Ristic A, et al: Guidelines on the diagnosis and management of pericardial diseases executive summary; The Task Force on the Diagnosis and Management of Pericardial Diseases of the European Society of Cardiology. Eur Heart J 25:587–610, 2004.

   This guideline document provides a comprehensive differential diagnosis of the causes of pericardial disease and criteria for diagnosis of cardiac tamponade and constrictive pericarditis. Detailed information on medical and surgical therapy for pericardial disease is provided. 245 references.

4. Ivens EL, Munt BI, Moss RR: Pericardial disease: what the general cardiologist needs to know. Heart 93:993–1000, 2007.

   The clinical presentation, echocardiographic findings, and clinical management of pericardial effusion, tamponade, constrictive pericarditis, transient constriction, and effusive-constrictive pericarditis are reviewed.

5. Little WC, Freeman GL: Pericardial disease. Circulation 113:1622–1632, 2006.

   This basic review of the etiology, pathophysiology, clinical presentation, and management of pericardial disease provides a useful overview of the topic.

6. Wann S, Passen E: Echocardiography in pericardial disease. J Am Soc Echocardiogr 21:7–13, 2008.

   This concise article provides a historical overview and summary of the echocardiographic findings in pericardial disease with 14 illustrations.

Pericardial Effusion

7. Markiewicz W, Brik A, Brook G, et al: Pericardial rub in pericardial effusion: Lack of correlation with amount of fluid. Chest 77:643–646, 1980.

   In 76 patients with a pericardial effusion, a rub was noted on auscultation in 4 of 13 (30%) with a small effusion, 23 of 40 (58%) with a moderate effusion, and 10 of 23 (43%) patients with a large effusion. These findings suggest that the size of the effusion cannot be predicted from the presence or absence of a rub.

8. Markiewicz W, Monakier I, Brik A, et al: Clinical-echocardiographic correlations in pericardial effusion. Eur Heart J 3:260–266, 1982.

   Of 100 patients with an effusion on echocardiography, 49 had a clinical course consistent with acute pericarditis (idiopathic in 23, post–radiation therapy in 7, Dressler's syndrome in 7, purulent in 4, and other in 7). In the 51 patients with chronic pericarditis, the etiology was carcinoma in 20, heart disease in 12, uremia in 7, rheumatoid arthritis in 5, chronic idiopathic pericarditis in 4, and other in 3 patients.

9. Cho BC, Kang SM, Kim DH, et al: Clinical and echocardiographic characteristics of pericardial effusion in patients who underwent echocardiographically guided pericardiocentesis: Yonsei Cardiovascular Center experience, 1993–2003. Yonsei Med J 45:462–468, 2004.

   Over an 11-year period, 272 patients underwent echo-guided pericardiocentesis. Pericardial effusion was due to malignancy in 46%, post–cardiac surgery or percutaneous intervention in 20%, and tuberculous in 15%. Overall procedural success rate was 99% with a major complication rate of only 0.7%. Complications included two RV free wall perforations that required emergency surgery.

Tamponade Physiology

10. Gillam LD, Guyer DE, Gibson TC, et al: Hydrodynamic compression of the right atrium: a new echocardiographic sign of cardiac tamponade. Circulation 68:294–301, 1983.

    RA free wall systolic inversion that persists for a third or more of the cycle length had a sensitivity of 94% and specificity of 100% for the diagnosis of tamponade physiology in 127 patients (19 with tamponade).

11. Leimgruber P, Klopfenstein HS, Wann LS, et al: The hemodynamic derangement associated with right ventricular diastolic collapse in cardiac tamponade: An experimental echocardiographic study. Circulation 68:612–620, 1983.

    In an experimental model, RV diastolic collapse occurred when intrapericardial pressure exceeded RV diastolic pressure and was associated with a 21% reduction in cardiac output (but no change in mean aortic pressure). Of note, RV diastolic collapse did not occur in the presence of RV hypertrophy.

12. Reddy PS, Curtiss EL, Uretsky BF: Spectrum of hemodynamic changes in cardiac tamponade. Am J Cardiol 55:1487–1491, 1990.

    The range of hemodynamic compromise that can be seen with tamponade physiology is emphasized in this study of 77 consecutive patients with >150 mL of pericardial fluid. In group I, intrapericardial pressures were less than RA and pulmonary artery wedge pressures. In group II, intrapericardial and RA pressures had equaled. In group III, intrapericardial, RA, and pulmonary artery wedge pressures were equal. All subjects improved after pericardiocentesis, with the greatest improvement seen in group III.

13. Gonzalez MS, Basnight MA, Appleton CP: Experimental pericardial effusion: Relation of abnormal respiratory variation in mitral flow velocity to hemodynamics and diastolic right heart collapse. J Am Coll Cardiol 17:239–248, 1991.

    Respiratory changes in LV diastolic filling are exaggerated in tamponade, with this variation occurring before equalization of intracardiac pressures and definite right-sided heart collapse. The presence of excessive respiratory variation, but not its magnitude, is predictive of tamponade physiology.

14. Himelman RB, Kircher B, Rockey DC, et al: Inferior vena cava plethora with blunted respiratory response: a sensitive echocardiographic sign of cardiac tamponade. J Am Coll Cardiol 12:1470–1477, 1988.

    Dilation of the inferior vena cava reflects an elevated RA pressure. Plethora (marked dilation without respiratory variation) of the inferior vena cava had a sensitivity of 97% but a specificity of only 40% for the diagnosis of pericardial tamponade. False-positive results occurred in patients with RV failure, tricuspid regurgitation, and pulmonary hypertension.

15. Eisenberg MJ, Schiller NB: Bayes' theorem and the echocardiographic diagnosis of cardiac tamponade. Am J Cardiol 68:1242–1244, 1991.

    Using Bayes' theorem, the predictive values of RV collapse, RA collapse, and inferior vena cava plethora for the diagnosis of tamponade were calculated (using published sensitivities and specificities for these variables). When the pretest probability of tamponade is high (>50%), both RA and RV collapse have high positive and negative predictive values. With a medium (10%) or low (1%) pretest likelihood, all three variables have a high (>97%) negative predictive value (i.e., tamponade can be excluded if absent) but a low positive predictive value.

Constrictive Pericarditis

16. Hatle LK, Appleton CP, Popp RL: Differentiation of constrictive pericarditis and restrictive cardiomyopathy by Doppler echocardiography. *Circulation* 79:357–370, 1989.

    Patients with constrictive pericarditis showed marked respiratory variation in LV and RV inflow velocities and IVRTs, while patients with restrictive cardiomyopathy did not have respiratory variation. With constrictive pericarditis, the first beat after inspiration showed a decrease in LV inflow velocity, an increase in RV inflow velocity, and an increase in LV IVRT. These changes resolve after pericardiectomy

17. Oh JF, Tajik AJ, Appleton CP, et al: Preload reduction to unmask the characteristic Doppler features of constrictive pericarditis: a new observation. Circulation 95:3799–3800, 1997.

    Increased filling pressures can mask the reciprocal changes in RV and LV diastolic filling seen in patients with constrictive pericarditis. If this diagnosis is suspected on clinical grounds, repeat recordings of ventricular filling after decreasing filling volumes is warranted (for example, in the sitting rather than supine position).

18. Oki T, Tabata T, Yamada H, et al: Right and left ventricular wall motion

velocities as diagnostic indicators of constrictive pericarditis. Am J Cardiol 81:465–470, 1998.

Doppler tissue imaging demonstrates an abrupt outward motion of the ventricular walls immediately after the early diastolic filling velocity in patients with constrictive pericarditis compared to normal subjects. This finding has potential value for diagnosis of constrictive pericarditis.

19. Abdalla AI, Murray RD, Lee JC, et al: Does rapid volume loading during transesophageal echocardiography differentiate constrictive pericarditis from restrictive cardiomyopathy? Echocardiography 19:125–134, 2002.

    Rapid intravenous infusion of normal saline during TEE in patients with suspected diastolic dysfunction was well tolerated and enhanced the respiratory variation in the pulmonary vein diastolic flow curve seen in patients with constrictive pericarditis.

20. Sohn D, Kim Y, Kim H, et al: Unique features of early diastolic mitral annulus velocity in constrictive pericarditis. J Am Soc Echocardiogr 17:222–226, 2004.

    Doppler tissue velocity data were evaluated before and after therapy in 17 patients with constrictive pericarditis and 8 patients with cardiac tamponade, compared to age- and sex-matched control subjects. Paralleling the findings of mitral inflow E velocities, tissue Doppler early-diastolic velocity is increased with constrictive pericarditis and reduced with tamponade physiology; both these changes resolved after pericardiocentesis or relief of constriction.

21. Sengupta P, Mohan J, Mehta V, et al: Accuracy and pitfalls of early diastolic motion of the mitral annulus for diagnosing constrictive pericarditis by tissue Doppler imaging. Am J Cardiol 93:886–890, 2004.

    Doppler tissue velocity imaging in 87 subjects with suspected constrictive pericarditis were compared to 35 age- and sex-matched controls. Constrictive pericarditis was confirmed at surgery in 45 subjects (52%); the remainder were diagnosed with restrictive cardiomyopathy (13%), cor pulmonale (23%), or old pericardial effusion. Mitral annular tissue Doppler early-diastolic velocity (E′) was normal (≥8 cm/s) in 89% of the subjects with constrictive pericarditis. In contrast, E′ was reduced in most patients with restrictive cardiomyopathy.

22. Sagrista-Sauleda J, Angel J, Sanchez A, et al: Effusive-constrictive pericarditis. N Engl J Med 350:469–475, 2004.

    Both pericardial effusion and constrictive pericarditis can coexist when there is excessive thickening and rigidity of the visceral pericardium (without adherence to the parietal pericardium). In a consecutive series of 1184 patients with pericarditis, 218 (18%) had tamponade physiology, and 15 (1.3% of total and 7% of those with tamponade) had effusive-constrictive pericarditis.

23. Yamada H, Tabata T, Jaffer S, et al: Clinical features of mixed physiology of constriction and restriction: Echocardiographic characteristics and clinical outcome Eur J Echocardiogr 8:185–194, 2007.

Echocardiographic findings consistent with combined constrictive pericarditis and restrictive cardiomyopathy were seen in 38 patients (mean age 57 ± 14 years, 8 females, 30 males). There was respiratory variation in LV and RV diastolic filling, but the degree of variation was only about 11% in those in sinus rhythm and 18% in those with an atrial arrhythmia. Pericardial thickening was present in all patients but was diffuse in only 24%; thickening was seen only adjacent to the right-heart chambers in 50% and the left heart in 26%. The cause of constriction/restriction was prior radiation therapy in 50%, coronary bypass surgery in 24%, and cardiac transplantation in 8%.

Valvular Stenosis

BASIC PRINCIPLES

Approach to Evaluation of Valvular Stenosis

Narrowing, or stenosis, of a cardiac valve can be due to a congenitally abnormal valve, a postinflammatory process (e.g., rheumatic), or age-related calcification. As the degree of valve opening decreases, the increasing obstruction to blood flow results in an increased flow velocity and pressure gradient across the valve. In isolated valve stenosis, clinical symptoms typically occur when the valve orifice is reduced to one quarter its normal size. In mixed stenosis and regurgitation symptoms can occur when each lesion, if isolated, would be considered only moderate in severity.

Secondary changes in patients with valvular stenosis include the response of the specific cardiac chambers affected by pressure overload. The ventricular response to pressure overload is hypertrophy; the atrial response is dilation. Chronic pressure overload also can lead to irreversible changes in other upstream cardiac chambers and in the pulmonary vascular bed (e.g., in mitral stenosis).

Complete echocardiographic evaluation of the patient with valvular stenosis includes:

- ❐ Imaging of the valve to define the etiology of stenosis
- ❐ Quantitation of stenosis severity
- ❐ Evaluation of coexisting valvular lesions
- ❐ Assessment of left ventricular (LV) systolic function
- ❐ The response to chronic pressure overload of other upstream cardiac chambers, and the pulmonary vascular bed

This echocardiographic evaluation then is integrated with pertinent clinical data for a complete evaluation of the patient.

Fluid Dynamics of Valvular Stenosis

High-Velocity Jet

The fluid dynamics of a stenotic valve are characterized by the formation of a laminar, high-velocity jet in the narrowed orifice. The flow profile in cross-section at the origin of the jet is relatively blunt (or flat) and remains blunt as the jet reaches its narrowest cross-sectional area in the vena contracta, slightly downstream from the anatomic orifice (Fig. 11–1). Thus, the narrowest cross-sectional area of flow (physiologic orifice area) is smaller than the anatomic orifice area. The magnitude of the difference between physiologic and anatomic area depends on orifice geometry and the Reynolds number (a descriptor of the inertial and shear stress properties of the fluid). The ratio of the physiologic to anatomic orifice area is known as the *discharge coefficient*.

The length of the high-velocity jet is dependent on orifice geometry as well and can be variable in the clinical setting with, for example, a very short jet across a deformed, irregular, calcified aortic valve and a longer jet across a smoothly tapering, symmetric, rheumatic mitral valve or a congenitally stenotic semilunar valve (Figs. 11–2 and 11–3).

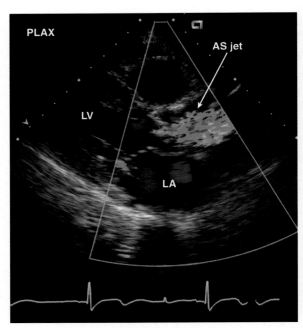

Figure 11–2 Color flow imaging in calcific valvular aortic stenosis in a parasternal long-axis view. The post-stenotic flow disturbance identifies the site of obstruction at the valvular level, but the laminar jet is short so that a jet direction is not clearly demonstrated.

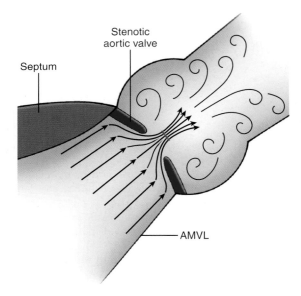

Figure 11–1 Schematic illustration of the fluid dynamics of the stenotic aortic valve in systole. The LV outflow tract is bounded by the septum and anterior mitral valve leaflet (AMVL). As LVOT flow accelerates and converges, a relatively flat velocity profile occurs proximal to the stenotic valve, as indicated by the *arrowheads*. Flow accelerates in a spatially small zone adjacent to the valve as blood enters the narrowed orifice. In the stenotic orifice, a high-velocity laminar jet is formed with the narrowest flow stream (vena contracta, indicated by the *blue line*) occurring downstream from the orifice. Beyond the jet, flow is disturbed, with blood cells moving in multiple directions and velocities. *(Reprinted with permission from Judge KW, Otto CM: Doppler echocardiographic evaluation of aortic stenosis. Cardiol Clin 8:203, 1990.)*

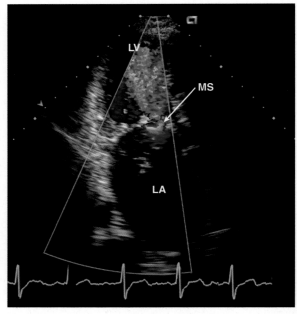

Figure 11–3 Color flow imaging of a mitral stenosis (MS) jet in an apical long-axis view. Note the long jet directed toward the LV apex with a well-defined proximal isovelocity surface area on the LA side of the valve.

Relationship between Pressure Gradient and Velocity

The pressure gradient across the stenotic valve is related to the velocity in the jet, according to the unsteady½ Bernoulli equation:

$$\Delta P = \tfrac{1}{2}\rho(v_2{}^2 - v_1{}^2) + \rho(dv/dt)dx + R(v)$$

$$\underset{\text{acceleration}}{\text{Convective}} \quad \underset{\text{acceleration}}{\text{Local}} \quad \underset{\text{resistance}}{\text{Viscous}} \qquad (11{-}1)$$

where ΔP is the pressure gradient across the stenosis (mm Hg), ρ is the mass density of blood (1.06×10^3 kg/m³), v_2 is velocity in the stenotic jet, v_1 is the velocity proximal to the stenosis, $(dv/dt)dx$ is the time-varying velocity at each distance along the flow stream, and R is a constant describing the viscous losses for that fluid and orifice. Historically, Daniel Bernoulli first described this equation in approximately 1738 from studies of steady water flow in rigid tubes. The concepts were later expanded and refined by Euler. Of note, these equations may not be strictly applicable to pulsatile blood flow in compliant chambers and vessels, although clinical studies have shown that remarkably accurate pressure gradient predictions can be made with this approach. This equation was first applied to Doppler data by Holen in 1976 for stenotic mitral valves and by Hatle in 1979 for stenotic aortic valves.

Eliminating the terms for viscous losses and acceleration, substituting known values for the mass density of blood, and adding a conversion factor for measuring velocity in units of meters per second (m/s) and pressure gradient in millimeters of mercury (mm Hg), the Bernoulli equation can be reduced to

$$\Delta P = 4(v_2{}^2 - v_1{}^2) \qquad (11{-}2)$$

If the proximal velocity is less than 1 m/s, as is commonly the case for stenotic valves, it becomes even smaller when squared (for example, $(0.8)^2 = 0.64$). Thus, the proximal velocity often can be ignored in the clinical setting so that:

$$\Delta P = 4v^2 \qquad (11{-}3)$$

This simplified Bernoulli equation allows highly accurate and reproducible calculation of maximum pressure gradients (from maximum velocity) and mean pressure gradients (by integrating the instantaneous pressure difference over the flow period).

Distal Flow Disturbance

Distal to the stenotic jet, the flow stream becomes disorganized with multiple blood flow velocities and directions, although fully developed turbulence, as strictly defined in fluid dynamic terms, may not occur. The distance that this flow disturbance propagates downstream is related to stenosis severity. In addition, the *presence* of a downstream flow disturbance can be extremely useful in defining the exact anatomic site of obstruction, for example, allowing differentiation of subvalvular outflow obstruction (flow disturbance on the ventricular side of the valve) from valvular obstruction (flow disturbance only distal to the valve).

Proximal Flow Patterns

Proximal to a stenotic valve, flow is smooth and organized (laminar) with a normal flow velocity. The spatial flow velocity profile proximal to a stenotic valve depends on valve anatomy, inlet geometry, and the degree of flow acceleration. For example, in calcific aortic stenosis, the acceleration of blood flow by ventricular systole coupled with a tapering outflow tract geometry results in a relatively uniform flow velocity (a "flat" flow profile) across the outflow tract just proximal to the stenotic valve. Immediately adjacent to the valve orifice there is acceleration as flow converges to form the high-velocity jet, but this region of proximal acceleration is spatially small. The flow profile differs slightly for congenital aortic stenosis in that the proximal acceleration region under the domed leaflets in systole is larger than with calcific stenosis. However, proximal flow patterns are similar regardless of disease etiology in that a relatively flat velocity profile is present at the aortic annulus.

In contrast, the flow pattern proximal to the stenotic mitral valve is quite different (Fig. 11–4). Here, the left atrial (LA) to LV pressure gradient drives flow passively from the large inlet chamber (the LA) abruptly across the stenotic orifice. Proximal flow

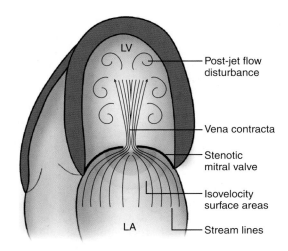

Figure 11–4 Schematic diagram of the fluid dynamics of rheumatic mitral stenosis. The stream lines of flow accelerate as they approach the stenotic orifice, with several curved proximal isovelocity surface areas indicated. The MS jet is long, with the post-jet flow disturbance occurring adjacent and distal to the laminar jet.

acceleration is prominent over a large region of the LA. The three-dimensional (3D) velocity profile is curved; that is, flow velocities are faster adjacent to and in the center of a line continuous with the jet direction through the narrowed orifice and slower at increasing radial distances from the valve orifice. The proximal velocity profile of an atrioventricular valve thus is hemielliptical, unlike the more flattened velocity profile proximal to a stenotic semilunar valve. Any 3D surface area proximal to a narrowed orifice at which all the blood velocities are equal can be referred to as a *proximal isovelocity surface area* (PISA).

The clinical importance of these flow patterns is that stroke volume can be calculated proximal to a stenotic valve based on knowledge of the cross-sectional area (CSA) of flow and the spatial mean flow velocity over the period of flow, as described in Chapter 6. This concept applies to the flat flow profile proximal to a stenotic aortic valve (used in the continuity equation), to the proximal flow patterns seen in mitral stenosis, and to the PISAs seen with regurgitant lesions (see Chapter 12).

AORTIC STENOSIS

Diagnostic Imaging of the Aortic Valve

Aortic valve stenosis in adults most often is due to

- ❑ calcific aortic stenosis,
- ❑ congenital valve disease (bicuspid or unicuspid), or
- ❑ rheumatic valve disease.

Calcific Aortic Stenosis

A frequent cause of valvular aortic stenosis in adults is age-related calcification of an anatomically normal trileaflet valve. Calcification occurs slowly over many years and initially presents on two-dimensional (2D) echo as aortic valve "sclerosis"—areas of increased echogenicity, typically at the base of the valve leaflets, without significant obstruction to LV outflow. Clinically significant obstruction tends to occur from age 70 to 85. When obstruction is present, 2D imaging shows a marked increase in echogenicity of the leaflets consistent with calcific disease and reduced systolic opening. When aortic stenosis is suspected, a systolic leaflet separation of 15 mm or more by 2D or 2D-guided M-mode echocardiography reliably excludes severe obstruction. When the leaflets are abnormal and systolic separation is less than 15 mm, the degree of obstruction may be mild, moderate, or severe, depending on the area of the narrowed orifice. Direct measurement of valve area on short-axis 2D imaging is possible in some patients either with excellent transthoracic (TTE) images or from a transesophageal (TEE) approach. However,

directly planimetered aortic valve areas should be interpreted with caution due to the complex 3D anatomy of the orifice in calcific degenerative stenosis. It is critical to ensure that the image plane is aligned at the narrowest orifice of the valve, although if the orifice is nonplanar, planimetry of apparent valve area may be misleading. Even when carefully performed, 2D or 3D valve area reflects anatomic valve area, whereas Doppler data provide functional valve area (Fig. 11-5).

Bicuspid Aortic Valve

A congenital bicuspid valve accounts for two thirds of cases of severe aortic stenosis in adults younger than 70 and one third of cases in those over age 70 years. Secondary calcification of a bicuspid aortic valve can be difficult to distinguish from calcification of a trileaflet valve once stenosis becomes severe; however, earlier in the disease course a bicuspid valve can be identified on 2D parasternal short-axis views by demonstrating that there are only two open leaflets in systole (Fig. 11-6). Long-axis views show systolic bowing of the leaflets into the aorta, resulting in a "domelike" appearance. M-mode recordings may help in identifying a bicuspid valve if an eccentric closure line is present but can be misleading in terms of the degree of leaflet separation if the M-mode is taken through the base, rather than the tips, of the bowed leaflets. Similarly, planimetry of valve area may be erroneous if the 2D image plane is not aligned with the narrowest point at the leaflet tips. Potentially, 3D imaging will provide more accurate visualization of anatomic valve area.

Typically, the two leaflets are unequal in size, with the anterior (if the leaflet opening is anteroposterior) or rightward (if the leaflet opening is lateromedial) leaflet being larger. Many bicuspid valves have a raphe in the larger leaflet, so that the closed valve in diastole appears trileaflet; accurate identification of the number of aortic valve leaflets can be made only in systole. Doppler interrogation of the aortic valve should be performed whenever a bicuspid valve is suspected to evaluate for stenosis and/or regurgitation. Bicuspid aortic valve disease often is associated with dilation of the aortic sinuses and ascending aorta.

Rheumatic Aortic Stenosis

Rheumatic valvular disease preferentially involves the mitral valve, so rheumatic aortic stenosis is diagnosed when aortic disease occurs concurrently with rheumatic mitral valve disease. The rheumatic disease process results in commissural fusion of the aortic leaflets, similar to the pathology seen in rheumatic mitral stenosis. Two-dimensional imaging may show increased echogenicity along the leaflet edges, commissural fusion, and systolic doming of the aortic leaflets. Often, however, the echocardiographic images appear similar

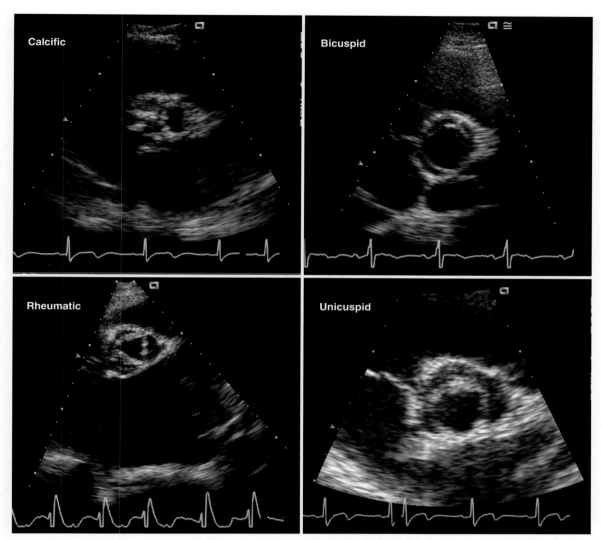

Figure 11–5 Parasternal mid-systolic short-axis views of the four most common causes of valvular aortic stenosis (AS). Calcific AS is characterized by calcific masses on the aortic side of the leaflet that result in increased leaflet stiffness without commissural fusion. Calcific shadowing and reverberations limit image quality. In a young patient with a congenital bicuspid valve, the two leaflets (with a raphe in the anterior leaflet) open widely in systole. Later in life, secondary calcific changes are seen that result in stenosis. The diagnostic features of rheumatic stenosis are commissural fusion and mitral valve involvement, with the characteristic triangular aortic valve opening in systole. The unicuspid valve, seen in young adults, has only one point of attachment (at the 6 o'clock position) with a funnel-shaped valve opening. Planimetry of valve area is inaccurate unless the image plane is at the narrowest segment of the doming valve in systole.

to those of calcific aortic stenosis (other than the presence of rheumatic mitral valve disease).

Congenital Aortic Stenosis

Congenital aortic stenosis usually is diagnosed in childhood, but some patients may not become symptomatic until young adulthood or may present with restenosis after surgical valvotomy performed in childhood or adolescence. These patients most often have a unicuspid valve with a single eccentric orifice and prominent systolic doming.

Differential Diagnosis

The differential diagnosis of LV outflow obstruction includes:

❒ Fixed subvalvular obstruction (a subaortic membrane or a muscular subaortic stenosis)
❒ Dynamic subaortic obstruction (hypertrophic cardiomyopathy)
❒ Supravalvular stenosis

In a patient with a clinical diagnosis of valvular aortic stenosis, the echocardiographic study should demonstrate whether the obstruction is, in fact,

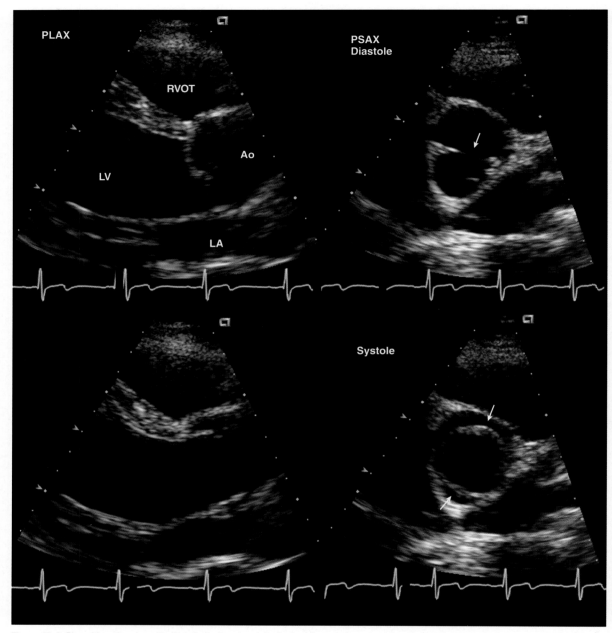

Figure 11–6 Bicuspid aortic valve with diastolic (*top*) and systolic (*bottom*) frames shown in parasternal long-axis (PLAX) (*left*) and short-axis (PSAX) (*right*) views. Note the diastolic sagging and systolic doming of the leaflets in the long-axis view. In the short-axis view only two leaflets (*arrows*) are seen to open in systole with the commissures at 4- and 10-o'clock positions.

valvular or if one of these other diagnoses accounts for the clinical presentation (Fig. 11–7).

A subaortic membrane should be suspected in young adults when the valve anatomy is not clearly stenotic, yet Doppler examination reveals a high trans-aortic pressure gradient. Since the membrane may be poorly depicted on a TTE study, TEE imaging should be considered when this diagnosis is suspected. The spatial orientation of the jet and the shape of the

CW Doppler velocity curve are similar for fixed obstructions, whether subvalvular, supravalvular, or valvular, but careful pulsed Doppler or color flow imaging allows localization of the level of obstruction by detection of the post-stenotic flow disturbance and site of increase in flow velocity.

In dynamic outflow obstruction the timing and shape of the late-peaking CW Doppler velocity curve are distinctive. In addition, the degree of obstruction changes

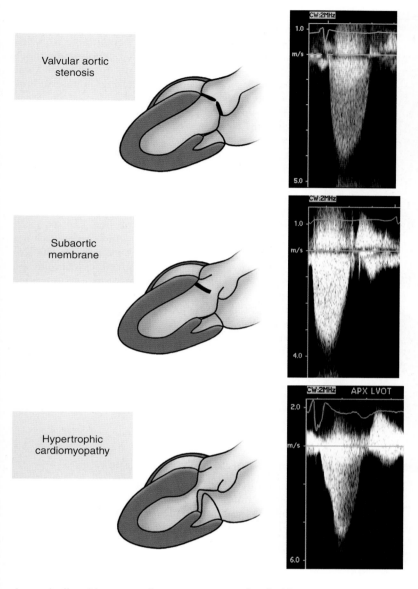

Valvular aortic stenosis

Subaortic membrane

Hypertrophic cardiomyopathy

Figure 11–7 Examples of the shape of the CW Doppler velocity curve in valvular AS, fixed subvalvular obstruction due to a subaortic membrane, and dynamic obstruction due to hypertrophic cardiomyopathy. Note that the CW curves for subvalvular and valvular AS are similar, although coarse fluttering of the valve with subvalvular obstruction results in a "rough" appearance of the systolic velocity curve. These can be distinguished by 2D and color flow imaging. The shape of the curve with dynamic obstruction is distinctly different, with the velocity peaking in late systole.

dramatically with provocative maneuvers, as detailed in Chapter 9. In the occasional patient with both subvalvular *and* valvular obstruction, high–pulse repetition frequency Doppler ultrasound can be helpful in defining the maximum velocities at each site of obstruction.

Quantitation of Stenosis Severity

The severity of valvular aortic stenosis can be determined accurately using equations derived from our understanding of the fluid dynamics of a stenotic valve. Standard evaluation of stenosis severity includes:

❑ Measurement of maximum aortic jet velocity
❑ Calculation of the mean transaortic pressure gradient
❑ Determination of continuity equation valve area

Pressure Gradients

Maximum transaortic pressure gradient (ΔP_{max}) can be calculated from the maximum aortic jet velocity (V_{max}) using the simplified Bernoulli equation (Fig. 11–8):

$$\Delta P_{max} = 4 V_{max}^2 \qquad (11\text{--}4)$$

Mean pressure gradient (ΔP_{mean}) can be calculated by digitizing the aortic jet velocity curve (where $v_1, \ldots, v_n$ are instantaneous velocities) and averaging the instantaneous gradients over the systolic ejection period.

$$\Delta P_{mean} = \frac{4v_1^2 + 4v_2^2 + 4v_3^2 + \ldots + 4v_n^2}{n} \qquad (11\text{--}5)$$

Interestingly, in native aortic valve stenosis transaortic pressure gradient correlates closely and linearly peak LV pressures do not occur simultaneously, so none of the instantaneous velocities recorded with Doppler ultrasound are strictly comparable with this clinical measurement. Potential confusion about Doppler pressure gradient data in an individual patient can be avoided by comparing only mean gradients (Fig. 11–9).

Physiologic changes in pressure gradient should be taken into consideration when comparing nonsimultaneous data recordings and in patient management decisions. Pressure gradients depend on volume flow rate, as well as the degree of valve narrowing, so in an individual patient the pressure gradient will rise when transaortic stroke volume increases (e.g., anxiety, exercise) and will fall when stroke volume decreases (e.g., sedation, hypovolemia).

The dependence of pressure gradients on volume flow rate can lead to erroneous conclusions about stenosis severity in adult patients with either a chronically elevated or depressed transaortic stroke volume. For example, a patient with coexisting aortic regurgitation will have a high transaortic pressure gradient with only a moderate degree of valve narrowing. Conversely, a patient with LV systolic dysfunction or coexisting mitral regurgitation may have a low transaortic pressure gradient despite severe aortic stenosis. These coexisting conditions are common in adults with valvular aortic stenosis, so determination of the stenotic orifice area is essential for complete evaluation of disease severity.

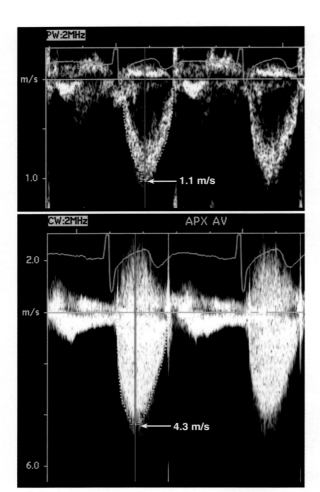

Figure 11–8 Pulsed Doppler recording of LV outflow tract velocity (*top*) and CW Doppler recording of an aortic stenosis jet (*bottom*). The CW Doppler was recorded from an apical approach with a dedicated non-imaging transducer after evaluation from several windows with careful angulation to identify the highest velocity jet. This represents the most parallel intercept angle between the direction of blood flow and the stenotic jet. The maximum pressure gradient is calculated as $\Delta P = 4v^2$, with mean pressure gradient determined by integrating the instantaneous gradients over the systolic ejection period. The velocity ratio is 0.26.

with maximum transaortic gradient, so that mean gradient can be approximated from published regression equations as:

$$\Delta P_{mean} = 2.4(V_{max})^2 \qquad (11-6)$$

With careful attention to technical details, Doppler-determined pressure gradients are accurate, as has been demonstrated in numerous in vitro and animal models and in clinical studies (Table 11–1). Although Doppler maximum gradients correspond to maximum instantaneous gradients by catheter measurement and Doppler mean gradients correspond to catheter-measured mean gradients, neither Doppler gradient correlates with the peak-to-peak gradient reported at catheterization. In fact, peak aortic and

Continuity Equation Valve Area

Aortic valve area can be calculated based on the principle of continuity of flow. Specifically, the stroke volume (SV) just proximal to the aortic valve (SV_{LVOT}) and that in the stenotic valve orifice (SV_{Ao}) are equal:

$$SV_{LVOT} = SV_{Ao} \qquad (11-7)$$

If flow is laminar with a spatially flat velocity profile,

$$SV = CSA \times VTI \qquad (11-8)$$

where CSA is the cross-sectional area of flow (cm^2), SV is stroke volume (cm^3), and VTI is the velocity-time integral (cm). Because flow both proximal to and in the aortic jet itself is laminar with a reasonably flat velocity profile,

$$CSA_{LVOT} \times VTI_{LVOT} = CSA_{Ao} \times VTI_{Ao} \qquad (11-9)$$

All the variables in this equation can be measured with 2D or Doppler echo except CSA_{Ao}, which is the stenotic aortic valve area (AVA) itself. Rearranging the equation,

$$AVA = (CSA_{LVOT} \times VTI_{LVOT})/VTI_{Ao} \qquad (11-10)$$

TABLE 11–1   Selected Studies Validating Doppler Pressure Gradients in Valvular Stenosis (in Vivo Simultaneous Data)

First Author and Year	N	Study Group/Model	R	Range (mm Hg)	SEE (mm Hg)
Callahan 1985	120	Supravalvular constriction (canines)	0.99 (ΔP_{max})	7–179	5.2
			0.98 (ΔP_{mean})	N/A	4.3
Smith 1985	88	Supravalvular constriction (canines)	0.98 (ΔP_{max})	5–166	5.3
			0.98 (ΔP_{mean})	5–116	3.3
Currie 1985	100	Adults with valvular aortic stenosis	0.92 (ΔP_{max})	2–180	15
			0.92 (ΔP_{mean})	0–112	10
Smith 1986	33	Adults with valvular aortic stenosis	0.85 (ΔP_{max})	27–138	N/A
Simpson 1985	24	Adults with valvular aortic stenosis	0.98 (ΔP_{max})	0–120	N/A
Burwash 1993	98	Chronic valvular aortic stenosis (canines)	0.95 (ΔP_{max})	10–128	8.4
			0.91 (ΔP_{mean})	5–77	5.3

N/A, not available.
Data from Callahan et al: Am J Cardiol 56:989–993, 1985; Smith et al: J Am Coll Cardiol 6:1306–1314, 1985; Currie et al: Circulation 71:1162–1169, 1985; Smith et al: Am Heart J 111:245–252, 1986; Simpson et al: Br Heart J 53:636–639, 1985; Burwash et al: Am J Physiol 265 (Heart Circ Physiol 34):H734–H1743, 1993.

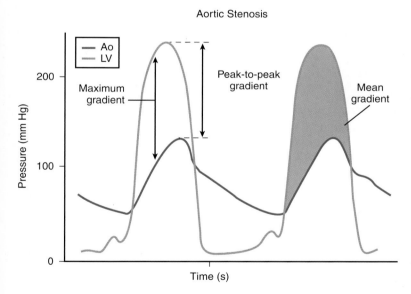

Aortic Stenosis

Figure 11–9 Example of LV and aortic pressures measured with fluid-filled catheters in a patient with severe valvular AS. Note that the maximum instantaneous gradient is greater than the peak-to-peak gradient. Mean gradient is indicated by the shaded area.

Thus, the measurements needed to calculate valve area with the continuity equation are (Fig. 11–10):

❏ LVOT diameter
❏ LVOT VTI
❏ Aortic jet VTI

LVOT diameter, measured on a 2D parasternal long-axis mid-systolic image, is used to calculate a circular outflow tract cross-sectional area. The VTI in the outflow tract is recorded with pulsed Doppler echocardiography from an apical approach. The VTI in the aortic stenosis jet is recorded with CW Doppler ultrasound from the window that yields the highest velocity signal.

For clinical use the continuity equation can be simplified by substituting maximum velocities (V) for VTIs. Since the shape and timing of outflow tract and aortic jet velocity curves are similar, their ratios are nearly identical:

$$\text{VTI}_{\text{LVOT}}/\text{VTI}_{\text{Ao}} \cong V_{\text{LVOT}}/V_{\text{Ao}} \qquad (11\text{--}11)$$

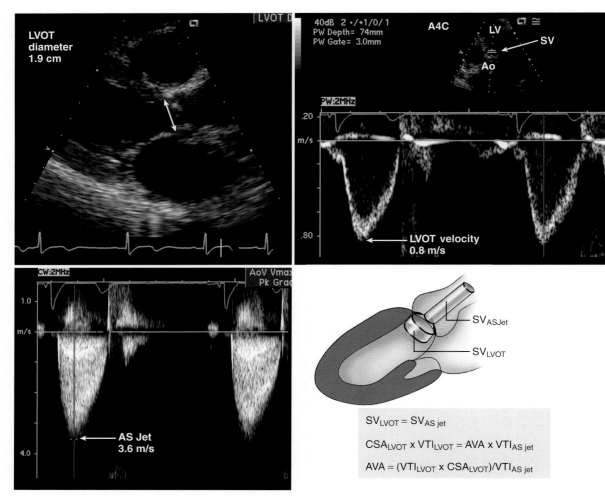

Figure 11–10 Continuity equation aortic valve area (AVA) calculations require measurement of LV outflow tract (LVOT) diameter from a parasternal long-axis view for circular cross-sectional area (CSA) calculation (*above, right*), pulsed Doppler recording of the LVOT velocity-time integral (VTI) from an apical approach (*above, left*), and continuous-wave Doppler recording of the AS-jet VTI from whichever window gives the highest velocity signal.

The simplified continuity equation then is

$$AVA = CSA_{LVOT} \times (V_{LVOT}/V_{Ao}) \qquad (11\text{--}12)$$

Outflow tract diameter must be measured in each patient for accurate valve area calculations. Although women tend to have smaller outflow tracts than men and outflow diameter correlates with body size when people of all ages from infancy to adulthood are considered; in the adult population, the relationship between gender or body size and outflow tract diameter is weak. On the other hand, outflow tract diameter tends to remain constant in a given adult patient over time. Apparent differences in diameter at follow-up visits are more likely to represent measurement error than an actual interval anatomic change. Thus, the ratio of outflow tract velocity to aortic jet velocity can be used to follow disease progression in individual patients.

Velocity Ratio

Although not strictly comparable to valve area, the velocity ratio also may be a useful measure of stenosis severity that, in effect, is "indexed" for body size. Obviously, normal valve area is dependent on body size; infants and children have smaller valve areas than adults and large adults are expected to have larger valve areas than small adults. One way to take the effect of body size into account is to "index" valve area by dividing it by body surface area (BSA) or some other measure of body size, such as height:

$$\text{Aortic valve index} = AVA/BSA \qquad (11\text{--}13)$$

An alternate approach is to define the "normal" valve area for that individual as the size of the outflow tract. Then, the increase in velocity from out-flow tract to aortic jet reflects stenosis severity regardless of body size. If the:

$$\text{"Normal"}AVA = CSA_{LVOT} \text{ and}$$
$$\text{Actual } AVA \cong \text{"normal" } AVA \times V_{LVOT}/V_{Ao},$$
$$\text{then Actual } AVA/\text{"Normal" } AVA \cong V_{LVOT}/V_{Ao}$$

$$(11\text{–}14)$$

A velocity ratio near 1 indicates little obstruction, a velocity ratio of 0.5 indicates a valve area that is one half normal, and a velocity ratio of 0.25 indicates a valve area reduced to about one fourth its normal value (see Fig. 11–8).

Technical Considerations and Potential Pitfalls

Continuity equation valve areas have been well validated in comparison with Gorlin formula valve areas calculated from invasive measurements of pressure gradient and cardiac output (Table 11–2). Some of the discrepancies between Doppler echo and invasive measurements of valve area are due to measurement variability for the invasive data and to limitations of the Gorlin formula itself. However, technical considerations in recording the Doppler and 2D echo data and the measurement variability of the noninvasive technique also are important (Table 11–3).

With careful attention to technical details, an experienced laboratory can obtain accurate noninvasive data for calculation of transaortic pressure gradients and valve areas in nearly all adults with valvular aortic stenosis. However, accurate noninvasive quantitation of aortic stenosis severity is a technically demanding procedure, and a significant learning-curve effect is seen in each laboratory for this clinical application. There are several potential pitfalls in the Doppler approach, as detailed below. Each laboratory should confirm the accuracy of its data by comparison with those of an experienced echocardiography laboratory or with other diagnostic tests.

THE AORTIC JET. Because of the high velocities seen in aortic stenosis (usually 3–7 m/s), CW Doppler ultrasound is needed for accurate measurement of the aortic jet signal. When aortic stenosis is suspected, the examination should include use of a non-imaging, dedicated CW Doppler transducer. The smaller "footprint" of the dedicated transducer allows optimal positioning and angulation of the ultrasound beam. In addition, a dedicated CW transducer has a higher signal-to-noise ratio than a combined imaging and Doppler transducer.

In recording the aortic jet velocity signal, a search is made for the highest frequency shift. This signal then is assumed to represent a near-parallel intercept angle (θ) between the ultrasound beam and the direction of the jet. With a parallel alignment, cosine θ

equals 1 and thus can be ignored in the Doppler equation (see Chapter 1). Any deviation from a parallel intercept angle will result in underestimation of jet velocity. For example, an intercept angle of 30° will result in a measured velocity of 4.3 m/s when the actual velocity is 5 m/s. Underestimation of velocity, which is squared in the Bernoulli equation, results in a large error in calculated pressure gradient. However, intercept angles within 15° of parallel will result in an error in velocity measurement of 5% or less.

The direction of the aortic jet often is eccentric relative to both the plane of the aortic valve and the long axis of the aorta and rarely can be predicted from the 2D images. Occasionally, jet direction can be visualized with color flow imaging, but, more often, the direction of the short jet of calcific stenosis cannot be identified. Even when jet direction is seen in a single tomographic plane, the orientation of the jet in the elevational plane remains unknown.

Pragmatically, the solution to the problem of aligning the ultrasound beam parallel to an aortic jet of unknown direction is to perform a careful search from several acoustic windows with optimal patient positioning and multiple transducer angulations. The highest velocity signal obtained then is assumed to represent the most parallel intercept angle. At a minimum, the aortic jet should be interrogated from an apical approach with the patient in a steep left lateral decubitus position on an examination bed with an apical cutout, from a high right parasternal position with the patient in a right lateral decubitus position, and from the suprasternal notch with the patient supine and the neck extended. Even then, the possibility of underestimation of jet velocity due to a nonparallel intercept angle cannot be excluded. In some cases, the highest velocity signal may be recorded from a subcostal or left parasternal window.

When the CW beam is aligned with the aortic jet, a smooth velocity curve is seen with a well-defined peak velocity and spectral darkening along the outer edge of the velocity curve. Audibly, the signal is high frequency and tonal. The spectral recording should be made with an appropriate velocity scale (at least 1 m/s higher than the observed maximum jet velocity), with wall filters set at a high level, and with gain adjusted to provide clear definition of the maximum velocity. Maximum velocity is measured at the edge of the dark velocity envelope. The VTI is measured by digitizing the velocity curve over systole.

Care is needed to correctly identify the origin of the high-velocity jet. Other high-velocity systolic jets (Table 11–4 and Fig. 11–11) may be mistaken for aortic stenosis if inadequate attention is paid to timing, shape, and associated diastolic flow curves. In some cases, 2D-"guided" CW Doppler may be helpful in correct identification of the jet, followed by recording with a nonimaging transducer for optimal signal quality.

TABLE 11–2   Selected Studies of Aortic Valve Area Determination

First Author and Year	Comparison	N	Study Group	R*	Range (cm²)	SEE* (cm²)
Hakki 1981	Simplified vs. original Gorlin formula	60	Aortic stenosis	0.96	0.2–2.0	0.10
Skjaerpe 1985	Cont eq vs. Gorlin	30	Aortic stenosis	0.89	0.4–2.4	0.12
Zoghbi 1986	Cont eq vs. Gorlin	39	Aortic stenosis	0.95	0.4–2.0	0.15
Otto 1986	Cont eq vs. Gorlin	48	Aortic stenosis	0.71	0.2–3.7	0.32
Teirstein 1986	Cont eq vs. Gorlin	30	Aortic stenosis	0.88	0.3–1.6	0.17
Oh 1988	Cont eq vs. Gorlin	100	Aortic stenosis	0.83	0.2–1.8	0.19
Danielson 1989	Cont eq vs. Gorlin	100	Aortic stenosis	0.96	0.4–2.0	—
Cannon 1985	Gorlin vs. videotape of valve opening	42	Porcine valves in pulsatile-flow model	0.87	0.6–2.5	0.28
	New formula vs. actual orifice area	42	Porcine valves in pulsatile-flow model	0.98	0.6–2.5	0.11
Segal 1987	Cont eq vs. actual valve area		In vitro pulsatile flow with orifice plates	0.99	0.05–0.5	0.016
	Gorlin formula vs. actual valve area			0.87		0.047
Cannon 1988	Gorlin vs. known valve area	135	Prosthetic aortic valves	0.39	0.6–2.3	—
Nishimura 1988	Cont eq vs. Gorlin	55	Pre-BAV	0.72	0.2–0.9	0.10
			Post-BAV	0.61	0.5–1.3	0.17
Desnoyers 1988	Cont eq vs. Gorlin	42	Pre-BAV	0.74	0.3–1.3	—
Tribouilloy 1994	TEE vs. cont eq	54	Aortic stenosis	0.96	0.3–2.0	0.11
	TEE vs. Gorlin			0.90		0.12
Cormier 1996	TEE vs. Gorlin	45	Aortic stenosis	0.74	0.5–1.4	—
Kim 1997	TEE vs. Gorlin	81	Aortic stenosis	0.89	0.4–2.0	0.04

BAV, balloon aortic valvuloplasty; Cont eq, continuity equation; Gorlin, Gorlin formula valve area; TEE, Planimetered 2D valve area on transesophageal echocardiography.

*If not stated in the publication, statistics were calculated from the raw data provided in tables. A blank indicates that data for this calculation were not available.

Data from Hakki et al: Circulation 63:1050–1055, 1981; Skjaerpe et al: Circulation 72:810–818, 1985; Zoghbi et al: Circulation 73:452–459, 1986; Otto et al: J Am Coll Cardiol 7:509–517, 1986; Teirstein et al: J Am Coll Cardiol 8:1059–1065, 1986; Oh et al: J Am Coll Cardiol 11:1227–1234, 1988; Danielson et al: Am J Cardiol 63:1107–1111, 1989; Cannon et al: Circulation 71:1170–1178, 1985; Segal et al: J Am Coll Cardiol 9:1294–1305, 1987; Cannon et al: Am J Cardiol 62:113–116, 1988; Nishimura et al: Circulation 78:791–799, 1988; Desnoyers et al: Am J Cardiol 62:1078–1084, 1988; Tribouilloy et al: Am Heart J 128:526–532, 1994; Cormier et al: Am J Cardiol 77:882–885, 1996; Kim et al: Am J Cardiol 79:436–441, 1997.

OUTFLOW TRACT DIAMETER. LVOT diameter is measured in mid-systole, just proximal to and parallel with the plane of the stenotic aortic valve, from the white/black interface of the septal endocardial echo to the white/black interface at the base of the anterior mitral leaflet. A parasternal long-axis view provides the most accurate measurement, because it depends on the axial (rather than lateral) resolution of the ultrasound beam. Outflow tract cross-sectional area (CSA) is assumed to be circular so that

$$CSA_{LVOT} = \pi (D/2)^2 \tag{11–15}$$

Note that small errors in outflow tract diameter measurement may lead to large errors in calculated area.

TABLE 11–3 Pitfalls in Echocardiographic Evaluation of Aortic Stenosis

Technical

Acoustic access
Intercept angle between AS jet and ultrasound beam
Outflow tract diameter imaging
Respiratory motion
Learning-curve effect

Interpretation

Identification of flow signal origin (AS vs. MR)
Beat-to-beat variability (AF, PVCs)
Intraobserver and interobserver measurement variability
Calculation errors

Physiology

Interim changes in heart rate or stroke volume
Dependence of velocity and ΔP on volume flow rate
Progression of AS severity

Standards of Reference

Maximum vs. peak-to-peak ΔP
Continuity vs. Gorlin formula valve areas

TABLE 11–4 Other High-Velocity Systolic Jets That May Be Mistaken for Aortic Stenosis

Subaortic obstruction (fixed or dynamic)
Mitral regurgitation
Tricuspid regurgitation
Ventricular septal defect
Pulmonic valve or branch PA stenosis
Peripheral vascular stenosis (e.g., subclavian artery)

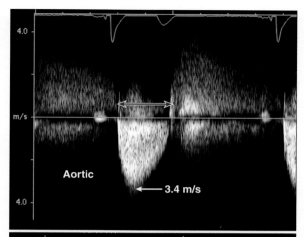
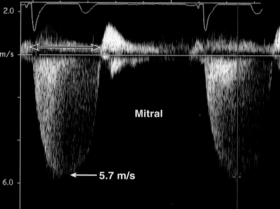
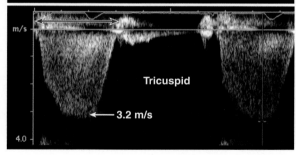

Figure 11–11 From an apical approach, three different high-velocity systolic jets directed away from the transducer were recorded in this patient with moderate aortic stenosis, mild mitral regurgitation, and severe pulmonary hypertension. These three flow signals can be differentiated based on timing, shape, and associated diastolic flow signals.

Furthermore, of the measurements made for evaluating aortic stenosis severity, outflow tract diameter shows the greatest intraobserver and interobserver variability. Several measurements should be averaged to minimize this potential source of error.

OUTFLOW TRACT VELOCITY. The outflow tract systolic velocity signal is recorded from an apical approach using pulsed Doppler echo. Either an anteriorly angulated four-chamber view or an apical long-axis view can be used. A sample volume 3 to 5 mm in length is positioned just proximal to the region of acceleration into the stenotic jet. Correct positioning is ensured by starting with the sample volume *in the* jet and slowly repositioning it apically until a smooth velocity curve with a well-defined peak velocity and little spectral broadening is seen. The presence of

an aortic valve closing (but not opening) click indicates that the sample volume is immediately adjacent to the valve. A transducer position is chosen initially that indicates a parallel alignment between the ultrasound beam and the long axis of the outflow tract on 2D imaging. Then, transducer position and angulation are adjusted, based on the audible Doppler signal and the velocity curve, to record the highest velocity signal proximal to the flow acceleration region. In addition, the sample volume is moved laterally across the outflow tract in each apical view to document a flat flow velocity profile.

The rationale for this protocol for sample volume positioning is that the outflow tract diameter and velocity signals need to be recorded *at the same* anatomic site for accurate transaortic stroke volume calculations. Necessarily, these two recordings are made nonsimultaneously from different acoustic windows because of the need for a parallel orientation between the Doppler beam and the direction of blood flow for accurate velocity measurement versus a perpendicular orientation between the 2D echo beam and the outflow tract for accurate diameter measurement. Measuring both immediately adjacent to the stenotic valve provides a reference point that ensures that both measurements are made at the same spatial location.

The maximum outflow tract velocity is measured at the edge of the most intense spectral signal. The VTI is measured by tracing the modal velocity of the systolic flow curve. Wall filters are set low enough that the systolic ejection period is clearly defined.

Coexisting Valvular Disease

A high percentage (~80%) of patients with predominant aortic stenosis also have aortic regurgitation, most often mild or moderate in severity. The degree of regurgitation can be evaluated as described in Chapter 12. Although coexisting aortic regurgitation results in an increase in the transaortic pressure gradient (due to increased transaortic volume flow), valve area calculations are accurate because the stroke volume in the continuity equation still represents transaortic stroke volume.

Coexisting mitral regurgitation also is common due to mitral annular calcification in adults with calcific aortic stenosis. Again, mitral regurgitant severity can be evaluated as described in Chapter 12. Particular attention should be directed toward AVA calculations when mitral regurgitation is present. Otherwise, severe aortic stenosis may be missed if the transaortic pressure gradient is low due to low transaortic volume flow.

Patients with rheumatic aortic stenosis may have significant mitral stenosis, mitral regurgitation, or mixed mitral disease. Evaluation of aortic stenosis severity is unaffected by these coexisting lesions other than the aforementioned potential for a low transaortic pressure gradient if the transaortic volume flow rate is depressed.

Response of the Left Ventricle

The LV response to the chronic pressure overload of valvular aortic stenosis is concentric hypertrophy—an increase in LV mass due to increased wall thickness

without chamber dilation. Hypertrophy tends to normalize LV wall stress, since

$$\text{Wall stress} \cong (R/Th) \times P \qquad (11\text{--}16)$$

where R is ventricular radius, Th is wall thickness, and P is LV pressure. The relative wall thickness (the ratio of wall thickness to radius) is a useful and simple measure of the degree of hypertrophy. LV mass (which can be indexed for body size) can be calculated from tracings of endocardium and epicardium at end-diastole, as described in Chapter 6.

In aortic stenosis, LV systolic function tends to be preserved until late in the disease course. When LV systolic dysfunction does occur, it may be due to the increased afterload of outflow obstruction and thus may be reversible after valve replacement. Ventricular systolic function can be evaluated qualitatively or quantitatively, as described in Chapter 6. Even a qualitative evaluation has significant prognostic implications in unoperated adults with aortic stenosis.

Clinical Applications

Decisions about Timing of Intervention

Doppler echocardiography is the diagnostic test of choice for adults with suspected aortic stenosis (Table 11-5). A complete echocardiographic examination includes evaluation of stenosis severity, assessment of LV systolic function, and evaluation of

---

TABLE 11–5   Echocardiographic Approach to Valvular Aortic Stenosis
Valve anatomy, etiology of stenosis
Exclude other causes of LV outflow obstruction
Stenosis severity
• Jet velocity
• Mean pressure gradient
• Continuity equation valve area
Left ventricle
• Dimensions/volumes
• Hypertrophy
• Ejection fraction
• Diastolic function
Aorta
• Aortic diameter at sinuses and mid-ascending aorta
• Evaluate for coarctation if bicuspid valve present
Aortic regurgitation
• Vena contracta width
• Quantitation if > mild
Mitral regurgitation
• Mechanism
• Severity
Pulmonary pressures

coexisting valvular lesions, as described previously. The presence of irregular focal thickening of the aortic valve leaflets without obstruction to outflow (a jet velocity <2.6 m/s) is called "aortic sclerosis." When aortic sclerosis is present, further evaluation of stenosis severity is not needed, although some of these patients have progressive disease over several years.

When obstruction to outflow is present, stenosis severity is categorized as mild, moderate, or severe (Table 11–6) based on jet velocity, mean gradient, and valve area. Mild stenosis is characterized by an aortic jet velocity between 2.6 and 3 m/s. Additional measures of stenosis severity are rarely needed, although caution is needed to ensure that the jet velocity measurement is accurate; a nonparallel intercept angle between the aortic jet and the Doppler beam can result in underestimation of jet velocity and the erroneous conclusion that severe stenosis is not present.

When aortic jet velocity is between 3 and 4 m/s, calculations of mean gradient and valve area are essential, because some of these patients have moderate, or even mild, stenosis, while others have severe stenosis with a relatively low cardiac output. Identification of severe stenosis is critical, because valve replacement is appropriate when symptoms are present and obstruction is severe (Fig. 11–12). A continuity equation valve area >1.5 cm^2 is consistent with only mild aortic stenosis. A valve area of 1.0 to 1.5 cm^2 is classified as moderate aortic stenosis, but the degree of obstruction may be only mild in smaller adults; consideration of the outflow tract to aortic velocity ratio or indexing valve area for body size may be helpful in this situation. With a valve area <1.0 cm^2, a jet velocity <4.0 m/s, and impaired LV systolic function, the possibility of "low-gradient low-output" aortic stenosis must be considered. Further evaluation includes the degree of valve calcification and, in selected cases, dobutamine stress echocardiography (see below).

A jet velocity >4.0 m/s confirms severe stenosis, but valve area calculation is recommended both to confirm this diagnosis and to identify patients with mixed stenosis and regurgitation. In clinical practice, valve area calculation probably is unnecessary when jet velocity is very high (>5.0 m/s), and the valve is severely calcified with reduced systolic opening. Adults with a jet velocity over 4.0 m/s but a valve area of 1.0 to 1.5 cm^2 may have symptoms due to aortic valve disease (and are candidates for valve replacement) if there is coexisting moderate or severe aortic regurgitation or if the patient has a large body size (Table 11–7). Decision making in these patients with mixed stenosis and regurgitation is based on multiple measures of stenosis severity (jet velocity and mean gradient in addition to valve area), quantitation of regurgitant severity, and careful assessment of clinical symptoms and functional status.

Disease Progression and Prognosis in Asymptomatic Aortic Stenosis

In observing individual patients over time, the reproducibility of a technique, as well as its accuracy, is important. Reproducibility of Doppler echo data includes:

❑ Recording variability (e.g., intercept angle, wall filters, signal strength, acoustic window)
❑ Measurement variability (e.g., identification of the maximum velocity, outflow tract diameter)
❑ Physiologic variability (e.g., interim changes in heart rate, stroke volume, or pressure gradient)

Aortic jet maximum velocity measurement is reproducible with an intraobserver variability of 3.2%

TABLE 11–6 Categories of Stenosis Severity

	Aortic Sclerosis	Mild	Moderate	Severe
Aortic Stenosis				
Aortic jet velocity (m/s)	<2.6 m/s	2.6–3.0	3–4	>4
Mean gradient (mm Hg)	—	<20 (30*)	20–40	>40 (50*)
AVA (cm^2)	—	>1.5	1.0–1.5	<1.0
Indexed AVA (cm^2/m^2)		>0.85	0.60–0.85	<0.6
Velocity ratio		>0.50	0.25–0.50	<0.25
		Mild	Moderate	Severe
Mitral Stenosis				
Mean gradient (mm Hg)		5	5–10	>10
MVA (cm^2)		>1.5	1.0–1.5	<1.0
Pulmonary systolic pressure (mm Hg)		<30	30–50	>50

AVA, aortic valve area; MVA, mitral valve area.
*ESC guidelines use higher mean gradient cutoffs as shown in parantheses.

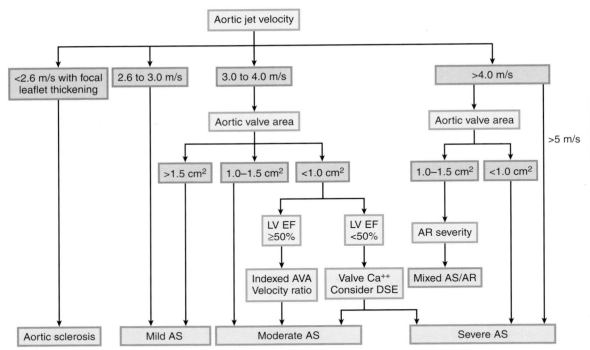

Figure 11–12 Flow chart of recommended approach for echocardiographic assessment of suspected aortic stenosis (AS) when imaging shows an anatomically abnormal valve. Yellow boxes indicate echocardiographic measurements, blue boxes indicate the measures of stenosis severity, and green boxes indicate the category of stenosis severity based on these quantitative measurements. AR, aortic regurgitation; AVA, aortic valve area; Ca^{++}, calcification; DSE, dobutamine stress echocardiography; EF, ejection fraction.

TABLE 11–7	Possible Causes of Discrepancies in Measures of Aortic Stenosis Severity

Severe AS by Velocity or Gradient But Not by Valve Area (AS velocity >4 m/s and AVA >1.0 cm²)

LVOT diameter overestimated
LVOT velocity recorded too close to valve
High transaortic flow rate due to:
- Moderate-to-severe aortic regurgitation
- High-output state
- Large body size

Severe AS by Valve Area But Not by Velocity or Gradient (AS velocity ≤4 m/s and AVA ≤1.0 cm²)

LVOT diameter underestimated
LVOT velocity recorded too far from valve
Small body size
Low transaortic flow volume due to:
- Low ejection fraction
- Small ventricular chamber
- Moderate-to-severe mitral regurgitation
- Moderate-to-severe mitral stenosis

AS, aortic stenosis; AVA, aortic valve area; LVOT, left ventricular outflow tract.

and an interobserver variability of 3.1%. Outflow tract velocity, recorded by two experienced sonographers, also is reproducible with intraobserver and interobserver variability of 3% and 3.9%. Measurement of outflow tract diameter shows the greatest variability, with intraobserver and interobserver mean coefficients of variation of 5.1% and 7.9%. These variabilities indicate that for values at the middle of the range, a change greater than measurement variability is greater than 0.2 m/s for maximum jet velocity, greater than 0.1 m/s for outflow tract velocity, greater than 0.2 cm for outflow tract diameter, and greater than 0.15 cm² for AVA.

Doppler echo has been used to follow disease progression in asymptomatic adults with valvular aortic stenosis. Several observations from these studies are noteworthy. First, prognosis depends on the presence or absence of clinical symptoms and not on hemodynamic severity per se. There is significant overlap in all measures of hemodynamic severity between symptomatic and asymptomatic adults, and it is not unusual to see asymptomatic individuals with a jet velocity greater than 4 m/s. Second, the rate of hemodynamic progression is variable from patient to patient. On average, jet velocity increases by 0.3 m/s per year, mean pressure gradient increases by about 7 mm Hg per year, and valve area decreases by about 0.1 cm² per year. Third, while hemodynamic

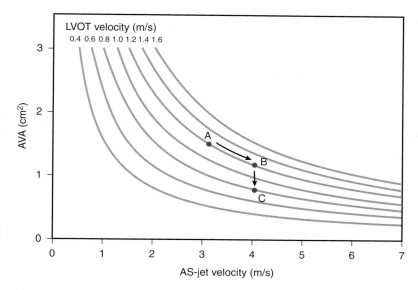

Figure 11–13 Graph of the relationship between aortic valve area (AVA) and AS-jet velocity for LV outflow tract (LVOT) velocities ranging from 0.4 to 1.6 m/s. In the example shown, a patient initially has a jet velocity of 3 m/s and a valve area of 1.5 cm^2 (**A**). As stenosis severity increases, jet velocity increases to 4.0 m/s and valve area decreases to 1.2 cm^2 (**B**). However, with further disease progression (**C**), jet velocity was unchanged at 4 m/s, but valve area decreased to 0.8 cm^2 in the setting of decreased transaortic volume flow (LVOT velocity 1.2 to 0.8 m/s).

progression may present as an increase in aortic jet velocity (and transaortic pressure gradient), disease progression can occur with no change in jet velocity if there is a concurrent decrease in transaortic volume flow rate (Fig. 11–13).

In patients with asymptomatic aortic stenosis, clinical outcome is highly dependent on Doppler jet velocity. In those with an initial jet velocity less than 3 m/s, the rate of symptom onset requiring valve replacement is 8% per year, compared to 17% per year for those with a jet velocity between 3 and 4 m/s and 40% per year for those with a jet velocity greater than 4 m/s (Fig. 11–14). Although it could be argued that once the baseline examination has established the diagnosis,

the patient can be followed clinically, because the timing of valve replacement is determined by symptom onset, adults with aortic stenosis often have significant comorbid disease, so that knowledge of hemodynamic severity can be important in patient management. Thus, in the clinically stable patient, repeat echocardiography every 2 to 3 years is indicated when the jet velocity is less than 3 m/s, with annual examinations appropriate in those with higher jet velocities.

Evaluation of Aortic Stenosis with Left Ventricular Systolic Dysfunction

In the patient with significant LV systolic dysfunction and aortic valve stenosis, evaluation of stenosis severity is problematic. Even with severe stenosis, pressure gradients may be low due to the low transaortic volume flow rate. Conversely, while valve area is less flow-dependent than pressure gradients, valve area can vary in parallel with flow rate and thus calculated valve area may appear to be reduced when ventricular dysfunction is present, even if stenosis is not severe. Even when LV ejection fraction is normal, the volume of transaortic flow may be small if there is a small ventricular size, for example, in older women or hypertensive patients.

Evaluation of low-output low-gradient aortic stenosis is challenging and includes evaluation for other causes of LV dysfunction, assessment of aortic valve anatomy (e.g., a bicuspid valve) and leaflet calcification, consideration of the therapeutic options, and comorbidities and the response to medical therapy. In selected cases, dobutamine stress echocardiography can be helpful. Aortic jet velocity, mean gradient, and continuity equation valve area are measured at baseline and with dobutamine infusion, up to a maximum dose of 20 µg/kg/min (Fig. 11–15). A

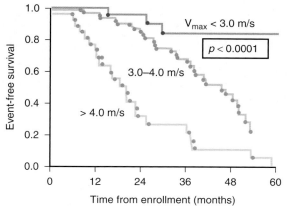

Figure 11–14 Cox regression analysis showing event-free survival in AS groups defined by aortic jet velocity at entry (p = 0.0001 by log rank test). *(From Otto CM, Burwash IG, Legget ME, et al: A prospective study of asymptomatic valvular aortic stenosis. Clinical, echocardiographic, and exercise predictors of outcome. Circulation 95:2262–2270, 1997. Used with permission.)*

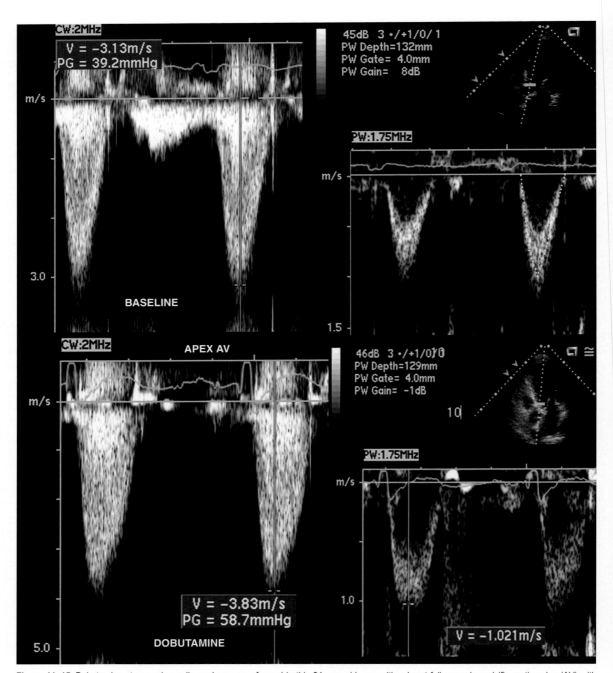

Figure 11–15 Dobutamine stress echocardiography was performed in this 84-year-old man with a heart failure and a calcific aortic valve (AV) with resting data (*top*) and stress data (*bottom*) for aortic jet velocity (*left*) and LV outflow velocity (*right*). At rest, his LV ejection fraction (EF) was 33% with an aortic jet velocity of 3.3 m/s and a continuity equation valve area of 1.0 cm². With dobutamine at 10 µg/kg/min, EF increased to 42% with an increase in transvalvular volume flow rate as evidenced by the increase in outflow tract velocity. Aortic jet velocity increased to 3.8 m/s, and continuity equation valve area showed no significant change at 1.0 cm². This response to dobutamine suggests fixed valve obstruction, as did the severe valve calcification seen on 2D imaging.

significant increase in valve area with an increase in transaortic volume flow rate reflects flexible leaflets (mild-moderate stenosis), whereas a fixed valve area indicates stiff leaflets that cannot open any further. Stress findings consistent with severe stenosis include a final valve area <1.0 cm² with a jet velocity >4.0 m/s or a mean gradient >40 mm Hg. Lack of contractile reserve—the failure of transaortic volume flow rate or LV ejection fraction to increase by at least 20% with dobutamine—is a poor prognostic sign. A more detailed discussion of this problem can be found in Suggested Readings 11–13.

MITRAL STENOSIS

Diagnostic Imaging of the Mitral Valve

Echocardiography in the patient with mitral stenosis includes evaluation of:

- ❑ Valve anatomy, mobility, and calcification
- ❑ Mean transmitral pressure gradient
- ❑ 2D echo mitral valve area
- ❑ Doppler pressure half-time ($T\frac{1}{2}$) valve area
- ❑ Pulmonary artery pressures
- ❑ Coexisting mitral regurgitation

Rheumatic Disease

Rheumatic disease predominantly affects the mitral valve and is almost always the cause of mitral stenosis. Rheumatic valvular disease is characterized by commissural fusion, which results in bowing or doming of the valve leaflets in diastole (Fig. 11–16). The base and midsections of the leaflets move toward the ventricular apex, while the motion of the leaflet tips is restricted due to fusion of the anterior and posterior leaflets along the medial and lateral commissures. Thickening at the leaflet tips occurs frequently, but the remainder of the leaflets can show variable degrees of thickening and/or calcification. If the base and mid-portions of the leaflets are relatively thin, leaflet mobility is normal other than the fused commissures. The rheumatic process also typically affects the subvalvular region with fusion, shortening, fibrosis, and calcification of the mitral chordae.

In rheumatic mitral stenosis, 2D echo allows detailed evaluation of mitral valve morphology, including assessment of leaflet thickness, leaflet mobility, the degree of calcification, and the extent of subvalvular involvement on TTE parasternal and apical views (Fig. 11–17). Occasionally, if TTE images are suboptimal, TEE imaging may be needed for evaluation of mitral valve anatomy, although definition of subvalvular disease may be limited due to shadows and reverberations from calcification of the mitral valve and annulus.

Mitral Annular Calcification

Mitral annular calcification is a common finding on echocardiography in elderly subjects. Mild annular calcification appears as an isolated area of calcification on the LV side of the posterior annulus, near the base of the posterior mitral leaflet. In more severe mitral annular calcification, increased echogenicity is seen in a hemielliptical pattern involving the entire posterior annulus. The area of fibrous continuity between the anterior mitral leaflet and the aortic root rarely is involved. The echocardiographic finding of mitral annular calcification, like aortic valve sclerosis, indicates a higher risk of adverse cardiovascular outcomes, even when valve function is relatively normal. Mitral annular calcification may result in mild-to-moderate mitral regurgitation due to increased rigidity of the mitral annulus. Occasionally the calcification extends into the base of the mitral leaflets themselves, rarely resulting in functional mitral stenosis due to narrowing of the diastolic flow area (Fig. 11–18). Calcific mitral stenosis can be distinguished from rheumatic disease by careful imaging techniques to demonstrate thin and mobile mitral leaflet tips without commissural fusion.

Differential Diagnosis

In patients referred for echocardiography with suspected mitral stenosis, the initial differential diagnosis includes other causes of pulmonary congestion. Standard echo Doppler evaluation will reveal whether LV systolic dysfunction, aortic valve disease, or mitral regurgitation is present. The possibility of diastolic LV dysfunction also should be considered. The rare case of an atrial myxoma or other atrial tumor obstructing LV inflow, thus mimicking the clinical presentation of mitral stenosis, can easily be diagnosed by 2D imaging (see Chapter 15). Rarely, a patient with mild obstruction due to cor triatriatum may present as an adult.

Quantitation of Mitral Stenosis Severity

Pressure Gradients

The mean diastolic transmitral pressure gradient (Fig. 11–19) can be determined from the transmitral velocity curve using the simplified Bernoulli equation:

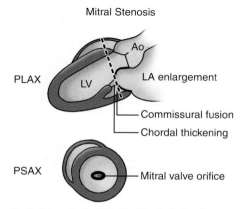

Mitral Stenosis

PLAX

Ao

LV

LA enlargement

Commissural fusion

Chordal thickening

PSAX

Mitral valve orifice

Figure 11–16 Schematic diagram of the 2D echo findings in mitral stenosis. In the parasternal long-axis view (PLAX), commissural fusion with diastolic doming of the mitral leaflets is seen, as well as chordal thickening and fusion. In a parasternal short-axis view (PSAX), at the mitral valve orifice level, the area of opening can be planimetered. The plane of the short-axis view is indicated by a *dashed line* on the long-axis image.

$$\text{Mean mitral } \Delta P = \frac{4v2_1 + 4v2_2 + 4v2_3 + ... + 4v2_n}{n}$$

$$(11\text{--}16)$$

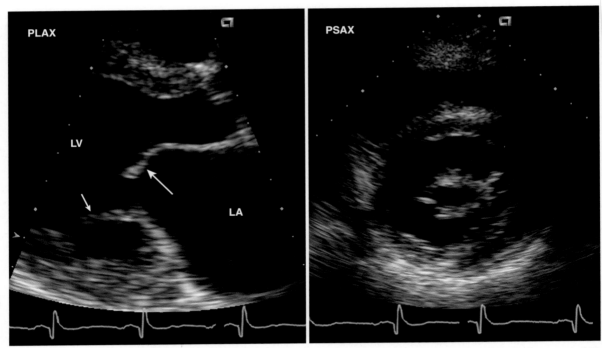

Figure 11–17 Parasternal long-axis (PLAX) view (*left*) of a patient with mild rheumatic mitral stenosis showing the typical doming (*long arrow*) of the anterior mitral leaflet due to commissural fusion. There is also chordal thickening and fusion (*small arrow*). LA enlargement is present. The parasternal short-axis (PSAX) view (*right*) allows accurate planimetry of the mitral orifice area if care is taken to identify the smallest opening by scanning slowly from apex toward the base.

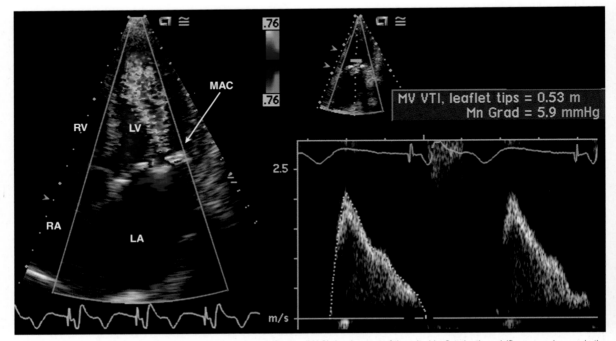

Figure 11–18 In an elderly patient with severe mitral annular calcification (MAC), involvement of the mitral leaflets by the calcific process in seen in the apical view with a narrow antegrade flow jet on color Doppler (*left*). The pulsed Doppler velocity curve across the valve shows an increased gradient (6 mm Hg) with a slightly prolonged pressure consistent with mild functional mitral stenosis.

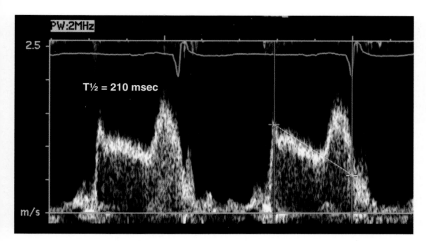

Figure 11–19 Transmitral flow curve in the same patient as in Figure 11–17. Using this velocity curve, pressure gradients can be calculated with the Bernoulli equation and valve area by the T½ method. Note the well-defined maximal velocity and the clearly defined, linear deceleration slope. An *A* velocity is seen because sinus rhythm is present.

With severe stenosis, the mean pressure gradient may be as high as 20 to 30 mm Hg but often is only 5 to 15 mm Hg. The variability in pressure gradients in severe mitral stenosis is due to the dependence of pressure gradients on volume flow rate as well as valve area. Severe mitral stenosis may be associated with a low stroke volume (due to the limitation of LV diastolic filling), resulting in a relatively low mean gradient. If volume flow rate increases, for example, with exercise, an increase in transmitral gradient is seen. As for other types of valvular stenosis, calculation of valve area, considering both pressure gradient and volume flow rate, is helpful in quantitation of mitral stenosis severity.

Mitral Valve Area

Two-Dimensional Echo Valve Area. Compared with valvular aortic stenosis, the 3D anatomy of rheumatic mitral stenosis is simpler with a planar elliptical orifice that is relatively constant in position in mid-diastole (Fig. 11–20). Thus, 2D short-axis imaging of the diastolic orifice allows direct planimetry of valve area. This approach has been well validated compared with measurement of valve area at surgery and in comparison with catheterization-determined valve areas. Because the shape of the mitral valve inflow region is similar to a funnel, with the narrowest opening at the leaflet tips, it is important to begin

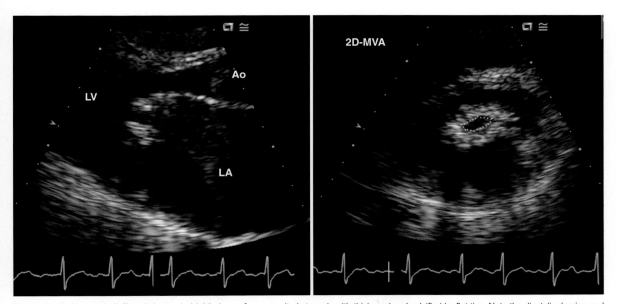

Figure 11–20 Long-axis (*left*) and short-axis (*right*) views of severe mitral stenosis with thickened and calcified leaflet tips. Note the diastolic doming and severe commissural fusion. Valve area by 2D planimetry is 0.6 cm^2. In addition, severe LA enlargement is present.

the 2D scan at the apex, slowly moving the image plane toward the mitral valve to identify the smallest orifice. With a low overall 2D gain setting, the inner edge of the black/white interface is traced. Given the accuracy of this technique, 2D echo mitral valve area (MVA) should be measured in patients with mitral stenosis whenever image quality is adequate.

PRESSURE HALF-TIME VALVE AREA. Calculation of mitral valve area by the *pressure half-time* ($T^{1/2}$) method is based on the concept that the *rate* of pressure decline across the stenotic mitral orifice is determined by the size of the orifice: The smaller the orifice, the slower the rate of pressure decline (Figs. 11–21 and 11–22). The influence of LA and LV compliance on the rate of pressure decline is assumed to be negligible—an assumption that is not always warranted, especially immediately after percutaneous commissurotomy.

The pressure half-time is defined as the time interval (in milliseconds) between the maximum early diastolic transmitral pressure gradient and the time point where the pressure gradient is half the maximum value. Initially, this concept was evaluated using invasive measurements of LA and LV pressure, which demonstrated a constant $T^{1/2}$ for a given individual, even with exercise-induced changes in volume flow rate, suggesting that this measurement is a constant measure of stenosis severity for a given valve area.

This concept then was adapted to transmitral Doppler flow velocity curves. Given the quadratic relationship between velocity and pressure gradients, the half-time is determined from a Doppler spectral velocity curve as the time interval from the maximum mitral velocity (V_{max}) to the point where the velocity has fallen to $V_{max}/\sqrt{2}$. Initial studies comparing Doppler half-time data with invasively determined Gorlin valve areas found a linear relationship, with a half-time of approximately 220 ms corresponding to a valve area of 1 cm^2. The empirical formula

$$MVA = 220/T^{1/2} \qquad (11–17)$$

was proposed and has been shown to correlate well with invasive valve areas in several clinical studies (Table 11–8).

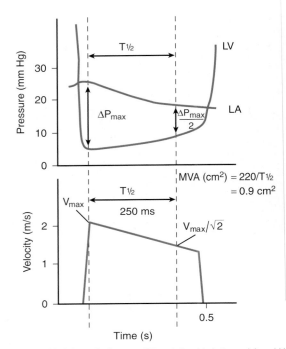

Figure 11–22 Schematic diagram of the relationship between LA and LV pressures and the Doppler velocity curve in mitral stenosis. Maximum velocity and the diastolic slope are identified as shown, yielding a $T^{1/2}$ of 250 ms corresponding to a MVA of 0.9 cm^2. There is no A velocity because atrial fibrillation is present.

CONTINUITY EQUATION MITRAL VALVE AREA. The continuity principle for calculation of valve area also can be applied to the mitral orifice:

$$MVA = transmitral\ SV/VTI_{MS\ jet} \qquad (11–18)$$

where SV is stroke volume (cm^3), VTI is the velocity-time integral (cm) in the mitral stenosis jet, and MVA (cm^2) is the mitral valve area. Stroke volume can be determined from the LVOT CSA and VTI (in the absence of aortic or mitral regurgitation) or from the pulmonary artery diameter and VTI. Note that stroke volume measured at either of these sites will represent transmitral volume flow accurately only if there is no significant mitral regurgitation.

Figure 11–21 $T^{1/2}$ measurement in the patient with severe MS shown in Figure 11–20. The $T^{1/2}$ of 302 ms corresponds to a valve area of 0.7 cm^2. The patient is in atrial fibrillation so no A velocity is seen.

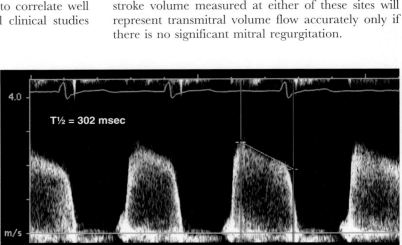

TABLE 11–8   Selected Studies of Mitral Valve Area Determination

First Author and Year	Comparison	N	Study Group	R	Range (cm²)	SEE (cm²)
Gorlin 1951	MVA by Gorlin formula vs. direct autopsy or surgery	11	MS	0.89	0.5–1.5	0.15
Libanoff 1968	T½ at rest vs. exercise	20	Mitral valve disease	0.98	20–340 ms	21 ms
Henry 1975	2D echo vs. direct measurement at surgery	20	MS patients undergoing surgery	0.92	0.5–3.5	—
Holen 1977	MVA by Doppler vs. Gorlin	10	MS	0.98	0.6–3.4	0.18
Hatle 1979	T½ vs. Gorlin MVA	32	MS	0.74	0.4–3.5	—
Smith 1986	2D echo vs. Gorlin	37	MS alone	0.83	0.4–2.3	0.26
		35	Prior commissurotomy	0.58		0.28
	T½ MVA vs. Gorlin	(37)	MS alone	0.85		0.22
		(35)	Prior commissurotomy	0.90		0.14
Come 1988	T½ MVA vs. Gorlin	37	Pre-MBC	0.51	0.6–1.3	—
			Post-MBC	0.47	1.2–3.8	—
	Gorlin vs. Gorlin		Repeat cath	0.74	0.4–1.4	—
Thomas 1988	Predicted vs. actual T½	18	Pre-MBC	0.93–0.96		
			Post-MBC	0.52–0.66		
Chen 1989	T½ MVA vs. Gorlin	18	Pre-MBC	0.81	0.4–1.2	0.11
			Immediately post-MBC	0.84	1.3–2.6	0.20
			24–48hr post-MBC	0.72	1.3–2.6	0.49
Faletra 1996	2D echo vs. direct measurement	30	MS undergoing surgical MVR	0.95	0.6–2.0	0.06
	T½ vs. direct measurement	30		0.80		0.09
	Cont eq vs. direct measurement	30		0.87		0.09
	Flow area vs. direct measurement	30		0.54		0.10

Cont eq, continuity equation; Gorlin, Gorlin formula valve area; MBC, mitral balloon commissurotomy; MS, mitral stenosis; MVA, mitral valve area; MVR, mitral valve replacement; T½, pressure half-time.
Data from Gorlin et al: Am Heart J 41:1–29, 1951; Libanoff et al: Circulation 38:144–150, 1968; Henry et al: Circulation 51:827–831, 1975; Holen et al: Acta Med Scand 201:83–88, 1977; Hatle et al: Circulation 60:1096–1104, 1979; Smith et al: Circulation 73:100–107, 1986; Come et al: Am J Cardiol 61:817–825, 1988; Thomas et al: Circulation 78:980–993, 1988; Chen et al: J Am Coll Cardiol 13:1309–1313, 1989; Faletra et al: J Am Coll Cardiol 28:1190–1197, 1996.

In theory, transmitral volume flow rate can be calculated accurately in mitral stenosis even when mitral regurgitation is present using the PISA method. The color Doppler flow parameters are adjusted to demonstrate a well-defined hemispheric aliasing surface area on the LA side of the mitral orifice. The velocity at this location equals the Nyquist limit (the "aliasing" velocity). The surface area of the aliased boundary can be calculated as the surface area of a hemisphere with diameter measured from the color flow image. Multiplying this area times the known velocity yields the volume flow rate, which then can be used in conjunction with the transmitral velocity-time integral in the continuity equation. One difficulty with this approach is that the volume flow rate must be integrated over the diastolic filling period; a single color image yields only the volume flow rate at one time point in diastole. Because of this problem, the proximal isovelocity method has not been widely applied in mitral stenosis.

Technical Considerations and Potential Pitfalls

As for any intracardiac blood flow, accurate pressure gradient calculations depend on accurate velocity measurements, which require a near-parallel intercept angle between the direction of blood flow and the Doppler beam (Table 11–9). The mitral stenosis jet nearly always can be recorded from an apical approach, but careful transducer positioning and angulation are needed to record an optimal signal. Color flow imaging may be helpful in defining the jet direction in a given tomographic plane. Depending on the maximum jet velocity, the velocity curve can be recorded with conventional pulsed, high–pulse repetition frequency, or CW Doppler ultrasound. Pulsed Doppler recordings may show better definition of the maximum velocity and early-diastolic slope than CW Doppler recordings because of a better signal-to-noise ratio.

Direct planimetry of mitral valve area on 2D short-axis images has proven to be a valid technique in most clinical situations. However, definition of valve area may be difficult if image quality is poor or if there is extensive distortion of the valve anatomy. Valve area can be underestimated if gain settings are too high and can be overestimated if the smallest area at the leaflet tips is not recorded. Low gain settings and careful scanning in a short-axis

plane from the apex toward the base help avoid these potential problems.

Pressure half-time valve area calculations have significant limitations in certain clinical settings. When coexisting aortic regurgitation is present, LV filling occurs both antegrade across the mitral valve and retrograde across the aortic valve (Fig. 11–23). This may result in a more rapid rise in LV diastolic pressure than if there were no aortic regurgitation, resulting in a shorter $T\frac{1}{2}$ measurement. Conversely, if severe aortic regurgitation impairs mitral leaflet opening, functional mitral stenosis may be superimposed on anatomic mitral stenosis, with lengthening of the $T\frac{1}{2}$ measurement. In clinical practice, if the 2D echo shows rheumatic mitral stenosis and only mild-to-moderate aortic regurgitation is present, the half-time method remains a useful approach for evaluation of stenosis severity. If aortic regurgitation is severe, or if the mitral valve anatomy is atypical, the potential influence of coexisting lesions should be considered.

A major assumption of the half-time method is that LA and LV compliances do not significantly affect the rate of pressure gradient decline across the stenotic orifice. While this assumption appears to be warranted in clinically stable patients with mitral stenosis, it is *not* justified in the period immediately after catheter mitral valvuloplasty. After relief of mitral stenosis, the fall in LA pressure and the

---

TABLE 11–9   Pitfalls in Evaluation of Mitral Stenosis Severity

Pressure Gradient

Intercept angle between mitral stenosis jet and ultrasound beam
Beat-to-beat variability in atrial fibrillation
Dependence on transvalvular volume flow rate (e.g., exercise, coexisting mitral regurgitation)

2D Valve Area

Image orientation
Tomographic plane
2D gain settings
Intraobserver and interobserver variability in planimetry of orifice
Poor acoustic access
Deformed valve anatomy post-valvuloplasty

T½ Valve Area

Definition of V_{max} and early-diastolic slope
Nonlinear early-diastolic velocity slope
Sinus rhythm with *a* wave superimposed on early-diastolic slope
Influence of coexisting aortic regurgitation
Changing LV and LA compliances immediately after commissurotomy

Continuity Equation Mitral Valve Area

Accurate measurement of transmitral stroke volume

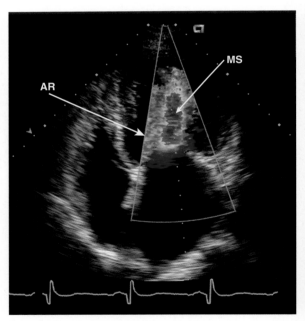

Figure 11–23 Color flow imaging in an apical four-chamber view shows the mitral stenosis (MS) jet and the aortic regurgitant (AR) jet in this patient with rheumatic disease. Although the AR usually does not affect LV pressures enough to invalidate the T½ method, care is needed to correctly identify the separate signals on pulsed and CW Doppler recordings.

increase in LV filling are accompanied by directionally opposite changes in LA and LV compliance. During the 24 to 72 hours after the procedure, equilibrium has not been reached, and the T½ may not be an accurate reflection of orifice area. After this adjustment period, compliances stabilize, and the half-time method again provides useful information.

Even under physiologically stable conditions, accurate T½ measurements require careful recording of the mitral stenosis velocity curve. It is important that the intercept angle be parallel to flow and *constant* throughout diastole to avoid artifactual distortion in the shape of the curve. The maximum early-diastolic velocity and the early-diastolic deceleration slope should be well defined. In addition, the half-time is most easily and reproducibly measured if the deceleration slope is linear. If a linear slope cannot be obtained even after careful adjustment of transducer position and angulation, the measurement should be made using the mid-diastolic slope of the curve.

In atrial fibrillation, several beats are averaged, since mean gradient will vary with the RR interval. While the half-time will be relatively constant despite variation in the length of diastole, only beats where the diastolic filling period is long enough to show the early-diastolic slope clearly are appropriate for measurement. Although the T½ method is accurate when sinus rhythm is present, the increase in velocity due to atrial contraction may obscure the early-diastolic slope, particularly at high heart rates, so that half-time measurements may not be possible unless a slow heart rate allows clear definition of the mid-diastolic slope.

Continuity equation mitral valve area determinations are most accurate in patients without significant coexisting mitral regurgitation. In this subgroup, continuity equation calculations provide a useful alternative to the half-time method, especially in situations of altered chamber compliances. The accuracy of the continuity equation method, as in aortic stenosis, depends on a parallel intercept angle between the mitral stenotic jet and the ultrasound beam and a careful stroke volume calculation from diameter and velocity recordings. Accurate pulmonary artery diameter measurement for stroke volume calculations can be difficult in adult patients due to poor acoustic access. LV outflow tract diameter nearly always can be depicted reliably. However, many patients with mitral stenosis have some degree of coexisting aortic or mitral regurgitation, so that transaortic stroke volume does not equal transmitral stroke volume.

Consequences of Mitral Stenosis

Left Atrial Enlargement and Thrombus

Chronic pressure overload of mitral stenosis leads to gradual enlargement of the LA, ranging from a mild increase with early or mild stenosis to a severe increase in atrial volume with long-standing severe

mitral stenosis. In conjunction with a low volume flow rate due to the stenotic valve, LA enlargement results in stasis of blood flow and thrombus formation. Thrombi are located preferentially in the LA appendage but also can occur in the body of the atrium as protruding or as laminated thrombus along the atrial wall or interatrial septum (Fig. 11–24). LA thrombi are most common when atrial fibrillation is present but may occur even in sinus rhythm.

TTE has a high specificity for detection of LA thrombus (i.e., if it is visualized, it most likely is a real finding), but the sensitivity is less than 50%. In part, this relates to the difficulty of imaging the LA appendage in adults. Sometimes the LA appendage can be visualized in a laterally angulated parasternal short-axis view at the aortic valve level or from an apical two-chamber view angulated slightly superiorly; however, often the atrial appendage cannot be visualized at all. When the atrial appendage is seen, image quality usually is too poor to allow reliable exclusion of atrial thrombus as a result of poor ultrasound tissue penetration and beam width artifact at the depth of the LA from surface imaging.

TEE has a high sensitivity (~99%) and specificity (~99%) for detection of LA thrombus. The LA appendage can be depicted well in multiple image planes using a multiplane probe. In addition, the higher transducer frequencies (5–7 MHz) and lower imaging depths result in high-resolution images. While thrombus in the appendage often protrudes into the chamber, laminated thrombus in the body

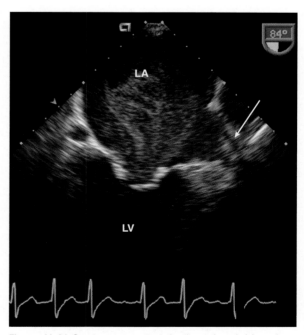

Figure 11–24 Spontaneous contrast in the enlarged LA and an echodensity suggestive of a thrombus in the atrial appendage of a patient with mitral stenosis, seen on TEE imaging.

of the atrium may be more difficult to recognize, especially along the interatrial septum.

Pulmonary Hypertension

In mitral stenosis, increased LA pressure results in pulmonary venous hypertension and consequent pulmonary artery hypertension. Initially, the increase in pulmonary artery pressure is "passive"; the pressure difference across the pulmonary bed (pulmonary artery minus LA pressure) is normal. In this situation, although pulmonary pressures are elevated, pulmonary vascular resistance is normal, and pulmonary pressures will fall toward normal after relief of mitral stenosis. With long-standing pulmonary venous hypertension, irreversible changes in the pulmonary vascular bed occur, leading to elevated pulmonary vascular resistance and persistent pulmonary hypertension after relief of mitral stenosis.

The presence of pulmonary hypertension can be suspected in mitral stenosis when there is mid-systolic partial closure (or "notching") of the pulmonic valve M-mode, a short interval between the onset of flow and maximum velocity, or mid-systolic abrupt deceleration in the right ventricular (RV) outflow velocity curve. With severe pulmonary hypertension, 2D echo may show RV hypertrophy and enlargement, paradoxical septal motion, and tricuspid regurgitation secondary to annular dilation.

The degree of pulmonary hypertension can be quantitated from the velocity in the tricuspid regurgitant jet and the appearance of the inferior vena cava. The simplified Bernoulli equation is used to calculate the right ventricular-to-right atrial (RV-RA) maximum systolic pressure difference from the CW Doppler tricuspid regurgitant jet recording. This difference is added to an estimate of RA pressure based on the size and respiratory variation of the inferior vena cava as it enters the RA as described in Chapter 6. Pulmonary hypertension out of proportion to the degree of mitral stenosis raises the possibility of a coexisting pulmonary disease process. Pulmonary vascular resistance also can be estimated as discussed in Chapter 6.

Exercise testing to evaluate the change in pulmonary pressure from rest to exercise is recommended when symptoms are greater than expected for the degree of stenosis. Pulmonary pressures are calculated from the tricuspid regurgitant jet measured at rest and immediately after exercise. Rapid data acquisition after exercise is essential for accurate estimation of the maximum exercise change.

Mitral Regurgitation

Some degree of coexisting mitral regurgitation is common in patients with mitral stenosis. Mitral regurgitant severity can be evaluated using standard techniques (see Chapter 12) and is an important factor in deciding on appropriate therapy. For example, significant mitral regurgitation is a contraindication to surgical or percutaneous commissurotomy. Coexisting mitral regurgitation elevates the transmitral pressure gradient (due to increased transmitral volume flow rate), but both 2D echo and $T\frac{1}{2}$ valve area measurements remain accurate.

Other Coexisting Valvular Disease

The rheumatic disease process also can affect the aortic valve (second in frequency to the mitral valve) and, less commonly, the tricuspid valve. Aortic valve involvement may result in stenosis and/or regurgitation that can be evaluated with appropriate 2D and Doppler echo techniques. Evaluation of aortic regurgitation by color flow imaging may be complicated in the presence of mitral stenosis due to merging of the two diastolic flow disturbances in the LV. Imaging the aortic regurgitant jet in short axis just proximal to the aortic valve and using other Doppler methods for evaluation of regurgitant severity will avoid this potential problem.

Rheumatic tricuspid stenosis may be difficult to appreciate on 2D imaging. Doppler flow patterns are similar to mitral stenosis, and the same quantitative methods for evaluation of stenosis severity can be applied. Even in the absence of rheumatic involvement of the tricuspid valve, significant tricuspid regurgitation is common (due to pulmonary hypertension and annular dilation) in patients with mitral stenosis. Careful evaluation of tricuspid regurgitation severity is especially important preoperatively in case tricuspid annuloplasty is needed at the time of mitral valve surgery.

Left Ventricular Response

The LV in mitral stenosis is small with normal wall thickness and normal systolic function, although diastolic function is impaired due to the restriction of flow across the mitral orifice. The presence of LV dilation suggests that significant coexisting mitral or aortic regurgitation or primary myocardial dysfunction (cardiomyopathy or ischemic disease) is present.

Clinical Applications

Diagnosis, Hemodynamic Progression, and Timing of Intervention

Echo Doppler is the standard clinical method for evaluation of the presence and severity of valvular mitral stenosis (Table 11–10). Disease progression can be followed and the timing of intervention can be determined using Doppler echo and clinical data alone. Evaluation by cardiac catheterization rarely is needed.

TABLE 11–10 Echocardiographic Approach to Mitral Stenosis

Valve morphology
Exclude other causes of clinical presentation
Mitral stenosis severity
- Mean transmitral pressure gradient
- 2D valve area
- T½ valve area
Coexisting mitral regurgitation
LA enlargement
Pulmonary artery pressure (from TR jet and IVC)
TEE for evaluation of LA clot if MBC is planned
Coexisting tricuspid regurgitation severity

MBC, mitral balloon commissurotomy; IVC, inferior vena cava; TR, tricuspid regurgitation.

TABLE 11–12 The French Three-Group Grading of Mitral Valve Anatomy

Echocardiographic Group	Mitral Valve Anatomy
Group 1	Pliable noncalcified anterior mitral leaflet and mild subvalvular disease (i.e., thin chordae ≥10 mm long)
Group 2	Pliable noncalcified anterior mitral leaflet and severe subvalvular disease (i.e., thickened chordae <10 mm long)
Group 3	Calcification of mitral valve of any extent, as assessed by fluoroscopy, whatever the state of subvalvular apparatus

Reprinted from Iung B, Cormier B, Discimetiere P, et al: J Am Coll Cardiol 27:407–414, 1996. Copyright 1996, with permission from American College of Cardiology Foundation.

Pre- and Post-percutaneous Commissurotomy

In the potential candidate for percutaneous balloon mitral commissurotomy, echo Doppler evaluation of mitral valve morphology is important in patient selection both in terms of predicted hemodynamic results and in terms of the risk of procedural complications. Mitral valve morphology may be described by a qualitative assessment, an additive scoring system (Tables 11–11 and 11–12), or quantitative measurements of leaflet mobility. Whatever approach is used, the important features to consider are leaflet mobility, leaflet thickness, leaflet and commissural calcification, and subvalvular involvement (Fig. 11–25). In general, the best hemodynamic results are seen with thin, mobile leaflets that have commissural fusion

TABLE 11–11 Mitral Valve Morphology by Two-dimensional Echocardiography

Grade*	Mobility	Thickening	Calcification	Subvalvular Thickening
1	Highly mobile valve has only leaflet tips restricted.	Leaflets near normal in thickness (4–5 mm)	A single area of increased echo brightness	Minimal thickening just below mitral leaflets
2	Leaflet middle and base portions have normal mobilty.	Mid-leaflets normal, considerable thickening of margins (5–8 mm)	Scattered areas of brightness confined to leaflet margins	Thickening of chordal structures extending to one third chordal length
3	Valve continues to move forward in diastole, mainly from the base.	Thickening extending through the entire leaflet (5–8 mm)	Brightness extending into the middle portions of the leaflets	Thickening extended to distal third of chords
4	No or minimal forward movement of the leaflets occurs in diastole.	Considerable thickening of all leaflet tissue (>8–10 mm)	Extensive brightness throughout much of leaflet tissue	Extensive thickening and shortening of all chordal structures extending down to papillary muscles

*The total echocardiographic score is derived from an analysis of mitral leaflet mobility, valvular and subvalvular thickening, and calcification, each of which is graded from 0 to 4 according to the above criteria. This gives a total score of 0 to 16.
From Wilkins GT, Weyman AE, Abascal VM et al: Br Heart J 60:299–308, 1988.

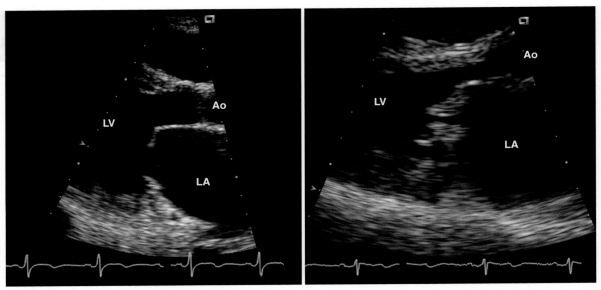

Figure 11–25 Parasternal long-axis views in two mitral stenosis patients, one with favorable *(left)* and one with unfavorable *(right)* mitral valve morphology for balloon valvuloplasty. The favorable valve morphology is characterized by relatively thin, flexible valve leaflets as evidenced by the "doming" of the anterior leaflet and little calcification or subvalvular involvement. The same view in *(right)* a different patient shows leaflets that are extensively calcified and immobile, with less diastolic doming and with extensive subvalvular involvement.

but little calcification or subchordal thickening. However, some patients with a relatively unfavorable morphology do have relief of mitral stenosis with percutaneous commissurotomy. It is noteworthy that patients with the most heavily calcified and deformed valves (and the most severe stenosis) are more likely to suffer procedure-related morbidity and mortality.

Another factor to consider in this patient population is the degree of coexisting mitral regurgitation, since percutaneous commissurotomy is contradicted if moderate or severe regurgitation is present. In addition, because any LA thrombi may be dislodged by the catheters during the procedure, TEE is needed to evaluate for LA thrombus before the procedure. TTE or TEE imaging may be used to monitor catheter and balloon position during the procedure (Fig. 11–26) as well as to assess hemodynamic results (Fig. 11–27).

After percutaneous commissurotomy, echo Doppler allows identification of complications, permits assessment of hemodynamic results, and provides a baseline for future disease progression. Potential complications include (1) an increase in the severity of mitral regurgitation and (2) the presence of an atrial septal defect (usually small) at the trans-septal catheter puncture site. Hemodynamic results can be evaluated with standard echo Doppler techniques, again with an awareness of the potential inaccuracies in the half-time method in the immediate post-commissurotomy period. Doppler

evaluation of post-procedure pulmonary artery systolic pressure also can be helpful. Predictors of long-term outcome after balloon mitral commissurotomy include valve area, severity of mitral regurgitation, and the mitral morphology score (Fig. 11–28).

Evaluation of the Pregnant Patient with Dyspnea

When echocardiography is requested in a pregnant patient with dyspnea, the possibility of valvular mitral stenosis should be considered. Symptoms due to mitral stenosis often occur initially during pregnancy due to increased metabolic demands and volume flow rate, and the murmur may not be appreciated on auscultation. Careful imaging of the valve and recording of the transmitral flow velocity curve allows exclusion or confirmation of this possibility.

TRICUSPID STENOSIS

Tricuspid stenosis is uncommon in adult patients; in nearly all cases it is due to rheumatic disease in association with rheumatic mitral involvement. Carcinoid heart disease affects both tricuspid and pulmonic valves and can lead either to stenosis or to regurgitation. RA tumors, large vegetations, or a large atrial

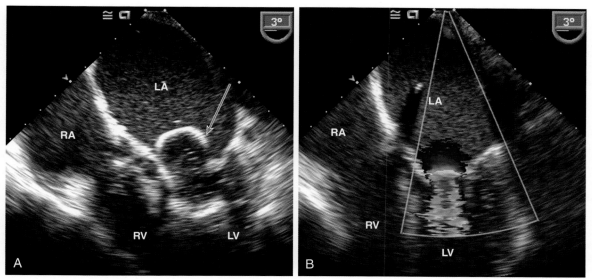

Figure 11–26 TEE performed during a percutaneous balloon mitral commissurotomy shows the balloon (*cyan arrow*) inflated during dilation of the mitral valve (**A**). The narrow midsegment of the balloon is positioned at the leaflet tips, and sequential inflations are used to open the fused commissures. Color Doppler (**B**) after the balloon is removed shows some residual MS with flow acceleration and signal aliasing at the leaflet tips. A catheter is present in the LA with a shadow artifact.

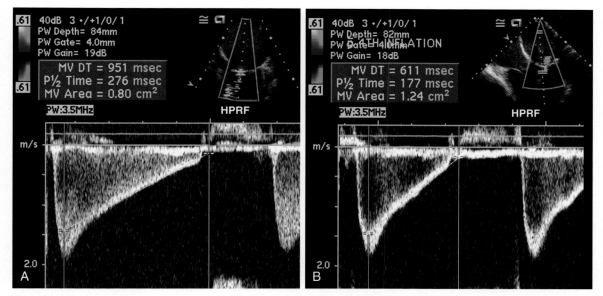

Figure 11–27 Doppler velocity curves across the stenotic mitral valve before (**A**) and after (**B**) percutaneous mitral valvuloplasty recorded from a TEE approach. T½ (or P½) decreased from 276 to 177 ms, indicating an increase in valve area from 0.8 to 1.2 cm². This is a suboptimal increase in valve area, but color flow also showed an increase in MR severity, which limited further dilation. Note that the T½ is measured from the linear mid-diastolic segment of the flow signal, extrapolating back to the onset of flow, ignoring the early-diastolic short steep deceleration.

thrombus (which may have embolized from the venous bed) can obstruct RV inflow and mimic tricuspid stenosis.

Two-dimensional echo images show thickening and shortening of the tricuspid valve leaflets (Fig. 11–29).

Commissural fusion and diastolic bowing indicate rheumatic disease. Doppler recordings of the transvalvular flow velocity allow calculation of mean gradient and T½ valve area as described for the mitral valve.

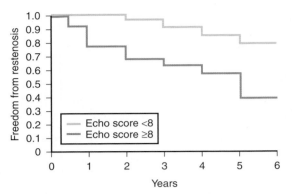

Figure 11–28 Freedom from restenosis in a series of 181 patients with initially successful mitral valvuloplasty and adequate echocardiographic data in those with an echo score less than 8 (*n* = 73) or ≥8. Restenosis was defined as a valve area less than 1.5 cm^2 and a 50% loss of the initial gain in valve area. *(From Wang A, Krasuski RA, Warner JJ, et al.: Serial echocardiographic evaluation of restenosis after successful percutaneous mitral commissurotomy. J Am Coll Cardiol 39:328–334, 2002.)*

PULMONIC STENOSIS

Pulmonic stenosis in adults is most often due to congenital disease, either residual stenosis after reparative surgery in childhood or clinically insignificant obstruction. Pulmonic stenosis may occur in conjunction with other congenital lesions such as ventricular inversion (congenitally corrected transposition of the great arteries) or tetralogy of Fallot.

Two-dimensional echo imaging of the pulmonic valve shows thickened leaflets with systolic bowing. On Doppler interrogation the antegrade velocity is increased with corresponding maximum and mean pressure gradients via the Bernoulli equation (Fig. 11–30). Pulmonic valve area is not usually calculated, but the continuity equation principle can be applied in this situation, using an appropriate intracardiac location for stroke volume determination. Post-stenotic pulmonary artery dilation may be present. Differentiation of valvular pulmonic stenosis from subvalvular or supravalvular obstruction can be difficult by 2D echo. Careful examinations with color flow and conventional pulsed Doppler can be very helpful in defining the site of the post-stenotic flow disturbance (and thus the site of obstruction).

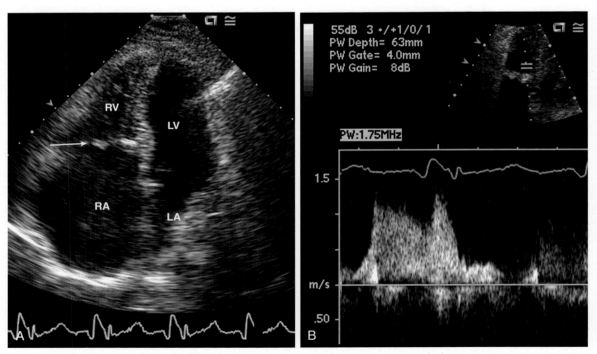

Figure 11–29 Rheumatic tricuspid stenosis with thickened valve leaflets (*arrow*) and RA enlargement in the apical four-chamber view (**A**) and the Doppler RV inflow velocity showing a slightly high mean gradient and prolonged deceleration time (**B**).

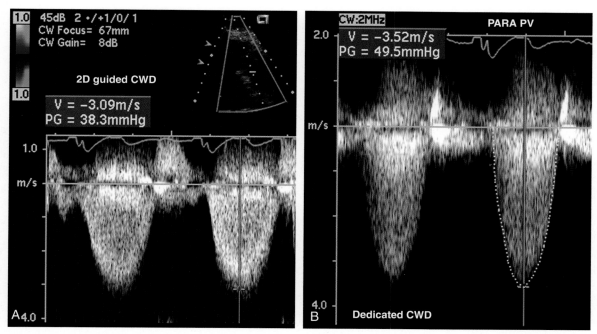

Figure 11–30 Residual pulmonic stenosis is present in a 26-year-old woman with a repaired tetralogy of Fallot. Using 2D-guided CW Doppler (CWD), a maximum velocity of 3.1 m/s is recorded from the parasternal window in an RV outflow view. However, with a dedicated CWD transducer a velocity of 3.5 m/s was recorded, because the smaller transducer can be angled to be more parallel to the jet and the non-imaging transducer has a better Doppler signal-to-noise ratio.

SUGGESTED READING

Guidelines

1. Baumgartner H, Hung J, Bermejo J, et al: Echocardiographic assessment of valve stenosis: ESE/ASE recommendations for clinical practice. J Am Soc Echocardiogr 22:1–23, 2009.

   This consensus document reviews approaches to evaluation of valve stenosis. Recommendations are provided for which measurements to use in clinical practice along with details on data acquisition and measurements. Tables summarize the formulas with advantages and limitations of each. A comprehensive list of references is included.

2. Bonow RO, Carabello BA, Chatterjee K, et al: ACC/AHA 2006 guidelines for the management of patients with valvular heart disease: a report of the American College of Cardiology/ American Heart Association Task Force on Practice Guidelines (Writing Committee to Develop Guidelines for the Management of Patients with Valvular Heart Disease). J Am Coll Cardiol 48:e1–e148, 2006.

   These detailed guidelines for management of adults with valvular heart disease include

definitions of hemodynamic severity for valve stenosis and valve regurgitation.

Fluid Dynamics

3. Garcia D, Kadem L, Savery D, et al: Analytical modeling of the instantaneous maximal transvalvular pressure gradient in aortic stenosis. J Biomech 39:3036–3044, 2006.

   The time dependence of the velocity in the vena contracta of a stenotic valve and the effects of volume flow rate are analyzed to describe the instantaneous pressure gradient across the valve in systole. References to the literature on fluid dynamics are provided.

Aortic Stenosis

4. Rosenhek R: Aortic stenosis: Echocardiographic evaluation of disease severity, disease progression and the role of echocardiography in clinical decision making. In Otto CM (ed): The Practice of Clinical Echocardiography, 3rd ed. Philadelphia: Saunders Elsevier, 2007, pp 516–551.

   Advanced discussion of the echocardiographic approach to evaluation of aortic stenosis severity with a review of the impact of

echocardiographic findings on the clinical decision-making process; 236 references. *Topics covered include stress echocardiography for detection of symptom onset and evaluation of low-output aortic stenosis, the effect of arterial hypertension on evaluation of aortic stenosis severity, other measures of stenosis severity, and the role of echocardiography in following progressive disease.*

5. Otto CM: Valvular aortic stenosis: disease severity and timing of intervention. J Am Coll Cardiol 47:2141–2151, 2006.

   This review summarizes the standard approach to clinical evaluation of aortic stenosis severity (velocity, gradient, and valve area) and explores the potential utility of more sophisticated echocardiography measures of disease severity, as well as other approaches including serum brain natriuretic peptide (BNP) levels and exercise testing. The effects of hypertension, aortic root dilation, coronary disease, LV dysfunction and atrial fibrillation on evaluation of stenosis severity are considered. A practical approach for clinical decision making is proposed.

6. Roberts WC, Ko JM: Frequency by decades of unicuspid, bicuspid, and tricuspid aortic valves in adults having isolated aortic valve replacement for

aortic stenosis, with or without associated aortic regurgitation. Circulation 111:920–925, 2005.

In adults undergoing aortic valve replacement for severe aortic stenosis, over 50% have a congenital bicuspid valve. In those age 50 to 70 years, about two thirds have a bicuspid valve, but even in those over age 70 years, a bicuspid valve is present in about 40%. When the number of leaflets cannot be determined with certainty on echocardiography due to leaflet calcification, a bicuspid valve is likely, especially in patients under age 70 years.

7. Goland S, Trento A, Iida K, et al: Assessment of aortic stenosis by three-dimensional echocardiography: An accurate and novel approach. Heart 93:801–807, 2007.

Aortic valve area was determined on TEE images by planimetry of valve from real-time 3D images, 2D images, and 3D-guided 2D images of the valve orifice. These three methods correlated with each other, but the 3D approaches showed less interobserver variability. Direct planimetry of valve area showed reasonable correlation with Doppler continuity equation and catheter-derived valve areas in this small series of patients. Further clinical experience with 3D guidance of 2D measurements is needed.

8. Kadem L, Dumesnil JG, Rieu R, et al: Impact of systemic hypertension on the assessment of aortic stenosis. Heart 91:354–361, 2005.

An animal model of aortic stenosis was used to examine the impact of systemic hypertension on measures of aortic stenosis severity. Hypertension resulted in about a 30% increase in valve area and a 40% decrease in maximum and mean pressure gradient, suggesting that concurrent hypertension might result in underestimation of stenosis severity by Doppler echocardiography. In this situation, re-evaluation after blood pressure control is appropriate.

9. Little SH, Chan KL, Burwash IG: Impact of blood pressure on the Doppler echocardiographic assessment of severity of aortic stenosis. Heart 93:848–855, 2007.

In 22 adults with aortic stenosis, blood pressure was increased acutely using handgrip exercise or phenylephrine infusion. An acute increase in blood pressure did not significantly change valve gradient, but valve area decreased in association with a decrease in mean transvalvular flow rate. Changes in blood pressure can result in an increase or decrease in measures of stenosis severity, even when the underlying severity of valve disease is unchanged.

10. Lancellotti P, Karsera D, Tumminello G, et al: Determinants of an abnormal response to exercise in patients with asymptomatic valvular aortic stenosis. Eur J Echocardiogr 9:338–343, 2008.

Exercise stress testing was abnormal in 60 of 128 asymptomatic adults with aortic stenosis. Multivariate predictors of an abnormal stress test were a greater increase in transaortic pressure gradient with exercise and limited contractile reserve (e.g., a smaller increase in ejection fraction from rest to exercise). See related articles in PubMed for other references on exercise testing in aortic stenosis patients.

11. Bergler-Klein J, Mundigler G, Pibarot P, et al: B-type natriuretic peptide in low-flow, low-gradient aortic stenosis: relationship to hemodynamics and clinical outcome: Results from the Multicenter Truly or Pseudo-Severe Aortic Stenosis (TOPAS) study. Circulation 115:2848–2855, 2007.

In 69 patients with low-flow aortic stenosis (indexed valve area $<0.6\ cm^2/m^2$, mean gradient ≤40 mm Hg, and LV ejection fraction $\leq40\%$), the dobutamine stress echocardiography (DSE) change in valve area versus change in flow rate was normalized to a flow rate of 250 mL/s to determine "projected valve area." A projected valve area $\leq1.0\ cm^2$ was defined as true severe aortic stenosis. Brain natriuretic peptide levels were higher in those with true severe aortic stenosis as compared with pseudo-aortic stenosis and also were a strong predictor of clinical outcome after valve replacement.

12. Bermejo J, Yotti R: Low-gradient aortic valve stenosis: Value and limitations of dobutamine stress testing. Heart 93:298–302, 2007.

This concise review of the role of dobutamine stress echocardiography (DSE) in clinical decision making discusses potential mechanisms for flow dependence of stenosis severity measures and summarizes the clinical literature. With severe aortic stenosis, outcome with medical therapy is very poor even when there is concurrent LV dysfunction, so that valve replacement should be considered in most of these patients unless the DSE shows that stenosis is not severe.

13. Hachicha Z, Dumesnil JG, Bogaty P, et al: Paradoxical low-flow, low-gradient severe aortic stenosis despite preserved ejection fraction is associated with higher afterload and reduced survival. Circulation 115:2856–2864, 2007.

In adults with severe aortic stenosis the transvalvular gradient and velocity may be low even with a normal LV ejection fraction if there is a low antegrade volume flow rate across the aortic valve. The cause of the low stroke volume typically is concentric LV hypertrophy with small ventricular volumes. Low-output aortic stenosis with a normal ejection fraction is associated with a poor clinical outcome.

14. Moss RR, Ivens E, Pasupati S, et al: Role of echocardiography in percutaneous aortic valve implantation. J Am Coll Cardiol Img 1:15–24, 2008.

Placement of an aortic valve prosthesis via a percutaneous approach requires careful guidance of the position of the valve in the aortic annulus. TTE is used for sizing of the device based on annular measurements. TEE is used during the procedure to guide device positioning and for early detection of complications.

Mitral Stenosis

15. Iung B, Vahanian A: Echocardiography in the patient undergoing catheter balloon mitral valvuloplasty: patient selection, hemodynamic results, complications and long term outcome. In Otto CM (ed): The Practice of Clinical Echocardiography, 3rd ed. Philadelphia: Saunders Elsevier, 2007, pp 481–501.

Review of the use of echocardiography in patient selection, prediction of hemodynamic results, diagnosis of complications, and long-term outcome after mitral valvuloplasty. Research applications and alternate approaches are also discussed. 120 references.

16. Carabello BA: Modern management of mitral stenosis. Circulation 112:432–437, 2005.

Contemporary review of the clinical presentation, diagnosis, natural history, and therapy for mitral stenosis.

17. Henry WL, Griffith JM, Michaelis LL, et al: Measurement of mitral orifice area in patients with mitral valve disease by real-time, two-dimensional echocardiography. Circulation 51:827–831, 1975.

Validation of 2D echo planimetry of MVA compared with measurements at operation. 2D echo valve area was within $0.3\ cm^2$ of surgical area in 12 of 14 (86%) patients.

18. Holen J, Aaslid R, Landmark K, et al: Determination of pressure gradient in mitral stenosis with a non-invasive ultrasound Doppler technique. Acta Med Scand 199:455–460, 1976.

Original description of Doppler measurement of transmitral pressure gradients.

19. Hatle L, Angelsen B, Tromsdal A: Noninvasive assessment of atrio-ventricular pressure half-time by Doppler ultrasound. Circulation 60:1096–1104, 1979.

Application of T½ concept to Doppler data.

20. Xie MX, Wang XF, Cheng TO, et al: Comparison of accuracy of mitral valve area in mitral stenosis by real-time, three-dimensional echocardiography versus two-dimensional echocardiography versus Doppler pressure half-time. Am J Cardiol 95:1496–1499, 2005.

In 30 patients with mitral stenosis, real-time 3D measurement of MVA correlated well with 2D planimetry and $T_{1/2}$ methods for valve area determination.

21. Pérez de Isla L, Casanova C, Almería C, et al: Which method should be the reference method to evaluate the severity of rheumatic mitral stenosis? Gorlin's method versus 3D-echo. Eur J Echocardiogr 8:470–473, 2007.

In 26 patients with mitral stenosis who underwent echocardiography and catheterization, 3D measurement of valve area correlated more closely than Gorlin formula valve area with the mean of three standard methods (2D planimetry, $T_{1/2}$, and PISA).

22. Messika-Zeitoun D, Meizels A, Cachier A, et al: Echocardiographic evaluation of the mitral valve area before and after percutaneous mitral commissurotomy: the pressure half-time method revisited. J Am Soc Echocardiogr 18:1409–1414, 2005.

In 120 patients undergoing balloon mitral commissurotomy, 2D valve area increased on average from about 1.0 to 1.8 cm² and mean gradient decreased from 10 to 5 mm Hg. The $T_{1/2}$ method underestimated the improvement in valve area and correlated poorly with 2D valve area. The $T_{1/2}$ approach should be used with caution in the first 24–48 hours after commissurotomy.

23. Kim HK, Kim YJ, Hwang SJ, et al: Hemodynamic and prognostic implications of net atrioventricular compliance in patients with mitral stenosis. J Am Soc Echocardiogr 21:482–486, 2008.

Net atrioventricular compliance (C_n) can be calculated from 2D planimetry of MVA (2D-MVA in cm²) and the deceleration slope of the transmitral E wave (E slope in cm/s²) in units of mL/mm Hg using the equation:

$$C_n = 1270(2D\text{-}MVA/E\ slope)$$

A C_n < 4 mL/mm Hg was associated with an increased likelihood of mitral valve commissurotomy or replacement during an average follow-up of 2 years.

24. Izgi C, Ozdemir N, Cevik C, et al: Mitral valve resistance as a determinant of resting and stress pulmonary artery pressure in patients with mitral stenosis: a dobutamine stress study. J Am Soc Echocardiogr 20:1160–1166, 2007.

The major hemodynamic effect of mitral stenosis is an excessive increase in pulmonary pressure with exercise. In 20 patients with isolated mitral stenosis (average valve area about 1.6 cm²), pulmonary systolic pressure increased from 39 to 60 mm Hg with dobutamine stress. Stress pulmonary pressure was the only independent predictor of exercise capacity.

25. Messika-Zeitoun D, Brochet E, Holmin C, et al: Three-dimensional evaluation of the mitral valve area and commissural opening before and after percutaneous mitral commissurotomy in patients with mitral stenosis. Eur Heart J 28:72–79, 2007.

Real-time 3D measurement of valve area correlates well with 2D planimetry of valve area and does not provide an advantage for experienced echocardiographers. However, with less experienced operators the real-time 3D measurement is more accurate than 2D planimetry. Real-time 3D echocardiography also allows evaluation of commissural opening in mitral stenosis before and after procedures.

Tricuspid Stenosis

26. Anwar AM, Geleijnse ML, Soliman OI, et al: Evaluation of rheumatic tricuspid valve stenosis by real-time three-dimensional echocardiography. Heart 93:363–364, 2007.

Tricuspid stenosis affects about 8% of patients with rheumatic mitral valve disease but may be underappreciated on standard 2D and Doppler approaches. This article describes the real-time 3D findings in five adults with rheumatic tricuspid stenosis. Unique measurements that are possible on real-time 3D imaging (and not standard 2D imaging) include commissural width and planimetry of valve area.

Pulmonic Stenosis

27. Lurz P, Coats L, Khambadkone S, et al: Percutaneous pulmonary valve implantation: impact of evolving technology and learning curve on clinical outcome. Circulation 117:1964–1972, 2008.

In 155 patients with pulmonic stenosis and/or regurgitation, percutaneous valve implantation resulted in an average reduction in the RV outflow gradient from 37 to 17 mm Hg. Survival at 83 months was 97%, and freedom from reoperation was 70% at 70 months. Echocardiography is a key element in patient evaluation before, during, and after the procedure.

E chocardiographic evaluation of the patient with valvular regurgitation includes assessment of valve anatomy, the severity of regurgitation, chamber dilation due to the imposed volume overload, ventricular function, and the degree of pulmonary hypertension. In some cases the clinical significance of valvular regurgitation is related to the *presence* of abnormal regurgitation, regardless of severity. For example, detection of aortic regurgitation (AR) in a patient with chest pain and an enlarged aorta heightens the suspicion of aortic dissection. In other situations (for example, mitral valve [MV] prolapse) the *severity* of regurgitation is an essential factor in clinical decision making regarding surgical intervention. In chronic regurgitation due to primary valve disease, regurgitant severity and the *response of the left ventricle (LV) to chronic volume overload* are the most important factors in deciding on the timing of valve surgery.

BASIC PRINCIPLES

Etiology of Valvular Regurgitation

Valvular regurgitation may be due to congenital or acquired abnormalities of the valve leaflets or to abnormalities of the associated supporting structures. For example, dilation of the ascending aorta or sinuses can result in AR even with anatomically normal valve leaflets. Similarly, LV dilation can result in mitral regurgitation (MR) even with normal valve leaflets and chordae. Echocardiographic examinations allow definition of the etiology of valvular regurgitation in most cases. Even when a single definite etiology is not evident, the differential diagnosis of the cause of regurgitation often can be narrowed to the few most likely possibilities. The examination also may provide clues as to whether regurgitation is acute or chronic in duration.

When transthoracic (TTE) images are not diagnostic for evaluation of aortic or mitral valve anatomy and the etiology of regurgitation, transesophageal (TEE) imaging may be helpful. With diseases of the aorta, visualization of the ascending aorta often is suboptimal on TTE imaging, so TEE imaging typically is needed to fully define the extent and severity of disease.

Fluid Dynamics of Valvular Regurgitation

The fluid dynamics of a regurgitant valve (Fig. 12–1) are in many ways similar to the fluid dynamics of a stenotic valve and are characterized by a:

- Regurgitant orifice area (ROA)
- High-velocity regurgitant jet
- Proximal flow convergence region
- Downstream flow disturbance
- Increased antegrade flow volume

Even though the anatomy of inadequate valve closure may be quite complex, the valve can be thought of as having a regurgitant orifice, which in simple physiologic terms is characterized by a high-velocity laminar jet (Table 12–1). The instantaneous velocity in this jet (v) is related to the instantaneous pressure difference (ΔP) across the valve, as stated in the simplified Bernoulli equation: $\Delta P = 4v^2$. Recording this high-velocity jet with continuous wave (CW) Doppler allows assessment of the time course of the difference in pressure between the two chambers on either side of the valve.

On the upstream side of the regurgitant valve, flow acceleration proximal to the regurgitant orifice is present, and a proximal isovelocity surface area (PISA) can be defined similar to that seen on the left atrial (LA) side of the stenotic MV. The PISA, multiplied by the aliasing velocity, provides a method for quantitative evaluation of regurgitant stroke volume. The narrowest segment of the regurgitant jet, the vena contracta, occurs just distal to the regurgitant orifice, with vena contracta diameter reflecting ROA.

As the high-velocity jet enters the chamber receiving the regurgitant flow, the flow pattern becomes disturbed with nonlaminar flow, multiple blood flow

TABLE 12–1	Relationship between Fluid Dynamics of Valvular Regurgitation and Diagnostic Approach
Fluid Dynamic Characteristic	**Diagnostic Approach**
Conservation of mass through the regurgitant orifice	Continuity equation for regurgitant orifice area
High-velocity jet in regurgitant orifice	Pressure-velocity relationship of CW Doppler curve
Proximal flow convergence	Proximal isovelocity surface area
Downstream flow disturbance	Jet area in chamber receiving regurgitant flow
Increased volume flow across valve	Stroke volume across regurgitant minus competent valve

velocities, and multiple blood flow directions. The *size* of the downstream regurgitant flow disturbance is affected by both physiologic and technical factors, and thus is less useful for quantitation of regurgitant severity (Table 12–2). In addition, the *shape* and *direction* of the regurgitant jet are affected by the anatomy and orientation of the regurgitation orifice, the driving force across the valve, and the size and compliance of the receiving chamber. Jets are "pulled" toward adjacent walls (e.g., MR in the LA) if within a critical distance from the wall at the entry site and also are "pulled" toward other flow streams (e.g., AR and mitral stenosis). Eccentric jets that adhere to the wall of the chamber will have a smaller color jet area on two-dimensional (2D) color flow imaging

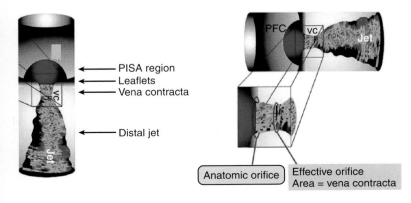

PISA region
Leaflets
Vena contracta

Distal jet

Anatomic orifice | Effective orifice Area = vena contracta

Figure 12–1 *Left,* The three components of a regurgitant jet: the proximal isovelocity surface area (PISA) region, also referred to as proximal flow convergence region; vena contracta (VC); and distal jet. *Right,* The effective regurgitant orifice area (ROA) is the orifice area defined by the narrowest regurgitant flow stream and typically occurs distal to the anatomic orifice defined by the valve leaflets. *(Adapted from Roberts BJ, Grayburn P: Color flow imaging of the vena contracta in mitral regurgitation: Technical considerations. J Am Soc Echocardiogr 16:1002–1006, 2003).*

TABLE 12–2   Factors That Affect Regurgitant Jet Size and Shape

Physiologic

Regurgitant volume
Driving pressure
Size and shape of regurgitant orifice
Receiving chamber constraint
Wall impingement
Timing relative to the cardiac cycle
Influence of coexisting jets or flow streams

Technical

Ultrasound system gain
Pulse repetition frequency
Transducer frequency
Frame rate
Image plane
Depth
Signal strength

(and a smaller three-dimensional [3D] volume), because entrainment of additional fluid elements into the jet occurs on only one side, instead of on all sides, as with a central jet.

Volume Overload

In patients with a regurgitant valve the term *total stroke volume* refers to the total volume of blood pumped by the ventricle on a single beat. *Forward stroke volume* is the amount of blood delivered to the peripheral circulation, and *regurgitant volume* is the amount of backflow across the abnormal valve (Fig. 12–2).

Mitral Regurgitation

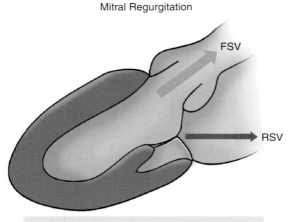

FSV

RSV

Total SV = Forward SV + Regurgitant SV

Figure 12–2 When mitral regurgitation is present, total stroke volume is the sum of the regurgitant and forward stroke volume (RSV and FSV).

Chronic valvular regurgitation results in progressive volume overload of the ventricle. Volume overload of the LV results in chamber dilation with normal wall thickness, so that total LV mass is increased. An important clinical feature of chronic LV volume overload is that an irreversible decrease in systolic function can occur in the absence of symptoms. In fact, an irreversible decrease in contractility can occur despite a normal ejection fraction due to the altered loading conditions of the ventricle when regurgitation is present.

Serial echocardiographic evaluation of LV size and systolic function is a standard method of clinical evaluation, but two factors potentially limit the reliability of this approach. First, suboptimal image quality or recording techniques may result in erroneous measurements. Care is needed to ensure that the dimensions are measured perpendicular to the long and short axes of the LV, and instrument settings must be adjusted for optimal endocardial definition. Accurate tracing of endocardial borders for calculation of ventricular volumes depends on clear endocardial definition, standard image planes without foreshortening of the long axis of the ventricle, and a trained and experienced individual tracing the borders at end-diastole and end-systole.

Second, the reproducibility of LV measurements must be considered. Overall reproducibility includes variation in *recording* the data, variation in *measuring* the data, and *physiologic* variation (such as heart rate and loading conditions) that may affect the measurement. Reproducibility of 2D-guided M-mode measurements of the LV suggests that an interval change of greater than 8 mm in end-systolic or end-diastolic dimensions represents a definite clinical change. Using 2D echocardiography, a change in ventricular volume or a change in ejection fraction greater than 10% on serial studies performed in the same laboratory indicates a significant change.

Detection of Valvular Regurgitation

Valvular regurgitation can be detected with either

- ❒ color flow imaging or
- ❒ continuous-wave (CW) Doppler ultrasound.

While 2D imaging provides detailed information about valve anatomy and chamber dilation and function, it provides only indirect evidence for the presence or absence of valvular incompetence. The finding of an anatomically abnormal MV in the presence of LA and LV dilation suggests that MR may be present, but Doppler examination is necessary for direct confirmation or exclusion of the diagnosis. Although a few M-mode findings have been shown to be specific for diagnosing valvular regurgitation (e.g., high-frequency fluttering of the anterior mitral leaflet in AR), these findings are not sensitive enough to reliably exclude regurgitation when suspected on clinical grounds.

With color flow imaging, detection of regurgitation is based on identification of the flow disturbance downstream from the regurgitant orifice. When instrument settings and examination technique are optimal, color flow imaging is extremely sensitive (>90%) and specific (nearly 100%) for detection of valvular regurgitation as compared with angiography. In fact, color flow imaging is so sensitive that regurgitation often is detected that is not audible by auscultation. These cases most often are true positives, as evidenced by angiographic confirmation. False-positive results can occur with color flow imaging when the origin or timing of the flow signal is mistaken. For example, normal pulmonary venous inflow into the LA may be mistaken for MR. False-negative results occur when signal strength is low due to poor acoustic access or attenuation due to the depth of interrogation. False-negative results also occur if color flow processing parameters are set incorrectly or if the examiner fails to evaluate the valve in more than one tomographic plane. Additional parameters important in detection of valvular regurgitation with color flow imaging include frame rate, Nyquist limit, color gain, and the color velocity/variance display.

CW Doppler detection of valvular regurgitation is based on identification of the high-velocity jet through the regurgitant orifice. An advantage of CW Doppler is that beam width is broad at the level of the valves when studied from an apical approach. Identification of the regurgitant signal uses the velocity, shape, timing, and associated antegrade flow signal to correctly identify the origin of the signal (Fig. 12–3).

Valvular Regurgitation in Normal Individuals

A small degree of regurgitation, often termed *physiologic*, is present in a high percentage of otherwise

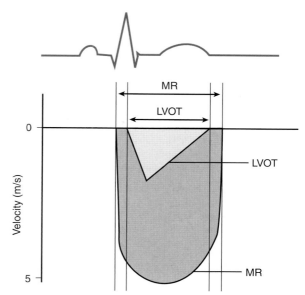

Figure 12–3 Relative timing of mitral regurgitation (MR) and LV outflow tract (LVOT) flow signals. MR extends from the onset of isovolumic contraction to the end of isovolumic relaxation. LV outflow is shorter, occurring only during ejection.

normal individuals (Fig. 12–4). Typically, physiologic regurgitation is:

☐ Spatially restricted to the area immediately adjacent to valve closure
☐ Short in duration
☐ Represents only a small regurgitant volume

When meticulously searched for, MR can be detected in 70% to 80%, tricuspid regurgitation in 80% to 90%, and pulmonic regurgitation in 70% to 80% of normal individuals. This small degree of regurgitation is normal and has no adverse clinical implications. AR is found in only a small percentage (5%) of young individuals with

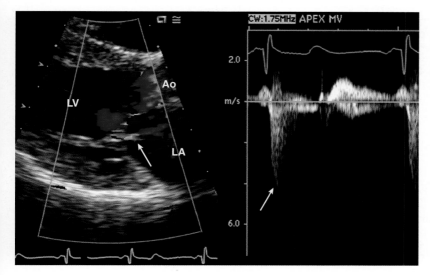

Figure 12–4 Example of "physiologic" mitral regurgitation recorded with color (*left*) and CW (*right*) Doppler in a normal individual. The color flow signal is localized to a small region adjacent to the valve coaptation point (*arrow*), and the intensity of the CW Doppler signal is low compared with antegrade flow with an incomplete waveform seen only in early systole (*arrow*).

an otherwise normal echocardiographic study, but the prevalence of detectable AR increases with age. The clinical significance of a small amount of AR is unknown.

APPROACHES TO EVALUATION OF THE SEVERITY OF REGURGITATION

The severity of valvular regurgitation typically is described using semiquantitative measures as mild, moderate, or severe; for example, using color jet area (Table 12–3). Other semiquantitative measures include:

❐ Vena contracta width
❐ Pressure half-time (for AR)
❐ Distal flow reversals

In addition, several quantitative measures of regurgitant severity have been well validated, including (Table 12–4):

❐ Regurgitant volume
❐ Regurgitant fraction
❐ Regurgitant orifice area (ROA)

Regurgitant volume (RV) is the retrograde volume flow rate across the valve, expressed either as an instantaneous flow rate in milliliters per second or (more correctly) averaged over the cardiac cycle in milliliters per beat. Regurgitant volume can be calculated by three different approaches:

❐ PISA flow rate,
❐ antegrade volume flow across the regurgitant valve minus across a competent valve, or
❐ 2D total LV stroke volume (SV_{total}) minus Doppler forward stroke volume.

Regurgitant fraction (RF) is

$$RF = RV/SV_{total} \qquad (12\text{–}1)$$

ROA is calculated, using the continuity equation, from regurgitant volume and the velocity-time integral of the regurgitant jet (VTI_{RJ}). Because the RV proximal to and *in* the regurgitant orifice are equal,

$$RV = ROA \times VTI_{RJ} \qquad (12\text{–}2)$$

so that, solving for ROA,

$$ROA = RV/VTI_{RJ} \qquad (12\text{–}3)$$

with RV in cm^3, VTI_{RJ} in cm, and ROA in cm^2.

Color Doppler Imaging

Jet Area

Screening for significant regurgitation often is based on the size of the flow disturbance in the chamber receiving the regurgitant jet. The size of the flow disturbance is evaluated using color flow imaging in at least two views. For each tomographic image plane it is noted whether an abnormal flow signal with appropriate timing (i.e., systole for MR, diastole for AR) is present or absent. The size of the jet, relative to the receiving chamber, provides a qualitative index of regurgitant severity on a 0 (mild) to 4+ (severe) scale. However, this index is most useful for identification of patients with mild regurgitation; there is substantial overlap in jet areas between patients with moderate and severe regurgitation (Figs. 12–5 and 12–6). Although the use of color flow imaging to define jet origin and direction is a useful qualitative descriptor in some cases, the length that a regurgitant jet extends

TABLE 12–3 Doppler Evaluation of Valvular Regurgitation

Method	Doppler Parameters	Limitations	Invasive Analog
Color flow imaging	Jet origin Jet direction Jet size	Variation with technical and physiologic factors	Angiography
Continuous-wave Doppler	Signal intensity Shape of velocity curve	Qualitative	Hemodynamics
Vena contracta width	Width of jet origin	Small values, careful measurement needed	None
Proximal isovelocity surface area (PISA)	Calculation of RV and ROA	Less accurate with eccentric jets Peak values only	None
Volume flow at two sites	Calculation of RV and ROA	Tedious	Invasive RV and RF
Distal flow reversals	Pulmonary vein (MR) or aorta (AR)	Qualitative, affected by LA pressure, AF (MR)	None

AF, atrial fibrillation; AR, aortic regurgitation; MR, mitral regurgitation; RF, regurgitant fraction; ROA, regurgitant orifice area; RV, regurgitant volume.

TABLE 12–4   Selected Studies Validating Quantitative Evaluation of Regurgitant Severity Using Doppler Echocardiography

First Author and Year	Method	Standard of Reference	N	R	SEE
Color Jet Area					
Spain 1989	Color jet area	Angio LV, TD CO	15 MR patients	0.62 (RF)	—
Tribouilloy 1992	Regurgitant jet width at origin	Angio LV, TD CO	31 MR patients	0.85 (RSV)	—
Enriquez-Sarano 1993	Color jet area	Doppler SV at two sites	80 MR patients	0.69 (RF)	4.4 cm^2
Vena Contracta					
Tribouilloy 2000	Vena contracta width	Doppler EROA and RV	79 AR patients	0.89 (EROA) 0.90 (RV)	0.08 cm^2 18 mL
Hall 1997	Vena contracta width	Doppler EROA and RV	80 MR patients	0.86 0.85 (RV)	0.15 cm^2 20 mL
PISA					
Recusani 1991	PISA (hemispherical)	Rotometer	In vitro, constant flow	0.94–0.99 (flow rate)	1–1.6 L/min
Utsunomiya 1991	PISA (hemispherical)	Actual flow rate stopwatch and cylinder	In vitro, pulsatile flow	0.99 (flow rate)	0.53 L/min
Vandervoort 1993	PISA	Actual flow rate	In vitro, steady flow	0.98–00.99 (flow rate)	—
Giesler 1993	PISA	LV angio, Fick CO	16 MR patients	0.88 (RSV)	17 mL
Chen 1993	PISA	Doppler SV at two sites	46 MR patients	0.94 (RSV)	18 mL
Continuous-wave Doppler					
Teague 1986	AR half-time	Angio LV, Fick CO	32 AR patients	~0.88 (RF)	11%
Masuyama 1986	AR half-time	Angio LV, ID CO	20 AR patients	~0.89 (RF)	—
Volume Flow at Two Sites					
Ascah 1985	Transmitral vs. transaortic SV	EM-flow	30 flow rates in canine model	0.83 (RF)	—
Kitabatake 1985	Transaortic vs. transpulmonic SV	Angio LV, TD CO	20 AR patients	0.94 (RF)	—
Rokey 1986	Transmitral vs. transaortic SV	Angio LV, TD CO	19 MR and 6 AR patients	0.91 (RF)	7%
Distal Flow Reversals					
Boughner 1975	Diastolic flow reversal in descending Ao	Angio LV, Fick CO	15 AR patients	0.91 (RF)	—
Touche 1985	Diastolic flow reversal in descending Ao	Angio LV, TD CO	30 AR patients	0.92 (RF)	8.8%

Ao, aortic; AR, aortic regurgitation; CO, cardiac output; EM-flow, volume flow rate measured by electromagnetic flowmeter; ID, indicator dilation; LV, LV; MR, mitral regurgitation; PISA, proximal isovelocity surface area method; RF, regurgitant fraction; RSV, regurgitant stroke volume; SEE, standard error of the estimate; SV, stroke volume; TD, thermodilution.

Data from Spain et al: J Am Coll Cardiol 13:585–590, 1989; Tribouilloy et al: Circulation 85:1248–1253, 1992; Enriquez-Sarano et al: J Am Coll Cardiol 21:1211–1219, 1993; Tribouilloy et al: Circulation 102:558–564, 2000; Hall et al: Circulation 95: 636–642, 1997; Recusani et al: Circulation 83:594–604, 1991; Utsunomiya et al: J Am Soc Echocardiol 4:338–348, 1991; Vandervoort et al: J Am Coll Cardiol 22:535–541, 1993; Giesler et al: Am J Cardiol 71:217–224, 1993; Chen et al: J Am Coll Cardiol 21:374–383, 1993; Teague et al: J Am Coll Cardiol 8:592–599, 1986; Masuyama et al: Circulation 73:460–466, 1986; Ascah et al: Circulation 72:377–383, 1985; Kitabatake et al: Circulation 72:523–529, 1985; Rokey et al: J Am Coll Cardiol 7:1273–1278, 1986; Boughner et al: Circulation 52:874–879, 1975; Touche et al: Circulation 72:819–824, 1985.

Figure 12–5 Color Doppler evaluation of mitral regurgitation (MR). The parasternal and apical views provide information on jet geometry and direction. The vena contracta is imaged in a parasternal view, when possible, but may be well seen from apical views as well. The proximal flow convergence region typically is measured from an apical approach. Multiple views allow identification of eccentric jets. The colors indicate mild, moderate, and severe regurgitation. Severe (4+) MR is associated with systolic flow reversal in the pulmonary veins (*red arrow*).

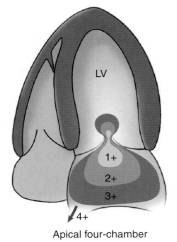

Apical four-chamber

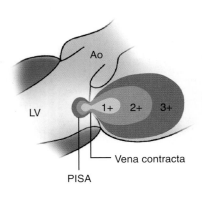

Parasternal long-axis

Figure 12–6 Evaluation of aortic regurgitant severity using color flow mapping in parasternal long-axis and short-axis views. The vena contracta can be imaged in a long-axis or short-axis view. In the clinical setting, multiple views are used because jets often are eccentric in direction and asymmetric in shape.

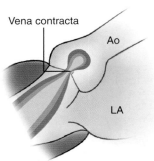

Long-axis

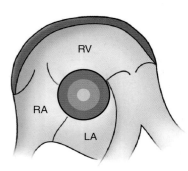

Short-axis just below aortic valve

into the receiving chamber is an unreliable indicator of disease severity and should no longer be used in patient management.

Because color flow imaging basically is pulsed Doppler ultrasound with somewhat different signal processing and display formats, it is important to remember that signal aliasing still occurs. However, flow imaging depends on the timing and spatial location of the Doppler signals and *not* absolute blood flow velocity. Thus, signal aliasing does not limit the utility of flow imaging and, in fact, may enhance the appreciation of abnormal flow patterns due to the presence of variance in the color flow signal. In addition, flow imaging can be performed from windows where the intercept angle between the ultrasound beam and the direction of regurgitant flow is nonparallel. Moreover, these windows often allow a shorter distance from the transducer to the flow region of interest, resulting in a better signal-to-noise ratio. For example, AR is best evaluated from the parasternal approach. Although the direction of an AR jet in the parasternal long-axis view is nearly perpendicular to the ultrasound beam, multiple flow directions within the jet allow detection of the

diastolic flow disturbance. Of course, an accurate blood velocity determination cannot be made both because of the nonparallel intercept angle and because the velocity exceeds the Nyquist limit of the pulsed Doppler mode.

The appearance of a regurgitant jet with color flow imaging will vary depending on the ultrasound system, transducer frequency, and specific instrument settings. Correct visual interpretation depends on experience with a particular instrument and knowledge of the influence of instrument settings on the visual display. On most systems, a "variance" color scale results in a green regurgitant signal superimposed on the normal red-blue flow patterns. A "velocity" scale results in a mosaic of red, blue, and white pixels in the regurgitant jet. Because the goal of this application is to identify the location and timing of abnormal flow signals in a tomographic format, the exact color scale used is not particularly important as long as it displays the boundaries of the flow disturbance accurately.

With either a variance or a velocity color flow scale, it is obvious that an abnormal color pattern is not synonymous with abnormal flow given the physics of pulsed Doppler color flow imaging. An abnormal color pattern can be seen even with normal intracardiac flow patterns. For example, the normal antegrade flow velocity of laminar flow across the aortic valve exceeds the Nyquist limit, resulting in aliasing and an "abnormal" color pattern. Conversely, abnormal flow signals may not demonstrate variance or a mosaic pattern if the flow velocities are within the Nyquist limit for that interrogation depth. For example, the low velocities seen in pulmonic regurgitation result in a uniform color display even though the flow pattern is abnormal. Interpretation of the color images will be most consistent from study to study if instrument settings and flow maps are standardized for each laboratory. Recommended instrument settings for color flow imaging are:

- ❒ Nyquist limit at the maximum for the imaging depth (60 to 80 cm/s)
- ❒ Color gain setting just below random speckle from nonmoving targets
- ❒ Maximum frame rate (e.g., narrow sector, shallow depth)
- ❒ Consistent color velocity/variance display scale

Evaluation of the exact timing of a flow signal in relation both to valve closing and to the QRS complex can be helpful in correct identification of the signal. With color flow imaging, temporal resolution is sacrificed for spatial resolution because frame rates are far lower than the sampling rate of pulsed or CW Doppler. Simultaneous recording of an electrocardiographic lead is essential for frame-by-frame analysis of the color flow images to verify the timing of the disturbance. If the timing of a color flow velocity signal is unclear, use of 2D-guided color "M-mode" may be helpful by providing higher time resolution. With color M-mode Doppler, the signal is displayed at each depth along a single line of interrogation (*y*-axis) versus time (*x*-axis) at a higher sampling rate (Fig. 12–7). Thus, the color M-mode tracing allows

evaluation of the timing of the flow disturbance in relation to valve opening and closing.

Vena Contracta

The vena contracta, the narrowest diameter of the flow stream, reflects the diameter of the regurgitant orifice with the advantages that it is independent of volume flow rate and driving pressure, and it is relatively unaffected by instrument settings. However, because vena contracta diameters have a narrow range of values, care is needed to obtain optimal images for measurement. In order to optimize both temporal and spatial resolution, the recommended approach to measurement of vena contracta is to use a view that is:

- ❒ Perpendicular to jet width
- ❒ In zoom mode
- ❒ Narrow sector
- ❒ Minimum depth

Angulation out of the standard image planes may be needed to depict both the proximal acceleration region and downstream flow expansion for accurate identification of the vena contracta (Fig. 12–8).

Vena contracta diameter may vary with dynamic changes in the regurgitant orifice, for example, with late-systolic MR due to MV prolapse. However, vena contracta width remains accurate in the setting of acute regurgitation, when jet area may be misleading.

Proximal Flow Convergence

Color flow imaging allows calculation of the retrograde volume flow rate based on measurement of the flow convergence region proximal to the regurgitant orifice. Acceleration of flow occurs proximal to the valve plane with, conceptually, a series of isovelocity "surfaces" leading to the high-velocity jet in the regurgitant orifice.

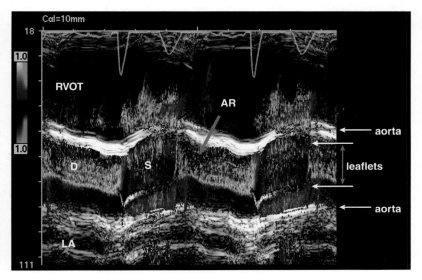

Figure 12–7 Color M-mode of aortic regurgitation (AR) recorded from the parasternal window, with the RV outflow tract (RVOT) anteriorly, and the anterior and posterior walls of the aorta as indicated. The M-color tracing shows the high time resolution of this approach with a mosaic of colors in diastole (D) due to AR and a relatively uniform blue color in systole (S) due to antegrade flow between the open aortic valve leaflets.

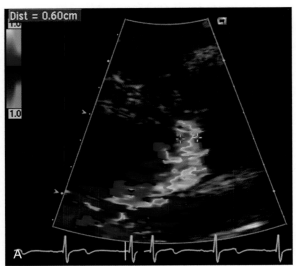

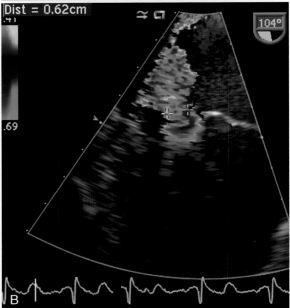

Figure 12–8 **A**, Vena contracta measurement for an eccentric aortic regurgitant jet in a parasternal long-axis view on TTE imaging. The long-axis view allows identification of the proximal flow convergence region and the downstream jet expansion, with the vena contracta identified as the narrowest segment joining them. Vena contracta width is measured perpendicular to the flow direction. **B**, On TEE imaging, the vena contracta width of a mitral regurgitant jet is measured as the narrow neck between the PISA and flow expansion in the LA. A view perpendicular to the jet direction is not feasible on TEE, but the image is still recorded using a narrow sector width and zoom mode to improve measurement precision.

Immediately adjacent to the orifice, these surfaces are small with higher flow velocities; at increasing distances from the orifice, areas are larger, and velocities are lower. Based on the principle of volume flow calculation by Doppler techniques, the volume flow rate (in

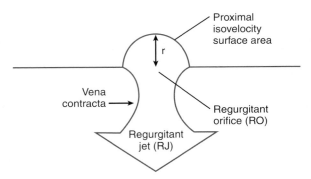

$$\text{Regurg. volume} = \text{PISA} \times \text{velocity}$$
$$\text{RO area} = \text{regurg. volume}/\text{VTI}_{RJ}$$

Figure 12–9 Proximal to a regurgitant orifice flow accelerates, resulting in concentric proximal isovelocity surface areas (PISAs). The radius (r) is used to calculate the PISA. The color Doppler aliasing velocity is used to calculate the instantaneous regurgitant flow rate based on the aliasing velocity. In combination with the maximum velocity (V_{MR}) of the CW Doppler recording of the regurgitant jet, regurgitant orifice (RO) area is estimated.

this case, regurgitant flow) for a PISA, when averaged over the temporal flow period, is (Fig. 12–9):

$$\text{Regurgitant flow rate} = \text{PISA} \times \text{aliasing velocity} \tag{12–4}$$

The velocity of the PISA can be determined from the color flow image as the aliasing velocity where a distinct red/blue interface is seen (Fig. 12–10). At this interface the velocity is known, being equivalent to the Nyquist limit on the velocity color scale. The size of the PISA can be maximized to allow more accurate regurgitant flow rate calculations by decreasing the velocity range and/or by shifting the velocity baseline.

The shape of the isovelocity surface proximal to a regurgitant valve typically is hemispherical with a tendency toward a hemielliptical shape closer to the orifice (Fig. 12–11). Assuming a hemispherical shape, the PISA is calculated from measurements of the distance from the aliasing velocity to the regurgitant orifice as the surface area of a hemisphere:

$$\text{PISA} = 2\pi r^2 \tag{12–5}$$

Note that the PISA method for calculating regurgitant volume is analogous to calculation of stroke volume proximal to a stenotic valve. The differences between these approaches are (1) the differing shapes of the proximal velocity stream lines; (2) the use of color flow, rather than pulsed Doppler, to measure velocity at a given location; and (3) the need for temporal averaging when color data from single images are used.

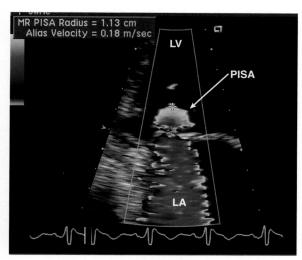

Figure 12–10 Mitral regurgitation (MR) showing the proximal isovelocity surface area (PISA) in a patient with a dilated cardiomyopathy. The PISA has been optimized by decreasing the depth, narrowing the sector, and using the zoom mode. In addition, the velocity color scale (no variance) has been adjusted to an aliasing velocity away from the transducer that maximizes the size of the PISA. The PISA radius of 1.1 cm (surface area $= 2\pi r^2 = 7.6$ cm^2) at an aliasing velocity of 18 cm/s indicates an instantaneous regurgitant flow rate of 137 mL/s. The maximum MR-jet velocity was 4.3 m/s, so that regurgitant orifice area (ROA) is 0.32 cm^2, consistent with moderate MR.

The PISA method can be combined with the VTI of CW Doppler flow through the regurgitant orifice to calculate ROA using Equation 12–3. Instead of averaging PISA over the duration of flow, most clinicians calculate the maximum instantaneous regurgitant orifice area (ROA_{max} in cm^2) based on the maximum regurgitant

(R_{FR}) flow rate (in mL/s) combined with maximum MR-jet velocity (V_{MR}) in cm/s:

$$\text{ROA}_{\text{max}} = R_{\text{FR}}/V_{\text{MR}} \qquad (12\text{–}6)$$

This approach assumes that R_{FR} and V_{MR} occur at the same time point in the cardiac cycle. The PISA should be recorded in a view parallel to the flow stream, typically an apical four-chamber view for MR, using a narrow sector and zoom mode, with the aliasing velocity adjusted to optimize visualization of a hemispherical aliasing boundary. If the PISA is hemielliptical or if the valve is nonplanar, an alternate approach should be used or appropriate corrections made in the calculations.

Continuous-wave Doppler Approach

Several types of information regarding the severity of valvular regurgitation can be derived from the spectral display of the CW Doppler signal:

❑ Signal intensity relative to antegrade flow
❑ Antegrade flow velocity
❑ Time course (shape) of the velocity curve

First, signal intensity is proportional to the number of blood cells contributing to the regurgitant signal. Because the ultrasound beam is relatively broad and signals from the entire length of the beam are recorded, much of the regurgitant jet can be encompassed in the beam with appropriate adjustment of beam direction. It is particularly helpful to compare the intensity of the regurgitant signal to antegrade flow across the same valve as a qualitative estimate

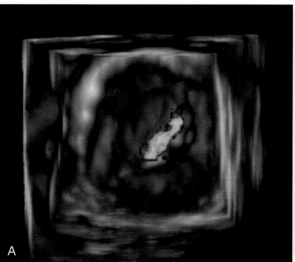

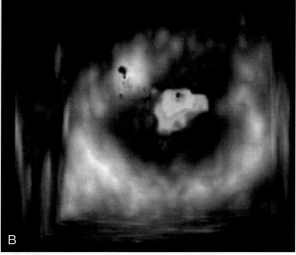

Figure 12–11 Three-dimensional echocardiography illustrates the variability in the shape of the proximal convergence zone in patients with mitral regurgitation. **A**, *En face* color 3D image from an LA perspective demonstrates an elongated and slightly curved PISA geometry along the entire leaflet coaptation line in patients with functional MR. **B**, In a patient with MV prolapse, a PISA more round in shape appears only in the region where the leaflet prolapses. *(From Matsumura Y, Fukuda S, Tran H, et al: Geometry of the proximal isovelocity surface area in mitral regurgitation by 3-dimensional color Doppler echocardiography: difference between functional mitral regurgitation and prolapse regurgitation. Am Heart J 2008;155:231–238).*

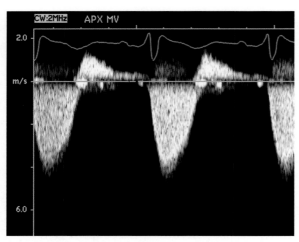

Figure 12–12 The CW Doppler mitral regurgitant signal, in the same patient as Figure 12–10, shows a dense signal, relative to antegrade mitral flow in diastole. The maximum velocity is only 4.3 m/s due to a low LV systolic pressure, and there is a rapid decline in velocity in late systole consistent with an LA *v*-wave.

of regurgitant severity (Fig. 12–12). A weak signal reflects mild regurgitation, whereas a signal nearly equal in intensity to antegrade flow reflects severe regurgitation. Moderate regurgitation has intermediate signal strength relative to antegrade flow.

Second, the associated antegrade velocity across the regurgitant valve provides useful information. Regurgitation results in an increase in the antegrade volume flow rate across the valve, which is reflected in an increase in the antegrade velocity across the valve. The greater the severity of regurgitation, the higher is the antegrade velocity. Of course, the possibility of coexisting valvular stenosis also must be considered.

Third, the shape of the velocity curve depends on the time-varying pressure gradient across the regurgitant valve. Each instantaneous velocity is related to the instantaneous pressure gradient across the valve, as stated in the Bernoulli equation. Normal LV systolic pressure is 100 to 140 mm Hg and normal LA pressure is 5 to 15 mm Hg, so the LV-to-LA pressure difference in systole is 85 to 135 mm Hg. Thus, the MR velocity curve typically shows a maximum velocity of 5 to 6 m/s. When ventricular function is normal, there is rapid acceleration to peak velocity, with a maintained high velocity in systole and with rapid deceleration prior to diastolic opening of the MV. An increase in end-systolic LA pressure (*v*-wave) results in a late-systolic decline in the instantaneous pressure gradient and in the instantaneous velocity (Fig. 12–13).

Similarly, the shape of the AR velocity curve depends on the time course of the diastolic pressure difference across the aortic valve. When LV end-diastolic pressure (EDP) is low and aortic EDP is normal or mildly reduced, a large pressure difference (and high velocity)

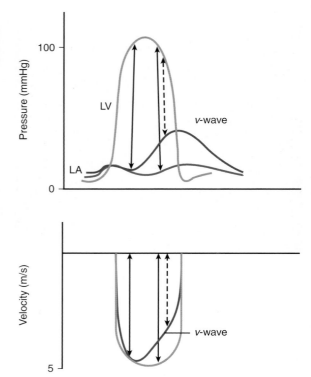

Figure 12–13 LV and LA pressures and the Doppler velocity curve in chronic (*yellow lines*) and acute (*blue lines*) mitral regurgitation are shown. Note that the shape of the velocity curve reflects the shape of the pressure difference between the LV and the LA, so that a late-systolic rise in LA pressure (*v*-wave) is seen as a more rapid decrease in velocity in late systole on the Doppler curve.

across the valve is present throughout diastole with a slow rate of pressure decline (Fig. 12–14). Acute or severe regurgitation results in more rapid equalization of LV and aortic pressures with a more rapid velocity decline in diastole.

The utility of the CW Doppler curve depends, in large part, on technical factors in data recording as well as on correct data interpretation. The high-velocity regurgitant signal is optimized by use of:

- ❏ Sweep speed of spectral display at 100 mm/s
- ❏ Velocity range adjusted so that signal of interest fits but fills the screen
- ❏ High-pass ("wall") filter set at the maximum level
- ❏ Gain and dynamic range adjusted to show dark outer edge of the velocity curve
- ❏ Examination from multiple acoustic windows
- ❏ Adjustment of transducer position and angulation

Optimal patient positioning, examination from multiple windows, and transducer angulation are needed to ensure a near-parallel intercept angle between the direction of the ultrasound beam and the regurgitant jet, to avoid underestimation of velocities. Use of a dedicated, small, CW transducer often facilitates the examination and provides a better signal-to-noise ratio

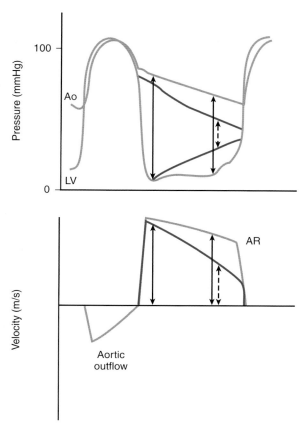

Figure 12–14 LV and central aortic (Ao) pressures and the corresponding Doppler velocity curve are shown for chronic (*green*) and acute (*blue*) aortic regurgitation (AR). Again, the shape of the velocity curve is related to the instantaneous pressure differences across the valve, as stated in the Bernoulli equation. With acute AR, aortic pressure falls more rapidly and ventricular diastolic pressure rises more rapidly, resulting in a steeper deceleration slope on the Doppler curve.

than 2D-guided CW Doppler. In addition, the 2D image may distract the examiner from searching for the highest velocity signal. Color flow imaging is of limited value for locating the best CW signal because it provides only 2D information; jet direction in the elevational plane remains unknown. Temporal factors also affect data quality, and caution is needed in interpreting the shape of the velocity curve if jet direction (and thus Doppler-jet intercept angle) varies during the regurgitant flow period.

Distal Flow Reversals

When atrioventricular valve regurgitation is severe enough that a significant volume of blood is displaced by the regurgitant jet, flow reversal is seen in the veins entering the atrium. With severe tricuspid regurgitation, the normal pattern of systolic inflow into the right atrium (RA) from the superior and inferior vena cava is reversed. This can be demonstrated with a pulsed Doppler sample volume positioned in

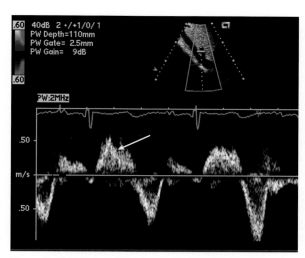

Figure 12–15 With the sample volume positioned in the central hepatic vein from a subcostal approach, systolic (*arrow*) flow reversal in the hepatic vein velocity curve is seen when severe tricuspid regurgitation is present. Forward flow into the RA in diastole also is seen.

the central hepatic vein (Fig. 12–15). Severe MR results in reversal of the normal patterns of systolic inflow into the LA from the pulmonary veins. This may be difficult to demonstrate on a TTE study due to signal attenuation at the depth of the pulmonary vein but is easily recorded from a TEE approach (Fig. 12–16).

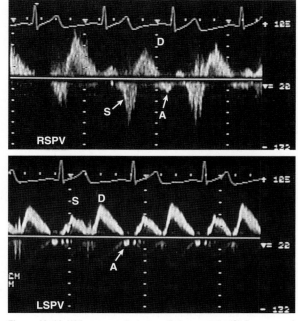

Figure 12–16 With severe mitral regurgitation, systolic (S) flow reversal in the right superior pulmonary vein (RSPV) Doppler velocity curve (*top*) and blunting of systolic flow in the left superior pulmonary vein (LSPV) (*bottom*) are seen on TEE imaging in a patient with an eccentric, anteromedially directed regurgitant jet. A, atrial reversal; D, diastolic flow.

Regurgitation of a semilunar valve results in reversal of flow in the associated great vessel as blood flows from the great vessel, across the incompetent valve, and into the ventricle. The distance from the valve plane that this flow reversal extends in the great vessel is proportional to regurgitant volume. For example, with severe AR, holodiastolic flow reversal is seen in the abdominal aorta. With moderate regurgitation, holodiastolic flow reversal only extends to the proximal descending thoracic aorta.

Volume Flow at Two Intracardiac Sites

Regurgitant stroke volume can be calculated using 2D diameter measurements in conjunction with pulsed Doppler flow velocities at two intracardiac sites. Total stroke volume is calculated from antegrade flow across the regurgitant valve as the cross-sectional area (CSA) of flow times the VTI of transvalvular flow. Forward stroke volume is calculated as antegrade flow across a different (and nonregurgitant) valve (Fig. 12–17).

For example, with AR, transaortic stroke volume (SV) represents total LV stroke volume and can be calculated as

$$SV_{total} = CSA_{LVOT} \times VTI_{LVOT} \qquad (12\text{--}7)$$

where CSA_{LVOT} is cross-sectional area of the LV outflow tract and VTI is the velocity-time integral of the LV outflow tract. Forward stroke volume is represented by LV inflow across the mitral annulus (MA), because the amount of blood filling the ventricle equals the amount of blood delivered to the body on each beat, and can be calculated as

$$SV_{forward} = CSA_{MA} \times VTI_{MA} \qquad (12\text{--}8)$$

With AR, alternate sites for measurement of forward stroke volume are the pulmonary artery and right ventricular (RV) inflow region. Regurgitant volume is

$$RV = SV_{total} \times SV_{forward} \qquad (12\text{--}9)$$

RF and ROA then are calculated with Eqs. 12–1 and 12–3. Alternatively, total stroke volume can be derived from 2D or 3D imaging of the LV with identification of endocardial borders at end-diastole and end-systole.

Calculation of regurgitant volume and regurgitant fraction from volume flow at two intracardiac sites has been shown to be accurate in animal models and in selected patient series. However, small errors in diameter measurement lead to large errors in area calculations due to the quadratic relationship between the two ($CSA = \pi r^2$). Other potential pitfalls in volume flow measurement are discussed in detail in Chapter 6. This method clearly can provide accurate quantitation of regurgitant severity when image quality is excellent; in other cases it is helpful to compare the antegrade VTI (or peak velocity) for the regurgitant valve to the antegrade flow across a competent valve as an indicator of their relative stroke volumes.

Limitations and Alternate Approaches

Echocardiography is the clinical standard for evaluation of valvular regurgitation. The diagnostic value of the echocardiographic study is increased when the interpretation integrates data from several potential measures of regurgitant severity into a summary statement. Rather than being redundant, the different approaches to regurgitant severity serve as cross-checks on each other. Errors or limitations of one approach will be recognized when other approaches, with better data quality, show discrepant results. Because valvular regurgitant is dynamic and varies with loading conditions, it is essential to record blood pressure at the time of the echocardiographic examination.

When TTE data are suboptimal, TEE is the next step. If further data are needed for clinical decision making, other approaches can be considered. Cardiac magnetic resonance (CMR) imaging provides quantitative measures of ventricular size and systolic function and of regurgitant volume and fraction (Fig. 12–18). Cardiac catheterization can be used to measure intracardiac pressures, angiographic visualization of regurgitation, and calculation of quantitative measures of regurgitant severity.

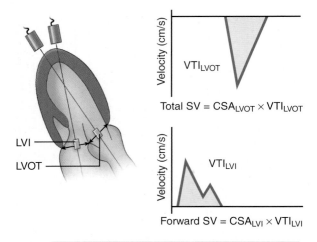

Figure 12–17 Calculation of aortic regurgitant stroke volume (SV) by measurement of transvalvular volume flow rate at two intracardiac sites is illustrated. Transaortic flow, representing total SV, is calculated from the cross-sectional area (CSA) and velocity time integral (VTI) of the LV outflow tract (LVOT). Transmitral flow, representing forward SV (FSV), is calculated from the CSA and VTI of LV inflow (LVI) across the mitral annulus. Regurgitant SV (RSV) is the difference between total SV and forward SV.

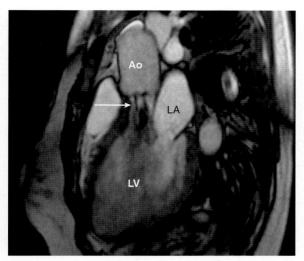

Figure 12–18 Cardiac magnetic resonance image showing aortic regurgitation due to a bicuspid aortic valve. The regurgitant flow appears as a black void in the lighter LV chamber using this pulse sequence.

AORTIC REGURGITATION

The echocardiographic approach to the patient with AR includes not only evaluation of the presence of regurgitation but also determination of the etiology and severity of regurgitation along with the effect of the regurgitant lesion on ventricular size and function and any other associated abnormalities.

Diagnostic Imaging of the Valve Apparatus

AR may be due either to abnormalities of the aorta or to abnormalities of the leaflets themselves (Table 12–5).

TABLE 12–5 Etiology of Aortic Regurgitation

Leaflet Abnormalities

Congenital bicuspid valve
Calcific valve disease
Rheumatic valve disease
Myxomatous valve disease
Endocarditis
Nonbacterial thrombotic endocarditis

Abnormalities of the Aorta

Marfan syndrome
Bicuspid aortic valve disease
Hypertensive aortic dilation
Cystic medial necrosis
Aortic dissection
Systemic inflammatory diseases

The disease processes that cause valvular aortic stenosis (*congenital bicuspid valve*, *calcific valve disease*, and *rheumatic disease*) also can result in AR due to alterations in leaflet flexibility or shape leading to inadequate diastolic coaptation of the leaflets. The 2D echocardiographic findings for these diagnoses are discussed in Chapter 11.

Other diseases that cause AR include *myxomatous valve disease*, which can affect the aortic valve as well as the MV. The leaflets are thickened and redundant on 2D echocardiography with slight sagging of the leaflets into the LV outflow tract in diastole. The normal hemicylindrical configuration of each leaflet in diastole is distorted so that the short-axis view intersects the center of the leaflet *en face*, resulting in the false appearance of an ill-defined echogenic "mass."

Endocarditis results in AR either by leaflet perforation due to the infectious process or to deformity of diastolic leaflet closure due to the presence of a vegetation (Fig. 12–19). Less common abnormalities of the aortic valve leaflets leading to AR include congenital leaflet fenestrations, nonbacterial thrombotic endocarditis (e.g. systemic lupus erythematosus), infiltrative diseases (e.g., amyloidosis), systemic inflammatory diseases (e.g., ankylosing spondylitis), mucopolysaccharidosis, and glycogen storage diseases.

Abnormalities of the aorta can result in AR, even when the leaflets themselves are normal, by alterations in the geometry of the structures supporting the leaflets. The aortic annulus is not a discrete planar ring of fibrous tissue but rather a complex crown-shaped structure where the leaflets attach to the aortic valve with the three "points" of the crown at the commissures and the three lowest points at the midsection of each leaflet. Dilation of this area at the base of the aorta—often termed *annular dilation*—results in AR due to inadequate coaptation of the stretched leaflets. Note that adjacent leaflets normally overlap (apposition zone), so that mild degrees of annular dilation may not result in valvular incompetence. Annular dilation may be due to a variety of causes, including *chronic hypertension*, *cystic medial necrosis*, or *Marfan syndrome*. Marfan syndrome is characterized by effacement of the normal sinotubular junction with dilation of the annulus and sinuses of Valsalva (see Chapter 16). In cystic medial necrosis, the sinotubular junction usually is identifiable, although dilation may involve the sinuses as well as the ascending aorta. *Bicuspid aortic valve disease* often is associated with significant dilation of the aortic sinuses and ascending aorta. AR due to *syphilitic aortitis* is rare in the United States. When present it typically is characterized by extensive calcification of the dilated ascending aorta. *Aortic dissection* can result in AR either by annular dilation resulting in inadequate coaptation or by the false channel of the dissection undermining the aortic annulus and resulting in a flail leaflet (see Chapter 16).

The *differential diagnosis* for the echocardiographer in evaluation of a patient referred for suspected AR depends on the specific indications for the

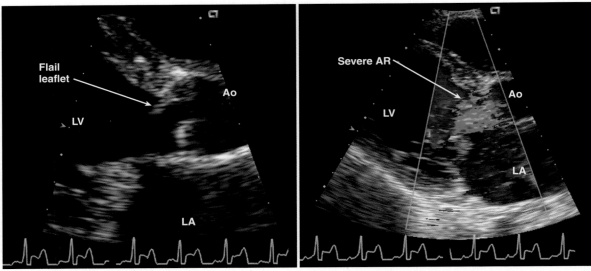

Figure 12–19 Flail aortic valve leaflet due to endocarditis (*left*) with a broad eccentric jet of aortic regurgitation (AR) on color flow imaging (*right*) in a parasternal long-axis view.

examination. If a diastolic murmur has been noted on auscultation, differential diagnoses include pulmonic regurgitation, mitral or tricuspid stenosis, and (rarely) a coronary arteriovenous fistula. In some cases only the diastolic portion of a continuous murmur (e.g., a patent ductus arteriosus) may have been appreciated. If AR is suspected because of a concern for aortic dissection, the differential diagnosis should focus on examination of the ascending aorta.

Left Ventricular Response

When exposed to chronic volume overload from AR, progressive dilation and increased sphericity of the LV occur. Initially, LV systolic function remains normal. With chronic gradually increasing AR, the LV remains compliant in diastole so that EDP remains normal. Typically, LV size slowly increases over a period of years without impairment of systolic function. However, LV systolic dysfunction eventually occurs in the presence of hemodynamically significant chronic volume overload, and in some individuals irreversible LV systolic dysfunction supervenes even in the absence of clinical symptoms.

In contrast to chronic regurgitation, in acute AR, the short interval from onset of volume overload to clinical presentation means that significant LV dilation has not yet occurred. The physiologic differences between acute and chronic AR are reflected both in the 2D echocardiographic findings and in the Doppler examination (Table 12–6).

Indirect Signs of Aortic Regurgitation

In addition to anatomic abnormalities of the aortic valve and the secondary LV dilation that occurs in

TABLE 12–6	Chronic versus Acute Aortic Regurgitation	
Parameter	**Chronic**	**Acute**
Etiology (examples)	Bicuspid valve Hypertension	Endocarditis Aortic dissection
LV size	Dilated	Normal
LV EDP	Normal	Elevated
Pulse pressure	Wide	Narrow
CW Doppler slope	Flat	Steep

CW, continuous-wave; EDP, end-diastolic pressure.

response to volume overload, several indirect signs may be seen in patients with AR:

- ❐ Increased E-point septal separation (EPSS)
- ❐ High-frequency fluttering of the anterior mitral leaflet
- ❐ "Reverse doming" of the anterior mitral leaflet
- ❐ Jet lesion on septum or MV

If the regurgitant jet impinges on the anterior MV leaflet, it causes impaired leaflet opening, resulting in an increased distance between the maximal anterior motion of the MV in early-diastole (the E-point) and the most posterior motion of the interventricular septum (e.g., increased EPSS). High-frequency fluttering of the anterior MV leaflet resulting from impingement of the regurgitant jet also may be

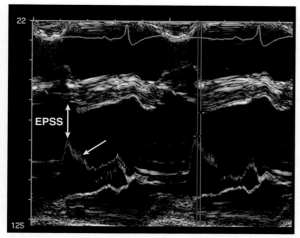

Figure 12–20 M-mode tracing showing increased *E*-point septal separation (EPSS) and high-frequency fluttering of the anterior mitral valve leaflet (*arrow*) due to impingement by an aortic regurgitant jet.

of the anterior leaflet is opposite to that seen in rheumatic mitral stenosis. With chronic regurgitation the focal blood flow disturbance impinging on the septum or anterior mitral leaflet may result in a raised fibrotic lesion—identifiable by the pathologist postmortem as a jet lesion—which appears as an area of increased echogenicity on 2D imaging.

While none of these indirect signs of AR provides quantitative data, their presence may suggest a previously unsuspected diagnosis and prompt a directed Doppler examination. Recognition of the impact of AR on mitral leaflet motion and the appearance of jet lesions avoids misinterpretation of these findings.

Evaluation of Aortic Regurgitant Severity

Screening Examination

appreciated on M-mode (with its high sampling rate), although it is rarely appreciated on 2D imaging (due to the relatively low frame rate) (Fig. 12–20).

On 2D long- and short-axis imaging, the anterior mitral leaflet may appear curved in diastole with the concavity toward the ventricular septum, with the region of abnormal curvature corresponding to the direction of the regurgitant jet. In short-axis views, a discrete area of reversed curvature corresponding to the spatial location of the regurgitant jet may be seen. This contrasts with the normal linear appearance of the anterior leaflet in diastole in long-axis views and the normal diastolic curvature toward the ventricular septum in the short-axis view. This observation has been termed *reverse doming*, because the curvature

Screening for AR with color flow imaging and CW Doppler ultrasound is part of a routine echocardiographic examination (Figs. 12–21 and 12–22). Parasternal views in both long and short axis are helpful and may allow identification of the exact origin of the regurgitant jet as well as assessment of its width and cross-sectional area. Mild AR fills only a small area of the LV outflow tract, whereas moderate-to-severe AR fills a larger percentage of the outflow tract diameter or area (Fig. 12–23). Eccentric jets may traverse the outflow tract obliquely, which makes measurement of jet size more difficult. A central jet that fills less than 25% of the outflow tract is consistent with mild regurgitation.

CW Doppler is used to record the antegrade aortic velocity signal from an apical approach with careful angulation to identify an AR signal, if present. A weak or absent diastolic signal confirms that significant regurgitation is not present.

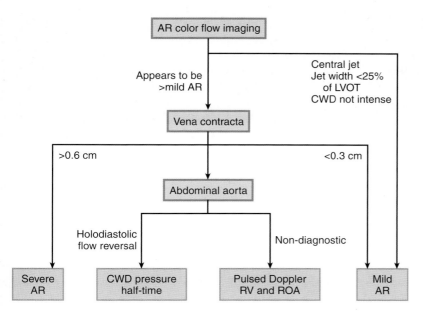

Figure 12–21 Approach to echocardiographic quantitation of aortic regurgitation (AR) severity; CWD, continuous-wave Doppler; LVOT, LV outflow tract; ROA, regurgitant orifice area; RV, regurgitant volume.

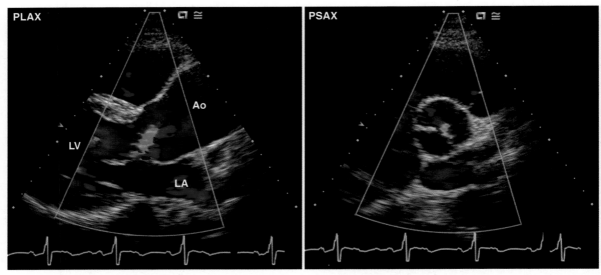

Figure 12–22 Color Doppler images in parasternal long-axis (PLAX) (*left*) and short-axis (PSAX) (*right*) views in a patient with mild aortic regurgitation. In long axis, a narrow eccentric jet is seen, which in short axis has a small cross-sectional area at the regurgitant orifice relative to the area of the outflow tract.

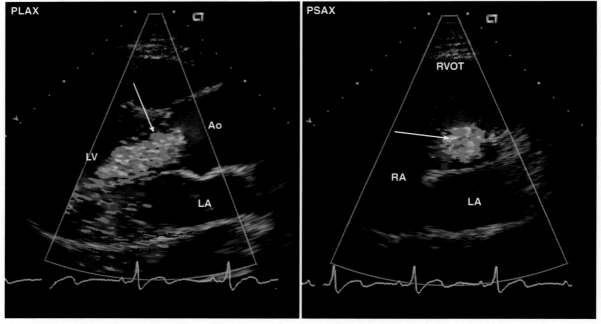

Figure 12–23 Color Doppler images in parasternal long-axis (PLAX) (*left*) and short-axis (PSAX) (*right*) views in a patient with severe aortic regurgitation. The flow disturbance fills the outflow tract in both views.

Vena Contracta

If the screening examination suggests more than mild AR, the next step is measurement of the vena contracta width, followed by further quantitation of regurgitant severity in some patients (Table 12–7). The vena contracta is visualized using color flow in a parasternal long-axis view in the zoom mode, with a narrow sector, to optimize temporal and spatial resolution. Careful angulation medially and laterally from the long-axis plane may be needed to clearly identify the narrowest segment of the regurgitant jet (see Fig. 12–8). A vena contracta width less than 0.3 cm is consistent with mild regurgitation, and no further evaluation is needed. A greater vena contracta width or poor data quality prompts further evaluation of regurgitant severity. With eccentric jets,

TABLE 12-7 Quantitative Evaluation of Aortic Regurgitant Severity (ASE Guidelines)

Parameter	Mild	Moderate	Severe
Jet width/LVOT (%)	<25	25–65	>65
Vena contracta (cm)	<0.3	0.3–0.6	>0.6
Pressure half-time (ms)	>500	200–500	<200
Regurgitant volume (mL/beat)	<30	30–60	>60
Regurgitant fraction (%)	<30	30–50	>50
Regurgitant orifice area (cm^2)	<0.10	0.1–0.3	>0.30

ASE, American Society of Echocardiography; LVOT, left ventricular outflow tract.

diameter is measured perpendicular to the long axis of the jet, not the long axis of the outflow tract.

Aortic Flow Reversal

With severe AR, holodiastolic flow reversal is seen in the proximal abdominal aorta, recorded from the subcostal window (Fig. 12–24). This observation is analogous to the physical examination finding of diastolic reversal in the femoral arteries (DeRosier's sign). Holodiastolic flow reversal in the abdominal aorta is sensitive (100%)

and specific (97%) for diagnosing severe AR. False-positive results may be due to the presence of a patent ductus arteriosus, where the diastolic flow is from aorta to pulmonary artery rather than to the LV. More proximal holodiastolic flow reversal, in the descending thoracic aorta, also is sensitive for detection of severe AR but is less specific, also being seen in some subjects with only moderate regurgitation (Fig. 12–25).

Continuous-wave Doppler

The CW Doppler spectral recording of AR has its onset at aortic valve closure (during isovolumic relaxation) with a rapid increase in velocity to a maximum of 3 to 5 m/s, followed by a gradual decline in velocity during diastole. The velocity abruptly decelerates during isovolumic contraction, reaching baseline at aortic valve opening. The intensity of the signal, relative to antegrade velocity, is an indicator of regurgitant severity. In moderate or severe regurgitation, the signal can easily be recorded throughout diastole, whereas mild regurgitation may not appear holodiastolic, with a recordable signal only at the beginning or end of diastole. This observation may be due to low signal strength or variation in jet direction during diastole resulting in significant intercept angle changes.

The shape of the CW Doppler time-velocity curve depends on the time-varying instantaneous pressure gradient across the valve in diastole, thus reflecting both severity and chronicity of regurgitation. Chronic severe AR results in an increased aortic pulse pressure with a low end-diastolic aortic pressure. The rapid rate of decline in aortic pressure is reflected in a more rapid decline in the Doppler velocity—that is, a steeper diastolic deceleration slope even if

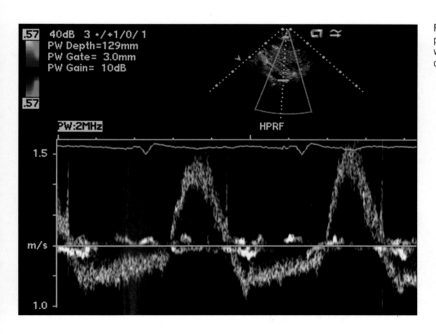

Figure 12–24 Doppler velocity curve in the proximal abdominal aorta from a subcostal window shows holodiastolic flow reversal consistent with severe aortic regurgitation.

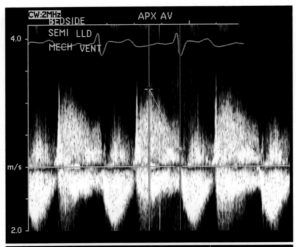

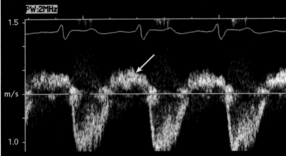

Figure 12–25 Severe acute aortic regurgitation with a dense CW Doppler signal with a steep deceleration slope (*top*) and holodiastolic flow reversal in the descending thoracic aorta recorded from a suprasternal notch window (*bottom*) in the same patient as in Figure 12–19.

with mild regurgitation, and a steep slope (pressure half-time < 200 ms) indicates severe regurgitation.

However, in addition to AR severity, other factors that affect either LV or aortic diastolic pressure also affect the course of the pressure difference (and velocity) across the regurgitant valve. With *acute* regurgitation, even if only moderate in severity, LV compliance has not yet adapted, as occurs in response to chronic volume overload, so a significant increase in end-diastolic pressure is seen. In extreme cases, aortic and LV diastolic pressure may equalize, resulting in a triangular-shaped CW velocity signal with a linear deceleration slope from maximum velocity to the baseline. Other factors that affect LV diastolic pressure (e.g., systolic dysfunction, ischemia) or aortic diastolic pressure (e.g., sepsis, patent ductus arteriosus) also will affect the shape of the AR velocity curve.

The CW signal for AR usually is best recorded from an apical window to obtain a parallel intercept angle between the jet and the blood flow direction. Occasionally, an eccentric jet, directed either anteriorly or posteriorly, will be best recorded from a parasternal approach. If signal strength from the suprasternal notch is adequate, a signal similar to that recorded from the apex (but, of course, inverted) is seen.

Regurgitant Volume and Fraction

Aortic regurgitant volume and fraction can be calculated as the difference between transaortic and transmitral volume flow. In addition, in the specific case of AR, both forward and total stroke volume can be calculated at a single anatomic site: the proximal descending thoracic aorta. When AR is present, significant systolic expansion of the aorta occurs, so the antegrade flow velocity integral must be multiplied by the systolic area of the aorta. The flow velocity integral of the reversed flow

end-diastolic LV pressure remains low (Fig. 12–26). Thus, diastolic deceleration slope provides a semi-quantitative measure of aortic regurgitant severity. A flat slope (pressure half-time > 500 ms) is consistent

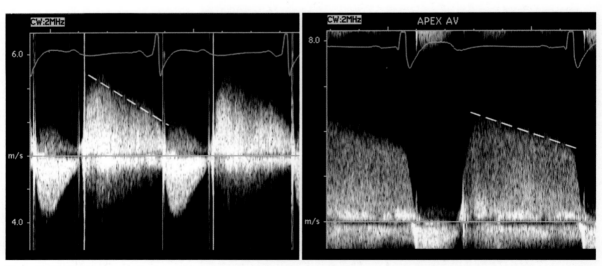

Figure 12–26 CW Doppler recording in two patients, one with acute aortic regurgitation due to aortic dissection (*left*) and one with chronic regurgitation due to calcific aortic valve disease (*right*) showing the differences in the deceleration slope in these clinical situations.

in diastole is multiplied by diastolic aortic area. Either 2D short-axis imaging or an M-mode through the aortic arch can be used for measurement of systolic and diastolic areas. Note that this quantitative approach is the logical extension of the semiquantitative approach, which relies on the *presence* and spatial extent of holodiastolic flow reversal in the aorta in patients with AR.

Clinical Utility

Diagnostic Utility for Aortic Regurgitation

An echocardiogram may be requested to either confirm or exclude a clinical diagnosis of AR. Given the high sensitivity and specificity of this approach, the resulting diagnostic data are highly reliable. In addition, information on the etiology of valve disease, associated conditions, and the degree of LV dilation is obtained. If AR is detected in the course of an echocardiogram ordered for some other indication, it is incumbent on the echocardiographer to search carefully for the etiology of regurgitation. The finding of regurgitation may be the first clue that aortic dilation or a disease process affecting the aortic leaflets is present.

Timing of Surgical Intervention for Chronic Asymptomatic Aortic Regurgitation

Timing of surgical intervention in the asymptomatic patient is a problem, because measures of LV systolic function are dependent on loading conditions, which are altered by the presence of valvular regurgitation. End-systolic volume or dimension provides a relatively load-independent measure of ventricular performance. Several studies examining outcome after valve replacement for AR have shown that an LV end-systolic dimension of less than 55 mm is predictive of preserved (or improved) LV systolic function and an excellent prognosis after valve replacement (Fig. 12–27). While a prospective, randomized trial of surgical intervention in the asymptomatic patient has not been performed, a consensus has developed that surgical intervention is indicated for progressive LV dilation or other evidence of decreased systolic function (see Suggested Readings 1 and 2). Annual echocardiography is recommended for evaluation of changes in LV size and systolic function and to optimize the timing of valve replacement in the asymptomatic patient with significant regurgitation.

MITRAL REGURGITATION

Diagnostic Imaging of the Mitral Valve Apparatus

Functionally, the MV apparatus consists of several components:

- □ LA wall
- □ Mitral annulus

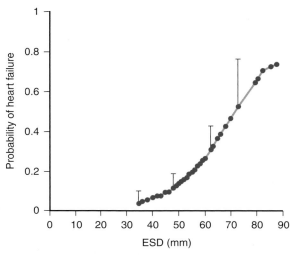

Figure 12–27 In a prospective study of 87 adults with aortic regurgitation, the probability of heart failure after aortic valve replacement (*y*-axis) plotted against preoperative end-systolic dimension (ESD) (*x*-axis). *(From Tornos MP, Olona M, Permanyer-Miralda G, et al: Heart failure after aortic valve replacement for aortic regurgitation: Prospective 20-year study. Am Heart J 136(Pt 1):681–687, 1998.)*

- □ Anterior and posterior leaflets
- □ Chordae
- □ Papillary muscles
- □ LV myocardium underlying the papillary muscles

Dysfunction or altered anatomy of any one of these components can result in MR (Fig. 12–28). Annular dilation may be due to either LA or LV dilation and results in MR because of incomplete leaflet coaptation. The normal mitral apparatus is a saddle-shaped ellipse with its most apical points seen in the apical four-chamber view and its most basal points seen in the long-axis view. As noted for the aortic valve, the mitral leaflets have a normal area of overlap (or apposition), so that some degree of annular dilation may be tolerated without significant regurgitation.

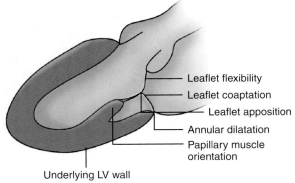

Mechanisms of Mitral Regurgitation

Leaflet flexibility
Leaflet coaptation
Leaflet apposition
Annular dilatation
Papillary muscle orientation
Underlying LV wall

Figure 12–28 Schematic diagram illustrating how abnormalities of any part of the complex mitral valve apparatus can result in mitral regurgitation.

The mitral annular area normally is smaller in systole than in diastole. Increased rigidity of the annulus, as seen with *mitral annular calcification (MAC)*, impairs systolic contraction of the annulus leading to MR. MAC has a typical appearance on 2D imaging as an area of increased echogenicity on the LV side of the annulus immediately adjacent to the attachment point of the posterior leaflet. Acoustic shadowing, due to the presence of calcium, is seen. In short-axis views the annular calcium may be focal or extensive, involving the entire U-shaped posterior annulus. The region of anterior mitral leaflet–posterior aortic wall continuity is involved only rarely. MAC is commonly seen in elderly subjects and in younger patients with renal failure or hypertension.

Diseases of the MV leaflets include myxomatous disease, rheumatic disease, endocarditis, Marfan syndrome, and rare disorders such as infiltrative diseases (amyloid, sarcoid, mucopolysaccharidosis) and systemic inflammatory disorders (systemic lupus erythematosus, rheumatoid arthritis). *Myxomatous* MV disease is characterized by thickened, redundant leaflets and chordae with excessive motion and sagging of portions of the leaflets into the LA in systole (Fig. 12–29). The severity of disease is variable, ranging from MV prolapse, in which there is only minimal displacement of the leaflets into the LA in systole, to severe involvement of both leaflets by myxomatous disease with frankly prolapsed or flail leaflet segments. *Chordal disruption* or *elongation* leads to MR because of inadequate tensile support of the closed leaflets in systole. Chordal elongation results in severe bowing of the leaflet, or leaflet segment, into the LA, with the tip of the leaflet still directed toward the ventricular apex. With chordal rupture there is a flail segment of the leaflet such that the leaflet is displaced into the LA in systole, with the tip of the leaflet pointing away from the ventricular apex (Fig. 12–30).

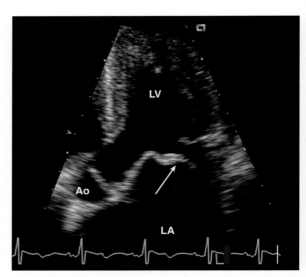

Figure 12–30 Apical four-chamber view demonstrating a partial flail anterior mitral valve leaflet in a young man with myxomatous mitral valve disease. Note that the tip of the flail segment (*arrow*) points away from the LV apex.

Rheumatic MR, like rheumatic mitral stenosis, is characterized by some degree of commissural fusion but chordal fusion and shortening are more prominent. *Endocarditis* results in MR by leaflet destruction, perforation, or deformity. *Marfan syndrome* is associated with a long redundant anterior leaflet that sags into the LA in systole. Infiltrative diseases result in irregular leaflet thickening and inadequate coaptation. Of note, *age-related degenerative changes* in the mitral leaflets often are seen (with or without associated MAC) and appear as irregular areas of thickening and increased echogenicity of the mitral leaflets.

Ischemic MR may be due to regional LV dysfunction with abnormal contraction of the papillary

Figure 12–29 Parasternal long-axis (*left*) and M-mode recording (*right*) in a young woman with mitral valve prolapse. Bileaflet prolapse is seen on 2D imaging (*arrows*), and the M-mode shows late-systolic posterior motion of the leaflets (*arrow*).

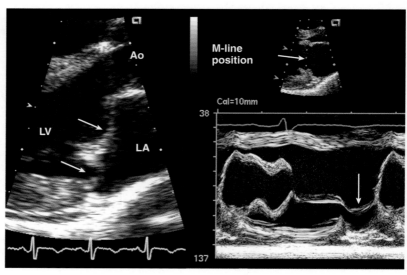

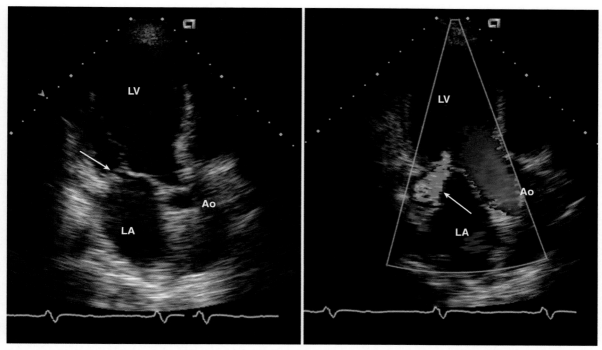

Figure 12–31 Ischemic mitral regurgitation (MR) with a posteriorly directed MR jet due to papillary muscle dysfunction seen in an apical long-axis view. Note the tethering of the posterior leaflet on the 2D image.

muscle or underlying ventricular wall. In patients with a myocardial infarction, myocardial scarring results in MR at rest. In patients with normal resting myocardial function but inducible ischemia with stress, MR may be intermittent. Ischemic MR is characterized by restricted leaflet motion, resulting in the appearance of "tenting" or tethering of the mitral valve in systole (Fig. 12–31).

Papillary muscle rupture can occur as a complication of acute myocardial infarction. If the entire papillary muscle is disconnected from the underlying LV wall, few patients survive due to acute severe mitral regurgitation. Echocardiographic evaluation in those who do survive shows a mass (the ruptured papillary muscle) attached to flail segments of anterior and posterior leaflets (since each papillary muscle attaches to both leaflets) (see Fig. 8–29). The ruptured papillary muscle head is seen in the LA in systole and in the LV in diastole. Severe mitral regurgitation is present on Doppler examination. Partial rupture of a papillary muscle, defined as rupture of one of several "heads" or as partial disconnection of the base of the papillary muscle, is seen more often than complete rupture, as patients are more likely to survive long enough to undergo diagnostic evaluation. In this situation the echocardiogram shows a thin, attenuated, excessively mobile papillary muscle and, if one head has ruptured, a mass attached to the leaflet with prolapse into the LA in systole.

MR due to LV dilation and systolic dysfunction, in patients with normal valve leaflets and chordae, often

is called *functional MR* (Fig. 12–32). The mechanism of functional MR remains controversial, with some studies suggesting abnormal orientation of the papillary muscles and others suggesting annular dilation.

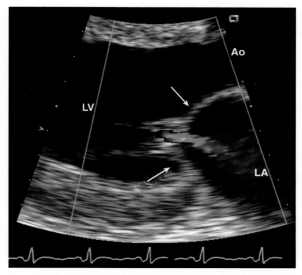

Figure 12–32 In parasternal long-axis view, a central mitral regurgitant (MR) jet due to dilated cardiomyopathy is seen. Because the leaflets and chordae are normal, this is often called *functional MR*. There is "tenting" of the leaflet closure plane (*arrows*) due to tethering of the leaflets as the mitral apparatus is distorted by the dilated ventricle.

Obviously, while MR due to conditions with unique anatomic features can be reliably diagnosed by echocardiographic imaging (rheumatic or myxomatous disease), there is considerable overlap in the anatomic features of other conditions (degenerative versus infiltrative leaflet abnormalities). In some cases, it is difficult to determine if MR is the cause or consequence of ventricular dilation and systolic dysfunction. When etiology is unclear, the echocardiographer can describe the valve anatomy and indicate possible reasons for the findings even though the specific tissue diagnosis remains unknown.

Response of the Left Ventricle, Left Atrium, and Pulmonary Vasculature

MR results in LV volume overload due to the increase in total LV stroke volume as blood is ejected both forward into the aorta and retrograde across the MV. With acute MR the LV empties more completely (e.g., ejection fraction increases), such that forward cardiac output is maintained. With compensated chronic regurgitation LV diastolic volume increases and ejection fraction is normal, such that end-systolic volume is within the normal range or only mildly increased. Although it might seem that afterload is decreased in patients with MR due to ejection into the low-pressure LA, the effect of decreased ejection force is counterbalanced by increased ventricular chamber size without an increase in wall thickness. Thus, with chronic MR, afterload is normal and ejection fraction typically is in the normal range (not increased).

With chronic regurgitation, progressive LV dilation eventually occurs as the regurgitant volume (and thus total LV stroke volume) increases. As with AR, an irreversible decline in LV contractility can occur in the absence of symptoms. The LA gradually dilates to accommodate the regurgitant volume while maintaining a normal LA pressure. LA compliance increases, that is, the LA pressure-volume relationship is shifted downward and to the right. With acute MR the regurgitant volume is delivered into a small, noncompliant LA, resulting in a significant increase in LA pressure and a v-wave in the LA pressure curve.

Pulmonary artery (PA) pressure increases passively in response to both the chronic mildly elevated LA pressure seen with chronic MR and the acute severe elevation seen with acute regurgitation. When LA pressure is chronically elevated, pulmonary vascular resistance may increase. Echocardiographic evaluation of the patient with MR includes noninvasive measurement of PA pressure from the tricuspid regurgitant jet velocity and an estimate of RA pressure.

Evaluation of Mitral Regurgitant Severity

Screening Examination

The basic screening examination for MR includes color flow imaging and CW Doppler ultrasound (Fig. 12–33). Color Doppler imaging allows detection of the presence of MR and separates mild regurgitation from moderate to severe disease. The shape and direction of the jet are helpful in diagnosis; an eccentric jet suggests pathologic regurgitation and provides clues about the mechanism of regurgitation. Abnormalities of the posterior leaflet tend to result in an anteriorly directed jet (Fig. 12–34), while anterior leaflet or papillary muscle dysfunction tends to result in a posteriorly directed jet (Fig. 12–35). Dilation of the LV or mitral annulus results in a central, symmetric regurgitant jet. In

Figure 12–33 Approach to quantitation of mitral regurgitation (MR) severity. Evaluation of systolic flow reversal in the pulmonary veins provides useful additional information in patients with sinus rhythm. TEE imaging often is needed for complete evaluation of MR severity in patients with moderate-to-severe disease. CWD, CW Doppler; PISA, proximal isovelocity surface area; ROA, regurgitant orifice area; RV, regurgitant volume.

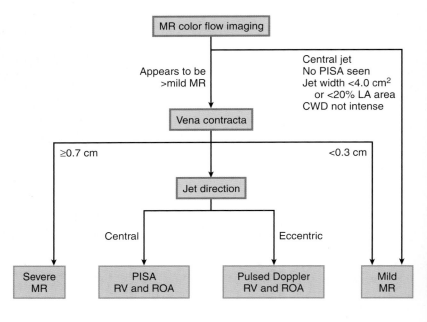

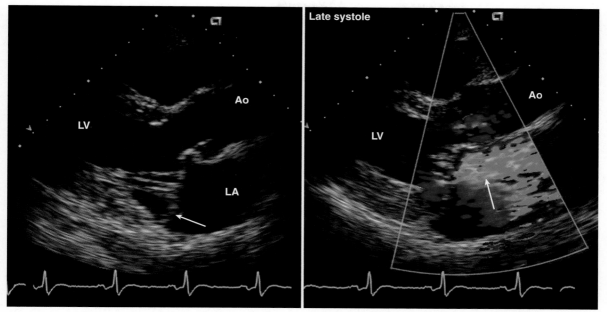

Late systole

Figure 12–34 This young woman with posterior leaflet prolapse (*left*) has an anteriorly directed mitral regurgitant (MR) jet (*right*). On frame-by-frame analysis and on CW Doppler, MR occurred only in the second half of systole.

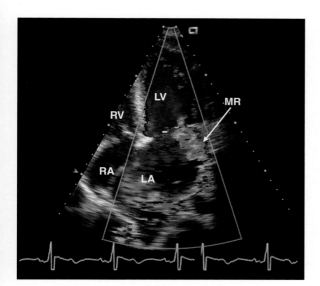

Figure 12–35 Eccentric posterior and laterally directed jet of mitral regurgitation (MR) (*arrow*) in the apical four-chamber view in the patient with a partial flail anterior leaflet, also shown in Figure 12–30.

addition to parasternal long- and short-axis views, apical four-chamber and long-axis views may be useful because they are nearly orthogonal to each other. However, signal attenuation at the depth of the LA may limit the utility of apical views if ultrasound penetration is suboptimal. A central jet with an area less than 4.0 cm^2 or less than 20% of the LA area in a non-oblique view, is consistent with mild MR.

The CW Doppler spectral recording of MR shows a rapid increase in velocity during isovolumic contraction (proportional to the rate of rise in LV pressure or dP/dt) from baseline to a maximum velocity of 5 to 6 m/s. The velocity stays high throughout systole with a curve paralleling the rise and fall of LV pressure given a normal LA pressure. During isovolumic relaxation the velocity rapidly returns to baseline. Signal intensity of the MR signal, in comparison with antegrade flow, is related to MR severity. In addition, significant regurgitation is associated with an increase in the antegrade velocity due to increased transmitral volume flow.

With acute MR (Table 12–8), an increase in LA pressure during late systole—a *v*-wave—may be present due to a steep pressure-volume relationship of the nondilated LA. In this situation, the pressure gradient between the LV and the LA is high initially but then begins to equalize in late systole as LA pressure rises. The corresponding Doppler velocity curve shows a high initial velocity with a more rapid fall in velocity in mid- to late-systole. This pattern of Doppler velocities also is termed a *v-wave* (see Fig. 12–13).

Vena Contracta

Vena contracta diameter should be measured if color Doppler imaging shows an eccentric or a large jet or if CW Doppler suggests more than mild MR (Table 12–9). In patients with MR, vena contracta width is optimally visualized in a parasternal long-axis view, although apical four-chamber and long-axis views may be used if parasternal images are inadequate. The apical two-chamber view is not reliable because the jet width may be broad in this

TABLE 12–8   Chronic versus Acute Mitral Regurgitation

Parameter	Chronic	Acute
Etiology (examples)	Myxomatous valve disease Annular dilation	Endocarditis Papillary muscle rupture Chordal rupture
LV size	Dilated	Normal
LV systolic function	Hyperdynamic early, may be normal or depressed with long-standing disease	Hyperdynamic
LA size	Enlarged	Normal
CW Doppler	High velocity throughout systole	Late-systolic velocity decline (v-wave)

TABLE 12–9   Quantitative Evaluation of Mitral Regurgitant Severity (ASE Guidelines)

Parameter	Mild	Moderate	Severe
Jet area (% of LA area)	<20%	20%–40%	>40%
Vena contracta (cm)	<0.3	0.3–0.7	>0.7
Regurgitant volume (mL)	<30	30–60	>60
Regurgitant fraction (%)	<30	30–50	>50
Regurgitant orifice area (cm^2)	<0.20	0.2–0.4	>0.40

image plane, even though regurgitation is not severe. Vena contracta width also can be measured with TEE imaging. A vena contracta width >0.3 cm indicates that further quantitation of regurgitant severity is needed.

Proximal Isovelocity Surface Area

With a central regurgitant jet, regurgitant volume and orifice area can be calculated by the PISA approach. The PISA is optimally imaged in an apical four-

chamber view using a narrow sector, minimal depth, and zoom mode. The PISA also can be imaged from a TEE approach. The aliasing velocity is adjusted to provide a clearly identified hemispherical PISA, typically at a Nyquist limit of 20 to 40 cm/s. Instantaneous regurgitant volume flow rate is calculated as indicated in Equation 12–4. The maximum velocity of the MR-jet on CW Doppler recording is then used in Equation 12–6 to determine ROA.

Regurgitation Volume and Orifice Area

The PISA approach is less accurate with eccentric jets or when the isovelocity surface area is not hemispherical. In these situations quantitation of MR by pulsed Doppler volume flow rates is more appropriate. Mitral regurgitant volume (RV_{mitral}) can be calculated from total LV stroke volume measured across the MV (SV_{mitral}) minus forward stroke volume measured in the LV outflow tract (SV_{LVOT}) (Fig. 12–36):

$$RV_{mitral} = SV_{mitral} - SV_{LVOT}$$

Alternate sites for measurement of forward stroke volume are the tricuspid valve and the PA. ROA then can be calculated (Eq. 12–3) using this regurgitant volume and the VTI of the CW Doppler MR jet.

Pulmonary Vein Flow Reversal

As the MR-jet enters the LA, it necessarily displaces blood that was already in the chamber. When severe regurgitation is present, systolic flow reversal in the pulmonary veins is seen. On TTE the flow pattern in the right inferior pulmonary vein can be recorded from the apical four-chamber view in most patients, although the signal-to-noise ratio may be suboptimal at this depth in some adult patients. On TEE the flow pattern in the pulmonary veins can be recorded at high resolution. Examination of all four pulmonary veins is especially helpful with an eccentric regurgitant jet, since the pattern of systolic flow reversal may not be uniform.

False-negative results (i.e., a normal pulmonary vein flow pattern despite severe regurgitation) occur when the LA is severely enlarged and compliant so that all the excess volume is contained in the LA without displacement into the pulmonary veins. False-positive results (i.e., blunted or reversed systolic pulmonary vein flow when regurgitation is not severe) occur when an eccentric jet is directed into a pulmonary vein, causing flow reversal in one vein even when regurgitation is not severe. False-positive results also may be seen in patients who are not in sinus rhythm, because the normal pattern of systolic atrial filling partly depends on the preceding emptying of the atrium due to atrial contraction. Other physiologic factors that affect the atrial inflow patterns include respiratory phase, cardiac rhythm, atrial and

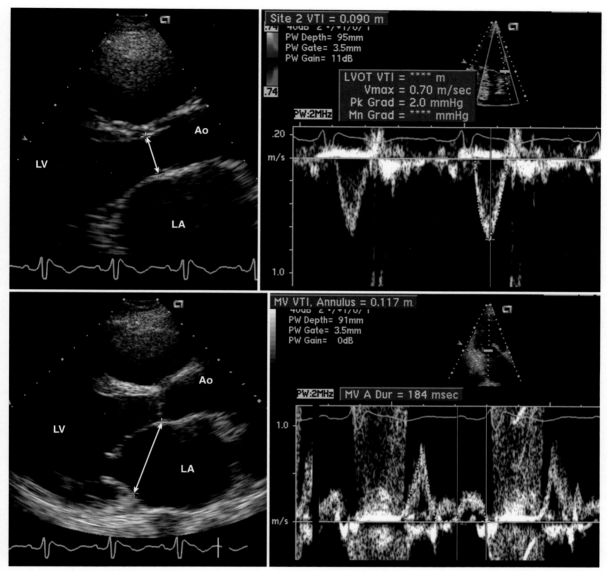

Figure 12–36 Quantitative evaluation of mitral regurgitation severity by calculation of transmitral and transaortic volume flow rates. Mitral annulus diameter and the velocity time integral (VTI) of flow across the annulus are used to calculate total stroke volume. Forward stroke volume is determined from the cross-sectional area and VTI of LV outflow tract flow.

venous compliance, ventricular diastolic filling, and age. Thus, while the presence and severity of venous systolic flow reversal is a useful adjunct in evaluation of atrioventricular valve regurgitant severity *in patients in sinus rhythm*, it certainly is not a pathognomonic finding.

Clinical Utility

Diagnosis and Severity of Mitral Regurgitation

Determination of the etiology of MR using 2D imaging often has important clinical implications. Evaluation of regurgitant severity also is of clinical importance, although a high degree of sophistication in echocardiographic interpretation is needed for this application (Fig. 12–37). In assessing the severity of regurgitation, the echocardiographer should first describe the individual findings and then integrate these findings into a consistent overall interpretation. In addition, the degree of pulmonary hypertension, LA size, LV size and systolic function, and any associated abnormalities are added to the Doppler findings before arriving at a final interpretation.

Examples of clinical situations in which decisions can be based on echocardiographic and Doppler data include acute MR after myocardial infarction, MV endocarditis, and chronic MR due to myxomatous MV disease. The decision whether or not to perform

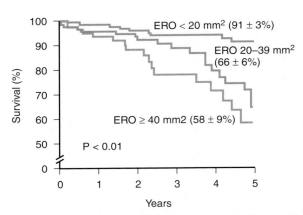

Figure 12–37 Kaplan-Meier estimates of the mean (±SE) rates of overall survival among patients with asymptomatic mitral regurgitation under medical management, according to the effective regurgitant orifice (ERO). *(From Enriquez-Sarano M, Avierinos JF, Messika-Zeitoun D, et al: Quantitative determinants of the outcome of asymptomatic mitral regurgitation. N Engl J Med. 2005;352:875–883).*

valve surgery (repair or replacement) usually can be made based on clinical and echocardiographic data without invasive studies in these patient groups. Only in cases where there is a discrepancy between the clinical impression and the echocardiographic findings (or when coronary angiography is indicated) are further diagnostic tests warranted.

Diagnosis of Mitral Valve Prolapse

MV prolapse or myxomatous MV disease is a pathologic condition characterized histologically by increased mucopolysaccharides, thickening, and disarray of the MV leaflet. Grossly, the leaflets and chordae are thick and redundant but with reduced tensile strength, so that they are prone to progressive elongation or rupture. 2D imaging demonstrates thick, redundant leaflets and chordae with systolic displacement of the leaflets into the LA in systole. Over time, a partial flail leaflet due to chordal rupture may develop. A subset of patients with this disease has a high incidence of significant MR and often goes on to require MV surgery. Patients with myxomatous MV disease also may have aortic or tricuspid valve involvement.

In contrast, other patients with MV prolapse have a more benign long-term outcome, suggesting that myxomatous MV disease encompasses a spectrum of disease severity. These patients have echocardiographic findings closer to the range of normal variation in MV anatomy and dynamics so that strict echocardiographic criteria must be used to avoid a false-positive diagnosis of MV prolapse. For example, in an apical four-chamber view, the closure plane of the mitral leaflets may appear "flat" relative to the MA even in subjects with normal valve leaflets, since the most apical points of the saddle-shaped annulus

are seen in this view. In addition, normal leaflet closure may appear displaced to the atrial side of the annulus if image planes are oblique relative to the annular plane. Displacement of the leaflets into the LA in systole is most reliably assessed in parasternal and apical long-axis views. In addition, it is helpful to describe valve anatomy (leaflet size, thickness, redundancy, chordal involvement) as well as the pattern of valve motion.

Follow-up of Chronic Asymptomatic Mitral Regurgitation

Sequential echocardiographic studies can be used to follow asymptomatic patients with MR. While regurgitation severity and valve anatomy provide the impetus for follow-up, the most important variables on serial studies are LV size and systolic function. Current data suggest that evidence of progressive ventricular dilation, an end-systolic dimension greater than 40 mm, or any reduction in LV systolic function should prompt consideration of surgical intervention, regardless of the symptomatic status of the patient, to prevent irreversible ventricular dysfunction postoperatively (Fig. 12–38).

Decision Making Concerning Mitral Valve Repair or Replacement

Once the decision has been made that surgical intervention is needed, the echocardiographic images are invaluable in considering whether MV repair or reconstruction is possible. The study should be reviewed with the surgeon, focusing on the exact etiology of MR, the degree of annular dilation, the relative involvement of anterior and posterior leaflets, the chordal and papillary muscle structural integrity, and overall ventricular size and systolic function. Typically, posterior leaflet prolapse and annular dilation are most amenable to repair, while more complex or extensive disease requires more complex procedures with a lower likelihood of successful repair. Often, TEE imaging is needed for preoperative evaluation when surgical intervention is contemplated. Patient selection for percutaneous valve repair also will depend on a detailed anatomic assessment.

Intraoperative Evaluation of Mitral Valve Repair

In the patient undergoing surgical MV repair, TEE is used to assess results after the procedure. Baseline TEE images are obtained in the operating room to reconfirm regurgitant severity under the loading conditions of general anesthesia and to serve as a baseline for comparison to the post-repair study, with blood pressure recorded with the echocardiographic images at both time points. After valve repair the patient is

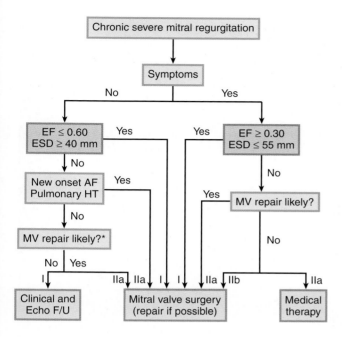

Figure 12–38 Clinical decision algorithm for timing of surgical intervention in patients with chronic severe mitral regurgitation. The Roman numerals refer to the ACC/AHA recommendation levels that the procedure should be performed (I), is reasonable (IIa), may be considered (IIb), or should not be done (III). AF, atrial fibrillation; EF, ejection fraction; ESD, end-systolic dimension; F/U, follow-up; MV, mitral valve; MVR, mitral valve replacement; PAP, pulmonary artery pressure; Rx, therapy. *(From Otto CM [ed]: Valvular Heart Disease, 3rd ed. Philadelphia: Elsevier/Saunders, 2007.)*

weaned from cardiopulmonary bypass, and valve anatomy and MR severity are reassessed. Preferably, regurgitant severity is evaluated under physiologic loading conditions with similar hemodynamics to those recorded during the baseline study (Fig. 12–39). If significant residual MR is present, a second bypass pump run may be done as part of the same procedure to allow a second attempt at repair or MV replacement. Other complications of the valve repair also may be identified, including dynamic LV outflow tract obstruction, functional mitral stenosis, and worsening of LV systolic dysfunction (see Chapter 18).

TRICUSPID REGURGITATION

Diagnostic Imaging of the Tricuspid Valve Apparatus

Tricuspid regurgitation occurs with abnormalities of the supporting structures (annulus, RV) or the leaflets themselves. Tricuspid regurgitation secondary to *annular dilation* often is due either to primary RV dilation and systolic dysfunction or to *pulmonary hypertension*. Left-sided heart disease leading to pulmonary hypertension—especially mitral stenosis or regurgitation—often results in significant tricuspid regurgitation, presumably based on RV dilation and systolic dysfunction.

Abnormalities of the tricuspid valve leaflets also are a cause of tricuspid regurgitation. *Rheumatic disease* involves the tricuspid valve in approximately 20% to 30% of cases, nearly always occurring in conjunction with mitral and aortic valve involvement. Rheumatic tricuspid disease typically is mild and may be difficult

to appreciate on 2D echocardiography unless careful attention is directed toward imaging the valve leaflets and searching for evidence of commissural fusion. Rheumatic tricuspid regurgitation is more common than rheumatic tricuspid stenosis.

Carcinoid heart disease is a rare condition, but the echocardiographic findings are pathognomonic. Carcinoid heart disease (seen with metastatic carcinoid tumor to the liver) is characterized by thickened, shortened, and immobile tricuspid valve leaflets with resultant tricuspid regurgitation or, less often, tricuspid valve stenosis (see Fig. 15–10). The pulmonic valve also may be involved. *Endocarditis* may involve the tricuspid valve, resulting in tricuspid regurgitation, and is most common in patients with a history of intravenous drug abuse.

Ebstein anomaly of the tricuspid valve is a congenital abnormality in which one or more leaflets of the tricuspid valve are displaced from the tricuspid annulus toward the ventricular apex (see Fig. 17–12). Most often the septal leaflet is involved, either in isolation or in association with apical displacement of posterior and anterior leaflets. The degree of apical displacement is extremely variable. While the normal tricuspid valve insertion plane is slightly more apical than the MV attachment plane, Ebstein anomaly should be considered when the separation between mitral and tricuspid valve planes is greater than 1 cm. The portion of the RV excluded from the pumping chamber is said to be *atrialized*, since it effectively functions as part of the RA. The RA may appear severely enlarged due to "atrialization" of the base of the ventricle *plus* dilatation of the atrium due to tricuspid regurgitation. RV enlargement is seen as well if significant tricuspid regurgitation is present.

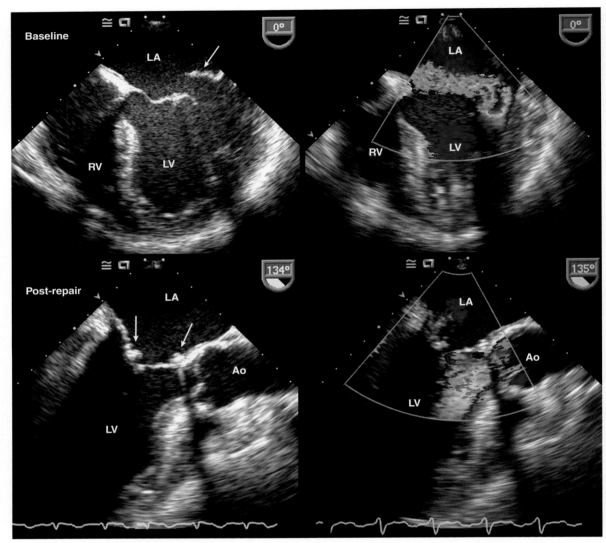

Figure 12–39 Two-dimensional (*left*) and color Doppler (*right*) intraoperative TEE images in a patient with myxomatous mitral valve disease before (*top*) and after (*bottom*) MV repair. Before repair, severe mitral prolapse with a partial flail leaflet segment and moderate-to-severe mitral regurgitation is seen in the four-chamber view. After repair, the long-axis view shows the annuloplasty ring (*arrows*). Regurgitation was not detected at similar loading conditions to the baseline study.

Right Ventricular and Right Atrial Dilation

Hemodynamically significant tricuspid regurgitation results in progressive RV and RA enlargement due to volume overload. This dilation may complicate assessment of the etiology of regurgitation because the dilation itself may further increase regurgitant severity.

RV volume overload is associated with a pattern of abnormal septal motion characterized on M-mode recording by posterior motion of the septum in diastole (since RV filling exceeds LV filling) and anterior motion of the septum in systole, often referred to as *paradoxical septal motion*. On 2D short-axis imaging the ventricular septum appears "flattened" in diastole as the increased trans-tricuspid stroke volume fills the RV. In systole the ventricular septum moves toward the center of gravity of the heart (normally toward the middle of the LV), which is the midline of the RV if severe RV dilation is present.

The differential diagnosis of 2D findings of RV dilation and paradoxical septal motion includes other causes of RV volume overload such as an atrial septal defect, partial anomalous pulmonary venous return, pressure overload due to pulmonic valve disease, or pulmonary hypertension due either to left-sided heart disease or intrinsic lung disease.

Evaluation of Tricuspid Regurgitation Severity

Tricuspid regurgitation can be evaluated with color Doppler imaging to assess vena contracta width or jet area. Vena contracta width is the most accurate approach; a jet width greater than 0.7 cm is sensitive (89%) and specific (93%) for severe tricuspid regurgitation. Using color jet area, mild regurgitation is characterized by a small systolic jet adjacent to the valve closure plane (jet area < 5 cm^2). Moderate regurgitation fills between 5 and 10 cm^2 of the RA, while severe regurgitation fills more than 10 cm^2 of an enlarged RA (Figs. 12–40 and 12–41). Useful views for evaluation of tricuspid regurgitation include parasternal short-axis view, the RV inflow view, and the apical four-chamber view. Mild-to-moderate tricuspid regurgitation often is directed along the interatrial septum and must be distinguished from normal caval inflow or from atrial septal defect flow. Calculation of regurgitant volume or orifice area by the PISA or pulsed Doppler methods is rarely performed for tricuspid regurgitation.

Severe tricuspid regurgitation results in systolic flow reversal in the inferior and superior vena cavae, analogous to the physical finding of a systolic pulsation in the neck veins. Inferior vena caval flow is best recorded in the central hepatic vein, which provides a flow channel parallel to the ultrasound beam from a subcostal approach and has no venous valves between the recording site and the RA (see Fig. 12–14). As with pulmonary vein flow reversal for severe MR, hepatic vein systolic flow reversal is specific for severe tricuspid regurgitation *only when sinus rhythm is present.* Normal systolic filling of the RA is partly dependent on the preceding phase of emptying with atrial contraction, so loss of atrial contraction affects the pattern of flow in systole.

The maximum velocity of the tricuspid regurgitant jet reflects the maximum pressure difference across the tricuspid valve and *not* the severity of regurgitation. Severe regurgitation with a normal RV systolic pressure (as seen with tricuspid valve endocarditis) has a low maximum velocity (Fig. 12–42). Mild tricuspid regurgitation in the presence of pulmonary hypertension (as seen with primary pulmonary hypertension) has a high maximum velocity. However, the *intensity* of the CW signals relative to the antegrade flow signal intensity does relate to regurgitant severity. In addition, the shape of the velocity-time curve indicates the time course of the instantaneous pressure differences across the valve; an RA *v*-wave seen in acute regurgitation results in a more rapid decline in velocity in late systole similar to that seen in acute MR.

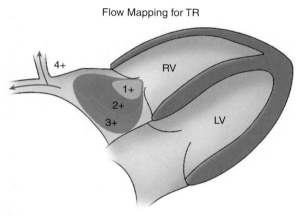

Flow Mapping for TR

Figure 12–40 Schematic diagram of flow mapping for semiquantitative evaluation of tricuspid regurgitation (TR) severity. Severe (4+) TR is associated with systolic reversal in the hepatic veins (*red arrows*).

Figure 12–41 In the parasternal RV inflow view, non-coaptation of the tricuspid valve leaflets is seen (*large arrow*), with a prominent eustachian valve (*small arrow*) at the entrance of the inferior vena cava into the RA. Color Doppler shows severe tricuspid regurgitation with a wide vena contracta (*arrow*) and a flow disturbance filling the RA.

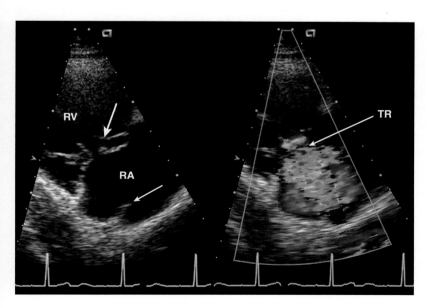

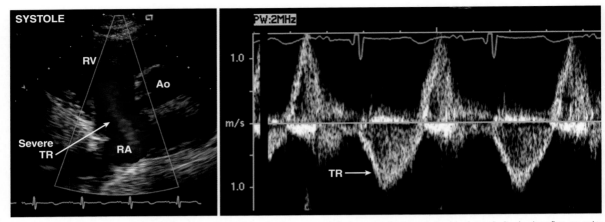

Figure 12-42 Severe tricuspid regurgitation with normal RV and pulmonary systolic pressures is characterized by low-velocity, laminar flow on color flow imaging (*left*) and on pulsed Doppler (*right*).

Clinical Utility

Evaluation of tricuspid regurgitation by Doppler echocardiography is the standard clinical approach to this problem. Even cardiac catheterization is of limited value, because the catheter placed across the tricuspid valve to perform the RV angiogram may itself induce regurgitation.

Evaluation of tricuspid regurgitant severity is particularly important in the patient undergoing MV surgery. Many of these patients have significant coexisting tricuspid regurgitation, and many of the clinical symptoms will persist postoperatively if this condition is not recognized and treated (with tricuspid annuloplasty) at the time of surgery.

In patients undergoing tricuspid valve repair or surgery for endocarditis, intraoperative TEE can be used to optimize the surgical approach and assess the functional consequences of the repair procedure.

PULMONIC REGURGITATION

Pulmonic regurgitation most often is an incidental benign finding, with a small amount of diastolic backflow across the pulmonic valve seen in most normal individuals (Fig. 12-43). Pathologic pulmonic regurgitation usually is a result of congenital pulmonic valve disease, either untreated mild disease or residual regurgitation after pulmonic valve surgery. The most common cause of significant pulmonic regurgitation in adults is previous surgery for tetralogy of Fallot. Acquired pulmonic regurgitation is rare, being due to endocarditis, carcinoid syndrome, or myxomatous valve disease.

Evaluation of pulmonic valve anatomy may be limited in adult patients by poor acoustic access. With congenital disease, thickened, deformed leaflets are seen. In endocarditis, a valvular vegetation may be identified, although the pulmonic valve is involved least often. Carcinoid syndrome results in shortening

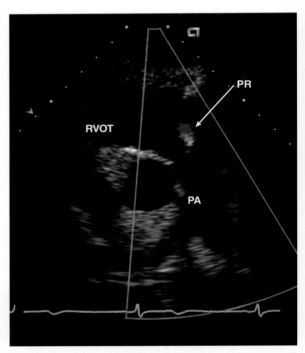

Figure 12-43 Color flow imaging in an RV outflow view showing a small amount of pulmonic regurgitation (PR).

and thickening of the pulmonic valve leaflet, similar to the involvement of the tricuspid valve, and may lead to stenosis and/or regurgitation. Myxomatous valve disease is rare, resulting in thickening, redundancy, and systolic sagging of the pulmonic valve leaflets.

Pulmonic regurgitation is diagnosed by documenting diastolic flow in the RV outflow tract with conventional pulsed or color Doppler flow imaging. The width of the diastolic flow on color imaging provides a semiquantitative index of pulmonic regurgitant severity. The intensity and shape of the CW Doppler signal also provide an indication of regurgitant severity, analogous to the findings in AR. Holodiastolic flow reversal may be noted in the main PA when significant regurgitation is present and must be distinguished from diastolic flow reversal due to a patent ductus arteriosus.

In adults, evaluation of pulmonic regurgitation is of most importance in patients with uncorrected or residual congenital heart disease (see Figs. 17–30 and 31). In these patients the severity of pulmonic regurgitation may be a factor in deciding whether to perform further surgical procedures and in the specific design of the surgical procedure.

The velocity in the pulmonic regurgitant curve reflects the PA-to-RV diastolic pressure difference. The instantaneous end-diastolic PA-to-RV gradient (calculated as $4v^2$) can be added to an estimate of RV diastolic pressure (from inferior vena cava size and respiratory variation) to provide an estimate of diastolic PA pressure. This approach to estimation of PA pressure complements systolic pressure estimation from the tricuspid regurgitant jet and serves as an internal validity check when both can be recorded accurately.

SUGGESTED READING

General

1. Otto CM: Timing of intervention for chronic valve regurgitation: the role of echocardiography. In Otto CM (ed): The Practice of Clinical Echocardiography, 3rd ed. Philadelphia: Elsevier/Saunders, 2007, pp 430–458.

   Comprehensive chapter discussing the key factors in clinical decision making and the pathophysiology of chronic valvular regurgitation in adults. The natural history, predictors of outcome after valve surgery, the echocardiographic approach, and alternate diagnostic approaches are discussed in detail for aortic and for mitral regurgitation.

2. Bekeredjian R, Grayburn PA: Valvular heart disease: Aortic regurgitation. Circulation 112:125–134, 2005.

   The combined LV pressure and volume overload due to AR account for the physical examination findings of a wide pulse pressure and bounding peripheral pulses. Echocardiography allows diagnosis of the cause and severity of AR and is one of the primary factors in determining timing of valve replacement. Potential future approaches to medical therapy are discussed.

3. Braverman AC, Beardslee MA: The bicuspid aortic valve. In Otto CM, Bonow RO (eds): Valvular Heart Disease, 3rd ed. Philadelphia: Elsevier/Saunders, 2009, Chapter 11.

   A bicuspid aortic valve occurs in about 1% of the population, and most of these patients will require surgical intervention for regurgitation, stenosis, or aortic root dilation during their lifetime. Familial occurrence is seen in 9% of first-degree relatives with an autosomal dominant inheritance pattern with incomplete penetrance.

4. Fedak P, McCarthy PM, Bonow RO: Evolving concepts and technologies in mitral valve repair. Circulation 117:963–974, 2008.

   A detailed review of normal and abnormal mitral valve anatomy and function is provided, followed by a summary of current (and potential future) approaches to valve repair for regurgitation.

Quantitation of Valvular Regurgitation

5. Hung J: Quantitation of valvular regurgitation. In Otto CM (ed): The Practice of Clinical Echocardiography, 3rd ed. Philadelphia: Elsevier/Saunders, 2007, pp 405–429.

   Advanced chapter on echocardiographic quantitation of valvular regurgitation. Both conventional and alternate methods for measurement are discussed, the literature validating these approaches is summarized, and technical aspects of data acquisitions are highlighted. 105 references.

6. Otto CM, Schwaegler RG: Valve regurgitation. In Echocardiography Review Guide. Philadelphia: Elsevier/Saunders, 2007, pp 201–230.

   This review guide summarizes basic principles, provides additional examples of images and Doppler data, reviews technical aspects of data acquisition and measurement, and demonstrates calculations for quantitation of regurgitant severity. Self-assessment questions with explanations of the answers are provided.

7. Zoghbi WA, Enriquez-Sarano M, Foster E, et al: Recommendations for evaluation of the severity of native valvular regurgitation with two-dimensional and Doppler echocardiography. J Am Soc Echocardiogr 16:777–802, 2003.

   Clear recommendations and detailed description of methods for quantitation of valvular regurgitation by echocardiography. Essential reading for all echocardiographers.

8. Robert BJ, Grayburn PA: Color flow imaging of the vena contracta in mitral regurgitation: technical considerations. J Am Soc Echocardiogr 16:1002–1006, 2003.

   Summary of the hemodynamics of valve regurgitation and the approach to recording and measuring the vena contracta. The authors emphasize the use of axial beam resolution, a narrow sector, fast frame rate, and zoom mode to improve accuracy of this approach.

9. Kim YJ, Jones M, Greenberg NL, et al: Evaluation of left ventricular contractile function using noninvasively determined single-beat end-systolic elastance in mitral regurgitation: Experimental validation and clinical application. J Am Soc Echocardiogr 20:1086–1092, 2007.

   The effects of chronic regurgitation on ventricular volumes and function area key element in clinical decision making. Measurement of end-systolic elastance (E_{ES} in mm Hg/mL) from a single beat using noninvasive data is proposed using the equations:

   $$E_{ES} = [DBP - 0.9 \times SBP + \alpha \times (DBP - EDP) \times ET/PEP]/SV$$

   where $\alpha = 1.171 \times EF + 0.022$

   Based on cuff measurement of diastolic (DBP) and systolic (SBP) blood pressure; 2D ejection fraction (EF) determination; and Doppler measurement of ejection time (ET), pre-ejection period (PEP), and stroke volume (SV). LV EDP was assumed to be 10 mm Hg for this estimate. In an experimental model, E_{ES} correlated well with invasively determined elastance. In a series of 105 patients undergoing valve repair for MR, preoperative E_{ES} and end-systolic volume correlated with postoperative EF. An $E_{ES} = 1.0$ mm Hg/mL predicted postoperative LV dysfunction with a sensitivity of 87% and specificity of 76%.

10. Foster E, Wasserman HS, Gray W, et al: Quantitative assessment of severity of mitral regurgitation by serial echocardiography in a multicenter clinical trial of percutaneous mitral

valve repair. Am J Cardiol 100: 1577–1583, 2007.

In a multicenter trial, 85% of required quantitative Doppler measures of regurgitant severity could be measured including vena contracta width, regurgitant volume, regurgitant fraction, and effective regurgitant orifice area (ROA). These data support the concept that quantitative assessment of valve disease severity is feasible in clinical trials and may help define mechanisms of benefit, in addition to serving as secondary endpoints.

11. Matsumura Y, Fukuda S, Tran H, et al: Geometry of the proximal isovelocity surface area in mitral regurgitation by 3-dimensional color Doppler echocardiography: Difference between functional mitral regurgitation and prolapse regurgitation. Am Heart J 155:231–238, 2008.

The 3D anatomy of the PISA was examined in 27 patients with functional MR and 27 with mitral valve (MV) prolapse. In functional MR the PISA is elongated with a horizontal length longer than in MV prolapse patients. The consequence of this non-hemispherical geometry is underestimation of ROA by the PISA approach by 24% with functional MR but not with MV prolapse.

12. Velayudhan DE, Brown TM, Nanda NC, et al: Quantification of tricuspid regurgitation by live three-dimensional transthoracic echocardiographic measurements of vena contracta area. Echocardiography 23:793–800, 2006.

In 93 consecutive patients, 3D measurements of tricuspid regurgitant vena contracta area correlated well with conventional 2D echocardiographic measures of regurgitant severity.

Anatomy and Mechanisms of Regurgitation

13. Levine RA, Schwammenthal E: Ischemic mitral regurgitation on the threshold of a solution: From paradoxes to unifying concepts. Circulation 112:745–758, 2005.

Ischemic MR is associated with worse outcomes in adults with ischemic heart disease and heart failure. Experimental and echocardiographic studies have provided insight into the mechanism of ischemic MR based on the balance of forces acting on the mitral leaflet in systole, with tethering of leaflet closure contributing to dynamic incompetence of valve closure. This review article discusses and illustrates these mechanisms and the implications for medical and surgical therapy.

14. de Waroux JB, Pouleur AC, Goffinet C, et al: Functional anatomy of aortic regurgitation: accuracy, prediction of

surgical repairability, and outcome implications of transesophageal echocardiography. Circulation 116(11 Suppl):I264–I269, 2007.

The mechanisms of AR, as assessed by TEE in 163 consecutive patients undergoing surgery for regurgitation, were aortic dilation in 25%, cusp prolapse in 38%, and restrictive cusp motion or endocarditis in 36%. The agreement between TEE and direct inspection was 93% for mechanism of regurgitation, and TEE correctly predicted the surgical procedure (repair vs replacement) in 88%. Repair was most often accomplished by valve resuspension in an aortic graft.

15. Sukmawan R, Watanabe N, Ogasawara Y, et al: Geometric changes of tricuspid valve tenting in tricuspid regurgitation secondary to pulmonary hypertension quantified by novel system with transthoracic real-time 3-dimensional echocardiography. J Am Soc Echocardiogr 20:470–476, 2007.

In a comparison of 17 pulmonary hypertension patients with tricuspid regurgitation to 13 control subjects, 3D echocardiography showed tenting of the tricuspid vale leaflets and annular dilation as the primary mechanisms of tricuspid regurgitation.

16. Song JM, Kim MJ, Kim YJ, et al: Three-dimensional characteristics of functional mitral regurgitation in patients with severe left ventricular dysfunction: A real-time three-dimensional colour Doppler echocardiography study. Heart 94:590–596, 2008.

Functional MR is associated with diverse leaflet anatomic configurations. The shape of the regurgitant orifice is determined by the shape and site of anterior leaflet bending. Several small regurgitant orifices may be present when the tenting area is small.

17. Gutiérrez-Chico JL, Zamorano Gómez JL, Rodrigo-López JL, et al: Accuracy of real-time 3-dimensional echocardiography in the assessment of mitral prolapse. Is transesophageal echocardiography still mandatory? Am Heart J 155:694–698, 2008.

Real-time 3D TTE was as accurate as multiplane 2D TEE imaging for determination of which scallops of the leaflets were prolapsing in a series of 41 patients. False negatives occurred with 2 cases each of prolapse of the A2 and P1 scallops. Accuracy was 100% for prolapse of the P2 scallop.

18. Veronesi F, Corsi C, Sugeng L, et al: Quantification of mitral apparatus dynamics in functional and ischemic mitral regurgitation using real-time 3-dimensional echocardiography. J Am Soc Echocardiogr 21:347–354, 2008.

Real-time 3D echocardiography was used to evaluated mitral annular dilation and papillary

muscle displacement in patients with MR due to dilated cardiomyopathy or ischemic disease. Dilated cardiomyopathy patients had a dilated annulus with symmetric papillary muscle alignment, whereas patients with ischemic disease had less annular dilation and greater asymmetry of the papillary muscles.

Clinical Applications

19. Reimold SC, Orav EJ, Come PC, et al: Progressive enlargement of the regurgitant orifice in patients with chronic aortic regurgitation. J Am Soc Echocardiogr 11:259–265, 1998.

In a prospective study of 59 patients with audible AR murmurs, aortic regurgitant jet width increased by 0.04 ± 0.01 cm/yr, and ROA increased by 0.01 ± 0.01 cm^2/yr. Rate of progression was not related to the cause of AR, gender, or baseline regurgitant severity.

20. Grigioni F, Enriquez-Sarano M, Zehr KJ, et al: Ischemic mitral regurgitation: long-term outcome and prognostic implications with quantitative Doppler assessment. Circulation 103:1759–1764, 2001.

Quantitative Doppler measures of MR severity, including regurgitant volume and ROA, are predictors of clinical outcome after myocardial infarction.

21. Monin JL, Dehant P, Roiron C, et al: Functional assessment of mitral regurgitation by transthoracic echocardiography using standardized imaging planes: Diagnostic accuracy and outcome implications. J Am Coll Cardiol 46:302–309, 2005.

With current instrumentation and harmonic imaging, TTE correctly predicted the likelihood of valve repair in 97% of 270 patients undergoing surgery for MR. TEE provided additional significant information in only 2 patients. Accuracy of standard 2D image planes on TTE imaging for localization of prolapsed segments was 91%, as compared to 93% for TEE in the 190 patients with MV prolapse.

22. Kerr AJ, Raffel OC, Whalley GA, et al: Elevated B-type natriuretic peptide despite normal left ventricular function on rest and exercise stress echocardiography in mitral regurgitation. Eur Heart J 29:363–370, 2008.

In 33 asymptomatic patients with significant MR and normal LV function, an elevated serum brain natriuretic peptide (BNP) level predicted an excessive rise in pulmonary pressure with exercise. The systolic PA pressure with exercise in those with an elevated BNP was 70 ± 20 mm Hg as compared to 48 ± 11 mm Hg in those with a normal BNP.

23. Enriquez-Sarano M, Avierinos JF, Messika-Zeitoun D, et al: Quantitative determinants of the outcome of asymptomatic mitral regurgitation. N Engl J Med 352:875–883, 2005.

This prospective study of 456 patients with chronic MR is the first to demonstrate that quantitative Doppler calculations of regurgitant severity predict long-term clinical outcome. Patients with an effective ROA ≥0.4 cm² had a 5-year survival rate of 58 ± 9%, as compared with 78% expected survival. As compared with patients with a ROA <0.2 cm², patients with a ROA ≥0.4 cm² had more than five times the risk of death from cardiac causes and cardiac events. Those with an orifice area of 0.20 to 0.39 cm² had intermediate outcomes.

24. Evangelista A, Tornos P, Sambola A, et al: Long-term vasodilator therapy in patients with severe aortic regurgitation. N Engl J Med 353:1342–1349, 2005.

In 95 adults with asymptomatic severe AR, randomization to treatment with nifedipine versus enalapril versus no treatment showed no beneficial effect of vasodilator therapy on the rate of LV dilation (assessed by echocardiography) or the need for aortic valve replacement.

25. Detaint D, Messika-Zeitoun D, Maalouf J, et al: Quantitative echocardiographic determinants of clinical outcome in asymptomatic patients with aortic regurgitation. J Am Coll Cardiol Img 1:1–11, 2008.

Quantitative measures of AR severity were strong predictors of clinical outcome in a prospective study of 251 asymptomatic adults with isolated AR and normal LV function. Survival at 10 years in those with severe AR (ROA = 0.3 cm² and RV = 60 mL) was 69 ± 9% as compared with a survival of 92 ± 4% in those with mild AR (ROA <0.1 cm² and RV <30 mL).

26. Vinereanu D, Turner MS, Bleasdale RA, et al: Mechanisms of reduction of mitral regurgitation by cardiac resynchronization therapy. J Am Soc Echocardiogr 20:54–62, 2007.

In 22 patients undergoing resynchronization therapy for severe heart failure, severity of MR improved with a decrease in vena contracta diameter from 5.2 ± 1.7 to 4.0 ± 1.7 mm with biventricular pacing. This improvement was associated with an increase in LV longitudinal function and reduction in subvalvular traction.

Alternate Approaches to Evaluation of Valvular Regurgitation

27. Shavelle DM: Cardiac catheterization and angiography for evaluation of valvular disease. In Otto CM, Bonow RB (eds): Valvular Heart Disease, 3rd ed. Philadelphia: Elsevier/Saunders, 2009, Chapter 6; and Garcia M: Cardiac magnetic resonance and computed tomography in valve disease. In Otto CM, Bonow RB (eds): Valvular Heart Disease, 3rd ed. Philadelphia: Saunders Elsevier, 2009, Chapter 7.

Chapters reviewing the role of cardiac catheterization, CMR imaging, and computed tomography in the evaluation of patients with valvular heart disease.

28. Cawley PJ, Otto CM: Cardiovascular magnetic resonance imaging for valvular heart disease: Technique and validation. Circulation 119:468–478, 2009.

This article reviews the literature validating the use of cardiac magnetic resonance (CMR) imaging for evaluation of valvular heart disease. Regurgitation can be quantitated based on differences in RV and LV stroke volume measured from anatomic images, using flow volumes based on velocity data in the great vessels (Q-flow) or a combination of these approaches. CMR may be useful in patients where echocardiographic data are nondiagnostic or discrepant with other clinical data.

13 Prosthetic Valves

E chocardiographic evaluation of prosthetic valves is similar in many respects to evaluation of native valve disease. However, there are some important differences. First, there are several types of prosthetic valves with differing fluid dynamics for each basic design and differing flow velocities for each valve size. Second, the mechanisms of valve dysfunction are somewhat different from those for native valve disease. Third, the technical aspects of imaging artificial devices—specifically the problem of acoustic shadowing—significantly affect the diagnostic approach when prosthetic valve dysfunction is suspected (Table 13–1).

Echocardiographers increasingly are asked to evaluate prosthetic valve function because of the increasing number of prosthetic valves implanted annually and the greater longevity of patients with prosthetic valves. Both an understanding of the basic approach to echocardiographic evaluation (as outlined in this chapter) and detailed knowledge of the specific flow dynamic for the size and type of prosthesis in an individual patient (see Suggested Reading) are needed for appropriate patient management.

BASIC PRINCIPLES

Types of Prosthetic Valves

The three basic types of prosthetic valves (Figs. 13–1 and 13–2) are:

- ❐ Tissue valves, or bioprostheses
- ❐ Homograft valves
- ❐ Mechanical valves

Bioprosthetic Valves

Tissue valves are composed of three biologic leaflets with an anatomic structure similar to the native aortic valve. With stented prosthetic valves, the leaflets (typically porcine) or pericardium (usually bovine or equine) shaped to mimic normal leaflets, are mounted on a cloth-covered rigid support that functions as the crown-shaped aortic annulus with a raised "stent" at each of the three commissures (Fig. 13–3). Variations in the support structure and leaflet types abound in commercially available valves; some include anticalcification

TABLE 13–1   Comparison of Different Valve Types

Normal	Native Valve	Bioprosthesis	Mechanical Valve
Fluid dynamics	Central orifice, laminar flow, blunt flow profile	Central orifice, laminar flow, blunt flow profile	Complex fluid dynamics depending on valve type
Antegrade velocity	Normal	Increased	Increased
Normal regurgitation	Mild, central	Mild, central	Mild, oblique jets
Mechanisms of dysfunction	Multiple	Tissue degeneration Endocarditis Pannus ingrowth Sewing ring dehiscence	Mechanical failure Endocarditis Pannus ingrowth Thrombus Sewing ring dehiscence
Technical aspects of imaging	Calcification may cause acoustic shadows in some cases	Acoustic shadow from sewing ring	Extensive reverberations and acoustic shadowing

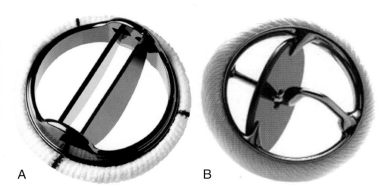

Figure 13–1 Two typical mechanical valves: **A,** A bileaflet valve (St. Jude Medical Regent valve) and **B,** a tilting-disk valve (Medtronic Hall valve). Images of other specific valve types can be found using a web search. *(A, Copyright St. Jude Medical Inc. St. Paul, Minnesota. B, Copyright Medtronic, Inc., Minneapolis, Minnesota.)*

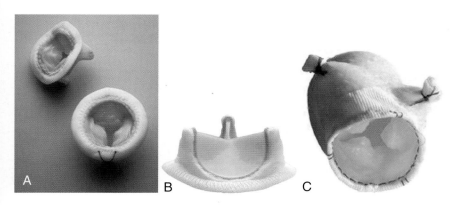

Figure 13–2 Examples of three tissue valve prostheses: Medtronic Mosaic stented valve (**A**), Carpentier Edwards Perimount aortic valve (**B**), and a Medtronic stentless freestyle valve (**C**). *(A and C, Copyright Medtronic, Inc., Minneapolis, Minnesota. B, Copyright Edwards Lifesciences LLC, Irvine, California.)*

treatments. Current-generation stented tissue valves include the Edwards Magna and the Medtronic Mosaic valve. Older examples of stented heterografts include Carpentier-Edwards porcine valves, Hancock porcine valves, and Ionescu-Shiley bovine pericardial valves.

"Stentless" tissue valves also have been developed that use a flexible cuff of fabric or tissue, instead of rigid stents, to support the valve leaflets. Stentless valves often are implanted as part of a composite tissue valve and aortic root, for example, the Medtronic freestyle valve and root.

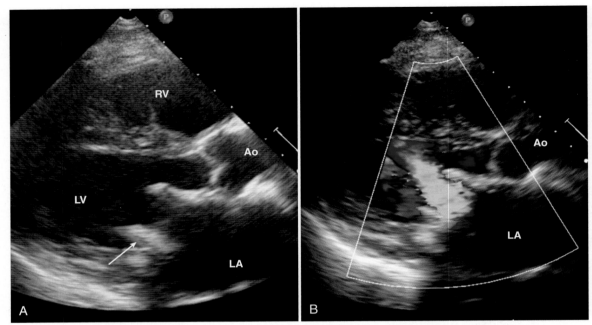

Figure 13–3 Parasternal long axis view of a stented mitral bioprosthetic valve. **A,** The valve struts (*arrow*) protrude into the ventricular chamber, with antegrade flow seen with color Doppler (**B**) directed toward the ventricular septum.

Typically bioprosthetic valves have been implanted surgically using cardiopulmonary bypass to support the circulation while the valve is implanted. Newer approaches to valve implantation include a transapical surgical approach and a nonsurgical percutaneous approach. The bioprosthetic valves used for catheter implantation are mounted on a compressible stent with a valve design similar to other stentless bioprosthetic valves (see Suggested Readings 34–36).

Homograft Valves

Homograft valves are cryopreserved human aortic or pulmonic valves harvested at autopsy. Typically, the valve and great vessel are preserved as a block, to be trimmed appropriately at the time of implantation in the aortic or pulmonic position. While the fluid dynamics of a homograft are similar to those of a native valve, flow velocities are slightly higher and valve areas slightly smaller than for a normal native valve due to the space occupied by the homograft annulus in the patient's outflow tract. Because of late severe tissue calcification with homograft valves, this approach is typically reserved for adults with complex aortic root abscesses.

Mechanical Valves

A variety of mechanical valves currently are available. In addition, several other types of valves, which were implanted in the past, are still in situ in some patients. The two basic types of currently implanted mechanical valves are

- A bileaflet valve wherein two semicircular disks hinge open to form two large lateral orifices and a smaller central orifice (Figs. 13–4 and 13–5)
- A tilting-disk valve wherein a single circular disk opens at an angle to the annulus plane, being constrained in its motion by a smaller "cage," a central strut, or a slanted slot in the valve ring

In the past, ball-cage mechanical valves also were used and may still occasionally be encountered. With a ball-cage valve, a spherical occluder is contained by a metal "cage" when the valve is open and fills the orifice in the closed position (like on a snorkel).

Valved Conduits

Valved conduits are used in congenital heart surgery and in ascending aortic repairs when both a new passageway for blood flow and a valve are needed. The conduit may be biologic (e.g., a homograft) or artificial (e.g., Gore-Tex or Dacron) material. A conduit may incorporate either a stented tissue or a mechanical valve with fluid dynamics similar to those for a valve implanted in the native annulus. The stentless valve and root prosthesis also is used in this situation.

Mechanisms of Prosthetic Valve Dysfunction

The types of disease processes that affect prosthetic valves are distinctly different from those seen with

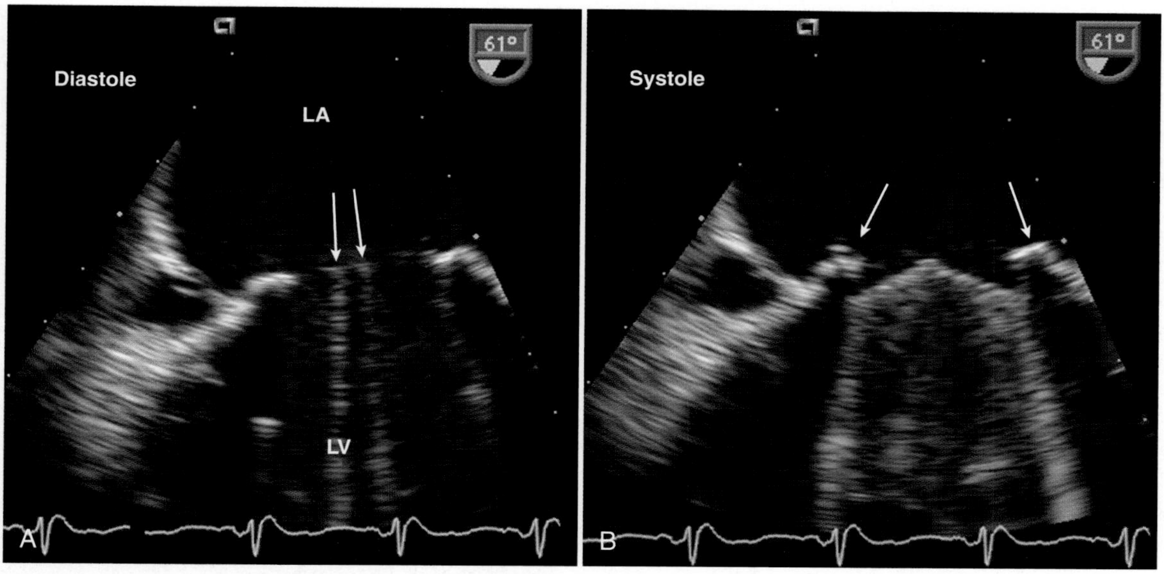

Figure 13–4 Bileaflet mitral valve prosthesis seen in diastole (**A**) and systole (**B**) from a TEE approach. In diastole, the sewing ring and two parallel open leaflets (*arrows*) are seen. In systole, the two leaflets close with a slightly obtuse closure angle, with reverberations from the leaflets and shadowing from the sewing ring (*arrows*) obscuring the LV side of the valve.

native valvular heart disease and can be classified into three groups:

- Structural failure
- Thromboembolic complications
- Endocarditis

Primary Structural Failure

Failure of a bioprosthetic valve to open or close properly (mechanical failure) usually is the result of slowly progressive tissue degeneration, with fibrocalcific changes of the leaflets resulting in increased resistance to opening (stenosis) or failure to coapt during valve closure (regurgitation). Typically, failure of tissue valves occurs 10 or more years after valve implantation. Acute bioprosthetic valve stenosis is rare. Acute bioprosthetic regurgitation can occur with a leaflet tear, usually adjacent to a region of calcification.

Failure of a mechanical valve can occur due to faulty design or wear and tear of the prosthetic

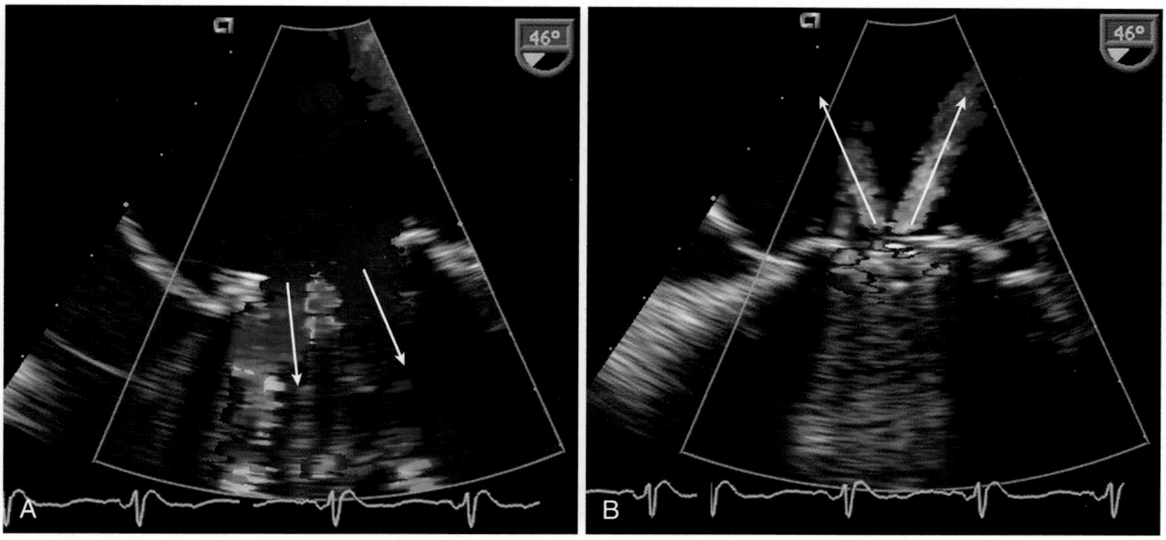

Figure 13–5 Color flow image of a bileaflet mitral valve prosthesis in diastole (**A**), showing flow across the valve with two large lateral orifices (*arrows*) and a small central orifice that appears red due to local flow acceleration. In systole (**B**), two normal jets of regurgitation (*arrows*) are seen.

material resulting in disk escape or incomplete valve closure. However, these complications were seen only with older generation valves (which may still be present in a few patients). Current-generation mechanical valves are reliable and very durable. More often, mechanical valve stenosis or regurgitation is due to thrombus formation or pannus ingrowth around the valve, impairing disk excursion or closure.

With both bioprosthetic and mechanical valves, paravalvular regurgitation can occur around the sewing ring due to loss of suture material postoperatively, most often related to fibrocalcific disease in the valve annulus. The new onset of paravalvular regurgitation late after surgery raises the possibility of an infectious process (endocarditis) resulting in valve dehiscence.

Thromboembolic Complications

Prosthetic valves, particularly mechanical valves, are prone to thrombus formation, which may result in systemic embolic events or valve dysfunction. Echocardiographic evaluation for prosthetic valve thrombus is limited, except with very large masses, due to shadowing and reverberations. In addition, clinical events may be associated with clots smaller than the limits of clinical ultrasound resolution. Thus, echocardiography cannot exclude the possibility of thrombus on a prosthetic valve; in patients with embolic events, the prosthetic valve itself is a cardiac "source of embolus."

Endocarditis

Infection of a valve prosthesis is a serious clinical problem, so suspected endocarditis is a frequent indication for echocardiography in patients with prosthetic valves. Endocarditis on a bioprosthesis may result in vegetations similar to those seen on a native valve. However, with a mechanical valve the infection often is paravalvular, and no discrete vegetation may be present.

Technical Aspects of Echo Evaluation

There are two major challenges in evaluating prosthetic valves by echocardiography. The normal fluid dynamics of the prosthetic valve must be distinguished from prosthetic valve dysfunction. However, the most technically limiting aspect of echocardiographic evaluation of prosthetic valves is the problem of acoustic shadowing. The sewing rings of both bioprosthetic and mechanical valves and the occluders of mechanical valves are strong echo reflectors, resulting in acoustic shadows and reverberations (Fig. 13–6). These reverberations and shadows obscure the motion of the valve structures themselves and block detection of imaging and Doppler abnormalities in

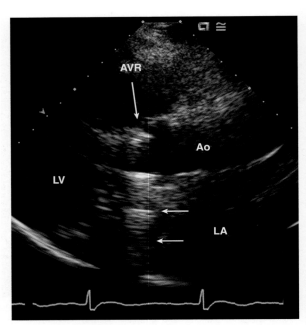

Figure 13–6 Parasternal long-axis view of a bileaflet mechanical aortic valve (AVR) in diastole. The valve leaflets are difficult to see because of shadowing and reverberations (*arrows*) from the valve sewing ring.

the acoustic shadow region. During the examination, considerable effort is directed toward utilizing windows and views that avoid these imaging artifacts. Transesophageal echocardiography (TEE) is particularly useful in evaluation of prosthetic mitral valves because it provides acoustic access from the left atrial (LA) side of the valve.

ECHOCARDIOGRAPHIC APPROACH

Imaging

Bioprosthetic Valves

Aortic homografts appear similar to native aortic valves except for some increased thickness in the left ventricular (LV) outflow tract (LVOT) and the ascending aorta at the proximal and distal suture sites. Typically, the homograft is implanted using the mini-root technique, with the homograft replacing a segment of the native aorta. This approach necessitates reimplantation of the coronary arteries. In the past, the aortic homograft sometimes was positioned inside the patient's native aorta with appropriate trimming to maintain patency of the coronary ostia. In patients with endocarditis the attached anterior mitral leaflet of the homograft may be used to patch a ventricular septal defect or abscess cavity. The echocardiographic appearance of a homograft is very similar to that of a native aortic valve, except for the associated surgical changes. Standard parasternal long- and

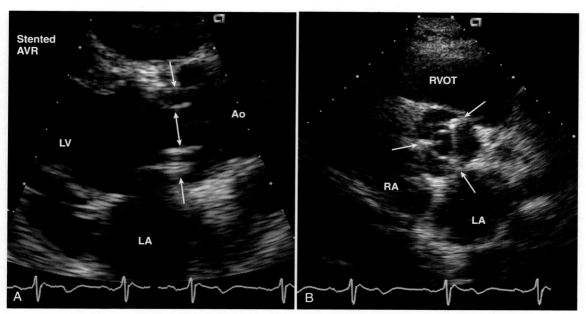

Figure 13–7 A, Parasternal long axis view of a normal stented aortic valve replacement (AVR). The orifice (*white double arrow*) between the thin open leaflets is seen, with the struts of the stent (*arrows*) seen within the sinuses. **B,** In the short-axis view, the triangular opening of the three leaflets is seen, with the three struts (*arrows*) located in the position of the native valve commissures.

short-axis image planes provide optimal visualization of valve leaflet anatomy and motion.

Stented tissue prosthetic valves have a trileaflet structure similar to a native aortic valve. An M-mode through the leaflets shows the typical "boxlike" opening in systole (for the aortic position) or diastole (for the mitral position) as is seen with a normal native aortic valve. However, with conventional valve designs, the echogenic sewing ring and struts may limit visualization of the leaflets, with the specific ultrasound appearance of the supporting structures depending on the specific model. Because there is marked variability in surgeons' valve preferences, it is helpful to review images or actual valves for the types most commonly encountered at your institution (Fig. 13–7). *Stentless bioprosthetic valves* have an echocardiographic appearance very similar to a native aortic valve, other than increased echogenicity in the aortic root in the early postoperative period (Fig. 13–8). This valve is best identified by reviewing the chart or asking the patient about any cardiac surgical procedures before beginning the study. Percutaneous valves (Fig. 13–9) appear similar to a native valve with increased para-annular thickness.

Improved images of prosthetic tissue valves can be obtained from a TEE approach, particularly for valves in the mitral position, since the ultrasound beam has a perpendicular orientation to the leaflets with no intervening structures from this approach. With aortic valve prostheses, TEE imaging is less rewarding, because the posterior part of the sewing ring shadows the valve leaflets. When images of the leaflets themselves are suboptimal, Doppler data can provide valuable information.

The longevity of bioprosthesis valves typically is limited by slowly progressive tissue failure with fibrocalcific changes resulting in leaflet deformity (leading to regurgitation) and/or increased stiffness (leading to stenosis). Echocardiographically, increased echogenicity and irregularity of the leaflets may be noted, although images of the leaflets often are suboptimal due to shadowing and reverberation.

Mechanical Valves

Ultrasound imaging of mechanical valves from a transthoracic (TTE) approach is frustrating because of severe reverberations and acoustic shadowing. While imaging may provide clues as to the type of valve prostheses (e.g., "low-profile" bileaflet or tilting-disk valve vs. "high-profile" ball-cage valve), obviously it is simpler to ascertain the exact valve type and size from the patient's medical record or valve identification card. Assessing motion of the valve occluder often is difficult. For example, the leading edge of a tilting-disk valve results in a strong reverberation across the image obscuring motion of the disk itself. In addition, an oblique image plane often is obtained relative to the prosthetic valve, since orientation of the prosthesis within the annulus is not standard. With a tomographic plane perpendicular to the open bileaflet valve, the two leaflets can be

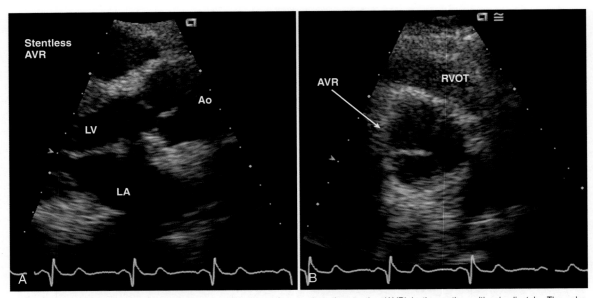

Figure 13-8 Parasternal long-axis (A) and short-axis (B) views of a stentless tissue valve (AVR) in the aortic position in diastole. The valve appearance is similar to a native trileaflet aortic valve other than slightly increased echogenicity in the aortic root.

identified clearly, an image plane that is best identified on multiplane TEE imaging.

Technical limitations make identification of prosthetic valve endocarditis or thrombosis problematic, because the abnormalities may be obscured by reverberations or hidden by acoustic shadowing. TEE imaging can be helpful in identifying thrombus or infected vegetations on the atrial side of a mitral prosthesis, because the LA is "masked" by the prosthetic valve from both parasternal and apical windows. In a patient with a mechanical aortic valve, the subaortic region can be evaluated well from a TTE approach from parasternal and apical windows. In this situation, TEE images are less helpful due to

shadowing of the outflow tract by the posterior aspect of the prosthesis.

Microcavitation

An incidental finding in some patients with a mechanical prosthetic valve is the phenomenon of *spontaneous contrast*. This phenomenon is similar to the spontaneous LA contrast seen in patients with an enlarged LA and low-velocity flow, which has been reported to be associated with a high propensity for thrombus formation. However, with a prosthetic valve there are only a few bright mobile echogenic particles that are seen downstream from the valve,

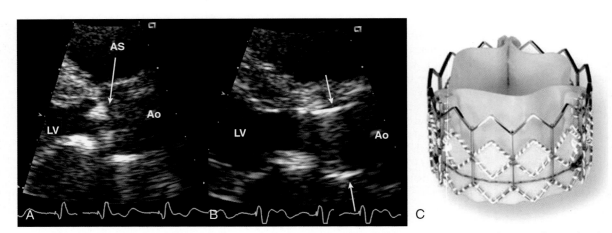

Figure 13-9 Parasternal long axis view zoomed to show calcific aortic stenosis (AS) (A) followed by percutaneous placement of an aortic valve prosthesis (B). The valve cage (*arrows*) is seen, corresponding to the photograph of the Edwards SAPEIN transcatheter heart valve (C). (C, Copyright Edwards Lifesciences LLC, Irvine, California.)

even in the absence of a low-flow state. The presumed mechanism of prosthetic valve spontaneous contrast is microcavitation due to impact of the occluder against the sewing ring.

Valved Conduits

Ultrasound imaging of a bioprosthetic or mechanical valve in a conduit (e.g., right ventricular to pulmonary artery) may be difficult due to ultrasound attenuation by the conduit prosthetic material. Of note, stenosis in a valved conduit can occur as a result of stenosis of the valve prosthesis or fibrotic ingrowth along the length of the conduit. In addition, residual or progressive stenosis at the proximal or distal anastomosis site can occur. Imaging the narrowing in the conduit often is difficult, but a careful Doppler examination may allow detection of the abnormal flow velocities. Continuous-wave (CW) Doppler is used to assess the maximum flow velocity, while pulsed Doppler or color flow imaging is used to localize the level of obstruction along the length of the conduit.

Normal Doppler Findings

Prosthetic Valve "Clicks"

The motion of the occluder of a mechanical valve (or the tissue leaflets of a biologic valve) creates a brief intense Doppler signal that appears as a dark narrow band of short duration on the spectral display (Fig. 13–10). Audibly, this signal is similar to the valve

"click" appreciated on auscultation. However, unlike auscultation, usually both opening and closing valve clicks are seen on spectral Doppler analysis. The Doppler signals associated with valve opening and closing are similar to those seen with native valves but are of greater intensity. The motion of the occluder also may result in color flow artifacts, with color signals covering large areas of the image that are inconsistent from beat to beat.

Antegrade Flow Patterns and Velocities

Bioprosthetic valves have a flow profile similar to a native aortic valve, with three leaflets that open to a circular orifice (in systole in the aortic position or in diastole in the mitral position), providing laminar antegrade flow with a relatively blunt flow profile. In the mitral position, the orientation of the bioprosthesis results in the inflow stream being directed anteriorly and medially toward the ventricular septum in most patients instead of toward the ventricular apex, as is seen for normal native valves. This results in a reversed vortex of blood flow in mid-diastole, as seen in an apical four-chamber view.

Flow profiles of different mechanical valves vary substantially, and none is analogous to flow across a normal native valve. Bileaflet mechanical valves have complex fluid dynamics that affect the Doppler echocardiographic evaluation of these valves. With the leaflets open, there are two large lateral valve orifices with a small narrow central "slitlike" orifice. The flow velocity profile shows three peaks corresponding to these three orifices, with higher velocities in the center of each orifice. The local acceleration forces

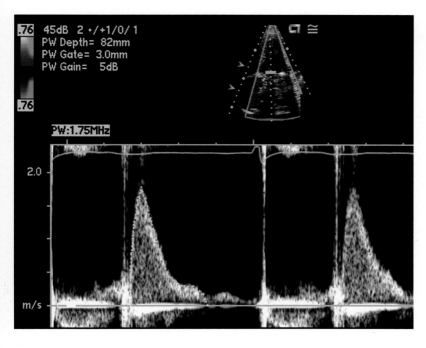

Figure 13–10 LV inflow across a mechanical mitral valve replacement showing an increased antegrade velocity (compared with a native valve) but a steep pressure half time indicating there is no significant stenosis.

within the narrow central orifice result in localized high-pressure gradients in this region of the valve that often are substantially higher than the overall pressure gradient across the valve.

The fluid dynamics of a tilting-disk valve are characterized by two orifices in the open position, one larger than the other (major vs. minor), with an asymmetric flow profile as blood accelerates along the tilted surface of the open disk. Subtle variations in this flow pattern depend on the shape of the disk (convex vs. concave surface) as well as the sewing ring design.

With a ball-cage valve in the open position, blood flows across the sewing ring and around the ball occluder on all sides. When the valve closes, a small amount of regurgitation is seen circumferentially around the ball as it seats in the sewing ring.

Prosthetic valve normal velocities, pressure gradients, and valve areas depend on the valve type, size, and position. However, compared with a normal native valve, all prosthetic valves are inherently stenotic to some extent. Specifically, the expected

antegrade velocities and pressure gradients across a normally functioning prosthetic valve are higher than the corresponding values for a native valve. Similarly, the effective orifice area of a prosthetic valve is smaller than the orifice area of a normal native valve. While manufacturers have data on in vitro flow characteristics for each valve, in vivo echocardiographic data are sparse because of the large number of valve types and sizes. Even in a large study, only a few patients have the same valve type, position, and size. In the available Doppler studies of normal prosthetic valves, data often are presented in various ways. Some studies report the mean ± 1 SD for each variable; others include the range as well. Expected normal velocities, pressure gradients, and valve areas for several commonly seen prosthetic valves are shown in Tables 13–2 and 13–3.

In general, larger valve sizes have lower velocities and gradients, and larger effective orifice areas. Mitral prostheses have lower velocities and gradients than aortic prostheses. Note that many of the smaller

TABLE 13–2 Normal Doppler Parameters for Selected Mechanical and Bioprosthetic Aortic Valves

Valve Type	Size (mm)	Peak Gradient (mm Hg)	Mean Gradient (mm Hg)	Peak Velocity (m/s)	Effective Orifice Area (cm²)
Mechanical					
Bileaflet (St Jude Medical)	19	35.17 ± 11.16	18.96 ± 6.27	2.86 ± 0.48	1.01 ± 0.24
	21	28.34 ± 9.94	15.82 ± 5.67	2.63 ± 0.48	1.33 ± 0.32
	23	25.28 ± 7.89	13.77 ± 5.33	2.57 ± 0.44	1.6 ± 0.43
	25	22.57 ± 7.68	12.65 ± 5.14	2.4 ± 0.45	1.93 ± 0.45
	27	19.85 ± 7.55	11.18 ± 4.82	2.24 ± 0.42	2.35 ± 0.59
	29	17.72 ± 6.42	9.86 ± 2.9	2 ± 0.1	2.81 ± 0.57
	31	16.0	10 ± 6	2.1 ± 0.6	3.08 ± 1.09
Tilting Disk (Medtronic-Hall)	20	34.37 ± 13.06	17.08 ± 5.28	2.9 ± 0.4	1.21 ± 0.45
	21	26.86 ± 10.54	14.1 ± 5.93	2.42 ± 0.36	1.08 ± 0.17
	23	26.85 ± 8.85	13.5 ± 4.79	2.43 ± 0.59	1.36 ± 0.39
	25	17.13 ± 7.04	9.53 ± 4.26	2.29 ± 0.5	1.9 ± 0.47
	27	18.66 ± 9.71	8.66 ± 5.56	2.07 ± 0.53	1.9 ± 0.16
Bileaflet (ATS Open Pivot)	16	47.7 ± 12	27 ± 7.3	3.44 ± 0.47	0.61 ± 0.09
	19	47 ± 12.6	26.2 ± 7.9	3.41 ± 0.43	0.96 ± 0.18
	21	25.5 ± 6.1	14.4 ± 3.5	2.4 ± 0.39	1.58 ± 0.37
	23	19 ± 7	12 ± 4	—	1.8 ± 0.2
	25	17 ± 8	11 ± 4	—	2.2 ± 0.4
	27	14 ± 4	9 ± 2	—	2.5 ± 0.3
	29	11 ± 3	8 ± 2	—	3.1 ± 0.3
Tilting Disk (Björk-Shiley)	17	—	—	4.1	—
	19	27.0	—	3.8	1.1
	21	38.94 ± 11.93	21.8 ± 3.4	2.92 ± 0.88	1.1 ± 0.25
	23	33.86 ± 11	17.34 ± 6.86	2.42 ± 0.4	1.22 ± 0.23
	25	20.39 ± 7.07	11.5 ± 4.55	2.06 ± 0.28	1.8 ± 0.32
	27	19.44 ± 7.99	10.67 ± 4.31	1.77 ± 0.12	2.6
	29	21.1 ± 7.1	—	1.87 ± 0.18	2.52 ± 0.69
	31	—	—	2.1 ± 0.14	—

TABLE 13–2—Cont'd

Valve Type	Size (mm)	Peak Gradient (mm Hg)	Mean Gradient (mm Hg)	Peak Velocity (m/s)	Effective Orifice Area (cm²)
Mechanical—Cont'd					
Bileaflet (Carbomedics)	17	33.4 ± 13.2	20.1 ± 7.1	—	1.02 ± 0.2
	19	33.3 ± 11.19	11.61 ± 5.08	3.09 ± 0.38	1.25 ± 0.36
	21	26.31 ± 10.25	12.68 ± 4.29	2.61 ± 0.51	1.42 ± 0.36
	23	24.61 ± 6.93	11.33 ± 3.8	2.42 ± 0.37	1.69 ± 0.29
	25	20.25 ± 8.69	9.34 ± 4.65	2.25 ± 0.34	2.04 ± 0.37
	27	19.05 ± 7.04	8.41 ± 2.83	2.18 ± 0.36	2.55 ± 0.34
	29	12.53 ± 4.69	5.8 ± 3.2	1.93 ± 0.25	2.63 ± 0.38
Bioprosthetic					
Stented Bioprosthesis (Carpentier-Edwards)	19	43.48 ± 12.72	25.6 ± 8.02	—	0.85 ± 0.17
	21	27.73 ± 7.6	17.25 ± 6.24	2.37 ± 0.54	1.48 ± 0.3
	23	28.93 ± 7.49	15.92 ± 6.43	2.76 ± 0.4	1.69 ± 0.45
	25	23.95 ± 7.05	12.76 ± 4.43	2.38 ± 0.47	1.94 ± 0.45
	27	22.14 ± 8.24	12.33 ± 5.59	2.31 ± 0.39	2.25 ± 0.55
	29	22.0	9.92 ± 2.9	2.44 ± 0.43	2.84 ± 0.51
	31	—	—	2.41 ± 0.13	—
Stented Bioprosthesis (Carpentier-Edwards Pericardial)	19	32.13 ± 3.35	24.19 ± 8.6	2.83 ± 0.14	1.21 ± 0.31
	21	25.69 ± 9.9	20.3 ± 9.08	2.59 ± 0.42	1.47 ± 0.36
	23	21.72 ± 8.57	13.01 ± 5.27	2.29 ± 0.45	1.75 ± 0.28
	25	16.46 ± 5.41	9.04 ± 2.27	2.02 ± 0.31	—
	27	19.2 ± 0	5.6	1.6	—
	29	17.6 ± 0	11.6	2.1	—
Stentless Bioprosthesis (CryoLife-O'Brien Stentless)	19	—	12 ± 4.8	—	1.25 ± 0.1
	21	—	10.33 ± 2	—	1.57 ± 0.6
	23	—	8.5	—	2.2
	25	—	7.9	—	2.3
	27	—	7.4	—	2.7
Stentless Bioprosthesis (Edwards Prima Stentless)	19	30.9 ± 11.7	15.4 ± 7.4	—	1 ± 0.3
	21	31.22 ± 17.35	16.36 ± 11.36	—	1.25 ± 0.29
	23	23.39 ± 10.17	11.52 ± 5.26	2.8 ± 0.4	1.49 ± 0.46
	25	19.74 ± 10.36	10.77 ± 9.32	2.7 ± 0.3	1.7 ± 0.55
	27	15.9 ± 7.3	7.1 ± 3.7	—	2 ± 0.6
	29	11.21 ± 8.6	5.03 ± 4.53	—	2.49 ± 0.52
Stentless Bioprosthesis (Medtronic Freestyle Stentless)	19	—	13.0	—	—
	21	—	7.99 ± 2.6	—	1.6 ± 0.32
	23	—	7.24 ± 2.5	—	1.9 ± 0.5
	25	—	5.35 ± 1.5	—	2.03 ± 0.41
	27	—	4.72 ± 1.6	—	2.5 ± 0.47
Stented Bioprosthesis (Medtronic Mosaic Porcine)	21	—	12.43 ± 7.3	—	2.1 ± 0.8
	23	—	12.47 ± 7.4	—	2.1 ± 0.8
	25	—	10.08 ± 5.1	—	2.1 ± 1.6
	27	—	9.0	—	—
	29	—	9.0	—	—

Data from Rosenhek R, Binder T, Maurer G, et al. Normal values for Doppler echocardiographic assessment of heart valve prostheses. J Am Soc Echocardiogr 16:1116–1127, 2003.
Data on additional valve types and references for these data are available in the original publication.

TABLE 13–3   Normal Doppler Parameters for Selected Mechanical and Bioprosthetic Mitral Valves

Valve Type	Size (mm)	Peak Gradient (mm Hg)	Mean Gradient (mm Hg)	Peak Velocity (m/s)	T½ (ms)	Effective Orifice Area (cm^2)
Mechanical						
Bileaflet (Carbomedics)	23	—	—	1.9 ± 0.1	126 ± 7	—
	25	10.3 ± 2.3	3.6 ± 0.6	1.3 ± 0.1	93 ± 8	2.9 ± 0.8
	27	8.79 ± 3.46	3.46 ± 1.03	1.61 ± 0.3	89 ± 20	2.9 ± 0.75
	29	8.78 ± 2.9	3.39 ± 0.97	1.52 ± 0.3	88 ± 17	2.3 ± 0.4
	31	8.87 ± 2.34	3.32 ± 0.87	1.61 ± 0.29	92 ± 24	2.8 ± 1.14
	33	8.8 ± 2.2	4.8 ± 2.5	1.5 ± 0.2	93 ± 12	—
Bileaflet (St Jude Medical)	23	—	4.0	1.5	160	1.0
	25	—	2.5 ± 1	1.34 ± 1.12	75 ± 4	1.35 ± 0.17
	27	11 ± 4	5 ± 1.82	1.61 ± 0.29	75 ± 10	1.67 ± 0.17
	29	10 ± 3	4.15 ± 1.8	1.57 ± 0.29	85 ± 10	1.75 ± 0.24
	31	12 ± 6	4.46 ± 2.22	1.59 ± 0.33	74 ± 13	2.03 ± 0.32
Tilting Disk (Medtronic-Hall)	27	—	—	1.4	78	—
	29	—	—	1.57 ± 0.1	69 ± 15	—
	31	—	—	1.45 ± 0.12	77 ± 17	—
Bioprosthetic						
Stented Bioprosthesis (Carpentier-Edwards)	27	—	6 ± 2	1.7 ± 0.3	98 ± 28	—
	29	—	4.7 ± 2	1.76 ± 0.27	92 ± 14	—
	31	—	4.4 ± 2	1.54 ± 0.15	92 ± 19	—
	33	—	6 ± 3	—	93 ± 12	—
Stented Bioprosthesis (Carpentier-Edwards pericardial)	27	—	3.6	1.6	100	—
	29	—	5.25 ± 2.36	1.67 ± 0.3	110 ± 15	—
	31	—	4.05 ± 0.83	1.53 ± 0.1	90 ± 11	—
	33	—	1.0	0.8	80	—
Stented Bioprosthesis (Medtronic Intact Porcine)	29	—	3.5 ± 0.51	1.6 ± 0.22	—	—
	31	—	4.2 ± 1.44	1.6 ± 0.26	—	—
	33	—	4 ± 1.3	1.4 ± 0.24	—	—
	35	—	3.2 ± 1.77	1.3 ± 0.5	—	—

Data from Rosenhek R, Binder T, Maurer G, et al.: Normal values for Doppler echocardiographic assessment of heart valve prostheses. J Am Soc Echocardiogr 16:1116–1127, 2003.
Data on additional valve types and references for these data are available in the original publication.

prosthetic aortic valves have hemodynamics that are consistent with clinical stenosis even with normal valve function. The lower velocities and pressure gradients with mitral valve prostheses are due in part to larger valve sizes but also to passive flow at a lower pressure gradient from the atrium into the ventricle in diastole compared with active ejection and a higher LV-to-aortic pressure gradient in systole for aortic prostheses.

The wide range of reported "normal" values for a given prosthetic valve type and size may relate to anatomic features and the details of implantation in each patient. However, the impact of transvalvular volume flow rate on transvalvular velocities and pressure gradients should not be underestimated. Even with a normally functioning prosthesis, a high cardiac

output (e.g., postoperative, pregnancy, or sepsis) results in a high velocity and pressure gradient. This variability in "normal" velocities can be compensated for by calculating effective orifice area to "correct" for volume flow rate.

A useful clinical approach is to obtain a baseline Doppler echo study in each patient after valve replacement (but not in the immediate postoperative period). The values obtained then serve as the "normal" reference for that patient. This facilitates detection of changes in prosthetic valve function over time, with each patient serving as his or her own control. Sometimes the implanted valve is relatively small for the patient's body size, resulting in "patient-prosthesis mismatch" (PPM) with baseline hemodynamics consistent with stenosis (high velocity, small valve area) despite normal valve function. A postoperative baseline study helps distinguish PPM from progressive stenosis due to mechanical valve failure.

Normal Prosthetic Valve Regurgitation

Normal prosthetic valve function implies a small degree of valvular regurgitation in virtually all mechanical valves and in a high percentage (30% to 50%) of bioprosthetic valves. The spatial patterns of regurgitation correspond to the fluid dynamics of each valve type. Bioprosthetic valves typically have a small amount of central regurgitation.

When a bileaflet valve closes, two crisscross jets of regurgitation are seen in the plane parallel to the leaflet opening plane (Fig. 13–5). In the perpendicular plane, two smaller diverging regurgitant jets are seen. With a tilting-disk valve, regurgitation occurs at the closure line with the major regurgitant jet directed away from the sewing ring at the edge of the major orifice. With a single-disk valve and a central strut (e.g., Medtronic-Hall), a small central jet of regurgitation also occurs around the central hole of the disk, as might be expected. The orientation of the prosthetic valve in the annulus can be variable, depending on surgical preference, so that the open disk position and the orientation of the regurgitant jet vary correspondingly. In addition, smaller regurgitant jets circumferentially around the annulus may be seen. However, the total volume of regurgitation is small with normal prosthetic valve function.

On a TTE study it may be difficult to separate normal from pathologic prosthetic regurgitation, especially for the mitral position. On color flow imaging, normal prosthetic regurgitation tends to be a uniform color with little variance, whereas pathologic regurgitation shows aliasing and variance with a "confetti-like" appearance to the flow pattern. On CW Doppler examination, normal prosthetic regurgitation has a low signal strength and may persist through only part of the cardiac cycle. On TEE imaging the normal patterns of prosthetic regurgitation for each valve type can be identified, keeping in mind that normal regurgitation tends to be relatively uniform in color, even though the jet area may appear relatively large. Physiologic regurgitation originates within the sewing ring, with typical patterns for each valve type. Pathologic regurgitation is typically characterized by:

- ❏ An eccentric or large jet
- ❏ Marked variance on the color flow display
- ❏ A jet that often originates around the valve sewing ring

- ❏ Visualization of a proximal flow acceleration region on the LV side of the mitral valve

Prosthetic Valve Stenosis

Pressure Gradients

The principles applied to evaluation of native valve stenosis also have been used for suspected stenosis of prosthetic valves. From a CW Doppler recording of the antegrade velocity across the valve, obtained at a parallel intercept angle, maximum instantaneous and mean pressure gradients can be calculated using the Bernoulli equation ($4v^2$). Although the maximum velocity across a prosthetic valve is higher than that for a native valve, the shape of the velocity curve is triangular (in contrast to the rounded contour seen in aortic stenosis). Thus, the calculated mean gradient typically is less for a prosthetic valve than for a native valve with the same maximum antegrade velocity (Fig. 13–11).

Maximum and mean pressure gradients across bioprosthetic valves calculated by Doppler echo compare well with directly measured pressure gradients (Table 13–4). The situation is more complex for mechanical valves because of the differing fluid dynamics of each type of prosthesis. In theory, the pressure gradient across a given degree of stenosis will be identical whether the stenosis consists of a single orifice or multiple orifices, with the Bernoulli

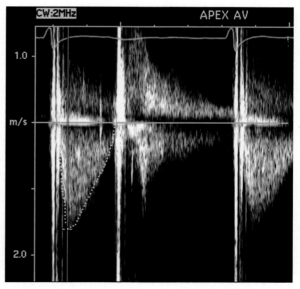

Figure 13–11 Antegrade velocity across a normal aortic valve replacement. The antegrade velocity is slightly increased compared with a native valve, but the triangular shape indicates a normal flow pattern. Prominent valve clicks are seen. The flow in diastole is transmitral flow, not aortic regurgitation based on timing, velocity, and shape of the diastolic signal. This patient also has a mechanical mitral valve (note the two valve clicks close together on the second beat).

TABLE 13–4   Validation of Doppler Echo Prosthetic Mean Valve Gradients Compared with Invasive Data (Selected Series)

First Author and Year	Valve Type (Position)	n	r	SEE (mmHg)	Mean Difference
Sagar 1986	Hancock & B.S. (mitral)	19	0.93	2.5	—
Sagar 1986	Hancock & B.S. (aortic)	11	0.94	7.4	—
Wilkins 1986	Mixed (mitral)	11	0.96	—	—
Burstow 1989	Mixed (aortic)	20	0.94	3	—
	Mixed (mitral)	20	0.97	1.2	—
Baumgartner 1990	St. Jude	In vitro	0.98	1.9	10 ± 3 mm Hg
	Hancock	In vitro	0.98	1.4	2 ± 1 mm Hg
Stewart 1991	Bioprosthetic (aortic)	In vitro	0.78–0.98	—	Overestimation by Doppler
Baumgartner 1992	St. Jude	In vitro	0.98	2.0	13 ± 8 mm Hg
	Medtronic-Hall	In vitro	0.99	0.5	0.8 ± 0.6 mm Hg
	Starr-Edwards	In vitro	0.97	2.0	8 ± 4 mm Hg
	Hancock	In vitro	0.99	1.5	1.9 ± 1.6

B.S., Bjork-Shiley tilting-disk mechanical valve; SEE, standard error of the estimate.
References as in Suggested Reading and Sagar et al: J Am Coll Cardiol 7:681–687, 1986.

relationship being valid for each orifice. Thus, a maximum pressure gradient of 36 mm Hg will correspond to a single or multiple 3-m/s jets across the valve. However, while this theory holds true when local acceleration and viscous forces can be ignored, local higher pressure gradients do occur with some valve types. This phenomenon has been studied most thoroughly for the bileaflet valve.

With the valve leaflets open, the bileaflet valve has a narrow, slitlike central orifice flanked by two larger semicircular orifices (Fig. 13–12). The walls of this

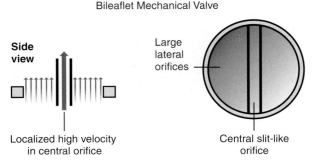

Bileaflet Mechanical Valve

Side view

Localized high velocity in central orifice

Large lateral orifices

Central slit-like orifice

Figure 13–12 Schematic drawing of a bileaflet mechanical valve in the open position in side (left) and frontal (right) views. Two large lateral orifices flank a central slitlike orifice that is associated with localized high-velocity flow (and a localized pressure gradient).

narrow central orifice are formed by the parallel valve disks, which are nearly perpendicular to the sewing ring of the valve. Within this narrow central flow stream, acceleration forces result in a localized high-pressure gradient (and corresponding high velocity), with rapid pressure recovery distal to the valve. Therefore, the pressure difference measured between the upstream side of the valve and this central orifice is greater than the pressure difference between the upstream and downstream sides of the valve. Because CW Doppler ultrasound records the highest velocity along the length of the ultrasound beam, it is this higher localized velocity that is recorded. Although this high localized gradient is measured correctly, the gradient of interest is the upstream-to-downstream valve gradient. This explains the observation that even though the correlation between Doppler and invasive pressure gradient measurements is high, the slope of the regression line indicates that the Doppler approach consistently "overestimates" the overall transvalvular gradient. This overestimation is large enough that an erroneous diagnosis of severe stenosis might be made if the phenomenon of pressure recovery is not recognized.

Interestingly, the overestimation of pressure gradients across bileaflet valves becomes less significant in the presence of prosthetic valve stenosis. The proposed mechanism for this observation is a gradual reduction in the size of the central orifice as leaflet opening is reduced. Clinically, this poses a dilemma in that a high velocity across a bileaflet valve might represent overestimation of the pressure gradient with normal valve function or a correct estimate of a high gradient with a stenotic valve. Again, a baseline study in the postoperative period provides a standard of comparison when subsequent valve dysfunction is suspected.

Valve Areas

Even when accurately measured, the physiologic limitation of transvalvular velocities across prosthetic valves is that velocities vary with volume flow rate for a given orifice area. A normally functioning valve prosthesis in an individual patient may have

❏ a high transvalvular velocity if cardiac output is elevated (e.g., with exercise, anemia, fever), or
❏ a low transvalvular velocity if cardiac output is depressed (e.g., LV dysfunction).

For these reasons a flow-independent measure of prosthetic valve function is more useful clinically.

Aortic. Bioprosthetic aortic valves have fluid dynamics similar to those of a native aortic valve, and it is logical to assume that continuity equation valve area calculations are valid in this situation (Fig. 13–13). In fact, direct comparisons of Doppler echo aortic valve area (AVA_{prost}) and invasive valve areas in patients with suspected stenosis of bioprosthetic aortic valves have shown a reasonable correlation. As for a native aortic valve, the components of the continuity equation are the LV outflow tract velocity-time integral (VTI_{LVOT}), the LV outflow tract cross-sectional area (CSA_{LVOT}), and the aortic jet velocity-time integral (VTI_{Ao}). The continuity equation, then, is

$$AVA_{prost} = (CSA_{LVOT} \times VTI_{LVOT})/VTI_{Ao}$$

LVOT velocity is recorded from an apical approach using pulsed Doppler echo with the sample volume positioned proximal to the prosthetic valve, avoiding the small region of flow acceleration immediately adjacent to the valve. Aortic jet velocity is recorded with CW Doppler from whichever window gives the highest-velocity signal, as for native valve stenosis. LVOT diameter is measured in a parasternal long-axis view in mid-systole from the septal endocardium to the anterior mitral leaflet parallel to and immediately adjacent to the aortic valve (Fig. 13–14). Direct measurement of outflow tract diameter is preferable to use of the implanted prosthetic valve size, since valve size relates to the external diameter of the sewing ring, not the effective diameter of the subvalvular flow region. As usual, a circular cross-sectional LVOT area is calculated as $\pi(D/2)^2$ from this diameter measurement.

The use of the continuity equation for mechanical aortic valves is more problematic. Presumably, if the transvalvular velocity curve is an accurate reflection of transvalvular volume flow rate, then calculated valve areas should be accurate. Remember that the continuity equation assumes a flat flow velocity profile *in* the stenotic orifice (or vena contracta), as well as proximal to the valve. Clearly, this assumption is not true for bileaflet valves. The local high velocities in the central orifice will result in a significant error in measurement of volume flow rate across the valve orifice, with a consequent underestimation of valve area. However, for tilting-disk and ball-cage valves, limited data suggest that the continuity equation may be reasonably accurate, despite complex fluid dynamics, because the CW velocity signal provides an approximation of the spatial mean flow velocity across the valve (Table 13–5).

Another approach to evaluation of suspected prosthetic aortic valve stenosis is to measure the "step-up" in velocity across the valve. The ratio of the outflow tract velocity to aortic jet velocity reflects the degree of stenosis; if no obstruction is present, these velocities will be nearly equal with a ratio close to 1; as the degree of narrowing increases, the aortic jet velocity will increase with no change in outflow tract velocity, resulting progressively in a ratio of about 1. Since all prosthetic valves are inherently stenotic to some degree, the "normal" velocity ratio across an aortic prosthesis ranges from 0.35 to 0.50, compared with 0.75 to 0.90 for a normal native aortic valve.

The velocity ratio has several advantages because it:

❏ Takes volume flow rate into account
❏ Does not require an outflow tract diameter measurement

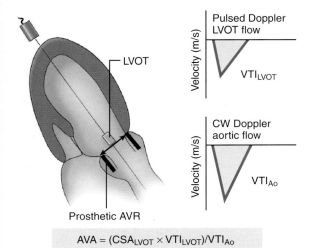

$$AVA = (CSA_{LVOT} \times VTI_{LVOT})/VTI_{Ao}$$

Figure 13–13 The continuity equation can be used for calculation of aortic valve area (AVA) for an aortic valve replacement (AVR). LV outflow tract (LVOT) flow is recorded from an apical approach using pulsed Doppler with the sample volume positioned just proximal to the prosthetic valve. LVOT diameter is measured from a parasternal long-axis view for calculation of a circular cross-sectional area (CSA) of flow. Continuous-wave Doppler is used to record the flow signal across the prosthetic valve from whichever window yields the highest velocity jet.

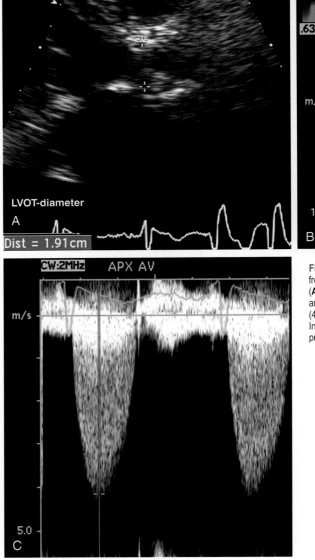

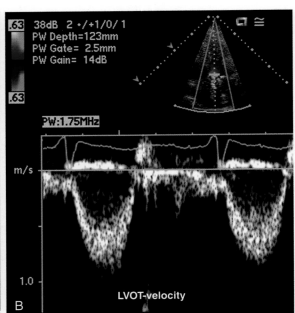

Figure 13–14 Continuity equation prosthetic valve area is calculated from a parasternal long-axis mid-systolic diameter (1.9 cm) measurement (**A**), the pulsed Doppler LV outflow tract velocity (0.75 m/s) recorded from an apical approach (**B**), and the CW Doppler signal of flow across the valve (4.1 m/s) recorded from whichever window gives the highest velocity (**C**). In this example the calculated valve area is 0.5 cm², consistent with severe prosthetic stenosis.

❑ Is easily measured and reproducible
❑ Serves as a baseline "normal" value for comparison on follow-up studies

Some investigators advocate measuring the velocity ratio with increases in flow rate (e.g., with exercise) to increase its specificity in excluding prosthetic valve stenosis. Pragmatically, even if Doppler velocities and continuity equation valve areas overestimate the degree of prosthetic valve stenosis, in an individual patient a *change* in velocity or valve area is valuable in patient management decisions.

MITRAL. Prosthetic mitral valve area (MVA) can be estimated using the pressure half-time ($T\frac{1}{2}$) approach as for native mitral valve stenosis. The expected normal half-time for a prosthetic valve is longer than for a native valve, with the specific value depending on valve type and size. For bioprosthetic mitral valves, valve area can be estimated from the same formula as for native valves:

$$MVA = 220/T\frac{1}{2}$$

where the pressure half-time ($T\frac{1}{2}$) is measured in milliseconds, as described in Chapter 11.

TABLE 13–5	Validation of Doppler Echo Prosthetic Valve Areas (Selected Series)						
First Author and Year	**Valve Type (Position)**	***n***	**Comparison**	***r***	**SEE**	**Mean Difference**	
Sagar 1986	Hancock and B.S. (mitral)	12	T½ vs. Gorlin	0.98	0.1 cm²	—	
Wilkins 1986	Porcine (mitral)	8	T½ vs. Gorlin	0.65	—	—	
Rothbart 1990	Bioprosthetic (aortic)	22	Cont eq vs. Gorlin at cath	0.93	—	—	
Chafizadeh 1991	St. Jude (aortic)	67	Cont eq vs. actual orifice area	0.83	—	Doppler effective orifice area less than actual orifice area	
Baumgartner 1992	St. Jude	In vitro	Cont eq vs. Gorlin	0.99	0.08	0.4–0.6 cm²	
	Medtronic-Hall	In vitro		0.97	0.10	0–0.25 cm²	
	Hancock (aortic)	In vitro		0.93	0.10	0–0.25 cm²	

B.S., Bjork-Shiley tilting-disk mechanical valve; Cont eq, continuity equation valve area with Doppler and 2D echo data; Gorlin, Gorlin formula valve area using invasive data; SEE, standard error of the estimate; T½, Doppler pressure half-time method.
References as in Suggested Reading and Sagar et al: J Am Coll Cardiol 7:681–687, 1986.

Somewhat surprisingly, the empirical constant 220 also appears to provide a reasonable approximation of MVA for mechanical prostheses. With a bileaflet valve the higher localized velocities in the central slit-like orifice affect the accuracy of pressure gradient calculations. However, the T½ measurement is less affected because it depends on the *time course* of the velocity decline relative to the maximum velocity rather than on the velocities themselves.

Continuity equation valve area also can be calculated for a mitral prosthesis (in the absence of mitral regurgitation) using the antegrade stroke volume across the aortic or pulmonic valve in the equation.

The antegrade velocity curve across a mitral bioprosthesis may be recorded from an apical approach using pulsed, high–pulse repetition frequency, or CW Doppler ultrasound. Care in positioning the transducer is needed, because inflow may be directed obliquely into the ventricular chamber. Some echocardiographers find it helpful to use the color flow image to aid in alignment of the Doppler beam parallel to the inflow stream. In many patients after mitral valve replacement, the inflow stream is directed anteriorly and medially toward the ventricular septum. In these patients, a low parasternal window may provide an optimal intercept angle for recording antegrade velocity. As for native mitral valve stenosis, Doppler acquisition parameters are adjusted to show a smooth velocity deceleration slope and a dark band of velocity signals along the edge of the curve.

Prosthetic Valve Regurgitation

Detection of Regurgitation

The echocardiographic approaches described for evaluation of native valve regurgitation in Chapter 12 also apply to evaluation of prosthetic valve regurgitation. The major differences between native or prosthetic valves are:

❏ The prosthetic valve has a higher antegrade velocity
❏ The degree of normal prosthetic regurgitation is greater than the trivial amounts of native valve regurgitation seen in normal individuals
❏ Acoustic shadowing, reverberations, and beam width artifact make evaluation of a prosthetic valve more difficult

These differences decrease the sensitivity of TTE imaging for detection of prosthetic regurgitation, so that TEE imaging is needed more frequently.

TTE color Doppler flow imaging for detection of prosthetic valve regurgitation can be helpful, particularly if a view can be obtained wherein the ultrasound beam has access to the chamber receiving the regurgitant flow without first traversing the valve prosthesis. For the aortic valve, both parasternal and apical views are helpful, because the ultrasound signal reaches the LV outflow tract region without intercepting the valve prosthesis, avoiding the problem of acoustic shadowing. For the mitral valve, the parasternal approach may be helpful if a view can be obtained wherein the LA side of the valve is not shadowed by the valve prosthesis. Apical views often are limited due to acoustic shadowing, but occasionally a paraprosthetic jet can be identified from this approach. In addition to acoustic shadowing, color artifacts are prominent in patients with prosthetic valves, which may obscure detection of abnormal flow signals.

CW Doppler also is helpful for detection of prosthetic regurgitation with the advantage of a wide beam size at the depth of a prosthetic valve and a high signal-to-noise ratio, enhancing the likelihood

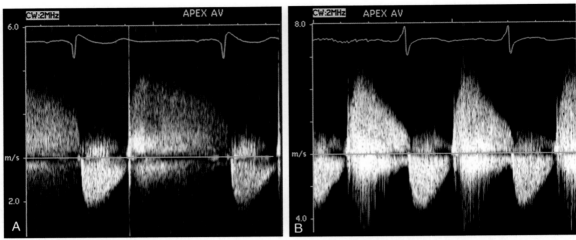

Figure 13–15 A, The continuous-wave (CW) Doppler signal in this patient with a bioprosthetic aortic valve shows mild aortic regurgitation (AR). **B,** One year later the patient presented with new heart failure symptoms (now 11 years after valve replacement). The CW Doppler signal now shows severe AR with a dense signal compared to antegrade flow and a steep deceleration time. The antegrade velocity is higher due to increased transaortic volume flow. Direct inspection at surgery showed a cusp tear adjacent to an area of calcification.

that a weaker signal or eccentric jet (i.e., paraprosthetic regurgitation) will be identified (Fig. 13–15). The timing of the presumed regurgitant signal is extremely important for correct identification of the origin of the Doppler signal. Many laboratories find it helpful to examine the prosthetic valve with CW Doppler starting with the ultrasound beam aligned in the flow direction of the valve and then slowly scanning in progressively larger circles to identify any potential paraprosthetic jets (Fig. 13–16).

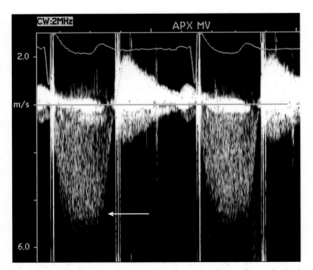

Figure 13–16 Continuous-wave Doppler recording of mechanical prosthetic mitral regurgitation obtained from an apical window. The regurgitant signal (*arrow*) starts immediately after the mitral closure click and continues up to the onset of antegrade flow across the prosthesis in diastole. The signal is not as dense as antegrade flow, suggesting regurgitation is not severe. However, TEE is preferred for evaluation of regurgitant severity of a mechanical mitral valve because shadowing may result in underestimation from the TTE approach.

Due to the problems of acoustic shadowing and reverberations, even the most carefully performed TTE examinations have a low sensitivity for detection and quantitation of prosthetic regurgitation. Especially for the mitral position, the TEE approach provides both improved image quality and the opportunity to interrogate the valve from the LA side; that is, the acoustic shadow now will obscure the LV rather than the LA. Thus, when prosthetic mitral valve regurgitation is suspected, a TEE study is recommended (Fig. 13–17). A TTE study showing prosthetic regurgitation can be clinically useful (high positive predictive value) but rarely allows for accurate quantitation of mitral regurgitant severity. A TTE study that does not show prosthetic regurgitation does not exclude this possibility (low negative predictive value).

Severity and Etiology of Regurgitation

When prosthetic regurgitation is detected, the first step in evaluation and interpretation is whether "normal" or pathologic prosthetic regurgitation is present. While the normal backflow across the valve represents a small volume of blood, the color jets on TEE imaging can be fairly large in area. Distinguishing features are the characteristic pattern for each valve type, a uniform color pattern rather than the mosaic flow disturbance seen with pathologic regurgitation, and the absence of other features (increased antegrade velocity, chamber sizes and function, pulmonary hypertension) to suggest significant regurgitation.

Pathologic regurgitation of bioprosthetic valves most often is due to degenerative changes of the leaflets. This can be slowly progressive, with gradually increasing severity of a central regurgitant stream, or can occur abruptly, with cusp rupture adjacent

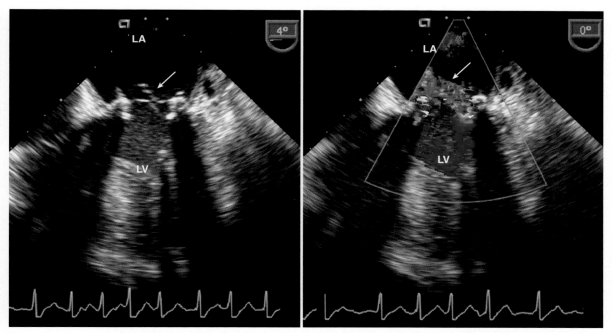

Figure 13–17 Transesophageal image showing a stented tissue mitral valve prosthesis with a flail leaflet (*arrow*), due to endocarditis, on 2D imaging (*left*). Color flow shows an eccentric jet of regurgitation through the valve with a wide vena contracta consistent with severe prosthetic regurgitation (*right*).

to a fibrocalcific nodule. The cause of mechanical valves regurgitation most often is incomplete closure resulting from pannus ingrowth around the sewing ring or from thrombus formation (Fig. 13–18).

Paraprosthetic regurgitation is most common with mechanical valves but also can occur with bioprosthetic valves. Distinguishing prosthetic from paraprosthetic regurgitation is difficult on TTE imaging; in most cases, TEE is needed. The etiology of paraprosthetic regurgitation may be a scarred and/or calcified annulus resulting in disruption of the sutures securing the valve or a paravalvular abscess with

tissue destruction (Fig. 13–19). The regurgitant jet originates external to the sewing ring, with an eccentric jet extending into the receiving chamber. A single or multiple paraprosthetic jet(s) may be present. Color flow imaging may show proximal flow acceleration (on the LV side of the mitral valve) into the regurgitant orifice, facilitating identification of the paraprosthetic origin of the signal. Immediately after implantation, a small degree of paraprosthetic regurgitation may be normal on intraoperative TEE imaging and usually does not have long-term adverse clinical consequences.

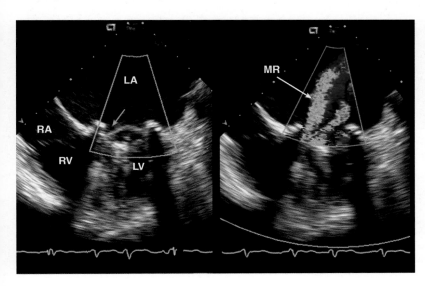

Figure 13–18 Transesophageal view of a patient with prosthetic mitral regurgitation (MR) seen on intraoperative imaging. The 2D image (*left*) shows incomplete closure of the medial valve disk (*arrow*), and color flow imaging (*right*) documented severe prosthetic MR (*arrow*) with a wide vena contracta. Incomplete closure was caused by retained native valve tissue, and normal valve function was restored by rotating the leaflet opening plane before completing the surgical procedure.

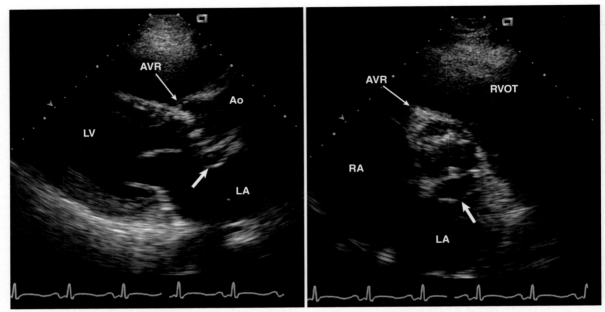

Figure 13–19 On transthoracic imaging in a patient with prosthetic valve endocarditis the cause of aortic regurgitation is evident, with an echolucent space (*arrows*) seen posterior to the tissue aortic valve prosthesis (AVR) in both long-axis (*left*) and short-axis views (*right*).

Evaluation of the severity of prosthetic regurgitation is more challenging than for a native valve, and TEE imaging usually is needed. However, the following approaches remain useful:

❒ The shape, origin, and orientation of the regurgitant jet

❒ Vena contracta diameter (if visualized)
❒ The intensity and shape of the CW Doppler signal
❒ Evidence for distal flow reversals (e.g., descending aorta diastolic flow in aortic regurgitation) (Fig. 13–20)

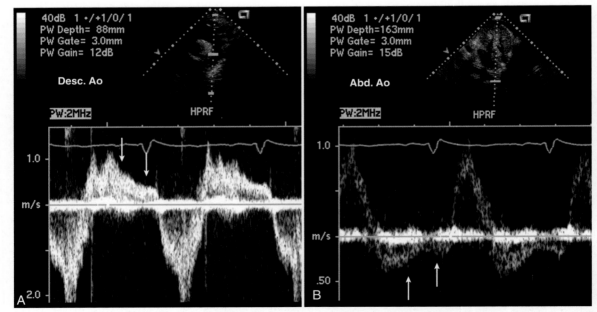

Figure 13–20 In a patient with a prosthetic aortic valve replacement, Doppler evaluation for distal flow reversal in the aorta is helpful. This example shows holodiastolic flow reversal both in the descending thoracic aorta from a suprasternal notch view (**A**), and in the proximal abdominal aorta from a subcostal view (**B**), consistent with severe prosthetic aortic regurgitation.

- The antegrade velocity across the prosthetic valve
- Estimated pulmonary pressures (particularly with mitral regurgitation)

Calculation of regurgitant volume and orifice area is more difficult because calculation of antegrade flow rates across a prosthetic valve is challenging and jets are usually eccentric, limiting the proximal isovelocity surface area approach. However, clinical decision making usually is based on the presence of pathologic prosthetic regurgitation and its clinical consequences (hemolysis, heart failure, etc.), not on exact measures of severity.

Other Echocardiographic Findings

In addition to direct imaging or Doppler evaluation of regurgitation, several other findings on the echocardiographic examination are integrated in the overall interpretation of prosthetic valve function:

- LV size, hypertrophy, and systolic function
- Antegrade prosthetic valve flow velocity
- Pulmonary artery pressures

For example, persistent LV hypertrophy after aortic valve replacement for aortic stenosis raises the possibility of prosthetic valve stenosis or patient-prosthesis mismatch (see below). In other cases, LV dilation may suggest aortic or mitral prosthetic regurgitation with resultant volume overload. A hyperdynamic (but previously normal) LV may indicate prosthetic mitral regurgitation. While it may be difficult in some patients to separate persistent postoperative abnormalities from new pathologic findings, a change between examinations is of concern.

An increase in antegrade velocity may be due to increased volume flow because of prosthetic regurgitation rather than prosthetic stenosis. In this case, while the calculated gradient will be higher, the valve area will be unchanged. Alternatively, an increased flow velocity across the prosthetic valve may be due to a high cardiac output state (such as fever, anemia, or anxiety). In this situation, antegrade velocities across the other cardiac valves will be increased proportionately.

Although pulmonary hypertension can persist after successful mitral valve surgery, *recurrent* pulmonary hypertension (after an initial postoperative decline) may relate to prosthetic valve dysfunction.

LIMITATIONS AND ALTERNATE APPROACHES

The major limitation of TTE for evaluation of prosthetic valves is technical, specifically reverberations, artifacts, and acoustic shadowing. The last of these problems can be circumvented to some extent with

the TEE approach by casting the shadow in the opposite direction. Reverberations and other ultrasound artifacts remain a problem with both approaches.

Other limitations are overestimation of transvalvular pressure gradients with bileaflet mechanical valves, limited validation of valve area calculations for mechanical valves, and the problem of differentiating "normal" from pathologic prosthetic valve regurgitation.

Importantly, the same factors that can lead to errors in evaluation of native valves also are significant limitations in evaluation of prosthetic valves. Most notably, these factors include ultrasound tissue penetration, Doppler intercept angle assumptions, accurate diameter measurement, correct image orientation, and correct identification of the origin of Doppler signals.

When the echocardiographic examination is negative or yields results discordant with other clinical findings, other diagnostic procedures may be indicated. Cardiac catheterization can be performed with direct measurement of intracardiac pressures to confirm the pressure gradient across the valve and measure pulmonary artery pressures. In combination with cardiac output measurement, Gorlin formula valve area and pulmonary vascular resistance can be calculated. Angiographic evaluation (LV for mitral regurgitation, aortic root for aortic regurgitation) is helpful in evaluating prosthetic regurgitation on a semiquantitative (0 to 4+) scale or for calculating regurgitant volumes and fractions in conjunction with other quantitative cardiac output data. Fluoroscopy is a simple approach to measure the angle of occluder opening with bileaflet and single-disk mechanical valves when valve thrombosis is suspected. Cardiac magnetic resonance imaging and computed tomographic imaging currently have limited utility for evaluation of prosthetic valves but may be helpful in selected cases.

CLINICAL UTILITY

Prosthetic Valve Stenosis

Echocardiography is the initial diagnostic approach to evaluation of suspected prosthetic valve stenosis. The antegrade velocity and mean gradient across the prosthetic valve, particularly in comparison with previous data in that patient, may be diagnostic. Valve area can be calculated by the continuity equation for valves in the aortic (Figs. 13–21 and 13–22) or pulmonic position and by the T½ method for valves in the mitral or tricuspid (Fig. 13–23) position. Despite the overestimation of the average transvalvular gradient that occurs with Doppler evaluation of bileaflet mechanical valves, this approach still is helpful in assessing changes over time in an individual patient.

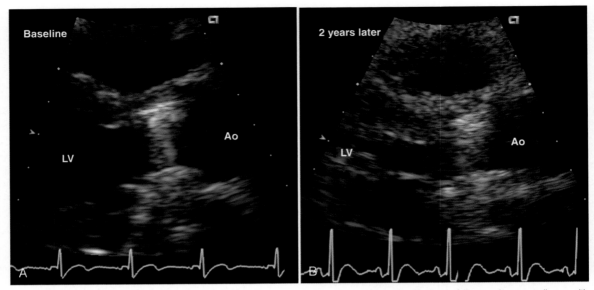

Figure 13–21 This 56-year-old man with a mechanical aortic valve replacement presented with heart failure and noncompliance with anticoagulation. Comparing the 2D parasternal long-axis images of the valve 2 years ago (**A**) and now (**B**), the septum appears more hypertrophied, but disk motion was not well seen on either study.

Figure 13–22 In the same patient as Figure 13–21, Doppler data was diagnostic, with the continuous-wave Doppler signal of transaortic flow (*top*) increasing from a baseline (*left*) of 2.8 m/s (maximum gradient 31 mm Hg) to 5.5 m/s (maximum gradient 123 mm Hg) 2 years later (*right*), concurrent decline in the LV outflow tract velocity (*bottom*) consistent with a decreased cardiac output. This patient has a mechanical mitral valve as well, as indicated by the two prosthetic valve clicks (*arrows*).

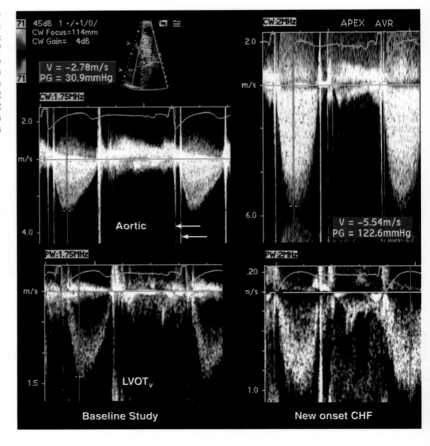

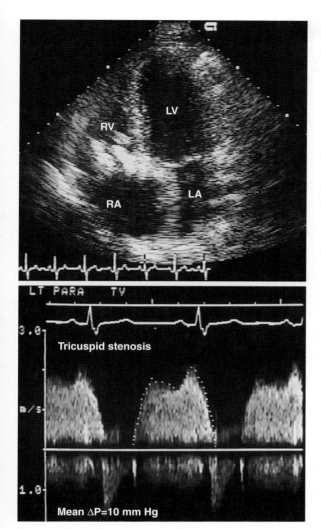

Figure 13–23 A 36-year-old man with a previous tricuspid valve replacement for endocarditis presented with right-sided heart failure. The apical four-chamber view showed a severely calcified porcine tricuspid valve replacement (*top*), with an increased antegrade velocity and prolonged pressure half-time (*bottom*).

in a conduit (typically right ventricle or right atrium to pulmonary artery). In this situation, the valve is difficult to image due to shadowing by the vascular graft, and it is difficult to obtain a window wherein the Doppler beam is parallel to flow across the prosthetic valve.

Patient-Prosthesis Mismatch

In some patients, the size of the prosthetic valve that can be implanted results in inadequate blood flow to meet the metabolic demands of the patient, even when the prosthetic valve itself is functioning normally. This situation, called "patient-prothesis mismatch (PPM)," is defined as an indexed effective orifice area of ≤ 0.85 cm^2/m^2 and is a predictor of a high transvalvular gradient, persistent ventricular hypertrophy, and an increased rate of cardiac events after aortic valve replacement. The impact of a relatively small valve area is most noticeable with severe PPM, defined as an orifice area <0.65 cm^2/m^2. PPM can be avoided by choosing a valve prosthesis that will have an adequate indexed orifice area, based on the patient's body size and annular dimension. In some cases, annular enlargement or other approaches may be needed to allow implantation of an appropriately sized valve or avoidance of a prosthetic valve.

Prosthetic Valve Regurgitation

TTE is accurate for the diagnosis of aortic prosthetic valve regurgitation and for the differentiation of normal from pathologic regurgitation (Figs. 13–24 and 13–25). However, because of acoustic shadowing, the sensitivity for detection of mitral prosthetic regurgitation is lower, and it is more difficult to distinguish normal from pathologic regurgitation. TEE imaging is needed when this diagnosis is suspected on clinical grounds. TEE has a high accuracy for detection of prosthetic regurgitation and reliably distinguishes transprosthetic from paraprosthetic regurgitation.

Prosthetic Valve Endocarditis

Detection of valvular vegetations on prosthetic valves is difficult with TTE due to reverberations and acoustic shadowing (Figs. 13–26 and 13–27). Features that might increase the suspicion of prosthetic valve endocarditis on a TTE examination include Doppler evidence of valve dysfunction (either regurgitation due to incomplete closure or stenosis due to an infected pannus on the inflow surface of the valve), evidence of valve instability (i.e., "rocking"), an unexplained increase in pulmonary artery pressures, or an interval change in chamber dimensions. Prosthetic valve endocarditis often involves the sewing ring and

The differential diagnosis of an increased antegrade velocity across the valve includes a high cardiac output state or coexisting valvular regurgitation, as well as prosthetic valve stenosis. A significant prosthetic or paraprosthetic regurgitant jet can increase the antegrade volume flow rate across the valve substantially, resulting in a high velocity and a high transvalvular gradient. Valve area, however, remains relatively normal.

With careful examination techniques, the antegrade velocity across the prosthetic valve can be recorded in nearly all patients. When signal strength is suboptimal, invasive evaluation may be required. This is most likely for evaluation of a prosthetic valve

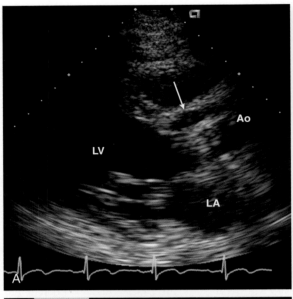

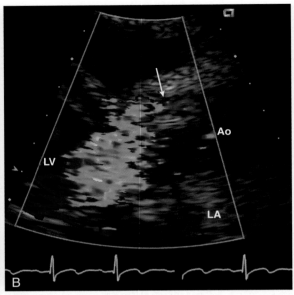

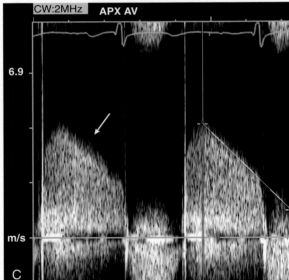

Figure 13–24 A, Parasternal long-axis view shows an echo-free space anterior to a mechanical aortic valve replacement. B, Color Doppler shows a diastolic flow disturbance originating in this space with flow into the LV chamber. C, Continuous-wave Doppler confirms that this flow is aortic regurgitation, showing the typical timing and velocity curve with a density and slope consistent with severe regurgitation.

annulus, resulting in formation of a paravalvular abscess ("ring" abscess) rather than the typical vegetation seen with native valve infection. Identification of an abscess may be limited on TTE.

Thus, given the technical and pathologic peculiarities of evaluation of suspected prosthetic valve endocarditis, TEE imaging is needed in the majority of these patients. TEE imaging has a high sensitivity for detection of prosthetic valve endocarditis and/or abscess formation. As for native valve endocarditis (see Chapter 14), cardiac abscesses may be echo-dense or relatively echo-free. Persistent infection also may result in an aneurysm instead of an abscess cavity (Fig. 13–28).

Prosthetic Valve Thrombosis

In patients with embolic events presumed secondary to prosthetic valve thrombosis, even TEE results may be negative if the thrombi are small or if new thrombus has not formed since the embolic event. When thrombi are documented on TEE, this finding may be important in patient management in some cases. However, an embolic event in a patient with a prosthetic valve (especially mechanical) presumably is related to the presence of a prosthetic valve even if TEE imaging is negative. Thus, the potential clinical implications of the study results should be considered *before* the examination. If the treatment and subsequent management

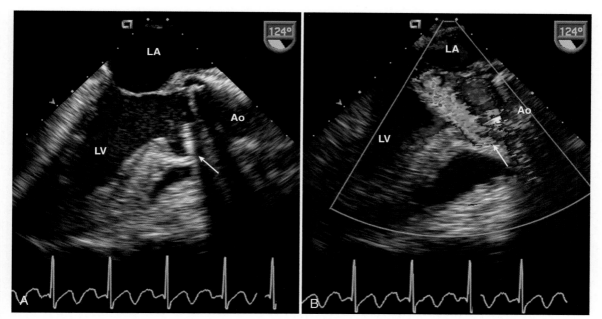

Figure 13–25 TEE imaging in the same patient as Figure 13–24 provides better definition of the area of valve dehiscence adjacent to the septum (*arrow*). The TEE probe has been positioned so the shadows from the valve prosthesis do not obscure the area of interest. Color Doppler shows aortic regurgitation originating from this site.

would be the same whether or not a thrombus is documented, then TEE may be unnecessary. If documentation of thrombus or exclusion of other possible abnormalities would affect patient management, then TEE examination is appropriate. Of course, infected pannus due to prosthetic valve endocarditis cannot be differentiated from thrombus on ultrasound imaging. Careful clinical and bacteriologic correlation is needed whenever an abnormal valve-associated mass is observed (Fig. 13–29).

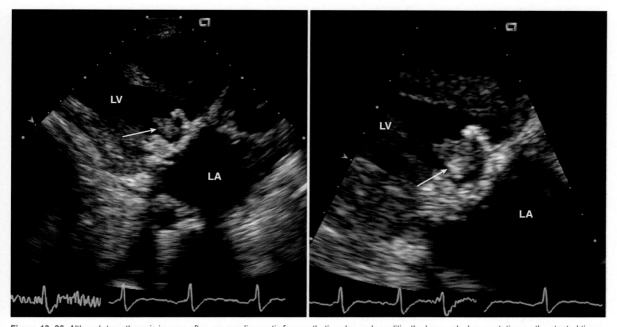

Figure 13–26 Although transthoracic images often are nondiagnostic for prosthetic valve endocarditis, the large valvular vegetation on the stented tissue mitral prosthesis in this patient is obvious (*arrow*) in a low parasternal long-axis view. In the image on the *right*, the depth has been decreased to improve image resolution showing the vegetation within the struts of the prosthetic valve.

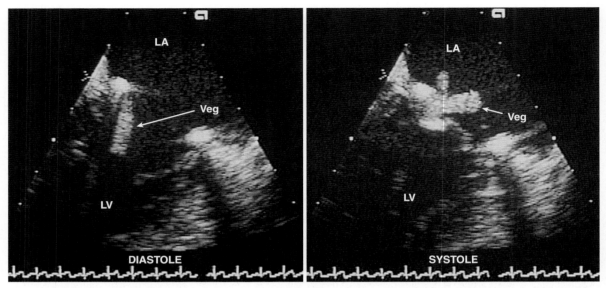

Figure 13–27 Prosthetic valve endocarditis of a mitral porcine valve seen on TEE imaging with a large vegetation prolapsing into the LV in diastole (*left*) and into the LA in systole (*right*).

Baseline Prosthetic Valve Function after Implantation

A baseline echocardiographic examination after implantation of a prosthetic valve is recommended in all patients. There is wide variability in normal antegrade velocities and in the degree of "normal" regurgitation across prosthetic valves even for a given size, type, and position. Establishing baseline Doppler findings in each patient soon after implantation serves as a reference point in case prosthetic valve dysfunction is suspected in the future. Approximately 6 to 8 weeks after surgery

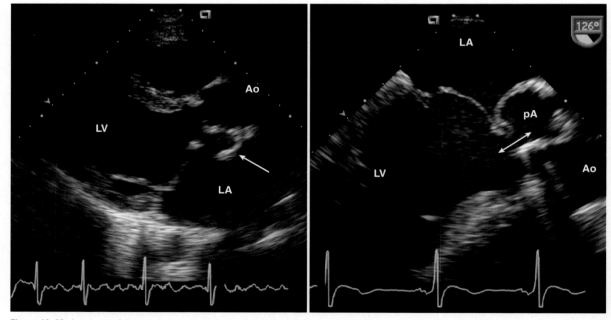

Figure 13–28 Aneurysm of the mitral aortic intravalvular fibrosa in a 28-year-old man with a mechanical aortic valve replacement. The transthoracic long-axis image (*left*) shows the pseudoaneurysm between the posterior aspect of the aortic prosthesis and the base of the anterior mitral leaflet (*arrow*). The corresponding transesophageal image (*right*) shows the narrow neck of the pseudoaneurysm (*double arrow*). Doppler color flow imaging showed flow into the pseudoaneurysm from the LV in systole (with flow back into the LV), and associated collapse of the pseudoaneurysm in diastole.

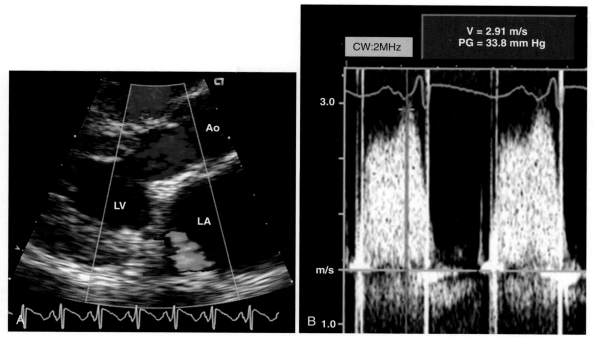

Figure 13–29 In a pregnant woman with a mechanical mitral valve, inadequate anticoagulation and severe pulmonary edema, the transthoracic parasternal long-axis view (**A**) shows only mild regurgitation. **B,** However, continuous-wave Doppler from the apex shows a very high antegrade velocity with a maximum pressure gradient (PG) of 34 mm Hg and a mean gradient of 25 mm Hg. *Pressure half time* is difficult to measure because the *a* wave is superimposed on the diastolic deceleration slope. *(From Stout KK, Otto CM: Pregnancy in women with valvular heart disease. Heart 93:552–558, 2007.)*

is a reasonable time to obtain this baseline study, because the patient has recovered from surgery, is returning to cardiology follow-up, and has stable hemodynamic status with a normal cardiac output. This timing of the examination also allows an initial evaluation of regression of LV hypertrophy or dilation, recovery of LV systolic function, changes in pulmonary artery pressures, and other long-term effects of the valve surgery.

SUGGESTED READING

General Reviews

1. Zabalgoitia M: Echocardiographic recognition and quantitation of prosthetic valve dysfunction. In Otto CM (ed): The Practice of Clinical Echocardiography, 3rd ed. Philadelphia: Elsevier/Saunders, 2007, pp 577–604.
   Advanced-level review and discussion of echocardiographic evaluation of prosthetic valve dysfunction. Numerous tables summarize normal values for prosthetic valves and findings reported with abnormal valve function. Excellent photographs and echocardiographic images of each valve type. Complications reviewed include mechanical failure, thrombosis, endocarditis, PPM, prosthetic stenosis, and regurgitation.

2. Dumesnil J, Pibarot P: Prosthetic heart valves: Selection of the optimal prosthesis and long-term management. Circulation 119:1034–1048, 2009.
   Review of the different types of prosthetic valves, clinical considerations in the choice of valve prosthesis, patient-prosthesis mismatch, long-term outcome, and recommendations for management. Tables of normal values for prosthetic valves are included.

3. Zoghbi WA: Echocardiographic recognition of unusual complications after surgery on the great vessels and cardiac valves. In Otto CM (ed): The Practice of Clinical Echocardiography, 3rd ed. Philadelphia: Elsevier/Saunders, 2007, pp 605–626.
   Discussion and examples of prosthetic valve complications including aortic pseudoaneurysms, LV pseudoaneurysm, aneurysm of the mitral-aortic intravalvular fibrosa, and intracardiac fistula after valve surgery.

4. O'Gara PT: Prosthetic heart valves: selection, management and outcomes. In Otto CM, Bonow RO (eds): Valvular Heart Disease, 3rd ed. Philadelphia: Elsevier/Saunders, 2009, Chapter 23.
   Clinical review of prosthetic heart valves with sections on hemodynamics and long-term outcome
for each valve type, medical management of patients with prosthetic valves, and evaluation and treatment of prosthetic valve dysfunction.

5. Van den Brink RB: Evaluation of prosthetic heart valves by transesophageal echocardiography: Problems, pitfalls, and timing of echocardiography. Semin Cardiothorac Vasc Anesth 10:89–100, 2006.
   Review of the TEE approach to evaluation of prosthetic valve function with algorithms for evaluation of abnormal findings. Clear summary with excellent illustrations.

Normal Doppler Flow Patterns

6. Yoganathan AP, Travis BR: Fluid dynamics of prosthetic valves. In Otto CM (ed): The Practice of Clinical Echocardiography, 3rd ed. Philadelphia: Elsevier/Saunders, 2007, pp 552–576.

Review of the basic principles of fluid dynamics and the application of fluid dynamics to evaluation of prosthetic heart valves. Extensive tables summarize in vitro data for each valve type and size. Illustrations show the flow patterns for each valve type. Mathematical descriptions of fluid dynamics are included.

7. Rosenhek R, Binder T, Maurer G, et al: Normal values for Doppler echocardiographic assessment of heart valve prostheses. J Am Soc Echocardiogr 16:1116–1127, 2003.
The article provides very detailed tables of the expected normal Doppler flow patterns for several valve types and sizes in the aortic and mitral positions. A useful reference table to have in the echocardiography laboratory.

8. Cheng R, Lai YG, Chandran KB: Three-dimensional fluid-structure interaction simulation of bileaflet mechanical heart valve flow dynamics. Ann Biomed Eng 32:1471–1483, 2004.
Flow dynamic analysis of mechanical valve closure shows that there are large wall shear stresses at the leaflet edge during impact, along with large negative pressure transients and vortical flow development. These factors can result in microcavitation adjacent to the valve, as frequently observed on clinical studies of patients with mechanical prosthetic valves.

Validation of Doppler Echo Pressure Gradients

9. Baumgartner H, Khan S, DeRobertis M, et al: Discrepancies between Doppler and catheter gradients in aortic prosthetic valves in vitro. A manifestation of localized gradients and pressure recovery. Circulation 82:1467–1475, 1990.
In vitro study emphasizing the importance of pressure recovery downstream from the valve as a cause of discrepancies between Doppler and invasive pressure gradient measurements, with an overestimation of 13% ± 11% for mean gradients across the Hancock bioprosthetic valve. High localized gradients in the narrow central orifice at the valve plane of the St. Jude (bileaflet) valve were measured accurately by Doppler echo. However, this localized gradient was greater than the gradient measured 30 mm downstream from the valve.

10. Wilkins GT, Gillam LD, Kritzer GL, et al: Validation of continuous-wave Doppler echocardiographic measurements of mitral and tricuspid prosthetic valve gradients: A simultaneous Doppler-catheter study. Circulation 74:786–795, 1986.
Simultaneous Doppler and catheter pressure gradients were measured across prosthetic mitral

valves in 12 patients, showing an excellent correlation for both porcine and mechanical valves.

11. Burstow DJ, Nishimura RA, Bailey KR, et al: Continuous wave Doppler echocardiographic measurement of prosthetic valve gradients. A simultaneous Doppler-catheter correlative study. Circulation 80:504–514, 1989.
Simultaneous Doppler and catheter pressure gradients were measured in 36 patients. Correlations for maximum and mean pressure gradients were excellent for both aortic and mitral prostheses and for bioprosthetic and mechanical valves.

12. Stewart SF, Nast EP, Arabia FA, et al: Errors in pressure gradient measurement by continuous-wave Doppler ultrasound: Type, size and age effects in bioprosthetic aortic valves. J Am Coll Cardiol 18:769–779, 1991.
Consistent overestimation of pressure gradients across prosthetic valves as measured by Doppler echocardiography was observed in detailed in vitro studies of four types of bioprosthetic valves. Pressure recovery downstream did not account for this overestimation. Instead, this error may be related to neglect of proximal velocities in the Bernoulli equation. For example, a mean proximal velocity of 0.66 ± 0.02 m/s at a mean flow rate of 5.6 L/min would result in an error of 1.74 ± 0.10 mm Hg for mean gradient and 3.48 ± 0.21 mm Hg for maximum gradient. These differences are even larger at higher flow rates.

13. Baumgartner H, Khan S, DeRobertis M, et al: Effect of prosthetic aortic valve design on the Doppler-catheter gradient correlation: an in vitro study of normal St. Jude, Medtronic-Hall, Starr-Edwards and Hancock valves. J Am Coll Cardiol 19:324–332, 1992.
This in vitro study shows that smaller valve sizes have higher antegrade velocities and pressure gradients than larger valve sizes. The 19-mm St. Jude and Hancock valves can have velocities as high as 4.7 m/s with a gradient of 89 mm Hg even with normal prosthetic valve function. Doppler gradients consistently overestimated catheter gradients for St. Jude and Starr-Edwards valves (differences as great as 44 mm Hg were seen). Agreement was closer for Hancock and Medtronic-Hall valves.

Prosthetic Valve Area

14. Chafizadeh ER, Zoghbi WA: Doppler echocardiographic assessment of the St. Jude medical prosthetic valve in the aortic position using the continuity equation. Circulation 83:213–223, 1991.
In 67 patients with recent implantation (and clinically normal valve function) of St. Jude

aortic valve prostheses, continuity equation valve areas (0.73–4.23 cm²) correlated well with the reported actual orifice area (r = 0.83). The Doppler velocity index—the ratio of LVOT to aortic jet velocity—provides a useful simple index of valve function and is less dependent on valve size.

15. Baumgartner H, Khan SS, DeRobertis M, et al: Doppler assessment of prosthetic valve orifice area: An in vitro study. Circulation 85:2275–2283, 1992.
Continuity equation valve areas correlated well with invasively derived Gorlin formula valve areas for St. Jude, Medtronic-Hall, and Hancock aortic valves in a pulsatile flow model. However, valve area of St. Jude valves was significantly underestimated due to the localized high velocities in the narrow central orifice. Valve areas decrease with low flow in Hancock valves consistent with incomplete opening of the leaflets at low flow rates.

16. Rothbart RM, Castriz JL, Harding LV, et al: Determination of aortic valve area by two-dimensional and Doppler echocardiography in patients with normal and stenotic bioprosthetic valves. J Am Coll Cardiol 15:817–824, 1990.
In 22 patients undergoing catheterization for suspected dysfunction of bioprosthetic aortic valves, Doppler continuity valve areas agreed well with invasively determined Gorlin valve areas.

17. Dumesnil JG, Honos GN, Lemieux M, Beauchemin J: Validation and applications of indexed aortic prosthetic valve areas calculated by Doppler echocardiography. J Am Coll Cardiol 16:637–643, 1990.
In 31 patients with a Medtronics Intact Bioprosthesis in the aortic position, both standard and simplified continuity equation valve areas correlated well with in vivo and known in vitro prosthetic valve areas (r = 0.86, standard error of the estimate = 0.16 cm²).

18. Chambers JB, Cochrane T, Black MM, Jackson G: The Gorlin formula validated against directly observed orifice area in porcine mitral bioprostheses. J Am Coll Cardiol 13:348–353, 1989.
In an in vitro pulsatile flow system, measured orifice area and the modified Gorlin relation (Q/Vmax) correlated well (r = 0.88). Maximum valve orifice area, measured by a high-speed video camera, decreased at low-flow rates for all four Carpentier-Edwards prostheses.

Natural History of Doppler Echo Findings

19. Palka P, Harrocks S, Lange A, et al: Primary aortic valve replacement with cryopreserved aortic allograft: An

echocardiographic follow-up study of 570 patients. Circulation 105:61–66, 2002.

Echocardiography was performed a mean of 6.8 years after aortic homograft valve replacement. Significant aortic regurgitation was present in 15% and aortic stenosis was present in 3%. The root replacement technique of homograft insertion was associated with the best long-term hemodynamics.

20. Bach DS, Goldman B, Verrier E, et al: Eight-year hemodynamic follow-up after aortic valve replacement with the Toronto SPV stentless aortic valve. Semin Thorac Cardiovasc Surg 13:173–179, 2001.

In 470 patients with stentless aortic valve replacements, a progressive decrease in LV mass and increase in LVOT diameter and valve area were seen over 8 years of follow-up. The prevalence of more than mild aortic regurgitation was only 2.5% at 6 years and 4.5% at 8 years.

21. Banbury MK, Cosgrove DM 3rd, Thomas JD, et al: Hemodynamic stability during 17 years of the Carpentier-Edwards aortic pericardial bioprosthesis. Ann Thorac Surg 73:1460–1465, 2002.

Echocardiography in 85 patients showed that valve area and mean gradient remained stable over 17 years of follow-up but there was a progressive increase in aortic regurgitation from none to 1–2+. However, at 17 years, less than 10% had developed 3 or 4+ aortic regurgitation.

22. Dellgren G, David TE, Raanani E, et al: Late hemodynamic and clinical outcomes of aortic valve replacement with the Carpentier-Edwards Perimount pericardial bioprosthesis. J Thorac Cardiovasc Surg 124:146–154, 2002.

Echocardiography was performed in about 50% of a group of 254 patients at a mean of 5.6 years after valve replacement. The peak prosthetic valve gradient was 23.2 ± 9.6 with a mean gradient of 12.3 ± 4.8 mm Hg. Trivial to mild aortic regurgitation was present in 94%, with moderate-to-severe aortic regurgitation in 4% of survivors.

Valve Stenosis and Patient-Prosthesis Mismatch

23. Pibarot P, Dumesnil JG: Prosthesis-patient mismatch: Definition, clinical impact, and prevention. Heart 92:1022–1029, 2006.

This article defines patient-prosthesis mismatch, describes the hemodynamics, and reviews the impact on short- and long-term clinical outcomes. Tables and charts provide reference data on expected orifice areas for different types of prosthetic valves, and algorithms for patient evaluation are proposed.

24. Bleiziffer S, Eichinger WB, Hettich I, et al: Prediction of valve prosthesis-patient mismatch prior to aortic valve replacement: which is the best method? Heart 93:615–620, 2007.

In a series of 383 patients who underwent aortic valve replacement, moderate PPM occurred in 33% and severe PPM in 6%. The best preoperative predictor of PPM was based on the predicted effective orifice area derived from echocardiographic studies. In comparison, in vitro data for geometric orifice area was unreliable for predicting PPM.

25. Baumgartner H, Schima H, Kuhn P: Effect of prosthetic valve malfunction on the Doppler-catheter gradient relation for bileaflet aortic valve prostheses. Circulation 87:1320–1327, 1993.

Malfunction of bileaflet mechanical valves was simulated in a pulsatile flow model by restricting opening of one leaflet. While Doppler and catheter gradients correlated well for each degree of prosthetic valve stenosis, the slope of the regression line progressively approached 1 with increasing stenosis. Thus, while Doppler overestimates bileaflet prosthetic valve gradients with normal valve function, the Doppler gradients are accurate when stenosis is present. The mechanism of this observation most likely is a reduction in the central orifice size. Clinically, these findings suggest that the development of stenosis of a bileaflet mechanical valve may not be reflected in increases in velocity across the prosthesis.

26. Roudaut R, Serri K, Lafitte S: Thrombosis of prosthetic heart valves: Diagnosis and therapeutic considerations. Heart 93:137–142, 2007.

The incidence of mechanical prosthetic valve thrombosis ranges from 0.3% to 1.3% per patient year, with thromboembolic complications occurring in 0.7% to 6% per patient year. The diagnosis is often made on TTE by demonstration of an increased transvalvular gradient and deceased effective orifice area. Visualization of the size of the thrombus on TEE is important, because decisions about surgical versus thrombolytic therapy are guided, in part, by thrombus size.

Prosthetic Valve Regurgitation

27. Vitarelli A, Conde Y, Cimino E, et al: Assessment of severity of mechanical prosthetic mitral regurgitation by transoesophageal echocardiography. Heart 90:539–544, 2004.

TEE evaluation of prosthetic mitral regurgitation was compared to cardiac catheterization in 47 patients. Severe prosthetic regurgitation was correctly identified, with the most useful Doppler measures being the vena contracta width and assessment of the proximal flow convergence region. Pulmonary vein systolic flow patterns were helpful only in those in normal sinus rhythm.

28. Rahko PS: Assessing prosthetic mitral valve regurgitation by transoesophageal echo/Doppler. Heart 90:476–478, 2004.

This editorial provides a concise overview of the key issues in TEE evaluation of prosthetic valve regurgitation. The TEE exam should be complete, including multiplane imaging at a minimum of 30 increments, measurement of vena contracta width, CW Doppler interrogation, and evaluation of the proximal flow convergence region. Regurgitant orifice area should be calculated when feasible. The final determination of regurgitant severity relies on integration of multiple imaging and Doppler parameters.

29. Baumgartner H, Khan S, DeRobertis M, et al: Color Doppler regurgitant characteristics of normal mechanical mitral valve prostheses in vitro. Circulation 85:323–332, 1992.

Patterns of normal regurgitation for bileaflet and tilting-disk mechanical mitral valves in a pulsatile flow model are described. Bileaflet valves showed two converging jets from the pivot points, a small central jet, and a variable number of peripheral jets. Normal bileaflet regurgitant jets showed little signal aliasing. Tilting-disk (with a central strut and hole) valves showed a large central jet and one or two small peripheral jets. The large central jet showed aliasing extending distally into the atrium.

30. Flachskampf FA, O'Shea JP, Griffin BP, et al: Patterns of normal transvalvular regurgitation in mechanical valve prostheses. J Am Coll Cardiol 18:1493–1498, 1991.

In an in vitro system, bileaflet valves showed peripheral convergent jets in a plane parallel to the two disk axes and several diverging jets in the orthogonal place. Tilting-disk (with central strut and hole) valves showed a prominent central jet with minor jets along the periphery of the disk.

31. Garcia MJ, Vandervoort P, Stewart WJ, et al: Mechanisms of hemolysis with mitral prosthetic regurgitation. Study using transesophageal echocardiography and fluid dynamic simulation. J Am Coll Cardiol 27:399–406, 1996.

In 27 patients with prosthetic regurgitation, echocardiographic factors associated with hemolysis (present in 16 patients) were examined. Hemolysis was associated with a paravalvular origin of the regurgitant jet (8/16 with hemolysis vs. 2/11 without hemolysis).

In addition, patterns of flow fragmentation, collision, or rapid acceleration were associated with hemolysis.

Exercise Studies with Prosthetic Valves

32. van den Brink RB, Verhuel HA, Visser CA, et al: Value of exercise Doppler echocardiography in patients with prosthetic or bioprosthetic cardiac valves. Am J Cardiol 69:367–372, 1992.

In 61 asymptomatic patients with an aortic (n = 24) or mitral (n = 39) prosthetic valve, postexercise Doppler data could be obtained within 60 seconds in 92%. In the mitral group, heart rate increased from 80 ± 12 to 116 ± 14 bpm, mean gradient from 6 to 14 mm Hg, and pulmonary artery systolic pressure from 34 to 57 mm Hg. In the aortic group, heart rate increased from 74 ± 0 to 105 ± 18 bpm and mean gradient from 24 (range 12–50) to 39 (range 18–100) mm Hg.

33. Pibarot P, Dumesnil JG, Briand M, et al: Hemodynamic performance during maximum exercise in adult patients with the Ross operation and comparison with normal controls and patients with aortic bioprostheses. Am J Cardiol 86:982–988, 2000.

Doppler echocardiography was used to evaluate rest and exercise hemodynamics in 20 adults after pulmonic autograft aortic valve replacement (Ross procedure) compared to 12 normal subjects. Aortic valve hemodynamics were similar in both groups, but the pulmonic homograft had a smaller valve area index at rest ($1.10 \pm 0.46 \, cm^2/m^2$ vs. $1.95 \pm 0.41 \, cm^2/m^2$). The peak exercise gradient across the pulmonic homograft was 21 ± 14 mm Hg in the Ross group.

34. Hobson NA, Wilkinson GA, Cooper GJ, et al: Hemodynamic assessment of mitral mechanical prostheses under high flow conditions: comparison between dynamic exercise and dobutamine stress. J Heart Valve Dis 15:87–91, 2006.

Both exercise and dobutamine stress studies were performed in 23 adults about 3 months after mechanical mitral valve replacement. Exercise stress resulted in a greater increase in transvalvular gradient, shorter diastolic filling, and higher transmitral volume flow rate. However, dobutamine resulted in a greater increase in effective orifice area, with a corresponding smaller increase in pressure gradient.

Percutaneous Valve Implantation

35. Munt B: Percutaneous aortic valve implantation. In Otto CM, Bonow RO (eds): Valvular Heart Disease, 3rd ed. Philadelphia: Elsevier/Saunders, 2009, Chapter 13.

This chapter reviews the literature on types of percutaneous valves, implantation techniques, patient selection, immediate hemodynamic results, and intermediate clinical outcomes. The role of echocardiography in patient selection, monitoring the procedure, and in follow-up is emphasized.

36. Grube E, Schuler G, Buellesfeld L, et al: Percutaneous aortic valve replacement for severe aortic stenosis in high-risk patients using the second- and current third-generation self-expanding CoreValve prosthesis: Device success and 30-day clinical outcome. J Am Coll Cardiol 50:69–76, 2007.

In 86 patients with severe symptomatic aortic stenosis and a very high surgical risk, percutaneous aortic valve replacement (CoreValve) was successful in 88%, with a 30-day mortality of 12%. Transvalvular mean gradient decreased from a average of 44 mm Hg to 9 mm Hg.

37. Webb JG, Pasupati S, Humphries K, et al: Percutaneous transarterial aortic valve replacement in selected high-risk patients with aortic stenosis. Circulation 116:755–763, 2007.

In 50 adults with severe symptomatic aortic stenosis but very high surgical risk, percutaneous aortic valve implantation (Cribier Edwards) was successfully performed in 86% with a 30-day mortality of 12%. Aortic valve area determined by echocardiography increased from 0.6 ± 0.2 to $1.7 \pm 0.4 \, cm^2$, and there was an increase in LV ejection fraction, decrease in mitral regurgitation, and improvement in functional class.

14 Endocarditis

E chocardiography is an essential component of the evaluation of a patient with infective endocarditis. In combination with clinical and bacteriologic data, the echocardiographic finding of a valvular vegetation allows an accurate diagnosis of endocarditis. In addition, echocardiographic assessment of the degree of valve dysfunction and detection of complications, such as a paravalvular abscess or fistula, are needed for optimal patient care.

While transthoracic echocardiography (TTE) is adequate in some cases, transesophageal echocardiography (TEE) is more sensitive and specific, both for the detection of valvular vegetations and for detection of complications. Furthermore, demonstration of normal valve anatomy and function on TEE imaging reliably excludes endocarditis in patients in whom this diagnosis is suspected.

BASIC PRINCIPLES

The diagnosis of endocarditis is most secure when there is pathologic confirmation of a valvular vegetation with active infection, local tissue destruction, and/or paravalvular abscess formation. In the clinical setting, endocarditis is diagnosed based on a combination of echocardiographic, laboratory, and physical examination findings as detailed in Table 14–1. The major criteria for the diagnosis of endocarditis are persistent bacteremia with typical organisms and echocardiographic evidence of endocardial involvement. Minor criteria include less specific bacteriologic and echocardiographic findings, factors predisposing to endocarditis (such as preexisting valve disease or intravenous drug use), vascular events (such as pulmonary or systemic emboli), immunologic phenomena (such as glomerulonephritis), and signs of systemic infection (such as fever).

The goals of echocardiography in a patient with infective endocarditis are to:

- Identify the presence, location, size, and number of valvular vegetations
- Assess functional abnormalities of the affected valve(s), especially valvular regurgitation
- Identify the underlying anatomy of the affected valve(s) and any coincident valvular disease
- Assess the impact of valvular disease on chamber dimensions and function, most importantly left ventricular (LV) size and systolic function
- Identify other complications of endocarditis (e.g., paravalvular abscess, pericardial effusion) and
- Provide prognostic data on the anticipated clinical course, risk of systemic embolization, and potential need for surgical intervention

TABLE 14–1 Modified Duke Criteria for Infective Endocarditis

Pathologic Criteria

Microorganisms: demonstrated by culture of histology in a vegetation, *or* in a vegetation that has embolized, *or* in an intracardiac abscess

Pathologic lesions: vegetation or intracardiac abscess present, confirmed by histology showing active endocarditis

Clinical Criteria

Definite endocarditis:	two major criteria *or* one major and three minor criteria *or* five minor criteria
Possible endocarditis:	one major plus one minor *or* three minor criteria

Major Criteria

Positive blood culture for infective endocarditis

- Typical microorganism for infective endocarditis from two separate blood cultures:
  Viridans streptococci*, *Staphylococcus aureus*, *Streptococcus bovis*, HACEK group, *or*
  enterococci, in the absence of a primary focus, *or*
- Persistently positive blood culture, defined as recovery of a microorganism consistent with infective endocarditis from:
  ○ Blood cultures drawn more than 12 hours apart, *or*
  ○ All of three or a majority of four or more separate blood cultures, with first and last drawn at least 1 hour apart
- Positive blood culture for *Coxiella burnetii* or anti–phase I IgG antibody titer >1:800

Evidence of endocardial involvement

- Positive echo for infective endocarditis
  ○ Oscillating intracardiac mass, on valve or supporting structures, *or* in the path of regurgitant jets, *or* on implanted
    material, in the absence of an alternative anatomic explanation, *or*
  ○ Abscess, *or*
  ○ New partial dehiscence of prosthetic valve, *or*
- New valvular regurgitation (increase or change in preexisting murmur not sufficient)

Minor Criteria

- Predisposition: predisposing heart condition *or* intravenous drug use
- Fever >38.0°C (100.4°F)
- Vascular phenomena: major arterial emboli, septic pulmonary infarcts, mycotic aneurysm, intracranial hemorrhage,
  conjunctival hemorrhages, Janeway lesions
- Immunologic phenomena: glomerulonephritis, Osler's nodes, Roth spots, rheumatoid factor
- Microbiologic evidence: positive blood culture but not meeting major criterion as noted previously[†] *or* serologic
  evidence of active infection with organism consistent with infective endocarditis

HACEK, *Haemophilus* spp., *Actinobacillus actinomycetemcomitans*, *Cardiobacterium hominis*, *Eikenella* spp., and *Kingella kingae*;
 IgG, immunoglobulin G.
*Including nutritional variant strains.
[†]Excluding single positive cultures for coagulase-negative staphylococci and organisms that do not cause endocarditis.
From Durack DT, Lukes AS, Bright DK: New criteria for diagnosis of infective endocarditis: utilization of specific echocardiographic findings.
 Duke Endocarditis Service. Am J Med 96:200–209, 1994. With a modification by Li JS, Sexton DJ, Mick N, et al: Proposed modification to
 the Duke criteria for the diagnosis of infective endocarditis. Clin Infect Dis 30:633–638, 2000.

In a patient with a lower likelihood of endocarditis on clinical grounds, an echocardiogram often is requested to "rule out" endocarditis. In this setting, the goals of the echocardiographic examination are:

❏ Identification of any valvular vegetations
❏ Assessment of valve anatomy and function with respect to anatomic or physiologic factors that increase the likelihood of endocarditis (e.g., bicuspid aortic valve, myxomatous mitral valve)

If an abnormality is identified, complete evaluation is directed toward the goals listed for clinical endocarditis.

ECHOCARDIOGRAPHIC APPROACH

Valvular Vegetations

Transthoracic Echocardiography

On two-dimensional (2D) echocardiography, the features that typify a valvular vegetation are:

Aortic Valve Vegetation

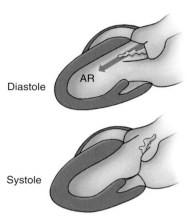

Figure 14–1 Schematic diagram of an aortic valve vegetation attached to the ventricular side of the leaflet with prolapse into the LV outflow tract in diastole. AR, aortic regurgitation.

❐ An abnormal echogenic, irregular mass
❐ Attachment on the upstream side of the valve leaflet and
❐ A pattern of motion that is dependent on, but more chaotic than, normal valve motion

For example, an aortic valve vegetation prolapses into the LV outflow tract in diastole and extends into the aortic root in systole (Fig. 14–1). The mass is attached to the LV side of the valve leaflet but shows motion in excess of normal valve excursion with rapid oscillations in diastole (best appreciated on M-mode recordings). A mitral valve vegetation is attached on the atrial side of the valve, prolapses into the left atrium (LA) in systole, and moves into the LV, beyond the normal range of mitral valve opening, in diastole (Fig. 14–2).

Mitral Valve Vegetation

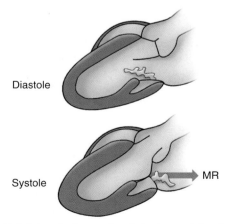

Figure 14–2 Schematic diagram of a mitral valve vegetation attached to the atrial side of the leaflet with prolapse into the LA in systole. MR, mitral regurgitation.

Valvular vegetations vary in size from so small as to be undetectable with current imaging techniques to greater than 3 cm in length. Vegetations may be attached at any area of the leaflet, although lesions at the coaptation line are most common. More than one valve can be involved, either by direct extension of infection or as a separate process, emphasizing the caveat that each valve requires careful examination even if a vegetation has been identified on another valve. In most but not all cases, endocarditis occurs on a previously abnormal valve.

Multiple acoustic windows and 2D views are needed for detection of a valvular vegetation. Because the vegetation is a discrete structure, it may be seen only in certain tomographic planes. Slow scanning between the standard image planes—for example, between the parasternal long-axis view and the right ventricular (RV) inflow view—increases the likelihood of identifying a valvular vegetation. Orthogonal views further ensure that all segments of the valve leaflets are examined. In a patient with suspected endocarditis, a complete examination is needed with scanning from parasternal, apical, subcostal, and suprasternal notch views for careful evaluation of each valve. The reported sensitivity of TTE for detection of valvular vegetations ranges from less than 50% to as high as 90% (Table 14–2). To some extent, the reported sensitivity of TTE increased between the advent of 2D instruments in the late 1970s and the improved image quality with advances in instrumentation in the 1980s. Possibly three-dimensional (3D) imaging will provide further improvements in the accuracy of TTE for detection of vegetations, but this has not yet been demonstrated.

AORTIC VALVE. Aortic valve vegetations most often are detected in parasternal long- and short-axis views. Careful angulation from medial to lateral in the long-axis plane and from inferior to superior in the short-axis plane is needed, because vegetations often are eccentrically located. Image quality is optimized by use of a minimum depth setting and adjustment of gain and processing parameters. An echogenic mass attached to the ventricular side of the leaflet with independent motion and prolapse into the outflow tract in diastole is diagnostic for a valvular vegetation (Fig. 14–3). Rapid oscillating motion may be best appreciated on an M-mode recording.

Less typically, a vegetation may be attached to the aortic side of the leaflet or may show little independent motion. A definitive diagnosis may be difficult if the underlying valve anatomy is abnormal. For example, a vegetation on a calcified aortic valve may be difficult to diagnose due to shadowing and reverberations by the leaflet calcification. In these cases, the findings of independent motion and prolapse into the LV in diastole are particularly helpful signs. Comparison with previous echocardiograms may allow recognition of recent changes, increasing the likelihood of valve infection, or may show no significant difference, decreasing the likelihood of an acute process.

TABLE 14–2   Accuracy of Echocardiographic Diagnosis of Valvular Vegetations (Selected Studies)

First Author and Year	Study Entry Criteria (Standard of Reference)	No. of Valves	Percentage Prosthetic	Transthoracic Echo		Transesophageal Echo	
				Sensitivity	Specificity	Sensitivity	Specificity
Mugge 1989	Definite endocarditis (surgery or autopsy)	91	24%	53/91 (58%)	—	82/91 (90%)	—
Jaffe 1990	Definite endocarditis (surgery or autopsy)	38	16%	38/44 (86%)	—	—	—
Burger 1991	Suspected endocarditis (clinical outcome)	101	—	35/39 (90%)	61/62 (98%)	—	—
Shively 1991	Suspected endocarditis (clinical outcome)	6	18%	7/16 (44%)	49/50 (98%)	15/16 (94%)	50/50 (100%)
Pedersen 1991	Suspected endocarditis (clinical outcome)	24	42%	5/10 (50%)	13/14 (93%)	10/10 (100%)	14/14 (100%)
Daniel 1993	Prosthetic valve (surgically confirmed endocarditis)	33	100%	12/33 (36%)	—	27/33 (82%)	—
Sochowski 1993	Suspected endocarditis with negative TTE (clinical outcome)	65	12%	—	—	Negative predictive value = 56/65 (86%)	
Shapiro 1994	Suspected endocarditis (clinical criteria)	68	—	23/34 (68%)	31/34 (91%)	33/34 (97%)	31/34 (91%)

Data from Mugge et al: J Am Coll Cardiol 14:631–638, 1989; Jaffe et al: J Am Coll Cardiol 15:1227–1233, 1990; Burger et al: Angiology 42:552–560, 1991; Shively et al: J Am Coll Cardiol 18:391–397, 1991; Pedersen et al: Chest 100:351–356, 1991; Daniel et al: Am J Cardiol 71:210–215, 1993; Sochowski, Chan: J Am Coll Cardiol 21:216–221, 1993; Shapiro et al: Chest 105:377, 1994.

Findings that may be mistaken for an aortic valve vegetation include beam-width artifact related to either a calcified nodule, a prosthetic valve, the normal leaflet apposition zone, or the normal leaflet thickening at the central coaptation region (the nodule of Arantius). Occasionally, a linear echo representing a normal variant called a *Lambl's excrescence* is seen. These small fibroelastic protrusions from the ventricular side of the leaflet closure zone occur with increasing frequency with age and are present in a high percentage of patients. As image quality improves, these normal structures are seen more frequently (Fig. 14–4).

Apical views of the aortic valve, both from an anteriorly angulated four-chamber view and from an apical long-axis view, may show an aortic valve vegetation. The finding of an abnormality in both parasternal and apical views decreases the likelihood of an ultrasound artifact, since the relationship of the ultrasound beam and aortic valve is entirely different from these two windows.

Two- or three-dimensional imaging of a definite or suspected aortic valve vegetation is accompanied by evaluation of the functional abnormalities due to valve destruction, as discussed in the following sections.

MITRAL VALVE. Mitral valve vegetations typically are located on the atrial side of the leaflets. Diagnostic features include rapid independent motion, prolapse into the LA in systole, and functional evidence of valve dysfunction. Parasternal long- and short-axis views with careful scanning across the valve apparatus in both image planes allows assessment of the presence, size, and location of any vegetation (Fig. 14–5). Apical four-chamber, two-chamber, and long-axis views again are helpful both in visualizing valve and vegetation anatomy and in distinguishing a true valve mass from an ultrasound artifact.

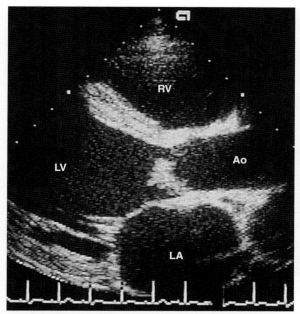

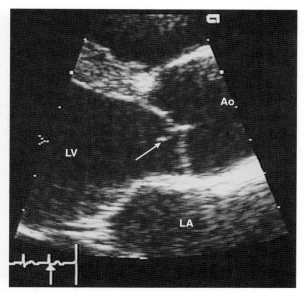

Figure 14–4 Lambl's excrescence at the aortic closure line that might be mistaken for a valvular vegetation.

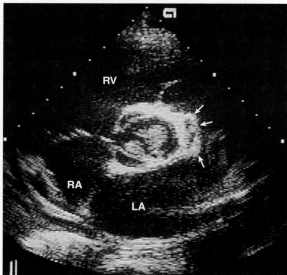

Figure 14–3 In a 29-year-old intravenous drug user with *S. aureus* endocarditis, aortic valve vegetations are seen in transthoracic parasternal long-axis (*top*) and short-axis (*bottom*) views. Irregularly shaped echogenic masses are attached to the ventricular side of the aortic valve leaflets, with prolapse into the outflow tract in diastole (seen in the long-axis view) and extension into the aortic root in systole (seen in the short-axis view). Severe aortic regurgitation was present. The short-axis view also shows a paravalvular abscess (*three arrows*).

As for the aortic valve, beam-width artifacts can be mistaken for a vegetation. A particular artifact to be aware of is the appearance of a "mass" on the atrial side of the anterior mitral leaflet in the apical four-chamber view due to beam-width artifact from a calcified or prosthetic aortic valve. Other types of mitral valve pathology may be difficult to distinguish from a valvular vegetation, including a severely myxomatous leaflet, a partial flail leaflet, or a ruptured papillary muscle. Comparison with previous studies may help differentiate an acute process from chronic underlying valve disease. Endocarditis also can occur on an anatomically normal valve (Fig. 14–6). With mitral valve endocarditis, mitral regurgitation often, but not invariably, is present.

TRICUSPID VALVE. Tricuspid valve endocarditis occurs most often in intravenous drug users and is associated with large vegetations due to *Staphylococcus aureus* infection. The RV inflow view often is diagnostic, showing a large, mobile mass of echoes attached to the atrial side of the leaflet with prolapse into the right atrium (RA) in systole (Fig. 14–7). Given the range of excursion and mobility of these vegetations, it is not surprising that septic pulmonary emboli are a frequent complication of tricuspid valve endocarditis. The apical and subcostal four-chamber views allow further evaluation of the presence and extent of tricuspid valve infection. Assessment of tricuspid regurgitant severity and consequent RA and RV dilation also can be performed from these windows.

Transesophageal Imaging

From the TEE approach the aortic valve is examined in multiple image planes including standard long-axis (typically at approximately 120° rotation) and short-axis (about 45° rotation) views. As with TTE imaging, careful scanning from medial to lateral in the long-axis view and from superior to inferior in the short-axis view is needed to fully evaluate valve

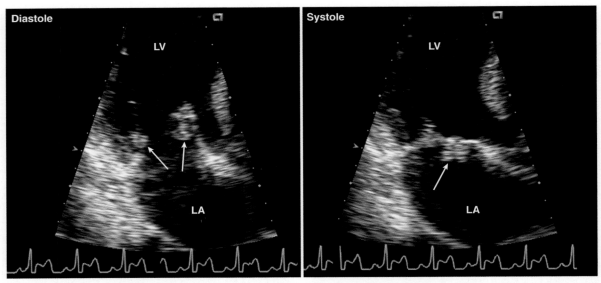

Figure 14–5 A typical-appearing mitral valve vegetation seen in an apical long-axis view in diastole attached to the atrial side of the anterior mitral valve leaflet (*left*). In systole (*right*) the mass prolapses into the LA with motion in real time independent of valve leaflet motion.

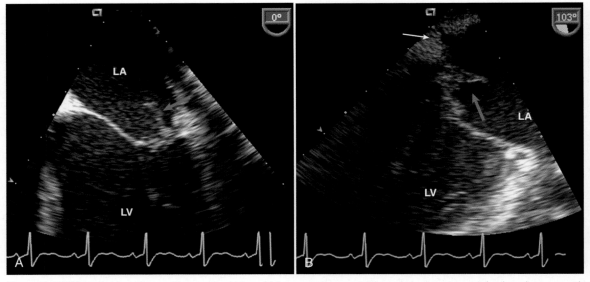

Figure 14–6 TEE imaging in a 22-year-old man with a history of intravenous drug use and bacteremia shows a vegetation (*arrow*) on a normal-appearing mitral valve (**A**). Rotation of the image plane to 103° (**B**) shows that the vegetative mass (*cyan arrow*) is attached at the base of the leaflet, raising concern for paravalvular abscess. The circular echolucency (*white arrow*) is the normal circumflex coronary artery.

anatomy and to achieve a high sensitivity for detection of valvular vegetations (Figs. 14–8 and 14–9). When the image plane is oblique, an aortic leaflet may be seen *en face*, mimicking an aortic valve mass. Evaluation in more than one image plane and assessment of the pattern of motion (rapid oscillating independent motion vs. motion *with* the valve) avoids this potential error. Image quality may be enhanced by use of a higher frequency transducer and magnification of the area of interest, but small normal variants of valve anatomy should not be interpreted as abnormalities. Sometimes the aortic valve can be evaluated from a transgastric apical view; however, image quality may be no better than from a TTE approach due to the distance of the aortic valve from the transducers.

The mitral valve is well seen from a high esophageal position. Since the mitral valve plane is

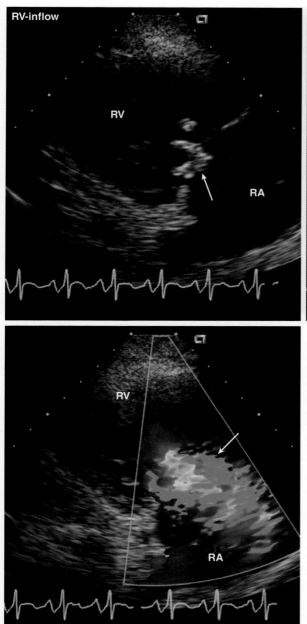

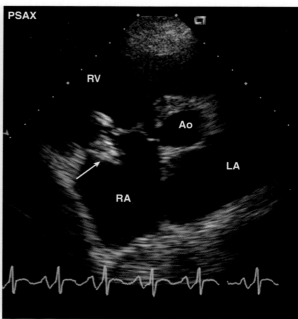

Figure 14–7 Transthoracic imaging in an RV inflow view of a patient with a history of intravenous drug use and *S. aureus* tricuspid valve (TV) endocarditis. In a parasternal short-axis view (*top right*), a mobile mass (*arrow*) is seen prolapsing into the RA attached to the TV leaflet. In an RV inflow view (*top left*) the mass again is seen at the leaflet coaptation (*arrow*). Color flow Doppler (*bottom left*) demonstrates a broad jet of reverse flow across the valve in systole (*arrow*), consistent with severe tricuspid regurgitation.

perpendicular to the ultrasound beam from this approach, excellent images can be obtained in multiple views by slowly rotating the multiplane transducer from 0 to 180°. Particular attention should be paid to standard four-chamber (at 0°), two-chamber (at 60°), and long-axis (at 120°) views. The degree of mitral regurgitation can be assessed with color flow imaging in these same views. Given the distance of the mitral valve from the chest wall in both parasternal and apical TTE views, TEE imaging often provides dramatically better images and important clinical data (Figs. 14–10 and 14–11).

The tricuspid valve is seen in the TEE four-chamber view and from a transgastric approach. Because the tricuspid valve lies closer to the chest wall than the mitral valve, TTE imaging often is diagnostic. TEE imaging is most valuable in these patients for detection of left-sided valve involvement. TEE also may be diagnostic when infection of a pacer lead is suspected (Fig. 14–12).

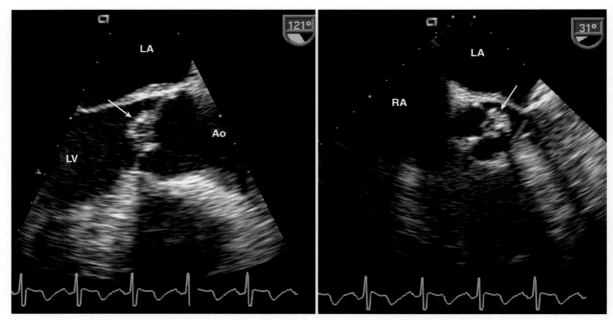

Figure 14–8 Transesophageal images of the aortic valve in a long-axis (*left*) and short-axis view (*right*) showing valvular vegetations (*arrow*).

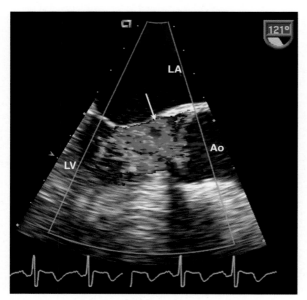

Figure 14–9 Color flow Doppler in the same patient as in Figure 14–8 in a TEE long-axis view shows acute severe aortic regurgitation (AR) due to the valve destruction in this patient.

Diagnostic Accuracy of Echocardiography for Detection of Vegetations

Numerous studies have evaluated the sensitivity of echocardiography for diagnosis of valvular vegetation by comparing the echo findings with subsequent surgical or autopsy findings. There are fewer data on specificity, because most studies include only subjects with a definite diagnosis of endocarditis. Thus, there are no subjects without the disease in the study group. Second, when surgical or autopsy inspection of the valve is the standard of reference, only patients who are sick enough to need surgery or who have died are included in the study group. Direct inspection of valves that appeared normal on echocardiography rarely is available.

A few studies (see Table 14–2) have circumvented these study design problems by including all patients with *suspected* endocarditis (some have the disease and some do not) and using clinical outcome rather than direct valve inspection as the standard of reference. All these studies demonstrate a high specificity of TTE (93% to 98%) and TEE (100%) imaging in excluding the diagnosis of endocarditis.

The specificity of echocardiography depends on distinguishing a valvular vegetation from other intracardiac masses and from ultrasound artifacts. Echocardiographic findings that may be mistaken for a vegetation include:

❏ Papillary fibroelastoma
❏ Myxomatous mitral valve disease
❏ Nonbacterial thrombotic endocarditis
❏ Systemic lupus erythematosus
❏ Thrombus (especially with prosthetic valves)
❏ Beam-width artifact and
❏ Normal valve variants such as a Lambl's excrescence or nodule of Arantius

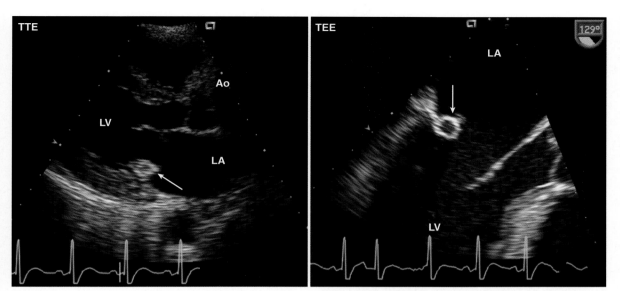

Figure 14–10 Transthoracic (TTE) (*left*) and transesophageal (TEE) (*right*) imaging in a patient with fungal endocarditis. The unusual-appearing valvular vegetation (*arrow*) is seen on TTE imaging but is better defined on TEE imaging, with a dense spherical mass with some small attached areas of independent motion (*arrows*).

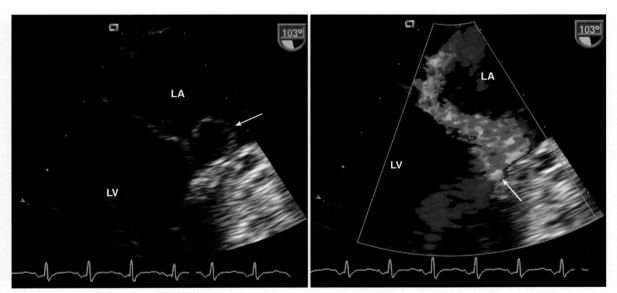

Figure 14–11 Transesophageal echocardiography in a 28-year-old man with systemic embolic events and blood culture results positive for *S. aureus*. There is an apparent prolapse of the lateral segment of the mitral leaflet in a two-chamber view (*left*). Color flow Doppler (*right*) shows an eccentric jet of severe mitral regurgitation through this region, with proximal flow acceleration and a wide vena contracta. These findings, in conjunction with the clinical symptoms and positive blood cultures, are consistent with a ruptured mitral valve pseudoaneurysm due to infective endocarditis.

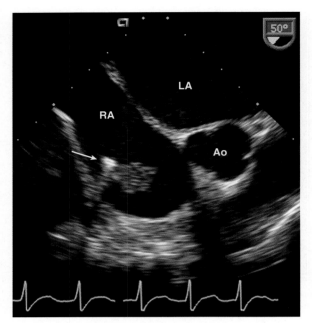

Figure 14–12 In a transesophageal short-axis view, a pacer lead (*arrow*) is seen in the RA with an attached mobile echo-density consistent with a vegetation or thrombus. Shadowing from the pacer lead is evident.

In a patient with abnormal valve leaflets (e.g., myxomatous, calcified), it may be difficult to distinguish the abnormal tissue from a valvular vegetation, particularly a partial flail leaflet or ruptured chord. A study performed before onset of the illness can provide a useful comparison. Mistaking ultrasound artifacts for a vegetation can be avoided by identification of the characteristic findings in more than one view. Note that not all valvular vegetations are "typical." Some may be on the downstream side of the valve or may show little independent motion. These atypical findings further decrease the sensitivity and specificity of echocardiography for valvular vegetations.

Functional Valvular Abnormalities Due to Endocarditis

Valve leaflet destruction by the infectious process and distortion of leaflet closure by the vegetation may result in valvular regurgitation. Regurgitation can occur at the closure line or through a perforation in the leaflet itself. The degree of regurgitation varies from none to mild, moderate, or severe. Assessment of valvular regurgitation in endocarditis is performed using the pulsed, color flow, and continuous-wave Doppler approaches described in Chapter 12 with careful attention to the features that distinguish acute from chronic regurgitation. Because endocarditis often affects a previously abnormal valve, acute regurgitation may be superimposed on chronic regurgitation, resulting in mixed findings on echocardiography.

Valve stenosis due to endocarditis is rare. Occasionally, a large vegetation will partially obstruct the orifice of the open valve, resulting in some degree of functional stenosis.

Although 90% of patients with endocarditis have a new murmur, approximately 10% do not, and a few have no regurgitation detectable on Doppler examination. This is most likely to occur if the vegetation is located at the base of the leaflet, resulting in little distortion of leaflet closure. Echocardiographic recognition of the diagnosis in this subgroup is all the more important in that endocarditis often is not suspected clinically with the echocardiogram having been ordered for other reasons.

Other Echocardiographic Findings

In addition to direct assessment of valvular disease, the examination includes evaluation of cardiac chamber size and function. Acute aortic regurgitation results in only mild LV dilation, but a subacute or acute course superimposed on mild-to-moderate chronic disease may result in significant ventricular dilation. Severe valve destruction may result in a flail aortic leaflet (see Figs. 14–8 and 14–9). Mitral regurgitation results in LA and LV enlargement. LV systolic dysfunction may be seen due to either long-standing valvular disease or the acute infectious process. Pulmonary pressures may be elevated due to mitral regurgitation directly resulting in an elevated LA pressure or to aortic regurgitation with a high end-diastolic LV pressure. A small pericardial effusion often is seen with endocarditis. A larger effusion raises the concern of purulent pericarditis due to direct extension from a paravalvular abscess.

Diagnosis of Paravalvular Abscess and Intracardiac Fistula

Unlike abscesses elsewhere in the body, a cardiac abscess may be either echolucent or echo-dense on ultrasound examination. Typically, abscesses occur in the valve annulus adjacent to the infected leaflet tissue and are more common with aortic than with mitral valve endocarditis. For diagnosis of aortic annular abscess, findings include increased echogenicity or an echolucent area in the base of the septum or increased thickness of the posterior aortic root (Fig. 14–13). Involvement of the aortic annulus may extend into the contiguous anterior mitral valve leaflet with evidence of increased thickness of the leaflet tissue, a valvular vegetation, and/or leaflet perforation (Fig. 14–14). A sinus of Valsalva aneurysm can occur due to infection of the aortic wall and may be detected by echocardiography, before rupture occurs, as a dilated and distorted sinus. In effect, this represents an abscess that is in direct communication with the bloodstream.

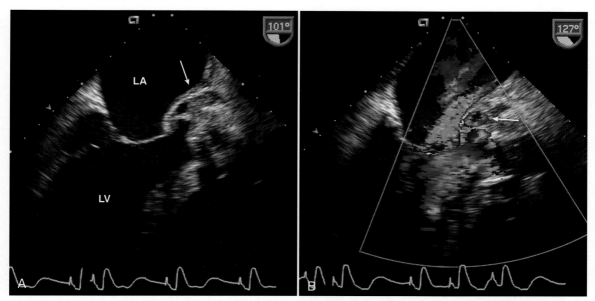

Figure 14–13 A, TEE long-axis image in a patient with aortic valve endocarditis and a vegetation seen on transthoracic imaging show irregular areas of echolucency and echo-density in the aortic annulus and sinuses (*arrow*). **B,** Color Doppler shows both mitral regurgitation and flow in the echolucent areas in the aortic annulus. At surgery, a paravalvular abscess was present.

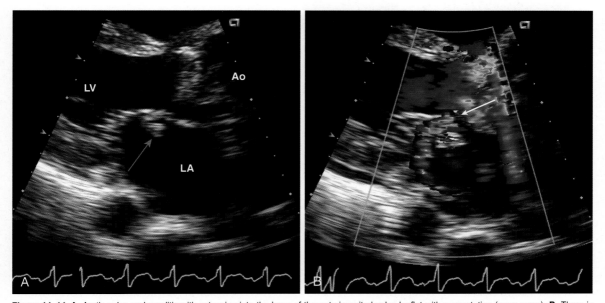

Figure 14–14 A, Aortic valve endocarditis with extension into the base of the anterior mitral valve leaflet with a vegetation (*cyan arrow*). **B,** There is associated leaflet perforation, demonstrated by color Doppler with a narrow eccentric jet originating from this point (*white arrow*).

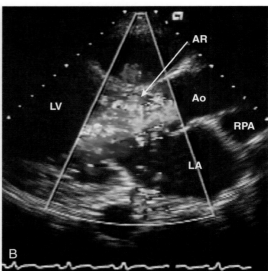

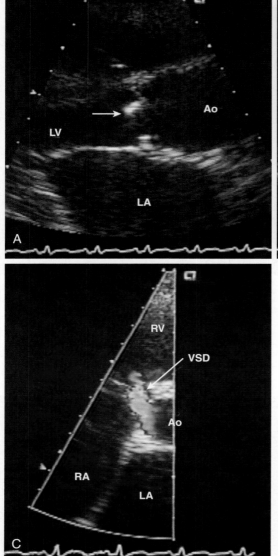

Figure 14–15 In a 50-year-old man with *S. aureus* endocarditis, echocardiography after 6 weeks of antibiotic therapy showed persistent aortic valvular vegetations (**A**) and severe aortic regurgitation (**B**). In addition, a ventricular septal defect was present just inferior to the aortic annulus, best seen in the parasternal short-axis view (**C**) with color flow from the LV outflow tract to RV immediately adjacent to the tricuspid valve.

Rupture of an aortic annular abscess can occur in several fashions. The region of the noncoronary cusp can rupture into the RV outflow tract either in the sinus of Valsalva (an aortic-to-RV connection) or from the LV outflow tract through the septum into the RV (a ventricular septal defect) (Figs. 14–15 and 14–16). An aortic-to-RV fistula shows both systolic and diastolic left-to-right flow on Doppler interrogation, while a ventricular septal defect shows predominantly systolic flow. Rupture also can occur from the LV into the mitral–aortic intervalvular fibrosa with flow into and out of the abscess cavity from the LV outflow tract (Fig. 14–17).

The right coronary sinus region can rupture into the RV or RA and can lead to involvement of the adjacent septal leaflet of the tricuspid valve. Again, rupture can occur either from the aorta or from the LV outflow tract into the right side of the heart. Note that a small segment of ventricular septum (the atrioventricular septum) actually separates the LV from the right *atrium*, so that a ventriculoatrial communication can occur. The left coronary sinus of the aortic valve can rupture into the LA or RA, or infection may extend directly into the interatrial septum.

A mitral annular abscess appears as increased thickening and echogenicity in the posterior aspect of the mitral annulus. Infection may extend into the basal segments of the ventricular myocardium or into the pericardial space. Again, identification may be difficult on TTE imaging, and the diagnosis should be pursued

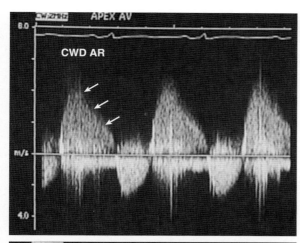

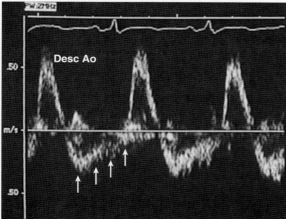

Figure 14–16 In the same patient as in Figure 14–15, evidence for acute severe aortic regurgitation is present, including a dense continuous-wave Doppler signal (*top*) with a steep deceleration slope (*arrows*) and holodiastolic flow reversal in the proximal abdominal aorta (*bottom*).

with TEE imaging when suspected on clinical grounds. An unusual complication of mitral valve endocarditis is a persistent contour abnormality, in effect a pseudoaneurysm, of the valve leaflet that persists even after the infection is treated.

Tricuspid valve endocarditis may be associated with a ring abscess, again manifested as increased thickening and echogenicity in the annulus region.

Diagnosis of paravalvular abscess by TTE imaging has a markedly lower sensitivity and specificity (Table 14–3), compared with TEE imaging, due to poor ultrasound tissue penetration resulting in suboptimal image quality. A high index of suspicion is needed by the echocardiographer, and subtle abnormalities that may suggest a valve abscess should not be ignored. However, even with careful imaging from several acoustic windows in multiple tomographic planes, a definite diagnosis may not be possible. TEE imaging is especially important in patients with prosthetic valve endocarditis, since paravalvular abscesses are common,

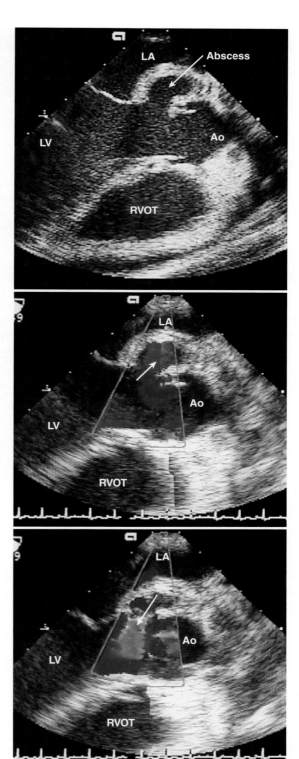

Figure 14–17 In this 26-year-old woman with a history of intravenous drug use and *S. aureus* endocarditis, TEE shows an abscess of the mitral-aortic intervalvular fibrosa (*top*). This cavity communicated with the LV outflow tract, with flow into the abscess in systole (*middle*) with diastolic regurgitation (*bottom*) into the LV.

TABLE 14–3   Accuracy of Echocardiographic Diagnosis of Paravalvular Abscess (Selected Series)

First Author and Year	Study Entry Criteria	No. of Valves	Percentage Prosthetic	Transthoracic Echo		Transesophageal Echo	
				Sensitivity	Specificity	Sensitivity	Specificity
Daniel 1991	Endocarditis with surgery or autopsy	137	25%	13/46 (28%)	90/91 (99%)	40/46 (87%)	87/91 (96%)
Jaffe 1990	Endocarditis with surgery or autopsy	7	–	5/7 (71%)	–	–	–
Karalis 1992	Endocarditis with surgery or autopsy	55	46%	13/24 (54%)	–	24/24 (100%)	–

Data from Daniel et al: N Engl J Med 324:795–800, 1991; Jaffe et al: J Am Coll Cardiol 15:1227–1233, 1990; Karalis et al: Circulation 86:353–362, 1992.

and shadowing and reverberations from the valve prosthesis compromise the examination (see Chapter 13).

The superior image quality of TEE imaging is associated with a higher sensitivity (87%) and specificity (96%) for diagnosis of paravalvular abscess. In addition to 2D findings of abnormal areas of increased echogenicity or abnormal echolucent areas adjacent to the valve, color flow imaging and conventional pulsed Doppler may allow demonstration of flow into and out of these abnormal areas consistent with an abscess that partially communicates with the bloodstream.

LIMITATIONS/TECHNICAL CONSIDERATIONS

Active versus Healed Vegetations

Sequential echocardiographic studies in a patient undergoing treatment for endocarditis may show a gradual reduction in size, decrease in mobility, and increase in echogenicity of the valvular vegetation. However, vegetations either may abruptly "disappear" from the heart due to embolization or may remain unchanged in size or appearance long after the acute episode. Thus, a patient with active endocarditis may have no visible vegetation if recent embolization has occurred. Conversely, a patient with prior endocarditis may have a persistent vegetation without active infection. Echocardiography, by itself, can neither exclude nor establish a diagnosis of endocarditis. Correlation of the echocardiographic findings with the patient's clinical presentation (fevers, systemic emboli, new murmur, and peripheral manifestation of endocarditis) plus the results of microbiologic cultures are needed for diagnosis as detailed in Table 14–1. Obviously, echocardiography provides no information regarding the causative organism. While certain etiologic agents (fungal endocarditis, *Haemophilus influenzae*) are associated with larger vegetations, this observation is not diagnostically useful in an individual patient.

Nonbacterial Thrombotic Endocarditis

The echocardiographic appearance of nonbacterial thrombotic endocarditis, as has been described in patients with malignancy and in patients with systemic lupus erythematosus, is similar to that of infectious endocarditis. Although the vegetations of nonbacterial thrombotic endocarditis tend to be smaller, to be located near the leaflet base, and to show variable echo density and less independent motion, again, clinical and bacteriologic correlation are needed for a correct diagnosis (Fig. 14–18).

Diagnosis of Vegetations with Underlying Valve Disease

Endocarditis most often occurs on a previously abnormal valve, because the local flow disturbance increases

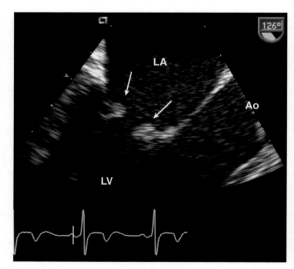

Figure 14–18 Transesophageal echocardiography in a 49-year-old woman with systemic lupus erythematosus shows mitral valve masses (*arrows*) consistent with nonbacterial thrombotic endocarditis.

the likelihood of bacterial deposition. When the underlying disease is anatomically straightforward, such as a bicuspid aortic valve, this poses little problem in diagnosing superimposed valvular vegetations. Often, however, the presence of an abnormal valve makes exclusion or confirmation of a valvular vegetation more difficult. For example, with calcific aortic stenosis, the irregular areas of increased echogenicity on the valve leaflets could represent a vegetation or chronic fibrocalcific changes. Findings of independent rapid motion and prolapse into the outflow tract in diastole increase the likelihood of a vegetation, but the absence of these findings does not allow a definite conclusion as to the absence of a vegetation.

Another example is myxomatous mitral valve disease, where an independently mobile mass of echoes attached to the leaflet and prolapsing into the LA in systole could represent either a valvular vegetation or a flail leaflet segment and attached chordae. When underlying valve disease is present, the improved images obtained by the TEE approach may increase the certainty of diagnosis. In any case, careful integration with other clinical findings usually leads to a correct diagnosis.

Endocarditis of Prosthetic Valves

Evaluation of prosthetic valves for suspected endocarditis is problematic for two reasons. First, infection often involves the area around the sewing ring of the prosthetic valve rather than resulting in a discrete valvular vegetation. Second, reverberations and shadowing by the prosthesis limit the ability of echocardiography to detect abnormalities. This is a particular problem with TTE imaging of mitral prostheses, wherein the LA side of the valve is "masked" by the prosthesis so that neither the paravalvular infection in the mitral annulus nor the resulting valvular incompetence can be detected (see Chapter 13). Acoustic shadowing is less of a problem with aortic valve prostheses, because aortic regurgitation can be evaluated from both apical and parasternal windows without "masking" by the valve prosthesis. However, since the anterior part of the valve prosthesis shadows the more posterior portions, images of the valve leaflets may be suboptimal.

With suspected prosthetic valve endocarditis, the TTE examination may provide clues that suggest the diagnosis even when definitive findings are not present. For example, if color flow imaging is nondiagnostic due to shadowing and color flow artifacts, a careful continuous-wave Doppler examination may show a regurgitant signal. (Figs. 14–19 and 14–20) Care is needed in assessment of the *severity* of regurgitation in this situation, and it may be prudent to state only that regurgitation is present but quantitation is not possible. Other clues to prosthetic valve dysfunction include an increased antegrade flow velocity across the prosthesis (reflecting

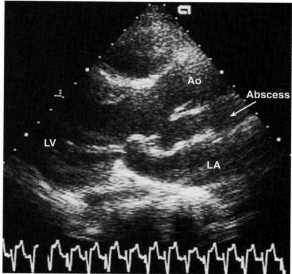

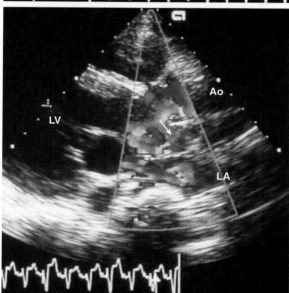

Figure 14–19 In a 24-year-old woman with an aortic homograft valve replacement for a previous episode of endocarditis, re-infection with *S. aureus* has resulted in a paravalvular abscess (or pseudoaneurysm) posterior to the homograft. The transthoracic parasternal short-axis view shows the proximity of the abscess cavity to the LA (*top*), and color flow Doppler shows a fistula from the abscess cavity into the LA (*bottom*).

increased antegrade volume flow due to prosthetic regurgitation) and an elevated tricuspid regurgitant jet velocity due to pulmonary hypertension.

Whenever prosthetic valve endocarditis is suspected, TEE imaging should be strongly considered (Figs. 14–21 to 14–23). If the TTE images are diagnostic, or if the results of TEE imaging will not change patient management, it may not be needed. Otherwise, this technique is warranted given its higher sensitivity and specificity for detection of

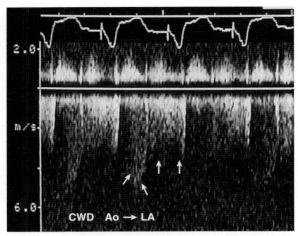

Figure 14–20 Continuous-wave Doppler in the same patient as in Figure 14–19 shows continuous high-velocity flow in systole and diastole (*arrows*) consistent with a fistula from a high-pressure (aorta) to low-pressure (LA) chamber.

prosthetic valve endocarditis, paravalvular abscess, and prosthetic mitral regurgitation.

Endocarditis rarely can result in prosthetic valve stenosis due to impingement of the infected mass on leaflet opening or to an infected pannus on the upstream side of the valve. Visualization of the infected mass may not be possible on TTE imaging. Prosthetic valve stenosis is recognized by findings of an increased transvalvular pressure gradient and a decreased valve area (by pressure half-time or by continuity equation).

In an individual patient, a *change* in the appearance or flow characteristics of a prosthetic valve is more diagnostic than an observation at one point in time. Review of previous studies (if available) performed

when the patient clinically was well can improve the diagnostic yield of echocardiography.

CLINICAL UTILITY

Suspected Endocarditis

Although TEE imaging is more sensitive than TTE for detection of valvular vegetations, TTE remains the initial procedure of choice in patients with a low pre-test likelihood of disease (the "rule-out-endocarditis" indication) due to the lower cost and risk of this approach (Fig. 14–24). Based on an average sensitivity of 80% and specificity of 98% for TTE echocardiographic detection of vegetations, the positive likelihood ratio of finding a vegetation is 40 (an excellent test), but the negative likelihood ratio is 0.20 (only a reasonably good test). Thus, in a patient with a pre-echo likelihood of disease of 50%, a normal TTE result reduces that likelihood to 10%. In contrast, using a sensitivity of 97% and specificity of 91% for TEE diagnosis of valve vegetations, the negative likelihood ratio is 0.03, indicating that a normal TEE result is reliable for excluding a diagnosis of endocarditis. A normal TEE result in the patient with a pre-echo likelihood of 50% reduces the likelihood of endocarditis to 1.5%. However, because more findings that may be mistaken for a vegetation are seen on TEE (lower specificity), the positive likelihood ratio of 10.7, while still consistent with an excellent test, is not as high as for TTE imaging.

TEE imaging is an appropriate initial test in patients at high risk of endocarditis and in situations wherein TTE imaging is likely to be nondiagnostic (Table 14–4). High-risk patients include those with prosthetic valves, congenital heart disease (CHD), previous endocarditis, new heart failure, new

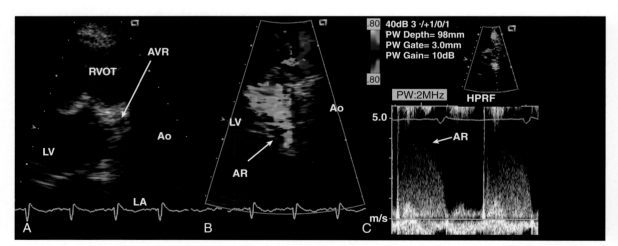

Figure 14–21 A, A mechanical aortic valve replacement (AVR) is not well seen in this transthoracic parasternal long-axis view. **B,** However, color Doppler shows a diastolic flow disturbance suggestive of an eccentric aortic regurgitation (AR) jet originating from the posterior aspect of the sewing ring. **C,** High pulse repetition frequency (HPRF) pulsed Doppler confirms a high-velocity signal consistent with AR originating from this site.

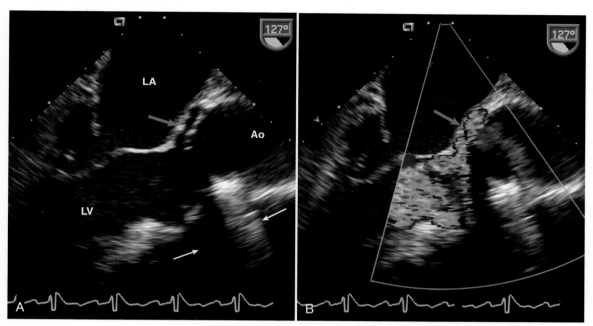

Figure 14–22 TEE imaging in the same patient as Figure 14–21 shows an echolucent space (*cyan arrow*) between the AMVL and aortic sewing ring in the long-axis view (**A**). Prominent shadows and reverberations (*white arrows*) from the valve now obscure the anterior aspect of the valve. **B,** Color Doppler shows diastolic flow in the abnormal echolucent area, suggestive of paravalvular regurgitation and valve dehiscence.

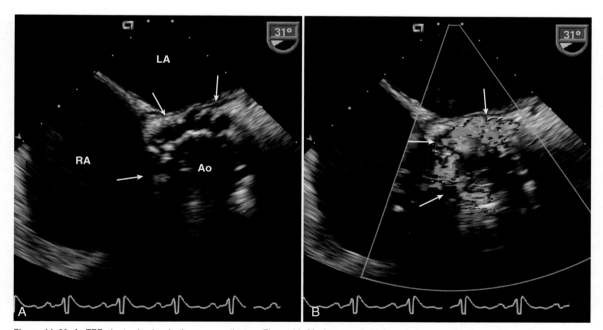

Figure 14–23 A, TEE short-axis view in the same patient as Figure 14–22 shows an irregular echolucent region (*arrows*) extending around the posterior aspect of the sewing ring. **B,** Color Doppler confirms valve dehiscence with paravalvular regurgitation.

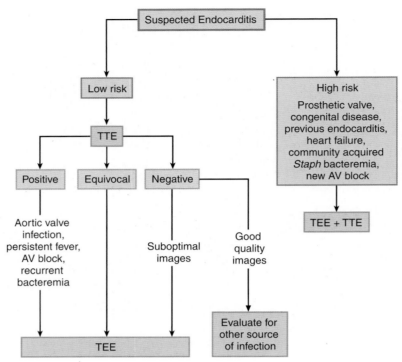

Figure 14–24 Flow chart for the suggested role of echocardiography in diagnosis of endocarditis.

atrioventricular block, and community acquired staphy-lococcal bacteremia. Typically, TTE imaging also is needed in these patients to allow parallel alignment for continuous-wave Doppler evaluation of high-velocity flows, standard measurement of chamber dimensions, quantitation of LV systolic function, and measurement of pulmonary artery pressures. In patients with definite vegetation on TTE imaging, TEE imaging often is reasonable, particularly when the aortic valve is involved, due to the risk or paravalvular abscess. TEE also is appropriate in patients with persistent fever, recurrent bacteremia, or new atrioventricular block—all signs of paravalvular abscess formation.

Cardiac Evaluation of the Patient with Endocarditis

In a patient with known endocarditis, an echocardio-gram is an invaluable adjunct to clinical decision making concerning potential surgical intervention and prediction of short- and long-term prognosis. Echocardiography often allows clear definition of which (and how many) valves are affected.

Diagnosis of acute severe valvular regurgitation or a paravalvular abscess is a clear indication for surgical treatment. Associated LV dysfunction, involvement of more than one valve, and secondary pulmonary hypertension as evaluated by echocardiography are important determinants of the surgical approach and timing of intervention.

Recurrent systemic embolic events generally are accepted as an indication for valve replacement; how-ever, the importance of vegetation size and appear-ance by echocardiography remains controversial. If patients with embolization before echocardiography are excluded, several studies have shown a trend toward a higher incidence of systemic embolization with a vegetation diameter greater than 1 cm (Fig. 14–25). However, other studies contest this con-clusion. Infection with *H. influenzae* and mitral valve involvement also have been shown to predict a higher rate of systemic emboli. Recent studies have sug-gested that sequential TEE echocardiographic evalu-ation of patients with endocarditis can predict whether antimicrobial therapy is effective by demon-strating progressive decreases in vegetation size. However, the cost-effectiveness (and patient accep-tance) of this approach is unclear.

In the current era, with aggressive and prompt sur-gical intervention, severe regurgitation and heart fail-ure do *not* predict mortality, since these patients undergo early valve replacement. With antibiotic therapy and appropriate surgical intervention, risk factors for in-hospital death are prosthetic valve infec-tion, systemic embolism, and infection with *S. aureus*. Long-term outcome in survivors is related to the residual degree of valve damage, the effects of chronic valvular regurgitation on ventricular function and pulmonary artery pressures, and the risk of recurrent episodes of endocarditis.

TABLE 14–4   ACC/AHA 2006 Recommendations for Echocardiography in Infective Endocarditis*

	TTE	TEE
Suspected Endocarditis:		
1. Detection of valvular vegetations (with or without positive blood cultures)	Recommended	
2. Known valve disease with positive blood cultures and nondiagnostic TTE		Recommended
3. Persistent staphylococcal bacteremia without a known source		Reasonable
4. Nosocomial staphylococcal bacteremia		May be considered
Known Endocarditis:		
1. Evaluation of valve hemodynamics	Recommended	Recommended if TTE nondiagnostic
2. Detect and assess complications (abscess, perforation, shunt)	Recommended	Recommended
3. Reassessment of valve function in high-risk patients (e.g., virulent organism, clinical deterioration, persistent or recurrent fever, new murmur, persistent bacteremia)	Recommended	
Prosthetic Valve Endocarditis:		
1. Diagnosis and complications	TEE preferred	Recommended
2. Patient with a prosthetic valve and a persistent fever without bacteremia or a new murmur.	Reasonable	
3. Reevaluation of prosthetic valve endocarditis during antibiotic therapy in the absence of clinical deterioration.	May be considered	
Perioperative Management:		
1. Preoperative evaluation in pts with known infective endocarditis		Recommended
2. Intraoperative TEE in pts undergoing valve surgery for infective endocarditis		Recommended

*Recommended, Class I; reasonable, Class IIa; may be considered, Class IIb.
TEE, transesophageal echocardiography; TTE, transthoracic echocardiography.
Derived from Bonow R et al.: Valve Disease Guidelines, 2006.
Table from Otto, Schwaegler: Echo Review Guide, Philadelphia: Elsevier/Saunders, 2007, p 260.

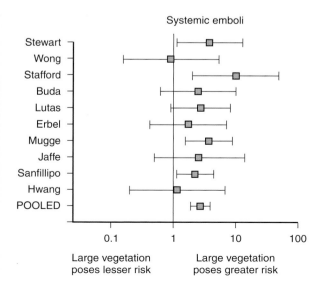

Figure 14–25 Meta-analysis of the relationship between risk of systemic embolization and echocardiographic vegetation size. Odds ratio with 95% confidence intervals for each of 10 studies and the pooled result. An odds ratio > 1 implies that larger vegetation size is associated with an increased risk of embolization. Data from Stewart et al: Circulation 61:374–380, 1980; Wong et al: Arch Intern Med 143:1874, 1983; Stafford et al: Br Heart J 53:310–313, 1985; Buda et al: Am Heart J 112:1291, 1986; Lutas et al: Am Heart J 112:107, 1986; Erbel et al: Eur Heart J 9:43–53, 1988; Mugge et al: J Am Coll Cardiol 14:631, 1989; Jaffe et al: J Am Coll Cardiol 12:1227, 1990; Sanfillipo et al: J Am Coll Cardiol 18:1191–1199, 1991; Hwang et al: Cardiology 83:250–257, 1993. *(Reprinted from Tischler MD, Vaitkus PT: The ability of vegetation size on echocardiography to predict clinical complications: a meta-analysis. J Am Soc Echocardiogr 10:562–568, 1997.)*

SUGGESTED READING

General

1. Cabell CH: Clinical decision making in patients with endocarditis: The role of echocardiography. In Otto CM (ed): The Practice of Clinical Echocardiography, 3rd ed. Philadelphia: Elsevier/Saunders, 2007, pp 501–515.

   Review of the current role of echocardiography in management of the patient with suspected or known endocarditis. In addition to a review of the literature, this chapter provides useful tips on the echocardiographic approach with clear illustrations.

2. Haldar SM, O'Gara PT: Infective endocarditis: diagnosis and management. Nat Clin Pract Cardiovasc Med 3:310–317, 2006.

   Concise review of the diagnostic criteria, imaging approach, antibiotic therapy, and management of complications in endocarditis. Indications for surgical intervention are discussed.

3. Bashore TM, Cabell C, Fowler V Jr: Update on infective endocarditis. Curr Probl Cardiol 31:274–352, 2006.

   A comprehensive review of the epidemiology, pathophysiology, and clinical outcomes with infective endocarditis is followed by a detailed discussion of clinical diagnosis, echocardiographic diagnosis, and therapy.

Clinical Diagnosis

4. Durack DT, Lukes AS, Bright DK: New criteria for diagnosis of infective endocarditis: Utilization of specific echocardiographic findings. Duke Endocarditis Service. Am J Med 96:200–209, 1994.

   Proposed criteria for the clinical diagnosis of endocarditis as detailed in Table 14–1 incorporate echocardiographic findings as a key factor in the diagnosis. Includes validation of sensitivity and specificity of this approach compared to older diagnostic approaches. The Duke criteria are used at many medical centers.

5. Li JS, Sexton DJ, Mick N, et al: Proposed modifications to the Duke criteria for the diagnosis of infective endocarditis. Clin Infect Dis 30:633–638, 2000.

   Modification of the Duke criteria to eliminate nonspecific echocardiographic findings, add evidence for Q-fever as a major criteria, and change the major criteria for S. aureus bacteremia to include any cause of bacteremia. Possible endocarditis is defined as one major plus one minor, or three minor criteria. Table 14–1 includes these modifications.

6. Dodds GA, Sexton DJ, Durack DT, et al: Negative predictive value of the Duke criteria for infective endocarditis. Am J Cardiol 77:403–407, 1996.

   In 405 episodes of suspected endocarditis, 52 were classified as "rejected" endocarditis based on the Duke criteria. With clinical outcome used as the standard of reference, none of these patients subsequently developed endocarditis, although one had possible endocarditis at autopsy, indicating a negative-predictive value of the Duke criteria of at least 92%.

Echocardiographic Diagnosis

7. Daniel WG, Mugge A, Grote J, et al: Comparison of transthoracic and transesophageal echocardiography for detection of abnormalities of prosthetic and bioprosthetic valves in the mitral and aortic positions. Am J Cardiol 71:210–215, 1993.

   Detection of prosthetic valve endocarditis was enhanced by TEE imaging. Of 148 prosthetic valves, 124 were abnormal at surgery or autopsy (33 endocarditis, 8 thrombi, and 83 degeneration). Endocarditis was correctly identified in 12 of 36 (36%) by TTE and 27 of 33 (82%) by TEE.

8. Lowry RW, Zoghbi WA, Baker WB, et al: Clinical impact of transesophageal echocardiography in the diagnosis and management of infective endocarditis. Am J Cardiol 73:1089–1091, 1994.

   In 93 consecutive patients undergoing TEE imaging for suspected endocarditis, the negative predictive value of TEE was 100% for native valves and 90% for prosthetic valves. TEE resulted in a change in the subsequent diagnostic or therapeutic plan in greater than 90% of patients.

9. Lindner JR, Case RA, Dent JM, et al: Diagnostic value of echocardiography in suspected endocarditis: an evaluation based on the pretest probability of disease. Circulation 93:730–736, 1996.

   This study suggests that echocardiography is not necessary in patients with a low pre-test likelihood of the diagnosis. In those with an intermediate or high pre-test likelihood (positive blood cultures plus new murmur or predisposing heart disease), TTE should be performed first. TEE is needed primarily when the TTE study is technically inadequate, indicates an intermediate probability of endocarditis, or a prosthetic valve is present.

10. Heidenreich PA, Masoudi FA, Maini B, et al: Echocardiography in patients with suspected endocarditis: A cost-effectiveness analysis. Am J Med 107:198–208, 1999.

    The effect of TTE and TEE imaging on quality-adjusted life years was evaluated using a decision tree and Markov model. With a pre-test likelihood between 4% and 60%, as commonly seen in clinical practice, TEE results in lower costs and improved outcomes compared with TTE. TTE alone was useful only in patients with a very low pre-test likelihood.

11. Chirillo F, Pedrocco A, De Leo A, et al: Impact of harmonic imaging on transthoracic echocardiographic identification of infective endocarditis and its complications. Heart 91:329–333, 2005.

    Detection of valvular vegetations on TTE imaging was improved with harmonic imaging. However, paravalvular abscess often was missed on a TTE examination, even with harmonic imaging, when compared to TEE diagnosis.

12. Kort S: Real-time 3-dimensional echocardiography for prosthetic valve endocarditis: Initial experience. J Am Soc Echocardiogr 19:130–139, 2006.

    The potential value of real-time 3D imaging for diagnosis of prosthetic valve endocarditis is illustrated in four case examples.

Paravalvular Extension of Infection

13. Daniel WG, Mugge A, Martin RP, et al: Improvement in the diagnosis of abscesses associated with endocarditis by transesophageal echocardiography. N Engl J Med 324:795–800, 1991.

    In 118 consecutive patients with endocarditis, 44 (37%) had surgical or autopsy evidence of abscess formation. Abscesses were more common with infection with Staphylococcus (52% of cases) and with aortic valve involvement. The hospital mortality rate in patients with an abscess was 23% versus 14% in the remainder of the study group. TEE imaging was much more sensitive than TTE for diagnosis of paravalvular abscess.

14. Karalis DG, Bansal RC, Huack AJ, et al: Transesophageal echocardiographic recognition of subaortic complications in aortic valve endocarditis: Clinical and surgical implications. Circulation 86:353–362, 1992.

    Detailed description (with illustrations) of the patterns of paravalvular and subaortic abscess formation in patients with aortic valve endocarditis. The authors note that eccentric jets of mitral regurgitation in patients with aortic valve endocarditis raise the possibility of involvement (perforation) of the anterior mitral leaflet by the infectious process.

15. Hill EE, Herijgers P, Claus P, et al: Abscess in infective endocarditis: the value of transesophageal echocardiography

and outcome: A 5-year study. Am Heart J
154: 923–928, 2007.

*In 115 endocarditis patients, abscess was found
at surgery in 44 (38%) patients. Of these 44
abscesses, only 21 (48%) were detected
preoperatively on TEE imaging. False-negative
TEE studies most often were related to
location of the abscess adjacent to mitral
annular calcification or with prosthetic valve
dehiscence.*

16. Anguera I, Miro JM, Vilacosta I, et al:
Aorto-cavitary fistulous tract formation
in infective endocarditis: Clinical and
echocardiographic features of 76 cases
and risk factors for mortality. Eur Heart
J 26:288–297, 2005.

*The prevalence of a fistula from the aorta to a
cardiac chamber was 1.6% in a series of
4681 adults with endocarditis, occurring in
0.4% of intravenous drug users, 1.8% of other
native valve endocarditis patients, and 3.5% of
prosthetic valve endocarditis cases. The fistula
was detected on TTE in only 53% of cases
but was seen on TEE in 97%. The fistula
was frequently accompanied by an abscess,
originated equally from all three aortic sinuses,
and entered all four cardiac chambers in equal
proportions. Overall mortality in patients with
an aorto-cavity fistula was 41% despite
surgical intervention in 87% of cases.*

Risk of Embolic Events

17. Steckelberg JM, Murphy JG, Ballard D,
et al: Emboli in infective endocarditis: The
prognostic value of echocardiography.
Ann Intern Med 114:635–640, 1991.

*In 207 patients with endocarditis, the
likelihood of first embolic events was 6.2 per
1000 patient days (95% confidence interval,
4.2–9.2). The risk of embolic events was
related to infection with Streptococcus viridans
infections but not to vegetation size. The
likelihood of embolization decreased over time,
falling to 1.2 per 1000 patient days after
2 weeks of therapy.*

18. Sanfilippo AJ, Picard MH, Newell JB,
et al: Echocardiographic assessment of
patients with infectious endocarditis:
prediction of risk for complications.
J Am Coll Cardiol 18:1191–1199,
1991.

*In 204 patients with endocarditis, multivariate
predictors of complications (persistent fever,
congestive heart failure, systemic emboli,
surgery, and mortality) were vegetation size,
extent, and mobility. The authors propose an
echo score for vegetation appearance to predict
the likelihood of complications.*

19. Di Salvo G, Habib G, Pergola V, et al:
Echocardiography predicts embolic
events in infective endocarditis. J Am
Coll Cardiol 37:1069–1076, 2001.

*In 178 patients with endocarditis, embolic
events occurred in 37% when a careful search
for both clinical and silent embolic events was
performed. On multivariate analysis, the only
predictors of embolic events were vegetation
length and mobility. In the 30 patients with
large (>15 mm) mobile vegetations, embolic
events occurred in 83%.*

20. Vilacosta I, Graupner C, San Roman
JA, et al: Risk of embolization after
institution of antibiotic therapy for
infective endocarditis. J Am Coll
Cardiol 39:1489–1495, 2002.

*In 217 episodes of left-sided endocarditis,
13% had embolic events after initiation of
antibiotic therapy (within 2 weeks in
65%). Risk factors for embolism were an
increasing vegetation size despite antibiotic
therapy, mitral valve involvement, infection
with Staphylococcus, and embolization before
the onset of antibiotic therapy.*

21. Thuny F, Di Salvo G, Belliard O, et al:
Risk of embolism and death in infective
endocarditis: Prognostic value of
echocardiography: A prospective
multicenter study. Circulation 112:
69–75, 2005.

*In 384 consecutive endocarditis patients,
embolism occurred in a total of 34%, with
7.5% having embolic events after initiation of
antibiotic therapy. The risk of total embolic
events was higher with infection with S. aureus
or Streptococcus bovis. However, vegetation
length > 1 cm and vegetation mobility were
independent predictors of embolic events on
antibiotic therapy. Vegetation length > 1.5 cm
also predicted higher 1-year mortality.*

22. Dickerman SA, Abrutyn E, Barsic B,
et al: The relationship between the
initiation of antimicrobial therapy and
the incidence of stroke in infective
endocarditis: an analysis from the ICE
Prospective Cohort Study (ICE-PCS).
Am Heart J 154:1086–1094, 2007.

*The incidence of stroke in adults with
endocarditis in the first week after diagnosis is
4.82/1000 patient days, but this incidence
falls to 1.71/1000 patient days after 1 week
of therapy and continues to decline with
further therapy. In the 1437 patients, only
3.1% suffered a stroke. These data suggest
surgical intervention is not appropriate solely
for prevention of embolic events.*

Prosthetic Valve and Device Infection

23. Lo R, D'Anca M, Cohen T, Kerwin T:
Incidence and prognosis of pacemaker
lead–associated masses: a study of 1,569
transesophageal echocardiograms. J
Invasive Cardiol 18:599–601, 2006.

*In a series of 1569 TEE studies, pacer leads
were visualized in the right heart in 125
patients. An echogenic mass was seen attached
to the pacer lead in 12% of these patients and
was probably due to endocarditis in 60%.
Treatment included antibiotics alone (6 of 9
cases) or antibiotics plus lead extraction (3
cases). In the 5% of patients with a pacer
lead–associated mass but no other clinical
evidence of endocarditis, management included
anticoagulation or watchful waiting; there
were no adverse outcomes in this subset of
patients.*

24. Habib G, Thuny F, Avierinos JF:
Prosthetic valve endocarditis: current
approach and therapeutic options. Prog
Cardiovasc Dis 50:274–281, 2008.

*This review summarizes the clinical
presentation, diagnosis and management of
prosthetic valve endocarditis. Diagnosis is more
difficult than in patients with native valve
disease, and TEE is needed in nearly all
patients to evaluate for prosthetic valve
periannular infection. Clinical outcomes
remain poor, and surgical intervention often
is needed.*

Nonbacterial Thrombotic Endocarditis

25. Roldan CA: Echocardiographic findings
in systemic disease characterized by
immune-mediated injury. In Otto CM
(ed): The Practice of Clinical
Echocardiography, 3rd ed. Philadelphia:
Elsevier/Saunders, 2007, pp 877–901.

*Excellent summary of echocardiographic
findings that might be mistaken for endocarditis
including findings in patients with systemic
lupus erythematosus, rheumatoid arthritis,
ankylosing spondylitis, scleroderma, and other
connective tissue disorders. Detailed tables and
illustrations. 172 references.*

26. Roldan CA: Valvular and coronary
disease in systemic inflammatory
diseases: Systemic disorders in heart
disease. Heart 94:1089–1101, 2008.

*A concise review of the cardiac findings in
patients with systemic lupus erythematosus,
rheumatoid arthritis, ankylosing spondylitis,
scleroderma, polymyositis/dermatomyositis,
and mixed connective tissue disease*

27. Roldan CA, Shively BK, Crawford
MH: An echocardiographic study of
valvular heart disease associated with
systemic lupus erythematosus. N Engl J
Med 335:1424–1430, 1996.

*Valvular abnormalities were seen on
echocardiography in two thirds of 69 patients
with lupus. Valve thickening was most
common, but vegetations were seen in 43% and
significant valvular regurgitation was seen in*

25%. Echocardiographic findings often changed on follow-up examination, with some patients having resolution of valvular abnormalities and others having increased valve dysfunction.

28. Edoute Y, Haim N, Rinkevich D, et al: Cardiac valvular vegetations in cancer patients: A prospective echocardiographic study of 200 patients. Am J Med 102:252–258, 1997.

    In 200 ambulatory patients with solid tumors, echocardiography showed valvular vegetations (most often on the aortic or mitral valve) in 19% of patients. Cardiac abnormalities were most common in patients with carcinoma of the pancreas and lung and with lymphoma. Systemic thromboembolism occurred in 11% of the total study group.

29. Asopa S, Patel A, Khan OA, et al: Non-bacterial thrombotic endocarditis. Eur J Cardiothorac Surg 32:696–701, 2007.

    In-depth review of the epidemiology, pathophysiology, clinical presentation, diagnosis, and management of nonbacterial thrombotic endocarditis. The role of echocardiography in patients with clinical findings suggesting endocarditis is emphasized. 41 references.

Long-term Outcome

30. Delahaye F, Alla F, Béguinot I, et al; AEPEI Group: In-hospital mortality of infective endocarditis: Prognostic factors and evolution over an 8 year period. Scand J Infect Dis 39:849–857, 2007.

    In 559 cases of definite endocarditis, in-hospital mortality was 17%. Multivariate predictors of mortality were heart failure, immunosuppression, diabetes, left-sided endocarditis, septic shock, coma scale score, cerebral hemorrhage, and C-reactive protein levels. Infection with S. aureus was not a predictor of outcome in this cohort.

31. San Román JA, López J, Vilacosta I, et al: Prognostic stratification of patients with left-sided endocarditis determined at admission. Am J Med 120:369.e1–369.e7, 2007.

    High-risk patients with left-sided endocarditis can be identified at admission as those with heart failure, S. aureus infection, or para-annular complications.

32. Hill EE, Herijgers P, Claus P, et al: Infective endocarditis: changing epidemiology and predictors of 6 month mortality: a prospective cohort study. Eur Heart J 28:196–203, 2007.

    In 193 patients with 203 episodes of definite endocarditis, 6-month mortality was 22%, but mortality was highest in those who had contraindications to surgical intervention (74%), lowest in those treated medically without a surgical indication (7%), and intermediate in the 63% of the total who underwent surgery (16%). The most common indications for surgery were heart failure, severe valve regurgitation, failure of medical therapy, perivalvular extension, and large vegetations with high embolic risk. Comorbidities that precluded surgical intervention included poor cardiopulmonary status and major cerebrovascular events. Predictors of 6-month mortality on multivariate logistic regressions analysis were age, causative organism, and treatment group. Compared with historical series, more patients now have prosthetic valve endocarditis or nosocomial sources of infection, and more patients undergo surgical intervention.

33. Yoshinaga M, Niwa K, Niwa A, et al: Risk factors for in-hospital mortality during infective endocarditis in patients with congenital heart disease. Am J Cardiol 101:114–118, 2008.

    In a retrospective, observational cohort study, 137 patients (mean age 12 years, range 1 month to 62 years) with congenital heart disease met criteria for definite endocarditis by the modified Duke criteria. Independent risk factors for mortality were vegetation size ≥ 20 mm, age <1 year, heart failure, and infection with S. aureus. Surgical intervention was associated with a lower in-hospital mortality (odds ratio 0.045, 95% confidence interval 0.003–0.70)

Clinical Guidelines

34. Baddour LM, Wilson WR, Bayer AS, et al: Infective endocarditis: diagnosis, antimicrobial therapy, and management of complications: A statement for healthcare professionals from the Committee on Rheumatic Fever, Endocarditis, and Kawasaki Disease, Council on Cardiovascular Disease in the Young, and the Councils on Clinical Cardiology, Stroke, and Cardiovascular Surgery and Anesthesia, American Heart Association: endorsed by the Infectious Diseases Society of America. Circulation 111:e394–e434, 2005.

    This comprehensive document reviews the literature and presents the American Heart Association scientific statement on diagnosis and management of endocarditis. The role of echocardiography is discussed in detail, including a flow chart of the use of TTE versus TEE imaging when endocarditis is suspected. Medical and surgical therapy also are reviewed. 281 references.

35. Wilson W, Taubert KA, Gewitz M, et al: Prevention of infective endocarditis: guidelines from the American Heart Association: a guideline from the American Heart Association Rheumatic Fever, Endocarditis, and Kawasaki Disease Committee, Council on Cardiovascular Disease in the Young, and the Council on Clinical Cardiology, Council on Cardiovascular Surgery and Anesthesia, and the Quality of Care and Outcomes Research Interdisciplinary Working Group. Circulation 116:1736–1754, 2007.

    Endocarditis prophylaxis is no longer recommended for most patients with native valvular heart disease undergoing dental or other procedures. Endocarditis prophylaxis continues to be recommended in high-risk patients, including those with:

    ❏ *Prosthetic cardiac valve or prosthetic material used for cardiac valve repair*

    ❏ *Previous infective endocarditis*

    ❏ *Congenital heart disease (CHD) as follows:*

        ❏ *Unrepaired cyanotic CHD including palliative shunts and conduits*

        ❏ *Completely repaired CHD with prosthetic material or device, whether placed by surgery or catheter intervention, during the first 6 months after the procedure*

        ❏ *Repaired CHD with residual defects at the site or adjacent to the site of a prosthetic patch or prosthetic device (which inhibit endothelialization)*

    ❏ *Cardiac transplant recipients who develop cardiac valvulopathy*

Cardiac Masses and Potential Cardiac "Source of Embolus"

A cardiac mass is defined as an abnormal structure within or immediately adjacent to the heart. There are three basic types of cardiac masses:

❐ Tumor
❐ Thrombus
❐ Vegetation

Abnormal mass lesions must be distinguished from the unusual appearance of a normal cardiac structure, which may be mistakenly considered as an apparent "mass." Echocardiography allows dynamic evaluation of intracardiac masses with the advantage, compared with other tomographic techniques, that both the anatomic extent and the physiologic consequences of the mass can be evaluated. In addition, associated abnormalities (e.g., valvular regurgitation associated with a vegetation) and conditions that predispose to development of a mass (e.g., apical aneurysm leading to left ventricular [LV] thrombus or rheumatic mitral stenosis resulting in left atrial [LA] thrombus) can be assessed. Disadvantages of echocardiography include suboptimal image quality in some patients, a relatively narrow field of view compared with computed tomography (CT) or cardiac magnetic resonance (CMR) imaging, and the possibility of mistaking an ultrasound artifact for an anatomic mass.

BASIC PRINCIPLES

The first step in assessing a possible cardiac mass is to ensure that the echocardiographic findings represent an actual mass rather than an ultrasound artifact. As discussed in detail in Chapter 1, artifacts can be caused by electrical interference, characteristics of the ultrasound transducer/system, or various physical factors influencing image formation from the reflected ultrasound signals. These include beam-width artifact, near-field "ring-down," and multipath artifact. Appropriate transducer selection, scanning technique, and evaluation from multiple examining windows will help to distinguish artifacts from actual anatomic structures.

Besides ultrasound artifacts, several normal structures and normal variants may be mistaken for a cardiac mass (Table 15–1). In the ventricles, normal trabeculae, aberrant trabeculae or chordae (ventricular "webs" or false tendons) (Fig. 15–1), muscle bundles (such as the moderator band), or the papillary muscles may be mistaken for abnormal structures.

Valve anatomy includes a wide range of normal variation, and the appearance of a normal (but often unrecognized) structure such as a nodule of Arantius on the aortic valve may be considered incorrectly to

TABLE 15–1	Structures That May Be Mistaken for an Abnormal Cardiac Mass
Left atrium	Dilated coronary sinus (persistent left superior vena cava) Raphe between left superior pulmonary vein and left atrial appendage Atrial suture line after cardiac transplant Beam-width artifact from calcified aortic valve, aortic valve prosthesis, or other echogenic target adjacent to the atrium IAS aneurysm
Right atrium	Crista terminalis Chiari network (eustachian valve remnants) Lipomatous hypertrophy of the IAS Trabeculation of RAA Atrial suture line after cardiac transplant Pacer wire, Swan-Ganz catheter, or central venous line
Left ventricle	Papillary muscles LV web (aberrant chordae) Prominent apical trabeculations Prominent MAC
Right ventricle	Moderator band Papillary muscles Swan-Ganz catheter or pacer wire
Aortic valve	Nodules of Arantius Lambl's excrescences Base of valve leaflet seen *en face* in diastole
Mitral valve	Redundant chordae Myxomatous mitral valve tissue
Pulmonary artery	Left atrial appendage (just caudal to PA)
Pericardium	Epicardial adipose tissue Fibrinous debris in a chronic organized pericardial effusion

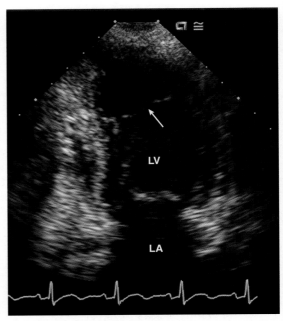

Figure 15–1 LV aberrant trabeculation or "web" seen in an apical four-chamber view in a 35-year-old woman with a normal echocardiogram.

represent a cardiac mass. The belly of a valve leaflet, if cut tangentially, may appear as a "mass" when it actually is a portion of the leaflet itself seen *en face*. In the atrium, normal ridges adjacent to the venous entry sites (Figs. 15–2 and 15–3), normal trabeculations (Fig. 15–4), postoperative changes (see Fig. 9–33 post-transplant), and distortion of the free wall contour by structures adjacent to the atrium (Fig. 15–5) all may be diagnosed erroneously as a cardiac mass.

Definitive diagnosis of an intracardiac mass by echocardiography is based on:

❑ Excellent image quality, which may require use of a high-frequency (5- or 7.5-MHz) short-focus transducer to evaluate the LV apex from the transthoracic (TTE) approach, and the use of transesophageal (TEE) imaging to evaluate posterior cardiac structures (e.g., LA, mitral valve)

❑ Identification of the mass throughout the cardiac cycle, in the same anatomic region of the heart, from more than one acoustic window. This decreases the likelihood of an ultrasound artifact.

❑ Knowledge of the normal structures, normal variants, and postoperative changes that may simulate a cardiac mass

❑ Integration of other echocardiographic findings (e.g., rheumatic mitral stenosis and LA enlargement in a patient with suspected LA thrombus) and clinical data in the final echocardiographic interpretation

Once it is clear that a cardiac mass is present, the next step is to determine whether that mass most likely is a tumor, vegetation, or thrombus. A definitive diagnosis generally cannot be made from the echocardiographic images alone, because the microscopic and bacteriologic characteristics of the structure cannot be determined. However, a reasonably secure diagnosis often can be made by integrating the clinical data, echocardiographic appearance, and associated echo Doppler findings.

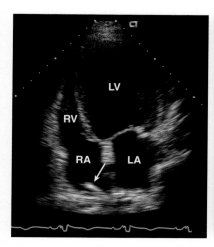

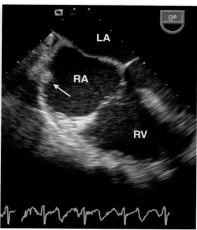

Figure 15–2 Normal appearance of the crista terminalis (*arrow*) in the RA in a transthoracic apical four-chamber view (*left*) and a transesophageal view (*right*).

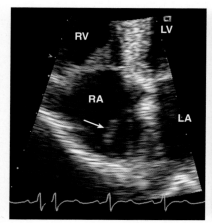

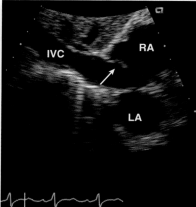

Figure 15–3 Prominent valve at the entrance of the inferior vena cava into the RA seen in an apical four-chamber view (*left*) might be mistaken for a cardiac mass. A subcostal view (*right*) shows the inferior vena cava (IVC) and valve (*arrow*) more clearly.

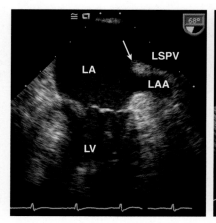

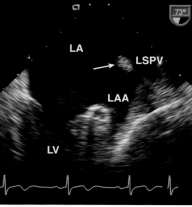

Figure 15–4 The normal ridge between the left atrial appendage (LAA) and left superior pulmonary vein (LSPV) may be mistaken for an abnormal mass. Transesophageal views of this ridge in two different patients are shown. Sometimes this ridge is evident on transthoracic parasternal short-axis or apical two-chamber views.

INFECTIOUS CARDIAC MASSES

Infectious cardiac masses include valvular vegetations, which are seen in patients with endocarditis (bacterial or fungal). Noninfectious vegetations also occur in patients with nonbacterial thrombotic endocarditis (or *marantic* endocarditis). Vegetations typically are irregularly shaped, attached to the upstream side of the valve leaflet (e.g., LA side of the mitral valve, LV side of the aortic valve), and exhibit chaotic motion that differs from that of the leaflets themselves (see Figs. 14–1 and 14–2). Valvular regurgitation is a frequent but not invariable accompaniment of endocarditis. Valvular stenosis

Figure 15–5 Persistent left superior vena cava resulting in a dilated coronary sinus (CS) posterior to the LA seen in a parasternal long-axis view (*left*). If there is ultrasound "dropout" from the wall of the CS, the abnormal contour of the LA may be mistaken for a mass. In the posteriorly angulated apical four-chamber view, the dilated CS is seen (*right*), which can be demonstrated to be connected to the RA by angulation back to a four-chamber view. DA, descending aorta.

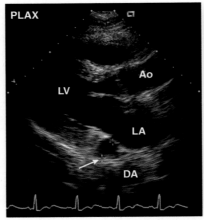 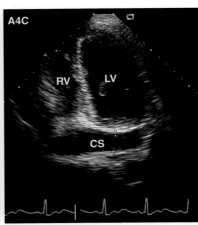

due to the vegetation is rare. Paravalvular abscess, which also presents as a cardiac mass, may be difficult to recognize on TTE imaging but can be diagnosed with a high sensitivity and specificity on TEE imaging. Infectious cardiac masses are discussed in detail in Chapter 14.

CARDIAC TUMORS

Nonprimary

Nonprimary cardiac tumors are approximately 20 times more common than primary cardiac tumors. Tumors can involve the heart by direct invasion from adjacent malignancies (lung, breast), by lymphatic spread, or by metastatic spread of distant disease (lymphoma, melanoma). In autopsy series of patients with a malignancy, cardiac involvement is present in approximately 10% of cases, although clinical recognition of cardiac involvement occurs less frequently. Melanoma has the highest rate of pericardial metastases, but since there are relatively few patients with melanoma, a cardiac tumor is more likely to represent a more prevalent malignancy, as shown in Table 15–2.

TABLE 15–2	Origin of Metastatic Cardiac Tumors in Adults (in Order of Frequency)
Lung	
Lymphoma	
Breast	
Leukemia	
Stomach	
Melanoma	
Liver	
Colon	

Data from Abraham KP, Reddy V, Gattuso P: Neoplasms metastatic to the heart: Review of 3314 consecutive autopsies. Am J Cardiovasc Pathol 3:195–198, 1990.

Almost three fourths of cardiac metastases are due to lung, breast, or hematologic malignancies. Lymphomas associated with acquired immunodeficiency syndrome have frequent and extensive cardiac involvement.

Nonprimary cardiac tumors can affect the heart by

❒ invasion of the pericardium, epicardium, myocardium, or endocardium;
❒ production of biologically active substances; or
❒ toxic effects of treatment on the heart (e.g., radiation therapy or chemotherapy).

Cardiac malignancies most often involve the pericardium and epicardium (approximately 75% of metastatic cardiac disease), presenting as a pericardial effusion, with or without tamponade physiology (Figs. 15–6 and 15–7). Because echocardiographic

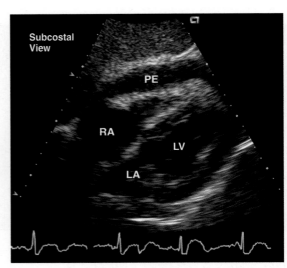

Figure 15–6 This 56-year-old man presented with symptoms of malaise and fatigue and was found to be in pericardial tamponade. The subcostal view shows a moderate-size effusion (PE) with compression of the right heart. Fluid sent for cytology at the time of therapeutic pericardiocentesis showed malignant cells, consistent with adenocarcinoma. Metastatic tumors most often involve an pericardium, although an initial presentation with tamponade is unusual.

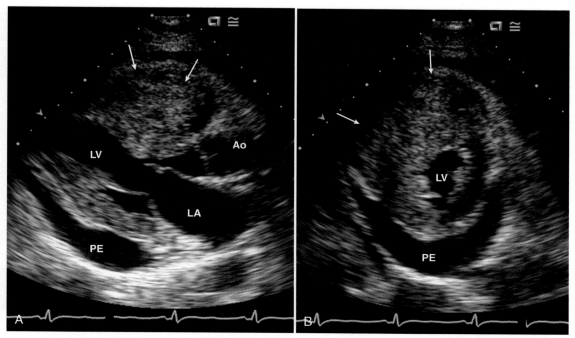

Figure 15–7 Metastatic hepatocellular carcinoma involving the myocardium with marked thickening of the RV free wall (*arrows*) and near obliteration of the RV cavity seen in parasternal (**A**) long- and (**B**) short-axis views. A pericardial effusion (PE) also is present.

diagnosis of the *cause* of a pericardial effusion rarely is possible, the diagnosis of a pericardial effusion (and particularly tamponade) in a patient with a known malignancy should alert the clinician to the possibility of cardiac involvement. Confirmation of the diagnosis requires examination of pericardial fluid and, if necessary, pericardial biopsy. The differential diagnosis of a pericardial effusion in a patient with a known malignancy includes radiation pericarditis and idiopathic pericarditis (which is common in patients with cancer), as well as metastatic disease. Repeat echocardiographic evaluation of patients with a malignant pericardial effusion often is needed after the initial diagnosis for assessment of therapeutic interventions and follow-up for recurrent effusion.

Myocardial involvement by metastatic disease is less common than pericardial involvement, but does occur, particularly with lymphoma or melanoma. Intramyocardial masses can project into or compress cardiac chambers, resulting in hemodynamic compromise. Endocardial involvement is rarely seen.

A specific type of cardiac involvement by tumor that should be recognized by the echocardiographer is extension of *renal cell carcinoma* up the inferior vena cava (Figs. 15–8 and 15–9). A "fingerlike" projection of tumor may protrude into the right atrium (RA) from the inferior vena cava, and the tumor can be followed retrograde (from a subcostal approach) back to the kidney. Correlation with other wide-view imaging techniques is needed for full delineation of

the tumor extent. *Uterine tumors* occasionally present in this fashion as well.

Tumors also can affect the cardiac structures indirectly, as is seen in *carcinoid heart disease* (Fig. 15–10). Metastatic carcinoid tissue in the liver produces biologically active substances, including serotonin, which cause abnormalities of the right-sided cardiac valves and endocardium. Typical changes include thickening, retraction, and increased rigidity of the tricuspid and pulmonic valve leaflets, resulting in valvular regurgitation or, less often, valvular stenosis. Left-sided valvular involvement is rarely seen, possibly due to a lower concentration of the active molecules after passage through the lungs. While metastatic carcinoid disease is rare, the echocardiographic findings are pathognomonic and may lead to the diagnosis in a patient in whom it was not considered previously. Although only one third of patients with carcinoid tumors have cardiac involvement, half the deaths in carcinoid patients are due to heart failure resulting from severe tricuspid regurgitation.

Primary

As for tumors elsewhere in the body, the distinction between benign and malignant primary cardiac tumors is based on pathologic examination of tissue and its tendency to invade adjacent tissue or metastasize to distant sites (Table 15–3). Although 75% of primary cardiac tumors are benign, a pathologically benign cardiac tumor can have "malignant" hemodynamic

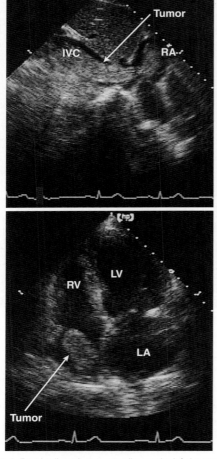

Figure 15–8 Renal cell carcinoma extending up the inferior vena cava is seen on a subcostal view (*above*) and in an apical four-chamber view (*below*) protruding into the RA and across the tricuspid valve into the RV. This tumor was resected en bloc at the time of surgery.

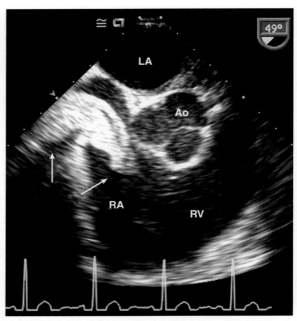

Figure 15–9 TEE imaging in a different patient with renal cell carcinoma showing the extension into the RA from the inferior vena cava without involvement of the atrial wall, septum, or valves.

consequences if it obstructs the normal pattern of blood flow. Thus, the echocardiographic examination includes definition of both the anatomic extent of a cardiac tumor and its physiologic consequences.

Benign Primary Cardiac Tumors

Myxomas account for 27% of primary cardiac tumors. Cardiac myxomas most often are single, arising from the fossa ovalis of the interatrial septum and protruding into the LA (in approximately 75% of cases) (Fig. 15–11). Other sites of origin include the RA (18%), the LV (4%), and the right ventricle (RV; 4%). More than one site can occur in an individual patient (5% of cases).

The clinical presentation of a cardiac myxoma can include constitutional symptoms (fever, malaise),

Figure 15–10 Carcinoid heart disease with thickening and shortening of the tricuspid leaflets (*arrows*) seen in an apical four-chamber view (*left*). Mild stenosis and severe regurgitation of the tricuspid valve were present as seen on color flow imaging, shown on an end-systolic frame (*right*).

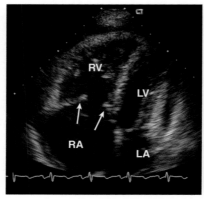
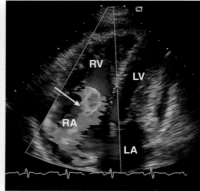

TABLE 15–3 Primary Cardiac Tumors in Adults	
Benign	
Myxoma	27%
Lipoma	10%
Papillary fibroelastoma	10%
Hemangioma	3%
Mesothelioma of the AV node	1%
Malignant	
Angiosarcoma	9%
Rhabdomyosarcoma	5%
Mesothelioma	4%
Fibrosarcoma	3%
Malignant lymphoma	2%
Extraskeletal osteosarcoma	1%
Cysts	
Pericardial	18%
Bronchogenic	2%

Data from McAllister HA, Fenoglio JJ: Tumors of the cardiovascular system. In Atlas of Tumor Pathology, Fascicle 15, 2nd Series. Bethesda, MD: Armed Forces Institute of Pathology, 1978.

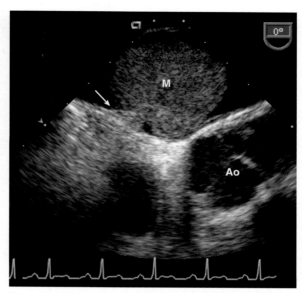

Figure 15–11 LA myxoma (M) arising from a thin stalk (*arrow*) attached to the fossa ovalis of the interatrial septum seen in a TEE view.

clinically evident embolic events, and symptoms of mitral valve obstruction. A myxoma also may be an unexpected finding on a study requested for other clinical indications.

An LA myxoma may nearly fill the LA chamber (Fig. 15–12), with prolapse of the tumor mass across the mitral annulus into the LV in diastole (accounting for the tumor "plop" on auscultation). The mass often has an irregular shape characterized by protruding "fronds" of tissue or a "grape cluster" appearance. The echogenicity of the mass may be nonhomogeneous, and sometimes areas of calcification are noted.

The degree to which the tumor causes functional obstruction to LV diastolic filling can be evaluated qualitatively by color flow imaging and quantitatively by the pressure half-time method. Careful echocardiographic evaluation from multiple views, often including

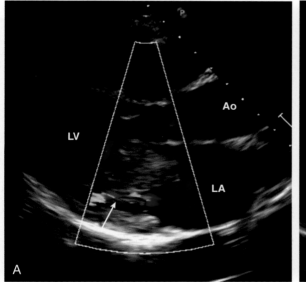

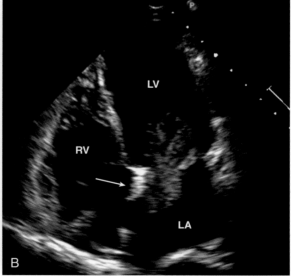

Figure 15–12 Large LA myxoma seen in a parasternal long-axis view (**A**) showing the tumor prolapsing into the mitral orifice in diastole, resulting in functional mitral stenosis with only a narrow flow stream (*arrow*) seen with color Doppler. In the apical view (**B**) the attachment to the septum (*arrow*) and the inhomogeneous echogenicity of the myxoma are seen.

Figure 15–13 Small mass, suggestive of a papillary fibroelastoma (*arrow*), attached to the septal leaflet of the tricuspid valve (with independent motion) as seen on TTE (*left*) and TEE imaging (*right*) in a 56-year-old woman referred for exercise echocardiography for atypical chest pain.

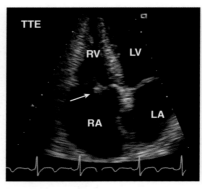
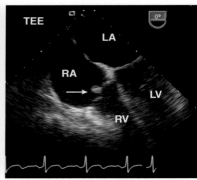

TEE, is needed in planning the surgical approach. Important goals of the echo examination are:

❑ To identify the site of tumor attachment
❑ To ensure that the tumor does not involve the valve leaflets themselves
❑ To exclude the possibility of multiple masses

Postoperatively, complete excision should be documented by echocardiography. Sequential long-term follow-up is indicated because recurrent myxomas have been reported, particularly with a familial form of this disease, with multiple myxomas, or with a less than full-thickness excision.

The echocardiographic approach to myxomas arising in other locations is similar to that described for LA myxomas, except that the imaging and Doppler examination are tailored toward evaluating the specific region of tumor involvement in that patient. Again, it should be emphasized that the diagnosis of a myxoma, based on the clinical features, anatomic location, and echocardiographic appearance of the tumor, is only presumptive until confirmed histologically. A "typical" myxoma may turn out to be a metastatic malignancy or a primary cardiac malignancy on pathologic examination. Hence the echocardiographic examination should be as complete as possible to exclude tissue invasion by the tumor, multiple sites of involvement, or atypical features.

A *papillary fibroelastoma* is a benign cardiac tumor that arises on valvular tissue, thus mimicking the appearance of a valvular vegetation. A papillary fibroelastoma appears as a small mass attached to the aortic or mitral valve with motion independent from the normal valve structures (Fig. 15–13). A papillary fibroelastoma also may be seen attached to the tricuspid or pulmonic valve or at nonvalvular sites. Unlike a vegetation, a fibroelastoma is more often found on the downstream side of the valve (LV side of mitral valve, aortic side of aortic valve). The histologic appearance is very similar to the smaller Lambl's excrescences, which can be seen on normal valves in the elderly. Usually a small papillary fibroelastoma is of no clinical significance; the relationship of larger benign valve tumors to embolic events is controversial. In addition, some cases of superimposed thrombus formation resulting in systemic embolic events have been described. Often these tumor are better visualized on TEE imaging.

Other benign cardiac tumors seen in adults include hemangiomas, and mesotheliomas of the atrioventricular node.

Lipomatous hypertrophy of the interatrial septum presents as a cardiac mass that may be mistaken for a tumor. Lipomatous hypertrophy typically involves the superior and inferior fatty portions of the atrial septum, sparing the fossa ovalis region (Fig. 15–14). However, symmetric ellipsoid enlargements of the interatrial septum also have been described. If the etiology of atrial septal hypertrophy is unclear on echocardiography, CT scanning may establish the diagnosis of lipomatous hypertrophy by showing the characteristic radiographic density of adipose tissue.

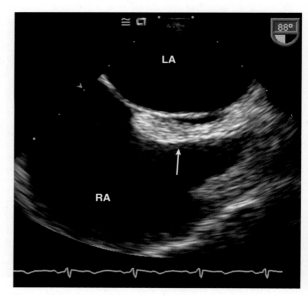

Figure 15–14 Lipomatous hypertrophy (*arrow*) of the interatrial septum seen on TEE imaging with typical sparing of the thin fossa ovalis.

Malignant Primary Cardiac Tumors

Malignant primary cardiac tumors are rare. In adults, angiosarcomas, rhabdomyosarcomas (Fig. 15–15), mesotheliomas, and fibrosarcomas are seen (see Table 15–2). The clinical presentation is variable, ranging from an "incidental" finding on echocardiography or nonspecific systemic symptoms (fever, malaise, fatigue) to signs and symptoms of cardiac tamponade. Because metastatic disease is far more likely than a primary cardiac origin, thorough evaluation must include a search for potential primary sites. Ultimately, the diagnosis depends on examination of tissue from the cardiac mass.

The echocardiographic examination focuses on:

❑ The anatomic location and extent of the tumor involvement

❑ The physiologic consequences of the tumor (e.g., valve regurgitation, chamber obliteration, obstruction)

❑ Associated findings (pericardial effusion, evidence of tamponade physiology)

Along with other imaging techniques, the echocardiographic examination may help guide therapy by determining whether the tumor is resectable or whether palliative cardiac procedures are likely to be beneficial. Specific attention also is directed toward possible involvement of the valves, coronary arteries, or conducting system.

Technical Considerations/Alternate Approaches

Although echocardiography has definite advantages for evaluating cardiac tumors, it has significant disadvantages as well. These include (1) poor acoustic access, resulting in suboptimal image quality, which limits the confidence with which tumor location and extent can be defined or results in a missed diagnosis (TEE imaging may obviate this limitation in some patients); (2) the need for a careful and meticulous examination to detect and fully evaluate the cardiac tumor (as for other applications, echocardiography is operator dependent, and a significant learning curve for obtaining optimal data can be observed); and (3) the limited "field of view" inherent in echocardiography (i.e., structures adjacent to the heart in the mediastinum and lung are difficult to evaluate). Other tomographic imaging techniques, specifically CT and CMR, have the advantage of a wide field of view so that the relationship between cardiac and extracardiac tumor involvement can be evaluated. Often judicious use of both echocardiographic techniques (to assess cardiac involvement in detail and to evaluate the physiologic consequences of the tumor mass) and CT or CMR (to assess potential extracardiac involvement) may be needed in an individual patient for optimal clinical decision making. Both CT and CMR may provide data on the tissue characteristics of the abnormal mass, which currently cannot be obtained with echocardiography (Fig. 15–16).

LEFT VENTRICULAR THROMBUS

Predisposing Conditions

Thrombus formation in the LV tends to occur in regions of blood stasis or low-velocity blood flow. The most familiar example of blood flow stasis in the LV is a ventricular aneurysm, in which low-velocity swirling blood flow patterns are seen. Stasis also may

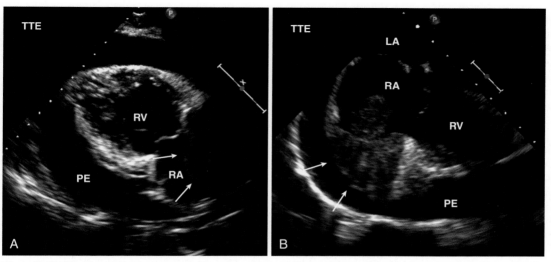

Figure 15–15 This 45-year-old man diagnosed with a primary cardiac angiosarcoma presented with a pericardial effusion. On a TTE RV inflow view (**A**), the pericardial effusion (PE) is seen and a mass in the RA is faintly visualized (*arrows*). **B**, TEE images show the tumor mass in the RA and demonstrate involvement of the RA wall (*arrows*).

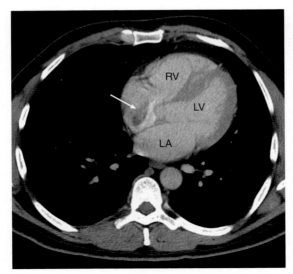

Figure 15-16 CT scan in the same patient as Figure 15-9 shows the tumor mass as a filling defect (*arrow*) in the contrast-filled RA. The wide field of view of CT allowed delineation of the full extent of the tumor as it extended from the kidney up the inferior vena cava and into the right heart.

TABLE 15-4	Sensitivity and Specificity of Diagnostic Tests for Intracardiac Thrombus Formation	
Test	**Sensitivity (%)**	**Specificity (%)**
LA Thrombus		
TTE*	53–63	95–99
TEE[†]	99	100
CT with contrast[‡]	36–100	72–94
Contrast angio[‡]	70	88
CMR[||]	100	94
LV Thrombus		
TTE[§]	92–95	86–88
TEE[¶]	40±14	96±3.6
LV angio**	26–31	—
Contrast-enhanced CMR[¶]	88–93	85–99

*Shrestha et al: Am J Cardiol 48:954–960, 1981; Chiang et al: J Ultrasound Med 6:525–529, 1987; Bansal et al: Am J Cardiol 64:243–246, 1989.
[†]Aschenberg et al: J Am Coll Cardiol 7: 163–166, 1986; Olson et al: J Am Soc Echocordior 5:52–56, 1992; Hwang et al: Am J Cardiol 72: 677, 1993.
[‡]Tang et al: J Interv Card Electrophysiol 22:199, 2008; Patel et al: Heart Rhythm 5:253, 2008; Gottlieb et al: J Cardiovasc Electrophysiol 19:247, 2008.
[§]Visser et al: Chest 83:228–232, 1983; Stratton et al: Circulation 66:156–165, 1982.
[¶]Srichai et al: Am Heart J 152:75, 2006.
[||]Ohyama et al: Stroke 34:2436, 2003.
**Reeder et al: Mayo Clin Proc 56:77, 1981.
CMR, cardiac magnetic resonance imaging; CT, computed tomographic imaging; TEE, transesophageal echocardiography; TTE, transthoracic echocardiography.

occur with less severe segmental wall motion abnormalities (e.g., apical akinesis) and with diffuse LV dysfunction (e.g., dilated cardiomyopathy). LV thrombus formation is extremely rare in the absence of an akinetic or dyskinetic apex or diffuse LV dysfunction. Thrombus formation also often accompanies an LV pseudoaneurysm. In this case, the thrombus lines an area of LV rupture that has been contained by the pericardium (see Fig. 8–27).

Even when a definite LV thrombus is not seen on an echocardiographic examination, the likelihood of thrombus formation remains high in patients with LV aneurysm, apical akinesis, or diffuse LV systolic dysfunction with an ejection fraction less than 20%. Doppler analysis of apical flow patterns has been suggested to help identify which of these patients are at highest risk of thrombus formation. Evidence of apical flow stasis or of continuous swirling of flow around the apex is thought to identify patients at particular risk for apical thrombus.

Identification of Left Ventricular Thrombi

The sensitivity of echocardiography for detecting LV thrombi is extremely operator dependent (Table 15–4). A careful and thorough examination requires not only standard views but also angulated apical views and the use of higher frequency short-focus transducers to improve near-field resolution. It is advantageous to use a 5- or 7.5-MHz transducer from the standard apical four-chamber window and also to move the transducer slightly laterally while angulating it medially to obtain an apical short-axis view. Scanning across the apex in

several views usually allows distinction of apical thrombi from prominent apical trabeculations or false tendons, which are bright linear structures that attach to mural trabeculae. Thrombus is often (though not always) somewhat more echogenic than the underlying myocardium, and has a contour distinct from the endocardial border.

The diagnosis of LV thrombus is most secure when an echogenic mass is seen with a convex surface that is not a "ring-down" artifact, is clearly distinct from the endocardium, and is located in a region of abnormal wall motion (Fig. 15–17). The diagnosis of laminated thrombus is more of a problem unless a clear demarcation between the thrombus and the underlying myocardium is seen, but it can be suspected when the apex appears "rounded" and akinetic with apparent excessively thick apical myocardium.

Clinical Implications

In some cases apical images are suboptimal despite careful examination technique. In this situation definite exclusion of apical thrombus may not be

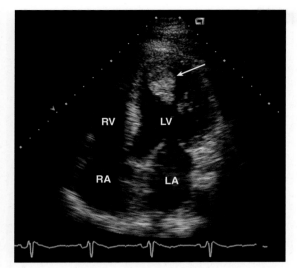

Figure 15–17 Protruding thrombus (*arrows*) in an akinetic apex in a patient with a dilated cardiomyopathy seen in an apical four-chamber view.

possible. Even so, clinical management (e.g., chronic anticoagulation) may depend more on assessment of overall LV function or the presence of an apical aneurysm than on the presence or absence of an echocardiographically documented thrombus.

The presence of an LV thrombus on echocardiographic examination is a strong predictor of subsequent embolic events, particularly when the thrombus protrudes into the ventricular cavity or shows independent mobility. Sessile, nonprotruding thrombi may have lower embolic potential.

Alternate Approaches

TTE is the clinical procedure of choice for identification of LV thrombi. TEE imaging rarely is helpful and is less sensitive, because the apex may not be depicted in standard image planes and the LV apex is at a considerable distance from the transducer, thereby limiting resolution of structural detail. LV contrast angiography and radionuclide ventriculography both have a low sensitivity and specificity for diagnosing LV thrombus. In the research setting, indium-114–labeled platelets with gamma-camera imaging have shown a high specificity, but this approach is not available for routine clinical use. Contrast-enhanced CMR imaging has a very high sensitivity and specificity for detection of LV thrombus and may be appropriate in selected patients.

LEFT ATRIAL THROMBUS

Predisposing Factors

LA thrombi tend to form when there is stasis of blood flow in the LA. In general, low-velocity flow in the LA is associated with:

- ☐ Atrial enlargement
- ☐ Mitral valve disease
- ☐ Atrial fibrillation

The highest incidence of LA thrombus is in patients with rheumatic mitral stenosis and atrial fibrillation. However, in the presence of mitral stenosis or poor LV function, even patients in sinus rhythm and those with only modest LA enlargement can have LA thrombi. LA thrombi are less common in patients with mitral regurgitation, presumably because the high-velocity regurgitant jet mechanically disrupts the area of blood stasis within the LA.

Identification of Left Atrial Thrombi

Visualization of LA thrombi using TTE imaging is limited by two factors:

1. The LA is in the far field of the image from both parasternal and apical windows, thus limiting resolution of LA structures and possible thrombi.
2. A large percentage of LA thrombi are found in the left atrial appendage, which is difficult to image from the TTE approach.

TEE imaging has a high sensitivity and a high negative predictive value for the diagnosis of left atrial thrombi. Hence, TEE evaluation is the appropriate procedure when the presence or absence of LA thrombus is important for patient management. From the TEE approach the LA lies close to the transducer, and the appendage can be visualized using 7.5-MHz transducer in at least two orthogonal views (Fig. 15–18). Optimally, the LA appendage is

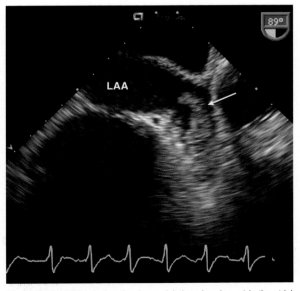

Figure 15–18 TEE imaging showing an LA thrombus (*arrow*) in the atrial appendage. This thrombus was visualized in two orthogonal views, using zoom mode and a high-frequency transducer (7 MHz).

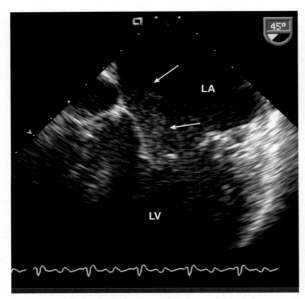

Figure 15-19 Spontaneous contrast in the LA seen on TEE in a patient with atrial fibrillation, and LV systolic dysfunction. Swirling echo densities (*arrow*) are seen in the LA on real-time images.

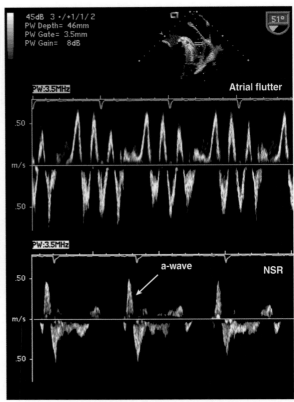

Figure 15-20 LA appendage blood flow pattern recorded on TEE in atrial flutter (*top*) and sinus rhythm (*bottom*). Notice that both the P wave in sinus rhythm and the flutter waves are associated with a flow velocity out of the atrial appendage greater than 40 cm/s. In contrast, when atrial fibrillation is present only very low flow velocities with an irregular pattern are seen, leading to stasis of blood in the atrial appendage. NSR, normal sinus rhythm.

evaluated by centering the appendage in the image plane at the 0° transducer position, using a small field of view and a high-frequency transducer. Then the image plane is slowly rotated through 180°, keeping the atrial appendage centered in the image, to evaluate for possible thrombus. In addition, the body of the LA and atrial septal region are evaluated using rotational scanning from 0° to 180° from a high esophageal position.

Stasis of blood flow may be seen on TEE imaging as "spontaneous" echo contrast, that is, echogenic reflections from the low-velocity blood flow appearing as white swirls on the echocardiographic image (Fig. 15–19). While the appearance of "spontaneous" contrast depends on technical factors such as transducer frequency and instrument gain, as well as the pattern of blood flow, this finding is associated with an increased risk of LA thrombus formation and embolic complications.

Doppler recordings of the pattern of blood flow in the LA appendage may be helpful in identifying patients at highest risk of thrombus formation (Fig. 15–20). With a pulsed Doppler sample volume positioned approximately 1 cm from the entry of the appendage into the body of the LA, a normal contraction velocity is about 0.4 m/s; values less than this are associated with an increased risk of thrombus formation.

In some patients the LA appendage can be imaged using a transthoracic parasternal approach, starting in the short-axis view at the aortic valve level and angulating the transducer inferiorly and laterally to demonstrate the triangular appendage just inferior to the pulmonary artery. From the apical two-chamber view, the LA appendage may be visualized by slight superior angulation of the transducer. If a discrete echogenic mass is seen in the LA of a patient with mitral stenosis and atrial fibrillation, the specificity of this finding for LA thrombi is high (Fig. 15–21). However, the sensitivity of TTE for detection of LA thrombus is very poor. If *no* LA thrombus is seen in a patient in whom the diagnosis is suspected, a TTE study certainly does *not* exclude this possibility.

Prognosis/Clinical Implications

The importance of an LA thrombus depends on the clinical setting. In a patient with new atrial fibrillation and an embolic stroke, the most likely cause of the stroke is an LA thrombus whether or not one is actually imaged, and thus the demonstration of an LA thrombus would be unlikely to change clinical management. In contrast, in a patient with rheumatic mitral stenosis the presence of an LA thrombus is a contraindication to mitral balloon commissurotomy. TEE evaluation for LA thrombus is routine prior to

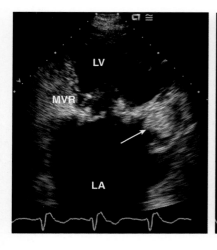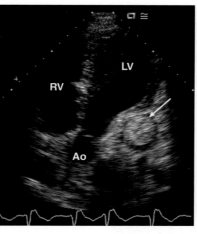

Figure 15–21 Transthoracic apical two-chamber view (*left*) showing a definite thrombus (*arrow*) in the LA appendage. The thrombus can also be seen in the atrial appendage in an anteriorly angulated apical four-chamber view (*right*). MVR, mitral valve replacement.

elective cardioversion and before interventional and electrophysiology procedures in which catheters or devices will be in the LA, for example, mitral valvuloplasty or atrial fibrillation ablation.

Alternate Approaches

While few direct comparisons of echocardiography versus CT or CMR have been performed, these imaging modalities have been reported to have a high sensitivity for detection of LA thrombus. Intracardiac echocardiography also can be used to evaluate for LA thrombus at the time of an invasive procedure.

RIGHT HEART THROMBI

Formation of thrombi in the right side of the heart is rare, although it has been reported in cases of severe RV dilation and systolic dysfunction. A more likely source of thrombi seen within the right side of the heart is venous thrombi that have embolized and become entrapped in the tricuspid valve apparatus or RV trabeculations during passage from the

peripheral veins toward the pulmonary artery (Fig. 15–22). Thrombi also can form on indwelling catheters or pacer wires. While thrombi in the right side of the heart can sometimes be demonstrated by meticulous TTE imaging (Fig. 15–23), TEE echo is better able to resolve the presence, extent, and attachment of right-sided heart thrombi.

When mobile echogenic targets are seen within the right heart chambers, it is important to distinguish thrombi from eustachian valve remnants, microbubbles, or reverberation artifacts. Eustachian valve remnants, which are persistent portions of the embryologic valves of the sinus venosus, are typically mobile, thin linear structures attached at the junction of the inferior or superior cavae and the RA cavity. They may be extensive and can cross the atrium, attaching to the fossa ovalis, sometimes referred to as a Chiari network. They do not extend antegrade to cross the tricuspid valve in diastole, however. Microbubbles, which are encapsulated gas bubbles that can be seen in patients with indwelling venous access, appear as discrete echogenic targets that are usually located in different parts of the heart during successive cycles.

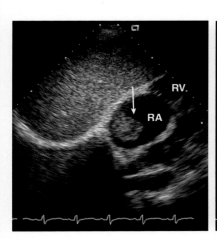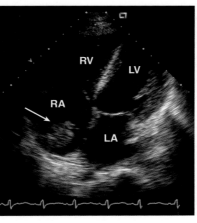

Figure 15–22 RA thrombus (*arrows*) seen on a subcostal (*left*) and apical four-chamber view (*right*). This may represent a thrombus-in-transit from a peripheral venous thrombosis.

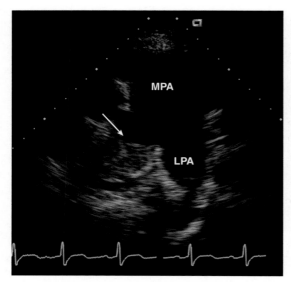

Figure 15–23 Transthoracic view of the main pulmonary artery (MPA) with bifurcation into the right and left pulmonary artery (LPA) demonstrates an echodensity nearly filling the right PA (*arrow*) in this 63-year-old woman with recurrent pulmonary emboli referred for surgical thrombectomy.

CARDIAC SOURCE OF EMBOLUS

Basic Principles

In a patient with a suspected cardiac origin of a systemic embolic event, echocardiographic evaluation is directed toward identification of:

- ❐ Abnormal intracardiac masses (e.g., LV thrombus, LA tumor, valvular vegetation)
- ❐ Abnormalities that may predispose the patient to development of intracardiac thrombi (e.g., LV aneurysm, mitral stenosis, atrial flow stasis)
- ❐ Cardiac abnormality that may serve as a potential conduit for systemic embolism (patent foramen ovale [PFO], atrial septal defect)
- ❐ Aortic atheroma, with or without protruding thrombus

Note that echocardiographic evaluation *after* an index embolic event may fail to demonstrate a cardiac thrombus even if it was the etiology of the clinical event, because now the thrombus has embolized and is no longer in the heart. Recurrent intracardiac thrombus formation may not yet have occurred.

Identifiable Cardiac Sources of Emboli

In patients with an abnormal intracardiac mass on echocardiography in the aftermath of a recent systemic embolic event, the likelihood is very high that a portion of the mass embolized, thereby causing the clinical event. Cardiac masses known to be associated with clinical systemic embolic events include:

- ❐ Valvular vegetations
- ❐ LV and LA thrombi
- ❐ Cardiac tumors (especially LA myxomas)

In patients with suspected systemic embolic events, a definite cardiac source is documented by TTE in approximately 10% to 15% of sequential cases. To some extent, the low prevalence of a definite source may relate to imaging *after* the event (when the mass is no longer in the heart). On the other hand, in many patients the source of embolus may have been outside the heart (e.g., atheromas with or without superimposed thrombus in the carotid arteries or ascending aorta), or the intracardiac thrombi may have embolized soon after formation. In this latter group it is especially important to search for conditions that predispose to intracardiac thrombus formation, even though an intracardiac thrombus is not identified at the time of the examination.

Predisposing Conditions

Apical aneurysms have a high incidence of associated thrombus formation. Other segmental wall motion abnormalities and diffuse LV systolic dysfunction also predispose to LV thrombus formation. An LV *pseudoaneurysm* is almost invariably accompanied by thrombus lining the pseudoaneurysm cavity.

Rheumatic mitral stenosis is associated with LA thrombus formation. *Atrial fibrillation*, even when it occurs without coexisting mitral valve disease, is strongly associated with systemic embolic events, presumably due to LA thrombi. In a patient with a systemic embolic event and either paroxysmal or sustained atrial fibrillation, LA thrombus formation is so likely that even if TEE imaging fails to demonstrate an LA clot, it still is appropriate to treat the patient with systemic anticoagulants to prevent recurrent atrial thrombus formation.

Intracardiac thrombi may occur in patients with *congenital heart disease*, particularly those with atrial dilation or ventricular dysfunction. Patients with a large atrial septal defect are at risk for "paradoxical" systemic embolization of peripheral venous thrombi. Thrombi can pass from the RA to the LA even when the shunt is predominantly left to right, due to streaming of flow or transient shifts in the RA-to-LA pressure gradient. Patients with Eisenmenger's complex and a large ventricular septal defect are at risk of systemic embolization from peripheral venous thrombus formation. However, paradoxical embolization is unlikely in adults with a small ventricular septal defect, because the high LV, compared with RV pressure, limits flow from right to left.

Prosthetic valves are another potential source of embolic events; the incidence of clinical events is higher with mechanical compared with tissue valves. Demonstration of small thrombi on prosthetic valves is difficult even with TEE imaging, due to shadowing and reverberations from the prosthetic leaflets and sewing ring. Hence, the diagnosis often is presumptive when there is evidence of suboptimal anticoagulation at the time of the event or when other causes for the clinical event have been excluded, even if the level of anticoagulation appears to have been adequate. In these patients the primary goals of the echocardiographic examination are to assess prosthetic valve function (because significant thrombus may result in stenosis and/or regurgitation) and to exclude other intracardiac sources of thrombus formation (e.g., associated LV systolic dysfunction).

TEE imaging provides imaging of atrial structures in more detail and has led to the recognition of other anatomic variants and disease processes that may be associated with systemic embolic events, although whether this association is a cause-effect relationship or whether the echo findings are a marker of increased risk is unclear:

- ❐ Patent foramen ovale
- ❐ Interatrial septal aneurysm
- ❐ Swirling pattern of blood flow in the LA in the absence of an exogenous "contrast" agent (thought to represent flow stasis and often called *spontaneous contrast*)
- ❐ Atherosclerosis in the aorta

A *PFO* is present in 25% to 35% of unselected patients at autopsy. During fetal development, incomplete closure of the interatrial septum shunts oxygenated placental blood from the RA to LA and then to the brain. This potential interatrial communication fuses within the first few days after birth in most individuals. If the flap valve covering the fossa ovalis remains unfused, there usually is no passage of blood across the interatrial septum. The "flap" is functionally closed, because LA pressure normally exceeds RA pressure. However, if RA pressure transiently exceeds LA pressure (as during a cough or the Valsalva maneuver), or if RA pressure chronically

exceeds LA pressure (e.g., after pulmonary embolization or with chronic lung disease), there can be right-to-left passage of blood (or thrombi) across the interatrial septum.

Echocardiographic demonstration of a PFO is possible with color flow Doppler imaging from a TEE approach in only about 5% to 10% of patients, with a lesser number detected by transthoracic color Doppler imaging. Detection of a patent foramen is enhanced by intravenous injection of echo contrast material (such as agitated saline solution), providing opacification of the right-sided heart structures. Passage of contrast across the interatrial septum is seen as bright echo contrast in the LA within one to three beats of its appearance in the RA (Fig. 15–24). It is important to use a view in which the contrast effect does not obscure identification of microbubbles in the left side of the heart. Often the site of origin of the contrast in the LA can be identified on frame-by-frame analysis. Using echo contrast, a patent foramen is detectable at rest in approximately 5% of the general population. When maneuvers to transiently increase RA pressure are performed simultaneously with contrast injection, the prevalence of detectable PFO by contrast TEE increases to approximately 25%—similar to the incidence at autopsy (Fig. 15–25).

Passage of very small microbubbles through the pulmonary capillaries can occur with a peripheral injection of agitated saline; microbubbles from transpulmonary passage typically appear in the LA via the pulmonary veins late after the appearance of contrast material in the RA. With an atrial septal defect or PFO, contrast material appears in the LA within three beats of its appearance in the right heart. With transpulmonary passage, contrast material is seen in the left heart after more than three beats.

In young patients (<45 years) with transient ischemic attacks or cerebrovascular events of unknown cause (called cryptogenic stroke), a higher incidence of PFO is found than in the general population, suggesting that passage of thrombi across the atrial

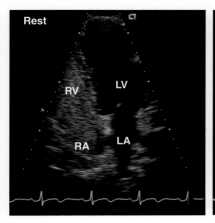
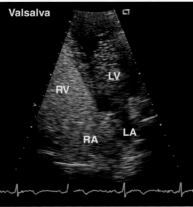

Figure 15–24 Patent foramen ovale on TTE. At rest (*left*), saline contrast fills the right heart with no evidence of contrast in the left heart. After a second contrast injection during Valsalva maneuver, contrast material is seen in the LA and LV within three beats of appearance of contrast material in the right heart.

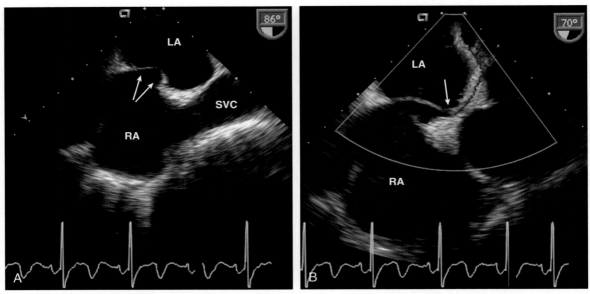

Figure 15–25 A, Atrial septal aneurysm (*arrows*) seen on TEE imaging in a long-axis view of the superior vena cava (SVC) and RA. This is a useful view to evaluation for patent foramen ovale (**B**), demonstrated with color Doppler in this patient showing a narrow jet across the patent foramen (*arrow*) from the RA to LA.

septum may be a significant cause of systemic embolic events in these patients. Often a peripheral venous source of thrombi is identified in these patients. Percutaneous device closure of a PFO is increasingly performed in patients with a systemic embolic event, although results of randomized trials have not yet been reported. Intracardiac or TEE imaging is used to monitor percutaneous device closure of a PFO or atrial septal defect (Fig. 15–26).

An *interatrial septal aneurysm* is defined as a transient bulging of the fossa ovalis region of the interatrial septum (total excursion from the septal plane) greater

than 15 mm in the absence of chronically elevated LA or RA pressure (Fig. 15–27). Septal aneurysms are associated with a high likelihood (up to 90%) of associated fenestration. Until recently the diagnosis rarely was made from TTE imaging due to suboptimal image quality, and this finding was thought to be of little clinical significance. The excellent views of the interatrial septum on TEE have resulted in an increasing recognition of this anatomic variant. Several investigators have suggested a possible relationship between the presence of an atrial septal aneurysm and an increased risk of systemic embolic events.

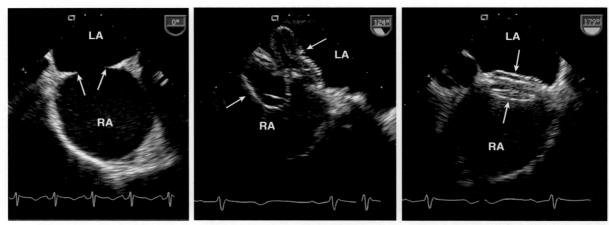

Figure 15–26 TEE imaging during placement of a percutaneous atrial septal defect closure device shows: (1) the secundum atrial septal defect (*left*), (2) the device across the defect with the LA side being pulled into position (*arrow*) and the RA side being deployed (*middle*), and (3) closure of the defect with full deployment of both the LA and RA sides of the device (*right*).

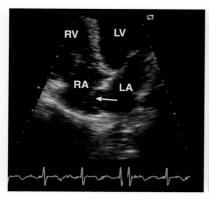 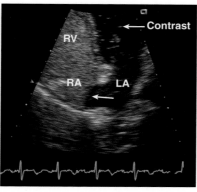

Figure 15–27 Incidental finding of an atrial septal aneurysm (*arrow*) in an elderly patient seen in a transthoracic apical four-chamber view (*left*). Peripheral venous injection of agitated saline to provide a contrast effect (*right*) shows opacification of the right heart with a few microbubbles seen in the left heart, consistent with an associated patent foramen ovale or fenestration in the atrial septal aneurysm.

"Spontaneous" contrast is seen in the LA when there is stasis of blood flow. It is seen more often on TEE than TTE imaging due to the higher transducer frequency and the closer proximity of the LA when interrogated from the esophagus but can be seen on TTE imaging in some patients. Spontaneous contrast is associated with LA enlargement and LA thrombus formation, and it may be a marker for a "prethrombotic" state when definite atrial thrombi are not seen. In extreme cases of spontaneous contrast in mitral stenosis patients, the jet of diastolic blood flow across the stenotic mitral orifice can be seen on two-dimensional imaging due to the contrast effect.

Spontaneous contrast can be seen in the LV when there is stasis of blood flow, such as in the region of an apical aneurysm. Spontaneous contrast also is observed frequently in patients with mechanical prosthetic valves. Here the mechanism of spontaneous contrast formation may be different, relating to the mechanical impact of the valve occluder during closure resulting in microcavitation or liberation of gas from solution. Of course, patients with mitral prosthetic valves also may also have stasis of blood flow in the LA if long-standing disease has resulted in LA enlargement and atrial fibrillation.

The presence of *atheroma* in the descending thoracic aorta is associated with an increased risk of stroke and transient ischemic attack. These are recognized as a focal area of increased thickness in the aortic endothelium with an irregular border and nonuniform echogenicity. An atheroma is considered "complex" if thickness is greater than 4 mm, there is evidence of ulceration, or areas of independent mobility are present. (See Suggested Readings 31 and 32 and Chapter 16).

Indications for Echocardiography in Patients with Systemic Embolic Events

Current understanding of potential cardiac etiologies for systemic embolism is incomplete, and there is considerable controversy as to the indications for TTE and TEE imaging in patients with suspected systemic embolic events. In patients with embolic events the prevalence of PFO is about 30%, as compared with a prevalence of 10% in control subjects. Aortic atheromas (see Chapter 16) are seen in 20% of patients with embolic events, as compared with 4% of control subjects. Other echocardiographic findings in patients with embolic events include LA thrombus in approximately 9%, spontaneous contrast in approximately 17%, and atrial septal aneurysm in 13%. The prevalence of these findings is highest in patients with cryptogenic stroke (e.g., no obvious primary cerebrovascular disease or other etiology). The potential cause-and-effect relationship between some of these echocardiographic findings and clinical embolic events remains controversial as discussed in the Suggested Reading section.

Current ACC/AHA guidelines recommend echocardiography in patients with neurologic or other vascular occlusive events:

- When there is abrupt occlusion of a major peripheral or visceral artery in patients of any age
- In younger patients (<45 years) with a cerebrovascular embolic event
- In older patients with a neurologic event without other evidence of cerebrovascular disease
- In patients in whom the clinical therapeutic decision would be altered based on the echocardiographic results

The use of echocardiography in older patients with cerebrovascular disease of questionable significance or with other evident causes for the cerebrovascular event remains controversial. When appropriate, if TTE studies are unrevealing, TEE imaging should be performed, given its higher sensitivity for diagnosis of a PFO, LA thrombus, interatrial septal aneurysm, valvular vegetation, and small intracardiac tumors.

SUGGESTED READING

General

1. Chen EW, Redberg RF: Echocardiographic evaluation of the patient with a systemic embolic event. In Otto CM (ed): The Practice of Clinical Echocardiography, 3rd ed. Philadelphia: Elsevier/Saunders, 2007, pp 806–828.

   Review of role of echocardiography in management of patients with systemic embolic events. Topics include LA thrombus, spontaneous echo contrast, atrial septal aneurysm, PFO, mitral valve strands, Lambl's excrescences, and aortic atheroma. Includes systematic review of the literature, examples of TTE and TEE findings, and 301 references.

2. McManus BM: Atlas of Cardiovascular Pathology for the Clinician, 2nd ed. Philadelphia: Current Medicine Group, 2008

   Useful pathology atlas with comprehensive coverage of cardiovascular disease, including cardiac tumors.

3. Chaowalit N, Somers VK, Pellikka PA, et al: Adipose tissue of atrial septum as a marker of coronary artery disease. Chest 132:817–822, 2007.

   Lipomatous hypertrophy of the interatrial septum is typically considered a benign incidental finding. However, this study suggests that atrial septal thickening is associated with increased severity of coronary artery disease, even after correction for the effects of age, gender, and body mass index.

4. Dujardin KS, Click RL, Oh JK: The role of intraoperative transesophageal echocardiography in patients undergoing cardiac mass removal. J Am Soc Echocardiogr 13:1080–1083, 2000.

   In 75 consecutive patients undergoing surgery for cardiac mass removal, masses were most often seen in the LA (46%), followed by the RA/inferior vena cava/superior vena cava (27%), LV (8%), and RV (7%), plus 12% that were attached to a valve. The most common causes of masses requiring excision were myxomas (41%), thrombi (16%), fibroelastoma (13%), and hypernephroma (9%). The baseline or post-procedure intraoperative TEE altered management in 16% of cases.

Cardiac Tumors

5. Bruce CJ: Cardiac Tumors. In Otto CM (ed): The Practice of Clinical Echocardiography, 3rd ed. Philadephia: Elsevier/Saunders, 2007, pp 1108–1138.

   This comprehensive textbook chapter includes sections on cardiac myxomas, papillary fibroelastoma, other benign cardiac tumors, malignant primary and secondary cardiac tumors, and the differential diagnosis of a cardiac mass. There are 27 illustrations and 197 references.

6. Shapiro LM, Shapiro LM: Cardiac tumours: Diagnosis and management. Heart 85:218–222, 2001.

   In adults, benign tumors of the heart in order of prevalence are myxoma (45%), lipoma (20%), and papillary fibroelastoma (15%), with fewer cases of angioma, fibroma, hemangioma, rhabdomyoma, or teratoma. However, in children the most common benign cardiac tumor is rhabdomyoma (45%), followed by myxoma, fibroma, and teratoma (15% each).

7. Sun JP, Asher CR, Yang XS, et al: Clinical and echocardiographic characteristics of papillary fibroelastomas: A retrospective and prospective study in 162 patients. Circulation 103:2687, 2001.

   In this series, the average diameter of a cardiac papillary fibroelastoma was 9 ± 4.6 mm; 83% occurred on valves and 44% were mobile.

8. Gowda RM, Khan IA, Nair CK, et al: Cardiac papillary fibroelastoma: A comprehensive analysis of 725 cases. Am Heart J 146:404–410, 2003.

   A comprehensive literature review was used to gather data on clinical and echocardiographic features of papillary fibroelastoma. The attachment site was described in 611 cases: 36% aortic valve, 29% mitral valve, 11% tricuspid valve, and 7% pulmonic valve. The most common attachment site for the 16% nonvalvular papillary fibroelastomas was the LV. The highest prevalence was in adults over age 70 years, with 55% of reported cases in men.

9. Acebo E, Val-Bernal JF, Gómez-Román JJ, Revuelta JM: Clinicopathologic study and DNA analysis of 37 cardiac myxomas: A 28-year experience. Chest 123:1379–1385, 2003.

   The risk of embolization (present in 27%) with a cardiac myxoma was higher with a villous surface. The likelihood of atrial fibrillation (present in 19%) is higher with larger LA tumors.

10. Abraham KP, Reddy V, Gattuso P: Neoplasms metastatic to the heart: Review of 3314 consecutive autopsies. Am J Cardiovasc Pathol 3:195–198, 1990.

    Autopsy study (n = 3314) with malignant disease in 24% (n = 806) and cardiac involvement in 12% of these cases (n = 95). The analysis of frequency of primary tumors was used the as the source of data for Table 15–2.

11. Silvestri F, Bussani R, Pavletic N, Mannone T: Metastases of the heart and pericardium. G Ital Cardiol 27:1252–1255, 1997.

    In a large autopsy series of patients with a malignancy (n = 1928), the rate of cardiac involvement was 8.4%. In men, the highest frequency of cardiac involvement was seen with mesothelioma, melanoma, and lung cancer. In women, melanoma, lung, and renal neoplasms had the highest rates of cardiac involvement.

Left Ventricular Thrombi

12. Stratton JR, Lighty GW Jr, Pearlman AS, Ritchie JL: Detection of left ventricular thrombus by two-dimensional echocardiography: Sensitivity, specificity, and causes of uncertainty. Circulation 66:156–165, 1982.

    In 78 patients with surgical, autopsy, or indium-111 platelet imaging evidence of LV thrombus, the two-dimensional TTE result was positive or equivocal in 21 of the 22 patients with a thrombus (sensitivity 95%) and was negative in 48 of 56 without a thrombus (specificity 86%). A definitely positive echo study had a positive predictive value of only 29%.

13. Srichai MB, Junor C, Rodriguez LL, et al: Clinical, imaging, and pathological characteristics of left ventricular thrombus: A comparison of contrast-enhanced magnetic resonance imaging, transthoracic echocardiography, and transesophageal echocardiography with surgical or pathological validation. Am Heart J 152:75–84, 2006.

    In 361 ischemic heart disease patients with surgical or pathologic confirmation in an LV thrombus was present in 29%. Sensitivity and specificity for contrast-enhanced CMR, TTE, and TEE were evaluated in 160 of these patients who had all three studies.

    Imaging

modality	Sensitivity	Specificity
CMR	88 ± 9%	99 ± 2%
TTE	23 ± 12%	96 ± 3.6%
TEE	40 ± 14%	96 ± 3.6%

   Compared with earlier echocardiographic studies (see Table 15–3), the sensitivity of TTE for detection of LV thrombus was low in this study.

Left Atrial Thrombi

14. Manning WJ, Weintraub RM, Waksmonski CA, et al: Accuracy of transesophageal echocardiography for identifying left atrial thrombi. A prospective, intraoperative study. Ann Intern Med 123:817–822, 1995.

In 231 consecutive patients undergoing intraoperative TEE before elective mitral valve surgery or excision of an LA tumor, the sensitivity (100%) and specificity (99%) of TEE detection of LA thrombus was determined compared to direct visualization by the surgeon.

15. Hwang JJ, Chen JJ, Lin SC, et al: Diagnostic accuracy of transesophageal echocardiography for detecting left atrial thrombi in patients with rheumatic heart disease having undergone mitral valve operations. Am J Cardiol 72:677–681, 1993.

In 213 consecutive patients with rheumatic heart disease undergoing surgery, atrial thrombi were present in 30 of 147 (20%) with predominant mitral stenosis, with 28 of these 30 patients in atrial fibrillation. The specificity of TEE detection of LA thrombus was 100%, with a sensitivity of 93% (two atrial thrombi were missed by imaging). Positive predictive value was 100%, negative predictive value was 99%, and diagnostic accuracy was 99%.

16. Ren JF, Marchlinski FE, Callans DJ: Left atrial thrombus associated with ablation for atrial fibrillation: Identification with intracardiac echocardiography. J Am Coll Cardiol 43:1861–1867, 2004.

Intracardiac echocardiography during ablation procedures allows prompt recognition of atrial thrombus formation, often in association with the ablation catheters. Risk factors for procedural thrombus formation include LA enlargement, persistent atrial fibrillation, and spontaneous echo contrast.

Management of Atrial Fibrillation

17. Manning WJ: The role of echocardiography in atrial fibrillation and flutter. In Otto CM (ed): The Practice of Clinical Echocardiography, 3rd ed. Philadelphia: Elsevier/Saunders, 2007, pp 999–1018.

Review of the literature on LA thrombus formation and the risk of embolic events with cardioversion. Summarizes the clinical approach to the use of echocardiography in management of patients with atrial fibrillation of prolonged or unknown duration. 139 references.

18. Manning WJ, Silberman DI, Gordon SPF, et al: Cardioversion from atrial fibrillation without prolonged anticoagulation with the use of transesophageal echocardiography to exclude the presence of atrial thrombi. N Engl J Med 328:750–755, 1993.

TEE imaging was performed in 119 patients with atrial fibrillation longer than 2 days in duration, who were not receiving long-term anticoagulant therapy and had no contraindications to the TEE procedure. LA thrombi were identified in 12 (13%) patients. In the 78 patients without detectable atrial thrombi and successful conversion to sinus rhythm, none had an embolic event. Most of these patients received short-term heparin therapy before cardioversion and warfarin for 1 month after cardioversion.

19. Goldman ME, Pearce LA, Hart RG, et al: Pathophysiologic correlates of thromboembolism in nonvalvular atrial fibrillation: I. Reduced flow velocity in the left atrial appendage (The Stroke Prevention in Atrial Fibrillation [SPAF-III] study). J Am Soc Echocardiogr 12:1080–1087, 1999.

In 721 patients with nonvalvular atrial fibrillation, an atrial appendage emptying flow velocity less than 20 cm/s was associated with dense spontaneous LA contrast, atrial appendage thrombus, and subsequent embolic events. Clinical predictors of a low atrial appendage emptying velocity include age, blood pressure, sustained atrial fibrillation, ischemic heart disease, and LA size.

20. Asinger RW, Koehler J, Pearce LA, et al: Pathophysiologic correlates of thromboembolism in nonvalvular atrial fibrillation: II. Dense spontaneous echocardiographic contrast (The Stroke Prevention in Atrial Fibrillation [SPAF-III] study). J Am Soc Echocardiogr 12:1088–1096, 1999.

Spontaneous LA echo contrast was present on TEE imaging in 55% of 772 patients with nonvalvular atrial fibrillation, and was dense in 13%. Multivariate predictors of dense spontaneous contrast were age, atrial appendage flow velocity, LA size, aortic atheroma, and a plasma fibrinogen level greater than 350 mg/dL.

21. Hart RG, Halperin JL, Pearce LA, et al, for the Stroke Prevention in Atrial Fibrillation Investigators: Lessons from the Stroke Prevention in Atrial Fibrillation Trials. Ann Intern Med 138:831–838, 2003.

Summary of the three Stroke Prevention in Atrial Fibrillation trials with treatment recommendations. The risk of stroke with aspirin therapy depends on clinical risk factors: about 7% per year in high-risk patients (previous embolic event, systolic blood pressure >160 mm Hg, heart failure, and women >75 years), 2% to 4% per year in moderate-risk patients (hypertension but no high-risk features), and in less than 2% per year low-risk patients (no hypertension or high-risk features).

22. Klein AL, Grimm RA, Jasper SE, et al; ACUTE Steering and Publications Committee for the ACUTE Investigators. Efficacy of transesophageal echocardiography-guided cardioversion of patients with atrial fibrillation at 6 months: A randomized controlled trial. Am Heart J 151:380–389, 2006.

TEE-guided cardioversion was compared to a conventional cardioversion strategy in a multicenter randomized trial of 1222 patients with atrial fibrillation longer than 2 days in duration. With the TEE-guided approach anticoagulation was started at the time of cardioversion and continued for 4 weeks after cardioversion. With the conventional strategy, patients received 3 weeks of therapeutic anticoagulation before and after cardioversion (with no TEE). At 6 months' follow-up there was no difference between groups in overall mortality (3% to 4%) or embolic events (1% to 2%). However, in the TEE-guided group there was a lower risk of hemorrhagic complications (4.4% vs. 7.5%) and a higher prevalence of sinus rhythm at 6 months (63% vs. 54%, p = 0.03).

Cardiac Source of Embolus

23. de Bruijn SF, Agema WR, Lammers GJ, et al: Transesophageal echocardiography is superior to transthoracic echocardiography in management of patients of any age with transient ischemic attack or stroke. Stroke 37:2531–2534, 2006.

In 231 consecutive patients with recent cryptogenic stroke or transient ischemic attack, a potential cardiac source of embolus was identified in 55%; 90 of these 127 findings (71%) were seen on TEE but not TTE. The most common major risk factors for embolic events was atrial appendage thrombus in 38/231(16%), with other major risk factors including dilated cardiomyopathy in 5 patients (2%) and LV thrombus in 2 patients(1%). Minor risk factors for embolic events were aortic atherosclerosis in 69 (30%), PFO in 15 (6%), spontaneous echo contrast in 7 (3%), and atrial septal aneurysm in 13 (5%). Cardiac sources were detected in both younger and older patients at equal rates.

24. Fatkin D, Kelly RP, Feneley MP: Relations between left atrial appendage blood flow velocity, spontaneous echocardiography contrast and

thromboembolic risk in vivo. J Am Coll Cardiol 23:961–969, 1994.

In 140 patients with atrial fibrillation, LA spontaneous contrast was present in 78 (56%) patients and LA thrombus was present in 15 (11%) patients. On multivariate analysis, spontaneous echo contrast was the only significant predictor for the presence of thrombus. LA appendage velocity was negatively associated with the degree of spontaneous contrast, and an appendage velocity less than 35 cm/s was associated with a 30 times higher risk of spontaneous contrast.

25. Homma S, Sacco RL, Di Tullio MR, et al, for the PFO in Cryptogenic Stroke Study (PICSS) Investigators: Effect of medical treatment in stroke patients with patent foramen ovale: Patent foramen ovale in cryptogenic stroke study. Circulation 105:2625–2631, 2002.

In a multicenter randomized trial, 630 stroke patients were randomized to treatment with aspirin or warfarin after evaluation by TEE. A PFO was present in 34%, but there was no difference in clinical events comparing those with and without a PFO, in those with large versus small PFOs, or PFOs associated with an atrial septal aneurysm. In patients with PFO there was no difference in clinical outcomes in those treated with aspirin versus warfarin.

26. Natanzon A, Goldman ME: Patent foramen ovale: Anatomy versus pathophysiology–which determines stroke risk? J Am Soc Echocardiogr 16:71–76, 2003.

In a retrospective study of 78 patients with a PFO detected on TEE, patients with a clinical embolic event (compared with those without) had greater contrast shunting from right to left and had less overlap between the septum primum and septum secundum (7.5 ± 3.4 mm vs. 9.9 ± 6.0 mm, p = 0.26). There was no difference in the size of the separation between the septum primum and secundum or in the presence of atrial septal aneurysm. Evidence for elevation of LA pressure was more common in

those without an embolic event, raising the possibility that hemodynamics, not anatomy, determines stroke risk in patients with a PFO.

27. Slottow TL, Steinberg DH, Waksman R: Overview of the 2007 Food and Drug Administration Circulatory System Devices Panel meeting on patent foramen ovale closure devices. Circulation 116:677–682, 2007.

Prospective randomized trials of PFO closure to prevent recurrent cryptogenic stroke are in progress, but enrollment has been slow, no study has been completed and no device is approved for this indication. The U.S. Food and Drug Administration convened a panel to discuss the obstacles to completion of a randomized trial. This article also provides a concise summary of the literature and a comprehensive list of references. The final recommendation of the panel was to support the AHS/ASA guideline that all eligible patients be encouraged to enroll in a randomized trial.

28. Di Tullio MR, Sacco RL, Sciacca RR, et al: Patent foramen ovale and the risk of ischemic stroke in a multiethnic population. J Am Coll Cardiol 49:797–802, 2007.

In the Northern Manhattan Study (NOMAS), PFO was present on TTE saline contrast echocardiography in 164/1100 (14.9%) adults over age 39 years, and an atrial septal aneurysm was present in 27 (2.5%) subjects (19 in association with PFO). The presence of PFO was not associated with an increased risk of ischemic stroke, which occurred in 68 subjects (6.2%) at a mean follow-up of 79.7 ± 28.0 months.

29. Handke M, Harloff A, Olschewski M, et al: Patent foramen ovale and cryptogenic stroke in older patients. N Engl J Med 357:2262–2268, 2007.

In 503 consecutive patients with stroke, the prevalence of PFO was higher in the 227 with cryptogenic stroke as compared with the 276 with stroke of known cause, both in the patient group younger and older than 55 years of age. On multivariate analysis the presence of a PFO was independently associated with stroke risk

with an odds ratio of 3.7 (95% confidence interval [CI] 1.42–9.65) in younger and 3.00 (95% CI 1.73–5.23) in older adults.

30. Roldan CA, Shively BK, Crawford MH: Valve excrescences: Prevalence, evolution and risk for cardioembolism. J Am Coll Cardiol 30:1308–1314, 1997.

Valve excrescences (thin, elongated, mobile structures attached near the leaflet closure line) are seen in approximately 40% of normal individuals on TEE and do not appear to be associated with an increased risk of thromboembolism.

31. Ward RP, Don CW, Furlong KT, et al: Predictors of long-term mortality in patients with ischemic stroke referred for transesophageal echocardiography. Stroke 37:204–208, 2006.

The only TEE finding predictive of long-term mortality (19% after about 3 years) after an ischemic stroke in 245 consecutive patients was the severity of aortic atherosclerosis. Other TEE findings were common, with a PFO in 19%, thrombus in 2.4%, spontaneous echo contrast in 3.7%, atrial septal aneurysm in 3.3%, valve masses in 7.8%; but none of these predicted long-term outcome. Complex aortic atheroma, present in 14.7%, was associated with a hazard ratio of 2.7 (95% CI 1.4–5.3) for long-term mortality. The definition of complex aortic atheroma was protrusion ≥4 mm into the aortic lumen, or plaque with evidence of ulceration or mobility.

32. Kronzon I, Tunick PA: Aortic atherosclerotic disease and stroke. Circulation 114:63–75, 2006.

This review article summarizes the literature on the association between aortic atheroma and stroke. Aortic atheroma also is associated with atherosclerosis in other vascular beds (carotid, coronary, renal, abdominal aorta), aortic stenosis, mitral annular calcification, and atrial fibrillation. The role of imaging with different modalities is summarized including TTE and TEE, epiaortic scanning, CMR, and CT.

16 Diseases of the Great Arteries

E chocardiographic evaluation of the aorta and main pulmonary artery is a routine part of the standard echocardiographic examination. For descriptive purposes, the aorta is divided into segments, beginning at the aortic valve, including the:

❐ Aortic annulus
❐ Sinuses of Valsalva
❐ Sinotubular junction
❐ Ascending aorta
❐ Aortic arch
❐ Descending thoracic aorta
❐ Proximal abdominal aorta

The base of the aorta at the origin from the left ventricle (LV) often is colloquially called the "aortic root." Unfortunately, "aortic root" has a variable definition so that this term can lead to errors in communication. In studies of genetic diseases of the great vessels, aortic root usually refers to the aortic sinuses, from the valve level to the sinotubular junction. However, a surgical aortic root replacement typically extends from the aortic annulus to the mid-ascending aorta. Thus, when the aorta is abnormal, more specific terms describing anatomic location are preferred.

Evaluation of the aortic annulus and sinuses is a routine component of an echocardiographic study. In addition, further evaluation of the ascending aorta, arch, and descending aorta can be performed when disease is suspected clinically. Transthoracic (TTE)

images often are suboptimal due to overlying or adjacent air-filled structures, so transesophageal (TEE) imaging greatly enhances the diagnostic utility of echocardiography for diseases of the aorta.

BASIC PRINCIPLES

Aortic abnormalities include:

❐ Dilation
❐ Aneurysm
❐ Dissection
❐ Sinus of Valsalva aneurysm
❐ Atherosclerosis

The most common abnormality of the aorta is *dilation*, or an increase in diameter greater than expected for age and body size. Dilation of the ascending aorta occurs in a variety of diseases. When aortic dilation is severe, the term *aneurysm* is used. Aneurysms can involve one or more segments of the aorta (ascending, arch, and descending) and may be tubular or saccular in configuration.

Aortic dilation due to hypertension or atherosclerosis is characterized by normal contours of the sinuses of Valsalva and narrowing at the sinotubular junction, with enlargement primarily in the ascending aorta. A bicuspid aortic valve (BAV) often is accompanied by dilation of the aortic sinuses or ascending aorta,

397

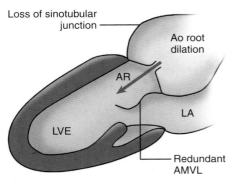

Figure 16–1 Schematic diagram of the typical 2D echo findings in Marfan syndrome as seen in a long-axis view. The proximal aorta is markedly dilated with effacement of the sinotubular junction. Aortic annular dilation results in inadequate aortic leaflet apposition with a central jet of aortic regurgitation (AR) and consequent LV enlargement (LVE). Often the anterior mitral leaflet (AMVL) is long and redundant.

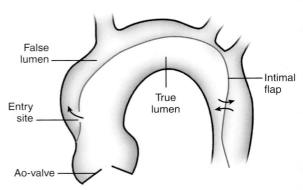

Figure 16–2 Schematic diagram of an aortic dissection showing an entry site above the sinotubular junction into a false lumen. In real time, the intimal flap shows rapid undulating motion, independent of the cardiac cycle. As indicated by the *arrows* across the intimal flap in the descending aorta, multiple flow communications between the true and false lumens may be seen with color flow imaging.

depending on the bicuspid valve leaflet orientation, but some narrowing at the sinotubular junction usually is preserved. Inherited connective tissue disorders that cause aneurysms of the ascending aorta, such as Marfan syndrome and Loeys-Dietz syndrome, are characterized by effacement of the sinotubular junction and enlargement of the sinuses of Valsalva, as well as dilation of the ascending aorta, resulting in a "water balloon" appearance of the proximal aorta (Fig. 16–1). Systemic inflammatory disease such as rheumatoid arthritis and ankylosing spondylitis are associated with aortic aneurysms and often affect the valve tissue as well. Aneurysms also may be seen in tertiary syphilis (with a characteristic pattern of calcification), aortic arteritis (such as Takayasu arteritis), and as a result of blunt or penetrating chest trauma. Large aortic aneurysms are prone to rupture, so prophylactic repair often is recommended.

An *aortic dissection* is a life-threatening situation in which an intimal tear in the aortic wall allows passage of blood into a "false" channel between the intima and the media (Fig. 16–2). This false channel may be localized or may propagate downstream, often in a spiral fashion, due to the pressure of blood flow in the channel. Complications related to the false lumen include:

❐ Expansion with compression of the true aortic lumen (which supplies major branch vessels)
❐ Propagation down major branch vessels
❐ Thrombosis
❐ Rupture

An accurate, rapid diagnosis of the presence or absence of aortic dissection and the site of the entry tear is crucial in the treatment of patients with suspected dissection.

In patients presenting with an aortic dissection, the most prevalent risk factors for aortic dissection are hypertension and atherosclerosis. However, patient

groups with the highest risk of aortic dissection include those with Marfan syndrome and other inherited connective tissue disorders, Turner's syndrome, aortitis, and vascular-type Ehlers-Danlos syndrome. There also is a fivefold increased risk of aortic dissection in patients with a congenital bicuspid or unicuspid aortic valve. Dissection is more likely in patients with a preexisting aneurysm, although dissection can occur in the absence of dilation in patients with Marfan syndrome.

Sinus of Valsalva aneurysms (Fig. 16–3) may be congenital or may be due to infection, Marfan syndrome, or previous surgical procedures. A sinus of Valsalva aneurysm protrudes into adjacent chambers and may be associated with a fistula. Specifically,

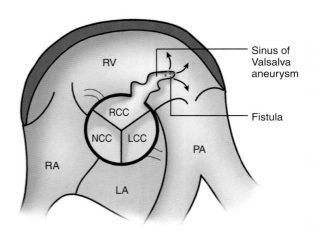

Figure 16–3 Schematic diagram of a congenital sinus of Valsalva aneurysm. A long "wind sock"–like membranous outpouching of the right coronary cusp (RCC) protrudes into the RV outflow tract. If there are fenestrations in the aneurysm, an Ao-to-RV fistula is seen. Note that an aneurysm of the left coronary cusp (LCC) would protrude into the LA, whereas an aneurysm of the right coronary cusp (RCC) would protrude into the RA.

an aneurysm of the right coronary sinus protrudes into the right ventricular (RV) outflow tract, the left coronary sinus into the left atrium (LA), and the non-coronary sinus into the right atrium (RA).

Atherosclerosis of the aorta may lead to dilation, aneurysm, or dissection. In addition, the presence of atheroma may be important as a marker for coexisting coronary artery disease and as a potential source of embolic cerebrovascular events.

ECHOCARDIOGRAPHIC APPROACH

Transthoracic Imaging of the Aorta

Two-dimensional and Doppler Echocardiography

On TTE imaging the *proximal ascending aorta* is well seen in parasternal long- and short-axis views (Fig. 16–4). Depending on ultrasound penetration, images of additional segments of the ascending aorta may be obtained by moving the transducer cephalad one or more interspaces. Image quality is enhanced by positioning the patient in a steep left lateral decubitus position, bringing the aorta in contact with the

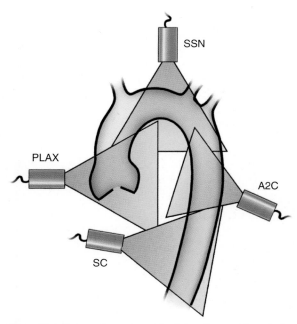

Figure 16–4 The use of several acoustic windows for complete evaluation of the aorta from a transcutaneous approach is shown. From a parasternal long-axis (PLAX) window, the sinuses and a segment of the ascending aorta are seen. From the suprasternal notch (SSN) window, the arch and proximal descending thoracic aorta are seen; from a posteriorly angulated apical two-chamber (A2C) approach, the midsegment of the descending thoracic aorta is seen; and from a subcostal (SC) approach, the distal thoracic aorta and proximal abdominal aorta are seen. In some individuals the segment of ascending aorta between the standard PLAX and SSN views can be imaged from a high parasternal position. However, in other patients, this segment of the aorta is "missed" on TTE imaging.

anterior chest wall (Figs. 16–5 and 16–6). Doppler interrogation of the ascending aorta from the parasternal approach is limited to qualitative evaluation of the flow pattern in the proximal aorta and assessment of aortic regurgitation severity (if present) given the non-parallel intercept angle from this position. The ascending aorta also may be imaged from the apical approach in an anteriorly angulated four-chamber view and in an apical long-axis view. While two-dimensional (2D) image quality may be limited at the depth of the ascending aorta from the apical approach, this view does allow a parallel intercept angle between the Doppler beam and the direction of blood flow. In some individuals, images of the ascending aorta can be obtained from the subcostal approach.

The *aortic arch* is imaged from a suprasternal notch or supraclavicular approach with the patient in a supine position with the neck extended. Both longitudinal (Fig. 16–7) and transverse views of the arch are obtainable in nearly all individuals. Usually only a short segment of the ascending aorta is visible from the suprasternal notch window, but this is variable among patients. Also note that the descending aorta appears to taper due to an oblique image plane with respect to its curvature (i.e., the descending aorta is only partially in the image plane).

Pulsed- or continuous-wave Doppler recordings of descending aortic flow from the suprasternal notch show systolic flow away from the transducer at a velocity of approximately 1 m/s. Normal flow in the descending aortic shows:

❏ Brief, low-velocity, early-diastolic flow reversal
❏ Low-velocity antegrade flow in mid-diastole
❏ Low-velocity flow reversal at end-diastole

The use of low wall filter settings is needed to appreciate this normal flow pattern (Fig. 16–8).

Although 2D imaging of the ascending aorta is suboptimal from the suprasternal approach, high-quality Doppler flow signals may be obtained because the Doppler beam is aligned parallel to flow. Antegrade flow toward the transducer in systole is seen, the reciprocal of the ascending aortic flow signal recorded from the apex.

The *descending thoracic aorta* is seen in cross-section posterior to the LA in the parasternal long-axis view. A longitudinal section of this segment of the descending aorta may be obtained by clockwise rotation and lateral angulation of the transducer. From the suprasternal notch approach, a small portion of the descending thoracic aorta is seen. From the apical two-chamber view a longitudinal section of a segment of the descending aorta is seen by lateral angulation and clockwise rotation of the transducer (Fig. 16–9). Doppler investigation of descending thoracic aortic flow is most easily performed from the suprasternal notch long-axis view. Flow abnormalities may be related to aortic disease

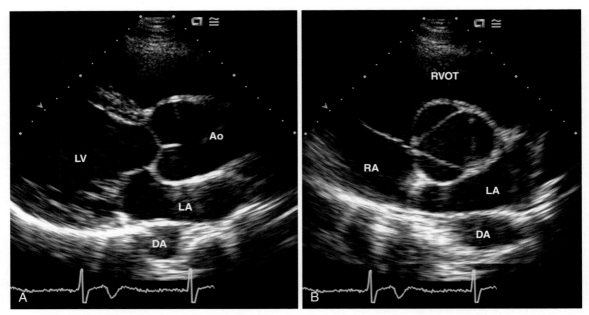

Figure 16–5 A, Parasternal long-axis view in a patient with Marfan syndrome showing dilated sinuses with effacement of the sinotubular junction. In short axis (**B**), the trileaflet valve in systole is stretched so the orifice is triangular, instead of the normal circular opening. DA, descending aorta; RVOT, RV outflow tract.

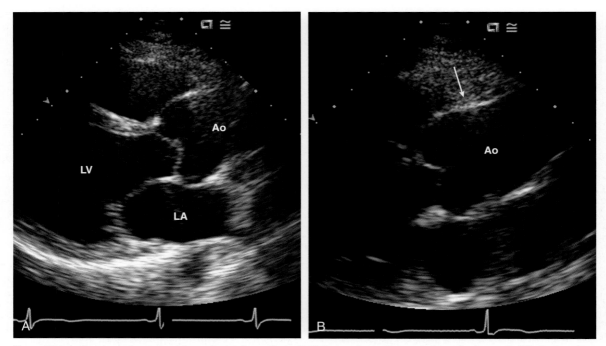

Figure 16–6 A, The standard parasternal long-axis view in a patient with Marfan syndrome shows only the aortic sinuses. **B,** With the transducer moved up one interspace, the loss of the normal contour of the sinotubular junction (*arrow*) and more of the ascending aorta are seen.

(e.g., coarctation), shunts (e.g., patent ductus arteriosus), or aortic valve disease (e.g., regurgitation).

From the subcostal approach the *distal thoracic* and *proximal abdominal aorta* is seen as it traverses the diaphragm. From this approach, the angle between the transducer and the aorta allows Doppler interrogation of antegrade flow (Fig. 16–10).

Thus, by combining images from multiple acoustic windows, visualization of much of the ascending aorta, arch, and descending thoracic aorta is possible

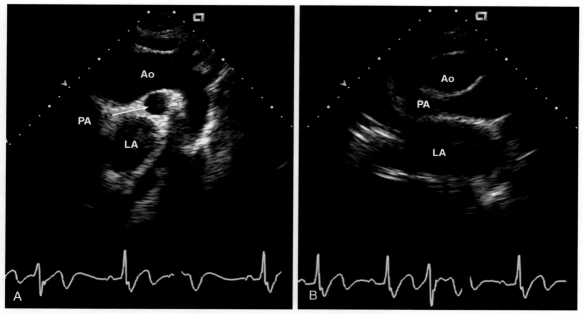

Figure 16–7 Suprasternal notch view in the long axis (*left*) of the Ao in a normal individual showing the ascending Ao, arch, and descending aorta with the right pulmonary artery (PA, *arrow*) in short axis and the LA inferiorly. The short-axis suprasternal notch view (*right*) shows the Ao arch, PA, and LA.

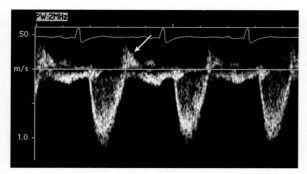

Figure 16–8 Normal pulsed Doppler recording of flow in the descending thoracic aorta from a suprasternal notch long-axis view. Antegrade flow in systole has a maximum velocity of 1.1 m/s with a normal systolic ejection curve. In diastole there is brief early-diastolic flow reversal (*arrow*), followed by low-velocity antegrade flow in mid-diastole and absence of flow (or low-velocity reversal) in end-diastole.

using TTE imaging. In patients with a left pleural effusion, images of the aorta can be obtained by imaging through the fluid from the left posterior chest (paraspinal) with the patient in a right lateral decubitus position.

Limitations of Transthoracic Imaging of the Aorta

The major limitations of the transthoracic approach to ultrasound evaluation of the aorta are acoustic access and image quality. In many individuals, acoustic access is suboptimal or minimal from one or more

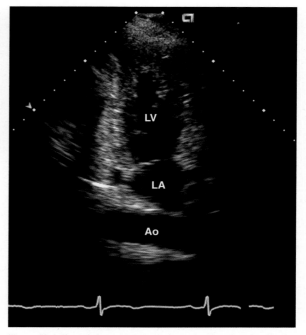

Figure 16–9 Posteriorly angulated apical two-chamber view showing the descending thoracic aorta (Ao) along its long axis in a patient with Marfan syndrome and prior aortic root replacement for type A dissection.

of the windows needed for full evaluation of the aorta, leaving "gaps" in the echocardiographic examination. Even when acoustic access is adequate, image quality often is poor due to beam width at

Figure 16-10 Subcostal view of the proximal abdominal aorta with color Doppler (*top*). The pulsed Doppler signal (*bottom*) shows normal antegrade flow toward the transducer in systole, followed by brief early-diastolic flow reversal and slight antegrade flow in mid-diastole.

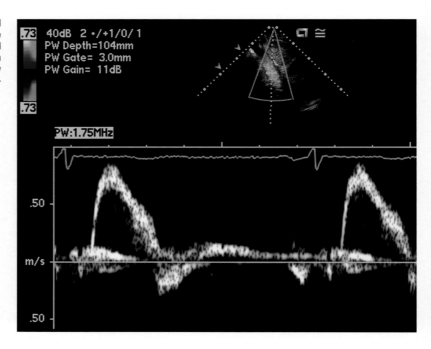

the depth of the aorta—particularly the descending thoracic aorta from apical and parasternal windows. Beam-width artifact, noise, and poor lateral resolution make differentiation of intraluminal defects from artifacts difficult. Because of these limitations, TEE is a more appropriate diagnostic test in patients with suspected aortic disease.

Transesophageal Imaging

Two-dimensional Echocardiography

The aortic valve, *sinuses of Valsalva*, and *ascending aorta* are seen in an oblique image plane with the transducer at 0° rotation from a high esophageal probe position. A short-axis view at the aortic valve level is obtained by rotating the image plane to approximately 45°, with a short-axis view of the proximal few centimeters of the ascending aorta obtained by slight withdrawal of the probe in the esophagus. In the short-axis plane, evaluation of more distal segments of the ascending aorta is obscured by the position of the air-filled trachea between the esophagus (and transducer) and the ascending aorta. However, by rotating the image plane to approximately 120°, a long-axis view of the aortic valve, sinus of Valsalva, and ascending aorta can be obtained in most patients (Fig. 16-11). More cephalad segments of the ascending aorta may be seen by slowly moving the transducer to a higher esophageal position.

The *aortic arch* is best imaged from a high esophageal position. Starting with a short-axis view of the descending thoracic aorta, the probe is withdrawn to the level of the arch and then the entire probe is turned toward the patient's right and angulated inferiorly to obtain a long-axis view of the arch. In some patients, images of the aortic arch may be suboptimal due to the positions of the trachea and bronchi. In many cases, transthoracic suprasternal notch views of the arch provide superior image quality.

The *descending thoracic* and *proximal abdominal aorta* are well seen by the TEE approach. The descending thoracic aorta lies immediately lateral and slightly posterior to the esophagus, so that posterior rotation of the probe provides excellent images in either a cross-sectional (transverse plane at 0°) or long-axis (at 90° to 120°) view (Figs. 16-12 and 16-13). Slight turning of the TEE probe is needed at different levels as the aorta curves relative to the esophagus. From a transgastric position, the proximal abdominal aorta is seen posterior to the stomach. Many examiners prefer to examine the length of the aorta in sequential cross-sectional views as the probe is slowly withdrawn from the stomach and esophagus, with imaging of the aortic arch just before probe removal. Any areas of abnormality can then be further examined in long-axis views.

Doppler Flows

Color flow imaging of the aorta shows the normal antegrade flow pattern in the ascending aorta and arch. Although from the TEE approach, the direction of blood flow in the descending aorta is nearly perpendicular to the direction of the ultrasound beam, flow signals often can be recorded from a long-axis plane

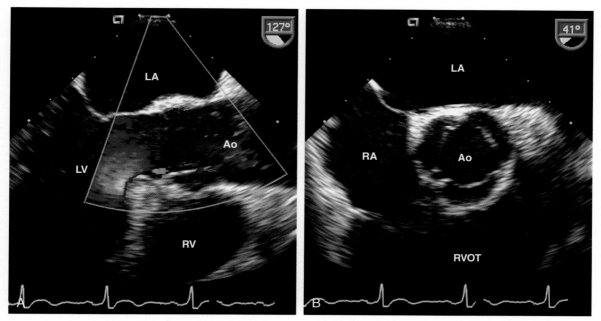

Figure 16–11 Normal ascending aorta seen on TEE imaging in long-axis view (**A**) at about 120° rotation and in the short-axis view (**B**) at about 30° to 40° rotation. Both image planes are aligned to the cardiac landmarks, analogous to TTE views, with the exact degree of rotation varying between patients.

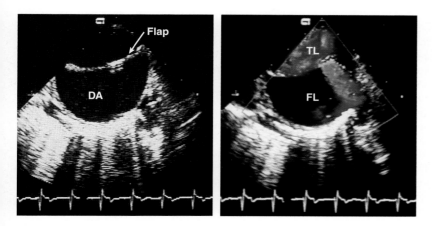

Figure 16–12 On TEE imaging, a 2D view (*left*) of the descending thoracic aorta (DA) shows a dissection flap (*arrow*), with flow between the true (TL) and false lumens (FL) seen on color flow imaging (*right*).

with the Doppler beam aligned at the distal end of the aorta. This approach probably underestimates velocity because of the nonparallel intercept angle but is useful to evaluate flow patterns, such as holodiastolic flow reversal with aortic regurgitation.

In short-axis views, normal aortic flow appears to show a hemicylindrical swirling pattern, with red in one half and blue in the other half of a cross-sectional view of descending aorta. Flow in the ascending aorta sometimes can be recorded from a transgastric "apical" view, but underestimation of flow velocity due to a nonparallel intercept angle should be considered. Alternatively, ascending aortic flow can be recorded from a very high TEE probe position looking down the ascending aorta.

CLINICAL UTILITY

Chronic Aortic Dilation

Aortic dilation often is first recognized on the chest radiograph or on an echocardiographic examination requested for other reasons. In specific clinical settings, such as Marfan syndrome, aortic dilation is an expected consequence of a systemic disease. In these cases, echocardiography is requested to assess the presence and degree of aortic abnormality. In patients with a bicuspid aortic valve, aortic dimension should be routinely measured (Fig. 16–14).

Measurements of aortic diameter on echocardiography are accurate and reproducible when care is

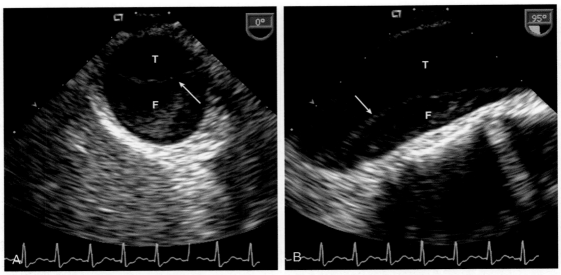

Figure 16–13 TEE images of the descending aorta show a dissection flap with spontaneous contrast in the false (F) lumen due to low flow in both short- (**A**) and long-axis (**B**) views. T, true lumen.

taken to obtain a true short-axis dimension (nonoblique), gain settings are appropriate, and standard measurement conventions (white-black interface on 2D images) are used. In patients with aortic dilation, it is important to measure aortic diameter at several locations and to specify the measurement site and timing in the cardiac cycle. The aorta is pulsatile with the change in dimension from end-diastole to end-systole depending on the aortic compliance. Aortic compliance may be significantly altered in different disease states, but a typical normal change in aortic diameter during the cardiac cycle is 2 to 3 mm. End-systolic measurements often are utilized in children. However, in adults, measurements are most reliable at end-diastole because timing in the cardiac cycle (onset of the QRS) is reproducible and because end-diastolic measurements are least affected by aortic compliance or loading conditions.

Measurements are made at *end-diastole* at the:

❏ Aortic annulus (the site used for LV outflow tract diameter measurement)
❏ Aortic sinuses leaflet tip level (the standard position of an M-mode of the aortic valve)
❏ Sinotubular junction
❏ Ascending aorta
❏ Aortic arch
❏ Descending thoracic aorta (Fig. 16–15)

While all these measurements are not needed in every patient, quantitative evaluation of the extent and severity of aortic dilation is extremely useful in follow-up and treatment of patients with chronic, progressive aortic dilation. Each measurement is made from the black/white interface on a freeze-frame end-diastolic image, averaging several beats to ensure a consistent measurement. Aortic annulus

diameter is measured at the insertion of the base of the valve leaflets in the long-axis view. The maximum aortic sinus dimension typically is measured in a long-axis view, but short-axis views also may be useful when anatomy is asymmetric. Note that M-mode sinus dimensions are measured at the tips of the aortic valve leaflets using a leading-edge–to–leading-edge convention. The sinotubular junction is measured at the point where the curved sinus contour meets the tubular ascending aorta. The ascending aorta is measured at the maximum dimension with notation of the distance from the aortic valve. The aortic arch is measured in its midsection and the descending aorta is measured in the midthoracic region.

The maximum aortic measurement is compared to the predicted (or expected) aortic dimension (Ao $D_{predicted}$) using empirically derived regression equations (Suggested Reading 19) to account for the effects of age and body surface area (BSA in m^2) on normal aortic dimensions:

Children (<18 years):
  Ao $D_{predicted} = 1.02 + (0.98 \text{ BSA})$

Adults (age 18–40 years):
  Ao $D_{predicted} = 0.97 + (1.12 \text{ BSA})$

Adults (>40 years):
  Ao $D_{predicted} = 1.92 + (0.74 \text{ BSA})$

The echo report includes the actual and expected measurements in millimeters; the ratio of the actual to expected aortic diameter (where 1.0 is normal) may also be included. In children, measurements are normalized for age and body size using Z-scores, based on the standard deviation from mean normal values.

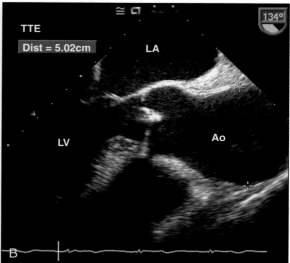

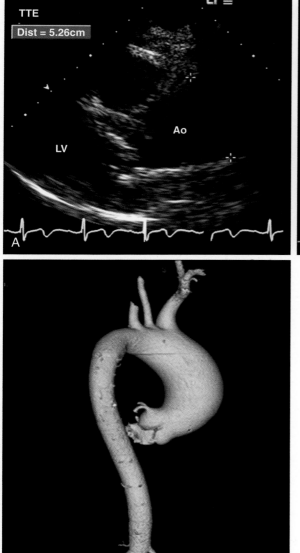

Figure 16–14 A, TTE imaging in a patient with a bicuspid aortic valve shows dilation of the ascending aorta with a maximum dimension at end-diastole of 5.26 cm. **B,** TEE images confirm dilation of the ascending aorta, although dimension is slightly underestimated due to a slightly oblique image plane. **C,** Three-dimensional reconstruction of the contrast CT images shows the location and severity of aortic dilation, but the timing of measurements during the cardiac cycle may not exactly match the echocardiographic data.

Sequential TTE studies of the degree of aortic dilation are used to observe patients with Marfan syndrome or other causes of aortic aneurysm. Prophylactic ascending aorta and valve replacement may be recommended when the degree of ascending aortic dilation reaches a critical range, typically in the range of 5.0 cm for aortic dilation associated with a bicuspid valve, 4.5 cm for Marfan syndrome, and even lower for some inherited conditions, such as Loeys-Dietz syndrome. Thus, careful measurements on sequential studies are needed to assess whether the dilation is progressive or stable over time and to determine the optimal timing of surgical intervention. TTE imaging is appropriate for nonurgent serial evaluation in most patients, although additional evaluation with computed tomography (CT) or cardiac magnetic resonance (CMR) imaging is also considered appropriate.

Aortic Dissection

Transthoracic Imaging

EVALUATION OF THE AORTA. A TTE examination for aortic dissection includes evaluation of the:

❑ Ascending aorta from the standard and high parasternal windows
❑ Aortic arch from the suprasternal notch window

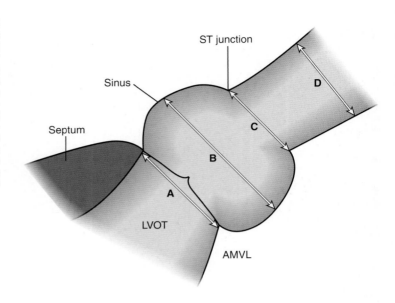

Figure 16–15 Schematic diagram of the sinuses and ascending aorta showing the possible sites for aortic diameter measurement. LV outflow tract (LVOT) diameter is measured in systole (**A**) when used for transaortic stroke volume calculations or for calculation of valve area in the continuity equation. Measurements of the aorta are made at end-diastole at the sinuses (**B**), the sinotubular (ST) junction (**C**), and in the mid-ascending aorta (**D**). The site of measurement should be specified in the echocardiographic report. Two-dimensional measurements are made from inner edge to inner edge of the white/black interface. M-mode measurements of the aorta usually correspond to the sinus diameter. The term *aortic root* may refer either to the sinuses or the entire aorta from the valve plane to the arch. AMVL, anterior mitral valve leaflet.

□ Descending aorta from parasternal and apical windows

□ Proximal abdominal aorta from a subcostal approach

When a left pleural effusion is present, the descending thoracic aorta can be imaged through the effusion with the transducer positioned on the left posterior chest wall.

The echocardiographic diagnosis of aortic dissection (Fig. 16–16) is most secure when there is:

□ A dilated aortic lumen

□ A linear, mobile echogenic structure with a pattern of motion different from the aortic wall

□ Different color Doppler flow patterns in the true and false lumen

When a definite, undulating intimal flap is seen, the specificity of TTE for diagnosis of dissection is high (Table 16–1). However, beam-width artifact and reverberations can be mistaken for intraluminal structures by an inexperienced observer, resulting in a specificity of less than 100%, particularly when the images are not "classic" or image quality is suboptimal.

Conversely, the sensitivity of TTE for aortic dissection is quite low (i.e., the inability to demonstrate an internal flap does not reliably exclude the diagnosis). This low sensitivity is due to poor image quality, particularly of the segment of ascending aorta between the sinotubular junction and the aortic arch, and the poor far-field resolution of the descending thoracic aorta from the transthoracic approach.

Even when the TTE does not show a dissection flap, indirect signs of aortic dissection may be present. These include aortic dilation, aortic regurgitation, a pericardial effusion, or a regional wall motion abnormality.

Figure 16–16 Transthoracic parasternal long-axis view (*left*) shows a dilated ascending aorta with a linear echo (*long arrow*) posterior to the aortic valve leaflets (*small arrows*), which showed motion independent of the aortic walls consistent with a dissection flap. Color flow Doppler (*right*) shows flow only in the true lumen, with no flow seen in the false lumen (FL) in this view.

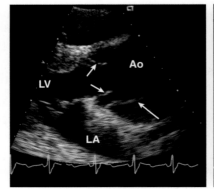
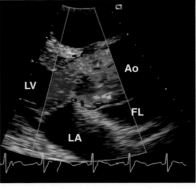

TABLE 16–1   Diagnosis of Aortic Dissection

First Author and Year	n	Approach	Sensitivity	Specificity	Standard of Reference
Victor 1981	42	TTE	80% (12/15)	96% (26/27)	Angio
Erbel 1987	21	TTE TEE	29% (6/21) 100% (21/21)	All had dissection	Surgery or angio
Hashimoto 1989	22	TTE TEE CT	71% (15/21) 100% (22/22) 100% (8/8)	All had dissection	Angio (17) and/or surgery (12)
Ballal 1991	61	TEE CT	97% (33/34) 67% (16/24)	100% (27/27) 100% (7/7)	Angio, surgery, or autopsy
Nienaber 1992	53	TTE TEE CMR	83% (26/31) 100% (31/31) 100% (31/31)	63% (14/22) 66% (15/22) 100% (22/22)	Surgery, autopsy, or angio
Nienaber 1993	110	TTE TEE CMR CT	59% (37/62) 98% (43/44) 98% (58/59) 94% (45/48)	83% (39/48) 98% (25/26) 87% (27/31) 83% (38/46)	Surgery (62), autopsy (7), and/or angio (64)

Angio, angiography; CMR, cardiac magnetic resonance; CT, computed tomography; MRI, magnetic resonance imaging; TTE, transthoracic echocardiography; TEE, transesophageal echocardiography.

Data from Victor et al: Am J Cardiol 48:1155–1159, 1981; Erbel et al: Br Heart J 58:45–51, 1987; Hashimoto et al: J Am Coll Cardiol 14:1253–1262, 1989; Ballal et al: Circulation 84:1903–1914, 1991; Nienaber et al: Circulation 85:434–447, 1992; Nienaber et al: N Engl J Med 328:1–9, 1993.

These abnormalities do not confirm a diagnosis of dissection, because there are many other causes for these findings. However, the presence or absence of these findings may weigh the clinical evidence toward or away from a diagnosis of dissection and may prompt additional imaging studies.

COMPLICATIONS OF AORTIC DISSECTION. Complications of aortic dissection can be recognized on echocardiography and have important clinical implications both for diagnosis and therapy. Complications of aortic dissection (Fig. 16–17) include:

❑ Acute aortic regurgitation
❑ Coronary ostial occlusion
❑ Distal vessel obstruction
❑ Pericardial effusion
❑ Aortic rupture (pleural effusion, mediastinal hematoma)

Aortic regurgitation is nearly always present, with either chronic regurgitation due to aortic dilation or associated valve abnormalities or acute regurgitation due to further aortic dilation or to inadequate leaflet support due to retrograde extension of the dissection. In extreme cases, a flail aortic leaflet may be seen due to the dissection disrupting the normal attachment of the commissure to the aortic wall.

Coronary artery ostial occlusion can occur as a result of the dissection flap separating the coronary artery from normal blood flow or by compression of

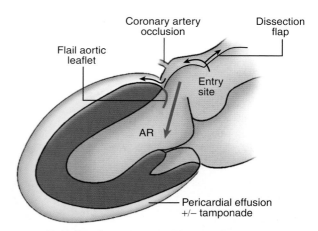

Figure 16–17 Potential complications of dissection of the ascending aorta are shown schematically. If the dissection proceeds retrograde (as well as antegrade) from the entry site, the false lumen can cause (1) occlusion in the coronary artery ostium with resultant myocardial infarction, (2) loss of support of an aortic leaflet with consequent severe aortic regurgitation (AR), or (3) rupture into the pericardium, which may result in tamponade physiology.

the vessel. The resultant wall motion abnormalities—inferior for right coronary obstruction, anterolateral for left main obstruction—are easily recognized on echocardiography. The diagnostic difficulty in this situation is recognizing that the wall motion abnormalities are a secondary event due to aortic dissection rather than the primary event (e.g., acute myocardial infarction due to coronary thrombosis).

Distal vessel obstructions rarely will be recognized during the cardiac ultrasound examination. However, the possibility of aortic dissection should be considered in patients with distal vessel obstructions referred for echocardiography to rule out a cardiac source of embolus. The correct diagnosis of distal vessel obstruction due to a dissection flap (rather than an embolus) may be made by the astute echocardiographer.

Aortic dissections can rupture in one of several ways. *External* rupture into the mediastinum or pleural space often results in exsanguination with acute hemodynamic collapse. If the rupture *thromboses*, the patient may exhibit a mediastinal hematoma and/or pleural effusion (more often left than right). Alternatively, the dissection can rupture at the aortic annulus into the pericardial space. Again, uncontrolled rupture leads to an acute pericardial effusion with tamponade and rapid hemodynamic collapse. However, a partial rupture or a leak may result in a smaller pericardial effusion. Obviously, the presence of any amount of pericardial fluid in a patient with an aortic dissection is an alarming sign and should prompt rapid intervention.

ECHOCARDIOGRAPHIC DIFFERENTIAL DIAGNOSIS. In most cases where TTE is requested to rule out aortic dissection, the differential diagnosis is broad, with aortic dissection being one of many (and often the least likely) possible diagnoses. Thus, if the echocardiographic appearance of the aorta is normal, echocardiographic examination for other possible etiologies of chest pain is needed, including:

❐ Coronary artery disease (e.g., wall motion abnormalities)
❐ Valvular disease (e.g., aortic stenosis)
❐ Pulmonary embolus
❐ Pericarditis

When the clinical suspicion of aortic dissection is low to intermediate, a normal aorta on echocardiography further decreases the post-test likelihood of disease, so other diagnoses might be pursued. However, when the clinical suspicion is moderate to high, a "negative" TTE does *not* substantially decrease the post-test likelihood of disease, so prompt further evaluation is needed. In fact, when the clinical suspicion is high, many clinicians would argue that TTE is inappropriate; either TEE, cardiac magnetic resonance imaging (CMR), or CT evaluation should be performed promptly.

Transesophageal Imaging

TEE images of the aorta are far superior to TTE images in most patients because of (1) the shorter distance between the transducer and aorta, (2) the use of a higher frequency transducer, and (3) better ultrasound tissue penetration (higher signal-to-noise ratio). The descending thoracic aorta can be examined in its entirety from the diaphragm to the arch in both long- and short-axis planes.

Features of aortic dissection seen on TEE imaging include any combination of:

❐ a dissection flap that appears as a linear, bright echogenic structure in the aortic lumen with erratic motion compared with normal systolic pulsations (Fig. 16–18);
❐ color Doppler evidence of blood flow in both the true (bounded by endothelium) lumen and false (bounded by media) lumen;
❐ the entry site into the false lumen;
❐ other communications between the two channels;
❐ thrombosis of the false lumen; or
❐ a hematoma in the wall of the aorta (instead of an initial flap).

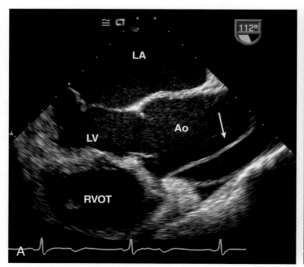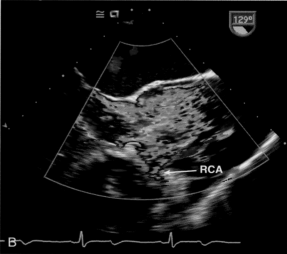

Figure 16–18 A, TEE showing a typical ascending aortic dissection in a long-axis view with linear flap (*arrow*) originating near the ostium of the right coronary artery (RCA). **B,** Color Doppler shows disturbed systolic flow in the true lumen and indicates the dissection flap may extend into the RCA.

An aortic wall hematoma has the same clinical implications as a classic intimal flap, so that careful evaluation for this possibility is needed. This area of hematoma appears as an echogenic mass adjacent to the aortic lumen and bounded by the bright adventitial echo signal (Figs. 16–19 and 16–20).

The proximal segment of the ascending aorta is seen on TEE imaging in the short-axis plane at the aortic valve level. However, evaluation of the ascending aorta depends on use of a long-axis view. Evaluation of the ascending aorta is particularly important, because the decision between emergency surgical intervention and medical therapy hinges on whether the dissection originates in (or involves) the ascending aorta. Note that even a localized dissection flap in the ascending aorta carries a grim prognosis and warrants surgical treatment. Again, color flow imaging may further define the entry site and demonstrate flow in true and false lumens.

The sensitivity of TEE imaging for the diagnosis of aortic dissection is high (>97%; see Table 16–1). Although specificity also is high, it is less than 100% due to misinterpretation of ultrasound artifacts, such as reverberations, beam-width artifacts, and oblique imaging planes. Careful evaluation from multiple views with adjustment of instrument settings helps avoid these false-positive diagnoses.

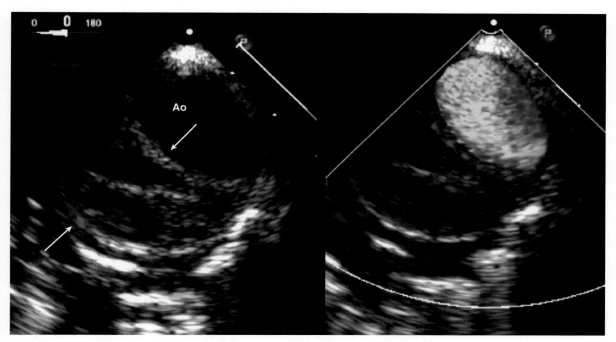

Figure 16–19 Intramural hematoma: In a transesophageal short-axis view of the descending thoracic Ao, the lumen is small with a large crescent shaped hematoma with areas of echo-density and echolucency (between *arrows*). Color Doppler shows flow in the true lumen.

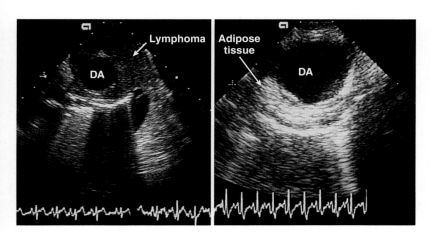

Figure 16–20 Potential false-positive echocardiographic findings with TEE imaging in two patients with no clinical evidence of aortic disease. On the *left*, lymphoma is seen surrounding the descending thoracic aorta (DA). On the *right*, prominent para-aortic adipose tissue is seen.

Alternate Approaches

Several centers have suggested that TEE imaging is the procedure of choice for evaluation of acute aortic dissections given its high sensitivity/specificity plus the ability to perform the study quickly at the patient's bedside (Table 16–2). However, there are several accurate alternate techniques (Figs. 16–21 and 16–22) available for evaluation of possible acute aortic dissection including:

- ❐ Chest computed tomography (CT)
- ❐ Cardiac magnetic resonance imaging (CMR)
- ❐ Contrast angiography

The choice of a particular procedure in an individual patient depends not only on availability of these tests but also on the differential diagnosis in the individual patient. Contrast angiography may be most appropriate when acute myocardial infarction is a likely diagnosis, since evaluation (and treatment) of coronary artery obstruction can be performed quickly if dissection is not present. Wide-angle tomographic imaging procedures (CT, CMR) may be most helpful in cases in which the differential diagnosis includes mediastinal tumor. Both CT and CMR approaches also allow three-dimensional (3D) visualization of the aorta, which may be helpful in clinical decision making. Echocardiography has the advantage of allowing evaluation of aortic valve anatomy and function, overall and regional LV systolic function, and the presence and significance of a pericardial effusion.

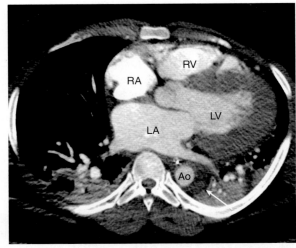

Figure 16–21 In the same patient as Figure 16–19, the chest CT shows contrast in the aortic lumen (Ao) with a marked thickening around the lumen consistent with an intramural hematoma.

TABLE 16–2	Diagnostic Imaging Procedures in Aortic Disease	
Imaging Approach	**Advantages**	**Disadvantages**
Transthoracic echo	Portable, rapid Inexpensive Evaluation of LV function Evaluation of aortic valve function Evaluation of PE	Moderate sensitivity/specificity due to poor acoustic access and suboptimal image resolution
Transesophageal echo	High sensitivity/specificity Portable, rapid Evaluation of LV function, valve function, PE Can assess proximal coronary arteries	Some risks (esp. if esophageal disease is present) Cannot evaluate distal coronary arteries
Computed tomography	High sensitivity/specificity Wide field of view	Site of intimal tear may not be well defined Not portable Ionizing radiation Few data on LV, aortic valve
Cardiac magnetic resonance	High sensitivity/specificity Wide field of view Evaluation of PE	High cost, not portable, limited availability Limited evaluation of valvular and ventricular function
Contrast aortography	High sensitivity/specificity Branch vessel anatomy Evaluation of AR Can assess and intervene for coronary artery disease	Expensive, invasive Ionizing radiation Limited availability Not portable No evaluation for PE

AR, aortic regurgitation; fx, function; PE, pericardial effusion.

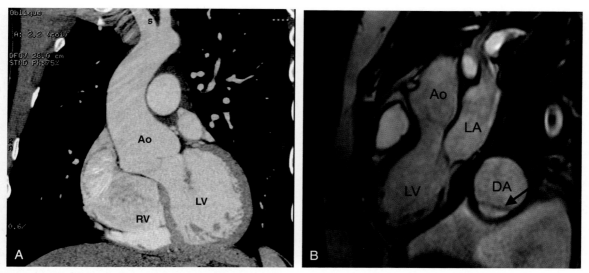

Figure 16–22 In a 24-year-old man with Marfan syndrome, chest CT (**A**) shows dilation of the ascending Ao and loss of the contour of the sinotubular junction. In a 32-year-old woman with Marfan syndrome, CMR imaging (**B**) in a long-axis plane shows mild dilation of the ascending Ao with marked dilation and a dissection flap (*arrow*) in the descending aorta (DA). Both these approaches provide a more complete evaluation of the aorta than the narrow imaging field seen with echocardiography. A combination of imaging approaches often is used in clinical practice.

Alternatively, the choice of imaging procedures may be driven by the specific additional information needed in an individual patient. Examples include distal vessel anatomy (angiography), adjacent mediastinal disease (CT or CMR), or valvular function (echocardiography).

Sinus of Valsalva Aneurysm

A sinus of Valsalva aneurysm can be due to:

☐ congenital disease,
☐ acute infection (e.g. endocarditis), or
☐ an inflammatory process.

Echocardiographically, a dilated and distorted sinus of Valsalva is seen both in long- and short-axis views at the aortic valve level either from a TEE or TTE approach. A congenital aneurysm often is complex in shape with a "wind sock" appearance of a mass of irregular, mobile echos protruding from the aortic sinus into adjacent cardiac structures (Fig. 16–23). If the aneurysm is not fenestrated, Doppler flow examination is unremarkable. More commonly, multiple fenestrations are present, with high-velocity turbulent flow from the high-pressure aorta to the low-pressure adjacent chambers detectable by continuous-wave, pulsed wave, and color flow Doppler techniques. Note that infection of a previously competent congenital

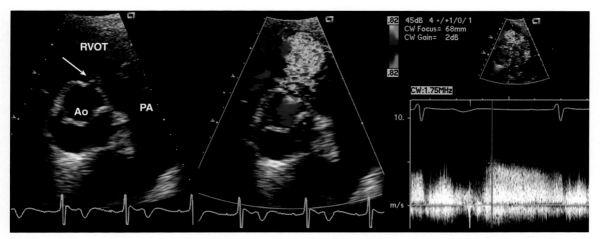

Figure 16–23 Transesophageal short-axis views in this 42-year-old man show (*left*) a small congenital sinus of Valsalva aneurysm of the right coronary cusp (*arrow*) (*center*), which has ruptured into the right ventricular outflow tract (RVOT). Continuous-wave Doppler (*right*) shows high-velocity (>4 m/s) flow from the Ao into the RV in both diastole and systole, confirming that the communication is from the Ao (not the LV).

sinus of Valsalva aneurysm may result in flow across a necrotic area of infection.

Acquired sinus of Valsalva aneurysms tend to be less irregular in shape. The dilation of the sinuses that occurs in Marfan syndrome symmetrically involves all three sinuses with a rounded, smooth pattern of dilation. Because of persistent sinus of Valsalva dilation in patients with Marfan syndrome, replacements of the ascending aorta are performed with a composite valve and graft (with reimplantation of the coronaries) to avoid sinus dilation and rupture with separate replacements of the aorta. A sinus of Valsalva aneurysm due to endocarditis tends to result in a more spherical, but still irregular-appearing dilation of the sinus. Again, the aneurysm protrudes and may rupture into adjacent cardiac structures depending on which sinus is involved.

Preoperative and Postoperative Evaluation of Aortic Disease

Preoperative Evaluation

In some cases, the suspicion of aortic dissection is so high that TEE examination may be performed initially in the operating room with the patient anesthetized and undergoing preparation for surgery. In these cases the echocardiographer aims to rapidly confirm or exclude the suspected diagnosis. If a dissection is present, evaluation of the entry site and extent of dissection is helpful in planning the surgical approach. Recognition of complications such as aortic regurgitation, coronary ostial occlusion, or pericardial effusion also may affect acute patient treatment.

Residual Dissection Flaps

TEE imaging may be used intraoperatively to assess for residual dissection following surgical repair. A residual dissection flap, with flow in both true and false lumens, persists in most patients (possibly as many as 70% to 80%) following emergency surgery for acute dissection. The usual operative procedure is to close the entry site by replacing a segment of the involved aorta with a prosthetic graft. At the distal graft anastomosis, the flap may persist. Often this persistence is intentional, because some branch vessels may be supplied by the false lumen and other vessels by the true lumen. Thus, the finding of a dissection flap in the aortic arch or descending aorta of a patient with a previous ascending aortic dissection and graft repair may represent stable residual disease or a second acute process. These conditions are differentiated by comparison with previous imaging studies (when available) and careful clinical evaluation. Some investigators have suggested that persistence of an intimal flap and flow in the false lumen are poor prognostic signs.

In patients with ascending aortic grafts, echocardiographic follow-up is warranted to assess for late

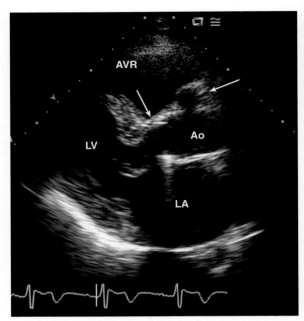

Figure 16–24 This 67-year-old man with Marfan syndrome underwent composite ascending aortic graft and bileaflet mechanical aortic valve replacement (AVR) 30 years ago. He has chronic stable dilation of the right coronary artery attachment to the graft (*arrow*).

complications. In patients with a valved conduit, a baseline study is indicated postoperatively to allow comparison with future studies in terms of prosthetic valve function (see Chapter 13). The prosthetic aortic graft itself appears as an echo-dense, cylindrical structure with a uniform diameter (Fig. 16–24). Although most surgeons now resect the native diseased aorta, in the past the native aorta often was "wrapped around" the prosthetic graft, resulting in irregular areas of thickening anterior and posterior to the graft on echocardiography. Even with resection of the native aortic segment, postoperative periaortic scar tissue may be prominent. The coronary arteries retain their normal insertions if a segment of the native aorta has been preserved. In these cases, careful examination for dilation of the remaining aortic tissue and the sinuses of Valsalva is needed. When the graft extends to the aortic valve level, the right and left coronary ostia are reimplanted into the graft along with a small "button" of native aortic tissue. Dilation or loss of structural integrity of this aortic tissue or dehiscence of the coronary reimplantation suture line results in myocardial infarction due to disruption of coronary blood flow. In addition, this complication can lead to aortic rupture or pseudoaneurysm formation.

Aortic Pseudoaneurysms

A pseudoaneurysm, escape of blood from the graft lumen into an area contained by surrounding scar tissue or the native aorta, can occur at the proximal or

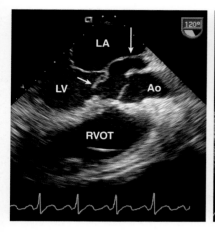 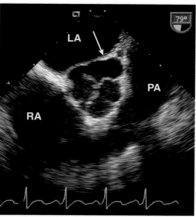

Figure 16–25 Echocardiography was requested for evaluation of cardiogenic shock in a 32-year-old man with *Pseudomonas* endocarditis. TEE imaging in a long-axis view (*left*) shows a flail noncoronary leaflet of the aortic valve (*small arrow*) in association with disruption of the posterior aortic sinus of Valsalva, resulting in a pseudoaneurysm (*large arrow*) between the Ao and LA. The normal right coronary cusp of the aortic valve is seen in a closed position. On color Doppler, flow into and out of the pseudoaneurysm from the Ao and severe aortic regurgitation were seen. The short-axis view (*right*) at the level of communication between the Ao and pseudoaneurysm (*arrow*) shows the distorted appearance of the aortic valve and sinuses. RVOT, right ventricular outflow tract.

the distal graft anastomoses to the aorta or at the coronary reimplantation sites. Rarer instances of rupture of the graft material itself have been reported. A pseudoaneurysm appears as an echolucent area adjacent to the aortic graft (Fig. 16–25). Flow into this region can be demonstrated with color flow imaging, although a TEE study often is necessary for adequate image quality. The pseudoaneurysm may rupture into the mediastinum or pleural spaces (both of which are likely to be fatal) or back across the aortic annulus into the LV. This pseudo-aortic regurgitation consists of flow from the pseudoaneurysm into the LV in diastole, with flow from the LV into the pseudoaneurysm in systole. The characteristics of this flow signal on pulsed and continuous-wave Doppler are similar to those of transvalvular aortic regurgitation. Color flow imaging shows the flow around, rather than through, the prosthetic aortic valve.

Atherosclerotic Aortic Disease

Aortic Atherosclerosis as a Potential Source of Embolus

The excellent-quality images of the aorta obtained by TEE imaging have led to the observation of extensive atherosclerotic plaque in many individuals, with mobile thrombus attached to the atheroma in some cases. These observations have generated the hypothesis that atherosclerosis of the ascending aorta and arch may serve as a nidus for embolic material, resulting in cerebrovascular events (see Suggested Readings 28 and 29 in Chapter 15). These areas of atherosclerosis rarely are seen on TTE imaging due to poor image quality related to acoustic access, the depth of the aorta from the transthoracic approach, and the use of a lower frequency transducer. Echocardiographic evaluation of the extent and severity of atheroma correlates well with histologic examination, and TEE is both sensitive and specific for detection of atheroma-related thrombus formation.

Aortic Atherosclerosis as a Marker of Coronary Artery Disease

The presence of detectable atherosclerotic plaques in the descending aorta on TEE (Fig. 16–26) indicates the presence of atherosclerosis and thus is a marker of coronary artery disease with a sensitivity of 90%. Conversely, the absence of detectable atherosclerosis in the descending thoracic aorta suggests that significant coronary artery disease is not present with a specificity of 90%.

Pulmonary Artery Abnormalities

Most abnormalities of the pulmonary artery are congenital, including poststenotic dilation, branch

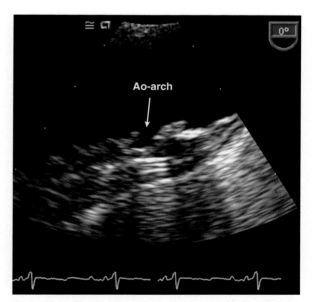

Figure 16–26 Transesophageal view of the Ao arch shows an ulcerated plaque (*arrow*) in a woman with a history of transient ischemic events. The atheroma protrudes into the lumen with areas of independent mobility suggesting thrombus. Shadowing from plaque calcification also is seen.

pulmonary artery stenosis, and an abnormal position of the pulmonary artery, as in transposition of the great vessels. However, the pulmonary artery may be involved by systemic diseases that affect the aorta, such as Takayasu arteritis. Pulmonary artery dissection is rare but has been reported in patients with chronic pulmonary hypertension.

The finding of a dilated pulmonary artery raises the possibility of:

❑ right-sided volume overload (e.g., atrial septal defect),
❑ pulmonary hypertension, or
❑ idiopathic dilation of the pulmonary artery.

The finding of a dilated main pulmonary artery mandates a careful evaluation for right-sided pressure or volume overload. Idiopathic dilation of the pulmonary artery is a rare diagnosis and should only be considered if there is no other cause for pulmonary artery dilation.

The pulmonary artery can be seen on TTE in a parasternal short-axis view at the aortic valve level or in an RV outflow view. In adults, it may be difficult to visualize the anterior pulmonary artery wall due to overlying lung tissue. In younger patients the pulmonary artery can be demonstrated from the anteriorly angulated apical four-chamber view by further anterior angulation. The subcostal short-axis view allows an alternate approach to visualize the pulmonary artery in most patients. From the suprasternal notch window, the right pulmonary artery is seen in cross-section in the long-axis view of the aortic arch and in its long axis in the orthogonal view (see Fig. 16–7). The left pulmonary artery can be imaged by slight lateral angulation and posterior rotation from the standard long-axis suprasternal notch view.

TEE images of the pulmonary artery can be obtained in a 0° image plane by slowly withdrawing the probe to an esophageal level superior to the LA. This view shows the long axis of the pulmonary artery and its bifurcation but may not be obtained in all patients due to interposition of the air-filled bronchus (Fig. 16–27). The pulmonary artery also can be imaged in the 90° plane (analogous to the transthoracic RV outflow view) by turning the transducer to the patient's right from the LV long-axis view. However, image quality may be suboptimal due to the distance of the pulmonary artery from the transducer in this view.

Alternate approaches to evaluation of the pulmonary artery include CT or CMR scanning and, rarely, contrast angiography.

LIMITATIONS/ALTERNATE APPROACHES

The major limitations of echocardiographic evaluation of diseases of the great vessels are acoustic access and image quality. From the transthoracic approach, images of each segment of the aorta can be obtained, but image quality depends on the body habitus of the patient, the skill of the sonographer, and careful attention to the technical details of image acquisition. Interpretation of the images obtained must consider

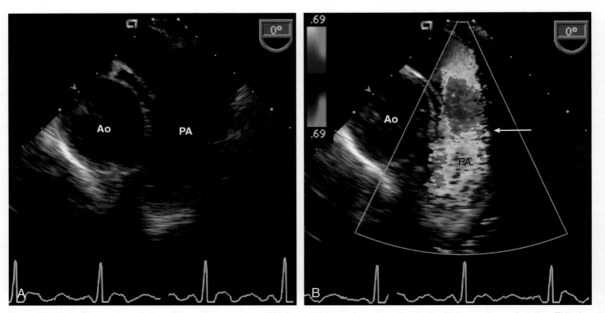

Figure 16–27 A, Transesophageal view of the pulmonary artery (PA) from a high esophageal position in the 0° image plane orientation. This view cannot be obtained in all patients due to interposition of the air-filled bronchus. **B,** Color Doppler shows flow in the PA directed toward the transducer. Aliasing from red to blue (*arrow*) occurs because the antegrade velocity exceeds the Nyquist limit of 69 cm/s.

the likelihood of false-positive findings from beam-width artifacts, reverberations, and oblique image planes, to false-negative findings due to limited acoustic access and poor resolution.

TEE imaging obviates many of these limitations by providing optimal acoustic access and excellent resolution. However, reverberations, beam-width artifacts, and oblique image planes still can result in apparent intraluminal "abnormalities," particularly in the ascending aorta, that in fact represent ultrasound artifacts. Use of a biplane or multiplane probe is essential, because the ascending aorta is visualized only at its base using the transverse image plane (single-plane probe). Even with a multiplane probe, a few centimeters of the ascending aorta at its junction with the arch may not be adequately demonstrated due to the interposed air-filled bronchial tree. Images of the ascending aorta are of particular importance in suspected aortic dissection, because the entry site (ascending or descending aorta), rather than the simple presence or absence of disease, determines therapy. Potentially 3D imaging may improve diagnostic accuracy, but this has not yet been demonstrated.

Alternate approaches provide excellent quality images of the aorta with sensitivities and specificities for diagnosis of aortic dissection at least comparable with those of TEE. Chest CT can be used to evaluate aortic disease with the advantages of a wide field of view, high accuracy, and wide availability. Disadvantages include the use of contrast, ionizing radiation, and the nonportable nature of the study device. Chest CT may identify associated pericardial effusion but is of limited value in evaluation of LV or aortic valve function. Three-dimensional reconstructions of CT scans enhance the ability to relate anatomic findings to each other.

CMR imaging of the aorta has the advantages of high resolution, high diagnostic accuracy, wide field of view, and the ability to orient the images along the long axis of the aorta. As with chest CT, CMR equipment is not portable, but contrast is not required for aortic imaging and there is no exposure to ionizing radiation. CMR also allows evaluation for aortic regurgitation, pericardial effusion, and LV function. Both chest CT and CMR provide data on branch vessel involvement, information that rarely is obtainable with echocardiography.

Contrast aortography allows accurate diagnosis of aortic disease, including aortic dissection, and may be the initial diagnostic procedure if the possibility of coronary artery disease is high on the differential diagnosis. Aortography allows evaluation of the degree of aortic regurgitation, involvement of branch vessels, and (by separate contrast injection) LV systolic function. Cardiac catheterization is the only diagnostic procedure that provides detailed coronary anatomy and allows rapid intervention if coronary artery obstruction is present. Disadvantages of contrast aortography are that it is not portable, uses ionizing radiation, is invasive, and is expensive.

SUGGESTED READING

Aortic Dilation and Dissection

1. Farah HH, Bolger AF: Aortic dissection and trauma: Value and limitations of echocardiography. In Otto CM (ed): The Practice of Clinical Echocardiography, 3rd ed. Philadelphia: Elsevier/Saunders, 2007, pp 793–815.
   Review of the pathophysiologic and clinical presentation of aortic dissection and the role of echocardiography both for the initial diagnosis, management at the time of surgery, and long-term follow-up. 132 references.
2. Bossone E, Evangelista A, Isselbacher E, et al; International Registry of Acute Aortic Dissection Investigators: Prognostic role of transesophageal echocardiography in acute type A aortic dissection. Am Heart J 153:1013–1020, 2007.
   In 522 patients with ascending aortic dissection, in-hospital mortality was 29%. Multivariate predictors of mortality were age > 70 years, pulse deficit, renal failure, and hypotension/shock. TEE findings of a dissection flap limited to the ascending aorta and thrombosis of the false lumen predicted a better survival rate.
3. Tsai TT, Nienaber CA, Eagle EA: Acute aortic syndromes. Circulation 112:3802–3813, 2005.
   Review of pathophysiology, classification, natural history, diagnosis, and medical and surgical management of aortic dissection.
4. Fedak PW, Verma S, David TE, et al: Clinical and pathophysiological implications of a bicuspid aortic valve. Circulation 106:900–904, 2002.
   A bicuspid aortic valve (BAV) is associated with aortic dilation in over 50% of patients and is associated with an increased risk of aortic dissection.
5. Schaefer BM, Lewin MB, Stout KK, et al: The bicuspid aortic valve: An integrated phenotypic classification of leaflet morphology and aortic root shape. Heart 94:1634–1638, 2008.
   A phenotypic classification of BAV disease is proposed that incorporates both leaflet morphology and aortic root shape. With fusion of the right and left coronary cusps (type I BAV) the aortic sinuses are larger than in those with fusion of the right and non-coronary cusps (type II BAV). Conversely, type II BAV is associated with dilation of the ascending aorta distal to the sinotubular junction and a higher prevalence (13% vs. 2.6%) of mitral valve prolapse.
6. Sachdev V, Matura LA, Sidenko S, et al: Aortic valve disease in Turner syndrome. Am Coll Cardiol 51:1904–1909, 2008.
   In women and girls with Turner syndrome (single X chromosome) a BAV is present in 30%, almost always with fusion of the right and left coronary cusps. Aortic dilation is present in 25% of those with a BAV.
7. Pape LA, Tsai TT, Isselbacher EM, et al; International Registry of Acute Aortic Dissection (IRAD) Investigators: Aortic diameter > or = 5.5 cm is not a good predictor of type A aortic dissection: Observations from the International Registry of Acute Aortic Dissection (IRAD). Circulation 116:1120–1127, 2007.
   In 591 patients with a type A aortic dissection, aortic diameter at the time of dissection was <5.5 cm in 59% and <5.0 cm in 40%. Only 5% of these patients had Marfan syndrome, 4%

had a BAV, and 12% had a history of aortic valve disease. Predictors of dissection with a smaller aortic diameter were a history of hypertension, radiating pain, and increasing age. With an aortic diameter >60 mm, annual risk of rupture or dissection is 15%.

8. Moore AG, Eagle KA, Bruckman D, et al: Choice of computed tomography, TEE echocardiography, magnetic resonance imaging, and aortography in acute aortic dissection: International Registry of Acute Aortic Dissection (IRAD). Am J Cardiol 89:1235–1238, 2002.

In a registry of 628 patients with acute aortic dissection, the first choice of imaging test was chest CT in 63%, echocardiography in 32%, aortography in 4%, and MRI in 1%. However, two thirds of patients had more than one imaging study, with TEE performed in 58% of those with a second study. Sensitivity of TEE for the diagnosis of ascending dissection was 90%, compared to 93% for CT.

9. Movsowitz HD, Levine RA, Hilgenberg AD, et al: TEE echocardiographic description of the mechanisms of aortic regurgitation in acute type A aortic dissection: Implications for aortic valve repair. J Am Coll Cardiol 36:884–890, 2000.

In 50 consecutive patients undergoing ascending aortic dissection repair, significant aortic regurgitation was present in 44%. Mechanisms of aortic regurgitation in patients with intrinsically normal leaflets included proximal aortic dilation with leaflet tethering, leaflet prolapse, and dissection flap prolapse through the aortic orifice. Identification of the mechanism of aortic regurgitation can assist the surgeon in optimizing the surgical procedure.

10. Dohmen G, Kuroczynski W, Dahm M, et al: Value of echocardiography in patient follow-up after surgically corrected type A aortic dissection. Thorac Cardiovasc Surg 49:343–348, 2001.

Residual abnormalities and complications were common after aortic dissection repair, with more than mild aortic regurgitation in 25%, a distal aneurysm greater than 5 cm in diameter in 33%, a residual distal dissection flap in 81%, and a new proximal aortic dissection in 10%. TEE imaging was optimal for evaluation of flow patterns and entry sites, whereas CT and MRI were better for visualization of aortic arch pathology.

Aortic Intramural Hemorrhage

11. Evangelista A, Mukherjee D, Mehta RH, et al; International Registry of Aortic Dissection (IRAD) Investigators. Acute intramural hematoma of the aorta: A mystery in evolution. Circulation 111:1063–1070, 2005.

In a series of 1010 patients with an acute aortic syndrome, an intramural hematoma (IMH) was present in only 5.7%. Patients with IMH tended to be older, were more likely to have distal aortic involvement, and often had a delay in diagnosis compared to those with aortic dissection. However, mortality was similar for patients with aortic dissection and those with IMH, and 16% of those with IMH progress to classic dissection on serial imaging studies.

12. Keren A, Kim CB, Hu BS, et al: Accuracy of biplane and multiplane TEE echocardiography in diagnosis of typical acute aortic dissection and intramural hematoma. J Am Coll Cardiol 28:627–636, 1996.

In a consecutive series of 112 patients undergoing TEE imaging for suspected aortic dissection, echocardiographic findings were compared to findings at surgery or autopsy. The sensitivity of TEE for the presence of aortic dissection was 98% with a specificity of 95%. The sensitivity of TEE for detection of intramural hematoma was 90% with a specificity of 99%. Echocardiography also was highly accurate for detection of associated aortic regurgitation and pericardial tamponade.

13. Pepi M, Campodonico J, Galli C, et al; Rapid diagnosis and management of thoracic aortic dissection and intramural haematoma: A prospective study of advantages of multiplane vs. biplane transoesophageal echocardiography. Eur J Echocardiogr 1:72–79, 2000.

The accuracy of multiplane TEE for detection of aortic dissection or intramural hematoma is high, and this approach also allows evaluation of the entry site, coronary artery involvement, aortic regurgitation, and pericardial effusion.

14. Pelzel JM, Braverman AC, Hirsch AT, Harris KM: International heterogeneity in diagnostic frequency and clinical outcomes of ascending aortic intramural hematoma. J Am Soc Echocardiogr 20:1260–1268, 2007.

IMH is reported in 32% of patients with an acute aortic syndrome in studies from Japan or Korea, compared with 11% in studies from North America or Europe. Early medical therapy is used in 78% of Japanese/Korean studies as compared with only 49% of North American/European studies. Overall mortality with IMH is lower (9.4%) in studies from Japan and Korea as compared with mortality (20.6%) in studies from North America and Europe.

Aortic Pseudoaneurysms

15. Zoghbi WA: Echocardiographic recognition of unusual complications after surgery on the great vessels and cardiac valves. In Otto CM (ed): The Practice of Clinical Echocardiography, 3rd ed. Philadelphia: Elsevier/Saunders, 2007, pp 605–626.

Review and discussion of complications after aortic surgery including pseudoaneurysms of composite aortic grafts and complications after composite valve and proximal aortic replacement. Excellent illustrations of the surgical techniques and echocardiographic findings.

16. Barbetseas J, Crawford ES, Sail HJ, et al: Doppler echocardiographic evaluation of pseudoaneurysms complicating composite grafts of the ascending aorta. Circulation 85:212–222, 1992.

Description of the echocardiographic appearance of pseudoaneurysm formation after ascending aortic graft surgery in eight cases. Periannular and coronary artery dehiscences were detected by echocardiography using both 2D imaging (TTE or TEE or both) and Doppler flow studies.

Inherited Connective Tissue Disorders

17. Keane MG, Pyeritz RE: Medical management of Marfan syndrome. Circulation 117:2802–2813, 2008.

The concept that aortic dilation in Marfan syndrome is due to structural weakness of microfibrils due to the fibrillin gene defect has been replaced by the concept that fibrillin affects transforming growth factor beta (TGFβ) signaling, leading to inflammation, fibrosis, and altered matrix metalloproteinase activity. In the future, this ongoing disease process may be amenable to therapy that interrupts these molecular pathways. This comprehensive review also summarizes clinical criteria for the diagnosis, cardiovascular features, pathophysiology, medical management, and recommendation for surgical intervention.

18. Judge DP, Dietz HC: Marfan's syndrome. Lancet 366:1965–1976, 2005.

Concise review article on the genetics, differential diagnosis, and clinical manifestations of Marfan syndrome. Nearly all patients with Marfan syndrome have (or develop) proximal aortic dilation as seen on echocardiography. Echocardiographic screening of first-degree relatives and periodic echocardiography to monitor aortic root size are recommended.

19. Roman MJ, Devereux RB, Kramer-Fox R, O'Loughin J: Two-dimensional echocardiographic aortic root dimensions in normal children and adults. Am J Cardiol 64:507–512, 1989.

Original article providing the data justifying the regression equations used to normalize aortic dimensions for body size and age.

20. Loeys BL, Schwarze U, Holm T, et al: Aneurysm syndromes caused by mutations in the TGF-beta receptor. N Engl J Med 355:788–798, 2006.

The Loeys-Dietz syndrome is an autosomal dominantly inherited aortic aneurysm syndrome due to mutations in the genes encoding TGFβ receptors. Characteristic clinical features are arterial tortuosity and aneurysms, hypertelorism, and a bifid uvula or cleft palate. Clinical outcomes are similar to vascular Ehlers-Danlos syndrome, including aortic dissection at a young age and a high rate of pregnancy-related complications; however operative mortality is much lower with Loeys-Dietz syndrome as compared with vascular Ehlers-Danlos syndrome. Most of these patients have aneurysms of the ascending aorta so may first be diagnosed by echocardiography.

21. Alizad A, Seward JB: Echocardiographic features of genetic diseases: Part 4. Connective tissue. J Am Soc Echocardiogr 13:325–330, 2000.

Review with illustrations of echocardiographic and clinical findings in Ehlers-Danlos and Marfan syndromes.

Aortic Atheroma

22. Thenappan T, Ali Raza J, Movahed A: Aortic atheromas: current concepts and controversies—a review of the literature. Echocardiography 25:198–207, 2008.

This review of the literature suggests that aortic atheromas seen on TEE reflect total atherosclerotic burden, but the relationship of specific aortic atheroma to cerebrovascular events remains unclear.

23. Sen S, Hinderliter A, Sen PK, et al: Aortic arch atheroma progression and recurrent vascular events in patients with stroke or transient ischemic attack. Circulation 116:928–935, 2007.

In 125 adults with a cerebrovascular event and evidence of aortic atheroma on TEE, progression of atheroma at 1 year was seen in 28%. Freedom from recurrent cardiac and vascular events was only 49% in those with atheroma progression compared with 89% in the no-progression group. The hazard ratio of atheroma progression for prediction of cardiac and vascular events was 5.8 (confidence interval 2.3–14.5).

24. Weber A, Jones EF, Zavala JA, et al: Intraobserver and interobserver variability of transesophageal echocardiography in aortic arch atheroma measurement. J Am Soc Echocardiogr 21:129–133, 2008.

The reproducibility of echocardiographic measurements of aortic arch atheroma thickness was evaluated in 160 TEE images recorded as part of a study of antithrombotic therapy to prevent cerebral events. The intraobserver mean measurement difference was 0.01 mm with an interobserver mean difference of 0.13 to 0.48 mm. Agreement for detection of a plaque thickness greater or less than 4 mm was 84% to 88%.

Traumatic Aortic Rupture

25. Smith MD, Cassidy JM, Souther S, et al: TEE echocardiography in the diagnosis of traumatic rupture of the aorta. N Engl J Med 332:356–362, 1995.

TEE imaging was attempted in 101 patients with possible aortic trauma and was successful in 93 patients. Aortic rupture was diagnosed on TEE images in 11 (12%) studies with confirmation by aortography, surgery, or autopsy showing a sensitivity of 100% and a specificity of 98% (one false-positive result). The typical appearance of aortic trauma on TEE is a mobile 2- to 3-cm intraluminal flap or mass just distal to the junction of the aortic arch and descending thoracic aorta.

26. Vignon P, Boncoeur MP, Francois B, et al: Comparison of multiplane transesophageal echocardiography and contrast-enhanced helical CT in the diagnosis of blunt traumatic cardiovascular injuries. Anesthesiology 94:615–622, 2001.

In a series of 110 consecutive patients with severe blunt chest trauma, TEE and chest CT were prospectively performed at presentation. Both TEE and CT identified the 11 subadventitial disruptions (10 at the isthmus just beyond the left subclavian artery, 1 in the ascending aorta) that required surgical repair. TEE missed a disruption of the innominate artery that was seen on CT. TEE (but not CT) also identified 11 cardiac lesions including acute aortic regurgitation, hemopericardium, and cardioc contusion.

27. Agostinelli A, Saccani S, Borrello B, et al: Immediate endovascular treatment of blunt aortic injury: Our therapeutic strategy. J Thorac Cardiovasc Surg 131:1053–1057, 2006.

Endovascular approaches to acute and chronic aortic disease are increasingly utilized. These approaches are often monitored by intraoperative TEE to guide positioning of the stent grafts, to ensure appropriate deployment, and to facilitate early detection of complications.

17

The Adult with Congenital Heart Disease

There are two basic categories of congenital heart disease in adults:

❐ The initial clinical presentation of previously undiagnosed and untreated congenital defects
❐ Survival into adulthood of patients with known congenital heart disease and previous surgical procedures

In adult patients with no previous diagnosis of heart disease, a congenital defect often is not considered as a potential cause of symptoms, and thus the initial diagnosis may be made at the echocardiographic examination. In these patients, the diagnostic challenge is to recognize and correctly evaluate the congenital abnormality. In patients with known congenital disease and previous surgical procedures,

the diagnostic challenge for the echocardiographer is to identify the postoperative anatomy and assess the physiologic consequences of residual defects in each patient. With "corrective" surgery, as well as with "palliative" procedures, many patients have significant residual or progressive abnormalities.

Both these challenges can be met by a logical and methodical approach to the echocardiographic examination with application of the basic principles of ultrasound imaging and Doppler data described throughout this text. Unusual imaging planes and careful integration of imaging and Doppler data may be needed for complete assessment of congenital heart disease. In addition, the physician and sonographer must have a thorough understanding of the three-dimensional (3D) anatomic relationships for each type of congenital defect.

Obviously, a comprehensive discussion of the echocardiographic findings in adult congenital heart disease is beyond the scope of this text. Instead, an overview of the echocardiographic approach to these patients and examples of the more common abnormalities is presented. The reader is referred to the specialized references listed at the end of the chapter for more detailed information. The goal of this chapter is to allow preliminary diagnosis of congenital heart disease; advanced training is recommended for definitive imaging and diagnosis of congenital heart disease.

ECHOCARDIOGRAPHIC APPROACH

Congenital heart disease in adults can be grouped into several categories (Table 17–1):

- ❑ Stenotic lesions
- ❑ Regurgitant lesions
- ❑ Intracardiac shunts
- ❑ Abnormal connections
- ❑ Combinations or complex congenital disease

TABLE 17–1   Unoperated Congenital Heart Disease Seen in Adults

Congenital Defect	Anatomic Findings	Doppler Findings
Bicuspid aortic valve	Bicuspid valve identified in systole (raphe seen in diastole)	Mild stenosis and/or regurgitation
Unicuspid aortic valve	Abnormal, deformed aortic valve with systolic doming; sometimes the unicuspid orifice can be imaged.	Aortic stenosis (may be severe) and/or aortic regurgitation.
Subaortic membrane	Membrane from anterior MV leaflet to ventricular septum; TEE may be needed for visualization.	High-velocity signal just proximal to aortic valve; AR due to nonsupport of aortic annulus or to a "jet lesion"
Pulmonic stenosis	Thickened pulmonic valve leaflets with systolic doming	Mild pulmonic stenosis (more severe stenosis is recognized and treated in childhood)
Aortic coarctation	Coarctation may not be easy to visualize since descending thoracic aorta goes out of the image plane from SSN; associated with bicuspid aortic valve; highly pulsatile aortic root and akinetic abdominal aorta	High-velocity systolic flow in descending thoracic aorta with extension of flow into diastole with severe obstruction; nonparallel intercept angle limits quantitation of severity in unoperated patients.
Marfan syndrome	Dilated aortic root with loss of the sinotubular junction; elongated, redundant anterior MV leaflet; dilation of ascending aorta, arch, and descending aorta may be present.	Aortic regurgitation
Sinus of Valsalva aneurysm	Dilated, thin sinus with "wind sock" type of projection into adjacent cardiac structures depending on sinus involved	May have fistula from aorta into RA, LA, RV, or LV depending on cusp involved
Coronary AV fistula	May not be able to visualize fistula, but coronary sinus may be dilated; proximal coronary artery may be dilated.	Disturbed flow in coronary sinus or in abnormal epicardial echolucent structures
Ebstein anomaly	Septal tricuspid valve leaflet is adherent to RV wall, appearing "apically displaced"; apparent RA enlargement (part of anatomic RV is physiologically part of RA); associated with WPW and with right-to-left atrial shunt	Tricuspid regurgitation
Myxomatous mitral valve disease	Thick, redundant, prolapsing mitral valve leaflets; LV and LA enlargement depending on severity of MR; tricuspid and aortic valves also may be affected.	Mitral regurgitation

Continued

TABLE 17–1—Cont'd

Congenital Defect	Anatomic Findings	Doppler Findings
Atrial septal defects	Right ventricular and right atrial volume overload with RVE, RAE, and paradoxical ventricular septal motion *Secundum ASD:* Absence of interatrial septum in fossa ovalis region best seen on parasternal views or subcostal four-chamber view *Primum ASD:* Defect in septum adjacent to central fibrous body; associated with atrioventricular valve abnormalities (cleft anterior MV leaflet) *Sinus venosus ASD:* Defect at vena cava-RA junction (may be associated with anomalous PVR); TEE helpful for imaging defect; suspect when $Q_p:Q_s$ is elevated without clear evidence of secundum or primum ASD	$Q_p:Q_s$ can be calculated from Doppler stroke volume measurements in LVOT (or Ao) versus PA. Color flow imaging of left-to-right flow across interatrial septum; IV echo contrast shows some right-to-left shunting. Color flow imaging of left-to-right flow across interatrial septum; may have associated mitral regurgitation TEE to visualize site of defect and left-to-right flow with color imaging
Partial anomalous pulmonary venous return	RVE, RAE, and paradoxical septal motion reflecting right-sided volume overload (may be associated with ASD)	Suspect when $Q_p:Q_s$, > 1 with no evidence for flow across interatrial septum
Ventricular septal defects	*Small VSD:* membranous, muscular, or outflow defects may be difficult to image; membranous defects may be partially or completely closed (ventricular septal aneurysm) by the septal leaflet of the tricuspid valve. *Eisenmenger VSD:* Large defect, often membranous or subaortic, with equal size and wall thickness of LV and RV	High-velocity jet from left to right in systole with pulsed or CW Doppler; color flow imaging shows flow disturbance on right ventricular side of the defect; normal PA pressures Low-velocity bidirectional flow across the ventricular defect; severe pulmonary hypertension
Patent ductus arteriosus	Mild LV and LA enlargement; duct itself rarely visualized in adults	Diastolic flow reversal in the pulmonary artery (typically along the anterior PA wall); diastolic flow reversal in the descending thoracic aorta
Corrected transposition (L-TGA)	In effect the ventricles are anatomically reversed with a physiologically normal blood flow path: RA to LV to PA; LA to RV to Ao Associated defects are common, including pulmonic stenosis, VSD, heart block, and Ebstein-type anomaly of the inverted tricuspid valve with systemic atrioventricular valve regurgitation.	Normal physiology in absence of associated defects; Doppler findings of pulmonic stenosis, VSD, atrioventricular valve regurgitation when present
Persistent left SVC	Dilated coronary sinus; absence of innominate vein on SSN view; small right SVC	Contrast injection from left arm opacifies coronary sinus first, then right atrium.
Hypertrophic cardiomyopathy	Asymmetrically hypertrophied LV with several patterns of involvement; 2D and M-mode signs of dynamic LVOT obstruction	Dynamic LVOT obstruction; mitral regurgitation; diastolic LV dysfunction
Tetralogy of Fallot	Large, overriding aorta, VSD, subvalvular or valvular pulmonic stenosis	High-velocity flow in RVOT and/or across pulmonic valve; bidirectional flow across VSD

AR, aortic regurgitation; ASD, atrial septal defect; LVOT, left ventricular outflow tract; PA, pulmonary artery; PVR, pulmonary venous return; $Q_p:Q_s$, pulmonic-to-systemic shunt ratio; RAE, right atrial enlargement; RVE, right ventricular enlargement; RVOT, right ventricular outflow tract; SSN, suprasternal notch; TEE, transesophageal echocardiography; TGA, transposition of the great arteries; VSD, ventricular septal defect; WPW, Wolff-Parkinson-White syndrome.

Congenital Stenotic Lesions

Congenital stenotic lesions are common, including obstruction to right ventricular (RV) or left ventricular (LV) outflow (subvalvular, valvular, or supravalvular), obstruction to LV inflow (congenital mitral stenosis, cor triatriatum), and narrowings in the great vessels (aortic coarctation, branch pulmonary artery [PA] stenosis).

The anatomy of a congenital stenotic lesion is specific for each, although images of the stenotic region may be suboptimal in adult patients. The physiology and fluid dynamics of congenital stenosis are identical to those seen in acquired disease. There is laminar, normal-velocity flow upstream and a flow disturbance downstream from the narrowing. In the narrowed region itself, a high-velocity laminar jet of flow is present, with velocity (V, in m/s) related to the pressure difference (ΔP, in mm Hg) across the narrowing as stated in the simplified Bernoulli equation:

$$\Delta P = 4V^2$$

When a parallel intercept angle can be obtained between the jet and the ultrasound beam, quantitative data on stenosis severity and intracardiac hemodynamics can be derived. For example, if the maximum velocity across a subpulmonic stenosis is 4.5 m/s, then the maximum RV-to-PA systolic pressure difference is approximately 80 mm Hg. Quantitative evaluation of stenosis severity for a congenitally

stenotic lesion includes calculation of maximum and mean pressure gradients as for acquired valve stenosis. Similarly, when possible, valve area calculations are performed either using the continuity equation (aortic valve) or the pressure half-time method (mitral valve).

Several significant differences between congenital and acquired stenosis should be noted. First, congenital stenosis of ventricular outflow, for both RV and LV, may involve the subvalvular or supravalvular region rather than (or in addition to) stenosis of the valve itself (Fig. 17–1). Careful evaluation with conventional pulsed Doppler or color flow imaging to identify the post-stenotic flow disturbance is helpful in determining the exact site of obstruction. Second, when serial stenoses are present, quantitation of the contribution of each level of obstruction to the overall degree of stenosis can be difficult using Doppler echo methods. Third, the proximal flow pattern in congenital stenosis often is characterized by a greater increase in velocity due to anatomic tapering of the proximal flow region (e.g., in aortic coarctation or in the congenitally stenotic pulmonic valve). In these situations, accurate pressure gradient calculations should include the proximal velocity (V_{prox}) as well as the jet velocity (V_{jet}) in the Bernoulli equation:

$$\Delta P = 4(V^2_{\text{jet}} - V^2_{\text{prox}})$$

Otherwise, evaluation of congenital stenosis is similar to evaluation of acquired stenosis in adults, and the methods described in detail in Chapter 11 can be applied in this patient group.

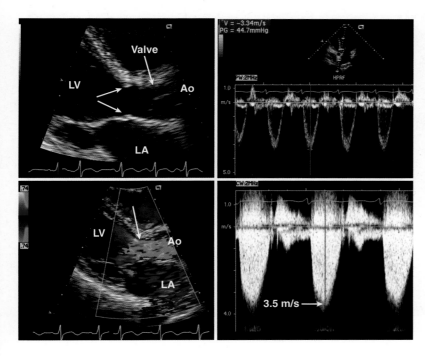

Figure 17–1 Parasternal long-axis 2D view (*top left*) in a patient with a systolic murmur showing a subtle ridge (*arrows*) in the LV outflow tract. Color Doppler (*bottom left*) shows an increased flow velocity in this region, suggesting the possibility of a subaortic membrane (*arrow*). High–pulse repetition frequency Doppler (*top right*) shows an increase in velocity to at least 3.3 m/s at this location, and CW Doppler shows a maximum outflow velocity of 3.5 m/s (*bottom right*).

Congenital Regurgitant Lesions

Careful imaging of a congenitally regurgitant valve may reveal the specific mechanism of regurgitation in that patient. For the atrioventricular valves, particular attention is focused on the number and position of papillary muscles; the chordal attachments (especially aberrant ones); leaflet size, shape, thickness, redundancy, and motion; and annulus size and shape. Malformations can include myxomatous changes of the leaflets, abnormal leaflet position (Ebstein anomaly), and abnormal chordal attachments (atrioventricular canal defect) (Fig. 17–2). The semilunar valves may be regurgitant due to great vessel dilation or a leaflet fenestration.

The physiology of congenital regurgitation is no different from that of acquired regurgitation. There is a flow disturbance in the chamber receiving the regurgitant flow with progressive dilation (and eventual dysfunction) of the volume-overloaded cardiac chambers. Evaluation of congenital regurgitation is similar to evaluation of acquired regurgitation, as detailed in Chapter 12.

Abnormal Intracardiac Communications (Shunts)

An abnormal intracardiac communication is characterized by blood flow across the defect, with the direction, timing, and volume of flow determined by the size of the orifice, the pressure gradient across the defect, and the relative resistance to flow of the vascular beds on each side of the defect. If left-sided heart pressures exceed right-sided pressures (pulmonary vascular resistance is low), left-to-right flow across the defect predominates. Small degrees of right-to-left shunting may be present briefly during the cardiac cycle, because right-sided pressures may transiently exceed left-sided pressures.

With conventional pulsed Doppler ultrasound or with color flow imaging, a flow disturbance is found downstream from the defect: on the right side of the interventricular septum for a ventricular septal defect (VSD), in the right atrium (RA) for an atrial septal defect (ASD), and in the PA for a patent ductus arteriosus.

Analogous to a stenotic or regurgitant orifice, the velocity of blood flow through the shunt orifice is related to the pressure gradient across the defect, as stated in the Bernoulli equation. Thus, a small VSD results in a high-velocity systolic flow signal (approximately 5 m/s), because LV systolic pressure greatly exceeds RV systolic pressure (by approximately 100 mm Hg) (Fig. 17–3). Conversely, flow across an ASD typically is low in velocity because only a modest left atrial (LA)-to-RA pressure difference is present.

A left-to-right intracardiac shunt imposes a chronic volume overload on the receiving chamber(s) with consequent dilation of the affected chamber(s). With an ASD, both RA and RV dilation, along with paradoxical septal motion, are seen. With a patent ductus arteriosus the volume overload is imposed on the LA and LV. Although it might seem that a VSD would cause RV volume overload, in fact, RV size usually is normal because the LV effectively ejects the shunt flow across

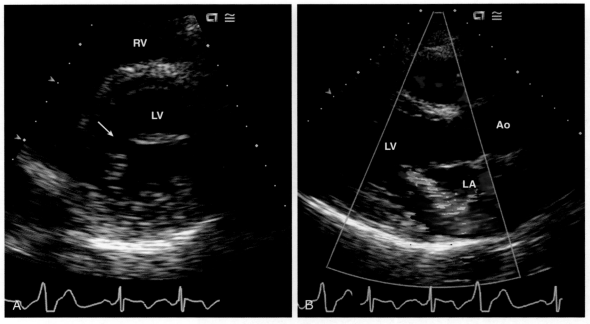

Figure 17–2 Cleft anterior mitral valve leaflet seen in a parasternal short-axis view (*left*). Discontinuity of the anterior leaflet is seen (*arrow*). On color flow imaging in a long-axis view (*right*), an eccentric regurgitant jet with proximal acceleration is present.

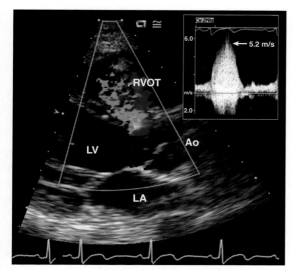

Figure 17–3 Small membranous ventricular septal defect seen in a parasternal long-axis view with color flow Doppler showing acceleration of flow in the orifice with a systolic flow disturbance in the RV outflow tract (RVOT). Continuous-wave Doppler from the parasternal window demonstrates a high-velocity (5.2 m/s) signal toward the transducer (with some channel cross-talk) corresponding to the high pressure difference between the LV and RV in systole. Because LV diastolic pressure is slightly higher than RV diastolic pressure, low-velocity flow from left to right also is seen in diastole.

the defect directly into the PA in systole. Instead, LA and LV dilation are seen, because these chambers receive the increased pulmonary blood flow as it returns to the left side of the heart via the pulmonary veins.

The volume of blood flow (Q) across an intracardiac shunt—the ratio of pulmonary to systemic blood flow ($Q_p:Q_s$)—can be determined by Doppler echo measurements of stroke volume at two intracardiac sites (Fig. 17–4). In the case of an ASD, transpulmonic volume flow (Q_p) is calculated from PA cross-sectional area (CSA) and velocity-time integral (VTI), while

systemic volume flow (Q_s) is calculated from measurements of LV outflow tract (LVOT) CSA and VTI:

$$Q_p = CSA_{PA} \times VTI_{PA}$$
$$Q_s = CSA_{LVOT} \times VTI_{LVOT}$$

so that

$$Q_p{:}Q_s = \frac{CSA_{PA} \times VTI_{PA}}{CSA_{LVOT} \times VTI_{LVOT}}$$

This approach is accurate when two-dimensional (2D) images are of adequate quality for precise diameter measurements (for calculation of a circular CSA) and when Doppler velocity data are recorded at a parallel intercept angle to flow. Potential errors in estimation of the $Q_p:Q_s$ ratio may arise as for any Doppler echo stroke volume measurement (see Chapter 6).

With significant left-to-right shunting, pulmonary pressures become elevated, and irreversible pulmonary hypertension may develop over time. When pulmonary vascular resistance equals or exceeds systemic vascular resistance, the direction of shunt flow reverses, resulting in decreased systemic oxygen saturation and cyanosis. Irreversible pulmonary hypertension with equalization of pulmonary and systemic pressures due to an intracardiac shunt is known as *Eisenmenger's physiology*. This phenomenon can occur in infancy, particularly with a large VSD, but also can occur later in life when the pulmonary-to-systemic shunt ratio chronically exceeds 2:1.

Abnormal Chamber and Great Vessel Connections

Echocardiographic diagnosis is more difficult when there are abnormal connections between the atrium and the ventricles and/or between the ventricles and great vessels. In adults, poor acoustic access may further compromise the examination. However,

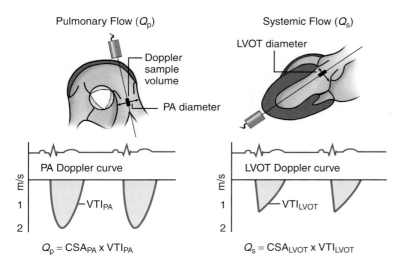

Figure 17–4 Schematic diagram of Doppler echo shunt ratio calculation. Pulmonary flow (Q_p) is calculated from transpulmonic stroke volume calculation using pulmonary artery (PA) diameter measured at the site of the Doppler sample position and the velocity-time integral (VTI) of PA flow. A circular cross-sectional area (CSA) is assumed. Similarly, systemic flow (Q_s) is calculated from LV outflow tract (LVOT) diameter and the VTI of LVOT.

with a systematic approach, a correct anatomic evaluation usually is possible.

Because the position of the heart in the chest may be abnormal, the echocardiographer cannot rely on the intrathoracic position of the chambers for correct identification of cardiac anatomy. *Dextroposition* is a rightward shift in the cardiac position with otherwise normal anatomy; for example, due to decreased right lung volume or severe scoliosis. Acoustic windows are shifted rightward, but image planes are similar to normal. With *dextroversion* the cardiac apex points to the right, but the right and left heart chambers are otherwise normally related. Long-axis views are obtained with the image plane aligned from the left shoulder to right hip, and the apical window is midline or right of the sternum. In contrast, with mirror-image *dextrocardia*, cardiac anatomy is a mirror image of normal (the right-sided chambers are left of the left-sided chambers) and the heart is located in the right hemithorax with the apex in the right midclavicular line. Thus, acoustic windows are on the right chest with image planes mirror images of normal. The term *situs inversus* refers to right-to-left reversal of thoracic and abdominal viscera.

Atrial situs refers to the position of the RA and LA in the chest. The inferior vena cava nearly always drains into the RA, allowing correct identification of this chamber by imaging the inferior vena cava from a subcostal approach and following it into the RA. Thus, the subcostal window often is a useful starting point for examination of a patient with complex congenital heart disease. The LA, then, is the "other" atrial chamber, because although the pulmonary veins normally drain into the LA, this is not always the case (e.g., partial or total anomalous pulmonary venous return).

The anatomic RV and LV can be distinguished from each other by several features (Fig. 17–5). The anatomic RV has:

- ❒ Prominent trabeculation
- ❒ A moderator band
- ❒ An infundibular region
- ❒ A more apical atrioventricular annulus than the LV
- ❒ A tricuspid valve

Fibrous continuity of the anterior mitral valve leaflet and the aortic valve occurs only with a normally related LV and aortic root. When the anatomic RV connects to the aortic root, a band of myocardium is seen between the base of the atrioventricular valve leaflet and the great vessel. When there are abnormal connections of the anatomic ventricles, the ventricle pumping blood to the pulmonary bed is called the *subpulmonary ventricle* and the ventricle pumping blood into the aorta is called the *systemic ventricle*.

The atrioventricular valves develop with the appropriate anatomic ventricle, so identification of the mitral valve is another feature that differentiates the LV from the RV. Caution is needed if a cleft anterior mitral valve leaflet is present because it may superficially resemble the tricuspid valve. In addition to the number of atrioventricular valve leaflets, the relative positions of the atrioventricular valve annuli are helpful, since the tricuspid valve annulus lies slightly closer to the apex than the mitral valve annulus. Note that ventricular size, shape, and/or wall thickness do not distinguish the two ventricles, because congenital lesions can result in dilation and hypertrophy of either chamber.

After identifying the atrium and ventricles, attention is directed toward the great vessels. The aortic

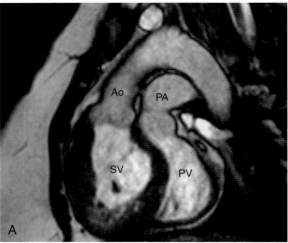
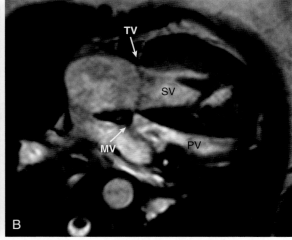

Figure 17–5 Cardiac magnetic resonance images in a patient with transposition of the great arteries demonstrate the anatomic relationships of the great arteries and ventricles. **A**, The longitudinal view shows the side-by-side orientation of the great arteries and the systemic (SV) and pulmonary ventricles (PV). The Ao is anterior to the pulmonary artery (PA). **B**, In a four-chamber view the systemic ventricle (SV) is an anatomic RV as demonstrated by the presence of a moderator band, prominent trabeculation, and the slightly more apical insertion of the tricuspid valve (TV) as compared with the mitral valve (MV). The SV is appropriately hypertrophied. The pulmonary ventricle (PV) is an anatomic LV.

root is best identified by following the vessel downstream to image the arch and head and neck vessels. Origins of the coronary arteries also may be seen, but anomalous origin of the coronary arteries from the PA must be considered. The PA is identified by its bifurcation into right and left branches.

The position of the great vessels within the thorax and relative to each other often is altered in congenital disease. Normally, the PA lies anterior and slightly medial to the aortic root at its origin and then courses posteriorly and laterally, with the right PA lying posterior to the ascending aorta. The aortic annulus normally lies posterior to the RV outflow tract, with the aortic root extending medially and anteriorly before turning posterolaterally to form the aortic arch. The normal relationship of the aortic and pulmonic valve planes is approximately perpendicular to each other, with the pulmonary valve slightly more superior within the chest than the aortic valve. With transpositions of the great vessels, these relationships are altered so that the semilunar valves lie in the same tomographic plane, and the aorta and PA lie parallel to each other instead of in their normal "crisscross" positions (Fig. 17–6). If the aorta is located anterior and to the left, L (for levo) transposition is present. An anterior and medial (rightward) aorta is termed D (for dextro) transposition.

Most patients with abnormal connections between the cardiac chambers and great vessels have associated abnormalities that require echocardiographic evaluation. These include intracardiac shunts, stenotic and regurgitant lesions, pulmonary hypertension, and ventricular dysfunction. The echocardiographic examination in these patients is facilitated by the following:

- ❑ Knowledge of the clinical history, including previous surgical procedures and diagnostic tests
- ❑ Formulation of specific clinical questions to be answered by the echocardiographic examination

During the examination, the physician and sonographer work together in:

- ❑ Identifying the cardiac chambers, great vessels, and their connections

- ❑ Identifying associated defects, and evaluating the physiologic consequences of each defect with appropriate Doppler modalities
- ❑ Identifying which clinical questions remain unanswered at the end of examination, and proposing appropriate alternate diagnostic tests that can provide answers to these questions

CONGENITAL DEFECTS SEEN IN ADULTS WITH OR WITHOUT PREVIOUS CARDIAC SURGERY

Congenital Aortic Valve Abnormalities

Although a congenital bicuspid aortic valve is the most common type of congenital heart disease (reported to occur in 1% to 2% of the general population), the bicuspid valve often is functionally normal until about age 50 to 60 years, when superimposed fibrocalcific changes lead to aortic valve stenosis. Significant regurgitation of a congenital bicuspid valve occurs somewhat less commonly but presents in young adulthood with a diastolic murmur and symptoms of exercise intolerance.

The presentation of significant LV outflow obstruction in a young adult should prompt consideration of abnormalities other than a bicuspid valve—specifically a unicuspid aortic valve, a subaortic membrane, or hypertrophic cardiomyopathy. A unicuspid aortic valve will appear as a thickened, deformed valve with systolic bowing of the valve on ultrasound imaging. A high parasternal short-axis view may show the eccentric unicuspid opening in systole, even allowing planimetry of the valve orifice. Doppler echocardiography can be used to determine the transvalvular gradient and valve area as for any type of aortic valve stenosis. Restenosis of the aortic valve in patients who previously underwent surgical valvotomy in childhood or adolescence is common. Restenosis occurs in up to 40% of patients a mean of 13 years after open surgical valvotomy.

Congenital subaortic obstruction can range anatomically from a muscular ridge to a thin membrane (Fig. 17–7). Although typically located 1 to 1.5 cm

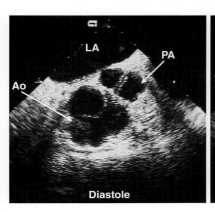
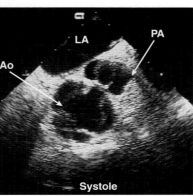

Figure 17–6 Transposed great arteries seen on a TEE view with an anterior Ao and a smaller posterior pulmonary artery with a bicuspid valve in a 42-year-old with congenital transposition of the great arteries, pulmonic stenosis, and a VSD.

Figure 17–7 TEE imaging in the same patient as in Figure 17–1 shows the subaortic membrane more clearly (*arrows*) in a long-axis view (*right*) with the flow disturbance demonstrated proximal to the aortic valve (*arrow*) on color Doppler (*left*).

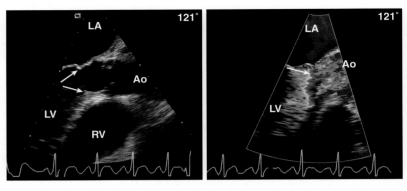

apically from the aortic valve plane, the membrane may be located immediately adjacent to the aortic valve. In either case a subaortic membrane can be difficult to see in adults due to poor acoustic access. The possibility of a subaortic membrane should be considered when high-velocity flow is recorded in the LV outflow tract, but the aortic valve leaflets appear normal. Transesophageal echocardiography (TEE) may allow direct imaging of the subaortic membrane, especially if multiple image planes are used to identify this thin structure. Conventional pulsed Doppler, high–pulse repetition frequency Doppler, and color flow imaging can be helpful from either transthoracic (TTE) or TEE approaches in demonstrating that, in contrast to valvular aortic stenosis, the increase in antegrade velocity and post-stenotic flow disturbance occur on the LV side of the aortic valve, indicating that subaortic obstruction is present. Coexisting aortic regurgitation may be present due to chronic exposure of the aortic valve leaflets to the high-velocity subaortic flow, resulting in a "jet lesion" on the aortic valve, or (rarely) due to fibrous attachments from the subaortic membrane to the aortic valve leaflets.

Congenital Obstructions to Right Ventricular Outflow

RV outflow obstruction may be subvalvular (in the muscular outflow tract), valvular, or supravalvular (either in the main PA or its major branches). Pulmonic stenosis can occur as an isolated anomaly but more often is part of a complex of abnormalities (for example, tetralogy of Fallot) or is associated with other abnormalities (for example, corrected transposition). The level of outflow obstruction can be determined using pulsed Doppler and color flow to identify the anatomic site at which the flow velocity increases and the post-stenotic flow disturbance appears. The obstruction itself may be seen on 2D echocardiography as a muscular subpulmonic ridge; as deformed, doming pulmonic valve leaflets; or as a narrowing in the PA. If significant obstruction is present, compensatory RV hypertrophy typically is seen.

The degree of obstruction can be measured by Doppler ultrasound using the Bernoulli equation (Fig. 17–8) with the proviso that only an estimate of

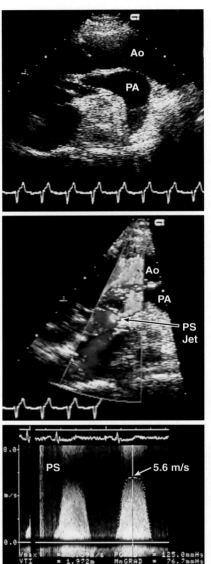

Figure 17–8 Two-dimensional parasternal long-axis view (*top*) of the same patient as in Figure 17–6 showing the transposed great vessels. Color flow imaging (*middle*) shows an eccentric jet with proximal acceleration across the stenotic bicuspid pulmonic valve. Note the proximal isovelocity surface area. Continuous-wave Doppler from a high right parasternal position (*bottom*) shows a maximum velocity of 5.6 m/s consistent with a maximum pulmonic stenosis (PS) pressure gradient of 125 mm Hg.

the total obstruction may be possible if serial stenoses are present. Note that in the presence of pulmonic stenosis, the tricuspid regurgitant jet velocity remains an accurate reflection of the RV-to-RA systolic pressure difference but no longer indicates PA systolic pressure. Instead, PA systolic pressure (PAP) can be estimated by:

(1) calculation of the right ventricular systolic pressure (RVSP) based on the tricuspid regurgitant jet velocity (V_{TR}) and right atrial pressure (RAP) estimated from the inferior vena cava size and respiratory variation:

$$RVSP = 4V_{TR}^2 + RAP$$

(2) calculating the RV-to-PA gradient (ΔP_{RV-PA}) from the pulmonic stenosis jet velocity(V_{PS}):

$$\Delta P_{RV-PA} = 4V_{PS}^2$$

(3) and then subtracting the transpulmonic gradient from the estimated RV systolic pressure:

$$PAP = (\Delta P_{RV-RA} + P_{RA}) - \Delta P_{RV-PA}$$

The end-diastolic velocity in the pulmonic regurgitation jet also may give useful data on PA pressure, because it reflects the diastolic pressure difference between the PA and the RV (high in patients with pulmonary hypertension, low in patients with pulmonic stenosis, and normal PA diastolic pressures).

Congenital Abnormalities of the Aorta

Aortic Coarctation

A congenital narrowing in the proximal descending thoracic aorta most often is located just upstream from the entry site of the ductus arteriosus. Less often, postductal coarctation is seen. The coarctation may be relatively discrete, with involvement of only a short segment of the aorta, or may be a long, tubular narrowing. Imaging of the coarctation site is difficult from transthoracic or suprasternal notch windows in adults. From the suprasternal notch approach, the descending thoracic aorta has a tapering appearance, even in normal individuals, due to the oblique tomographic view of the descending aorta obtained as the

descending aorta leaves the image plane. Adults with previous surgical repair of a coarctation may present with restenosis, depending on the specific surgical procedure used and the patient's age at the time of repair. For both operated and unoperated coarctations, TEE imaging with a long-axis view of the descending aorta may be helpful.

Doppler examination shows an increased velocity across the coarctation and, if the obstruction is severe, persistent antegrade flow into diastole (Fig. 17–9). If elevated, the proximal velocity should be included in the Bernoulli equation for pressure gradient estimation. The jet direction in an unoperated coarctation may be very eccentric, so it rarely is possible to achieve a parallel alignment between the ultrasound beam and jet direction, leading to underestimation of the severity of obstruction. In restenosis of a previously operated coarctation, the jet orientation tends to be more symmetrical, and a parallel intercept angle with correct estimation of the pressure gradient is more likely. In either case, other clinical methods for assessing severity of the coarctation are available (e.g., upper versus lower extremity blood pressure, cardiac catheterization, other imaging approaches).

Marfan Syndrome

Marfan syndrome is inherited in an autosomal dominant pattern with variable penetrance. It is characterized by a specific, but variable, gene defect coding for fibrillin resulting in musculoskeletal, ocular, and cardiovascular manifestations. Cardiovascular abnormalities of Marfan syndrome include dilation, aneurysm formation, and rupture of peripheral arteries, an abnormally redundant anterior mitral valve leaflet, and most important, dilation and dissection of the aorta. Echocardiography may be helpful in confirming or excluding a diagnosis of Marfan syndrome in patients with a suspected diagnosis. Examination also is indicated to screen first-degree relatives of an affected individual.

Characteristic echocardiographic findings include dilation of the aortic annulus, sinuses of Valsalva,

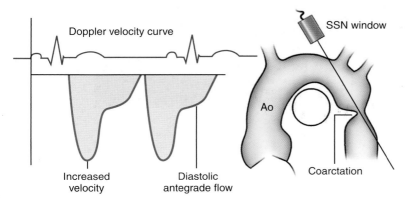

Increased velocity · Diastolic antegrade flow · SSN window · Ao · Coarctation · Doppler velocity curve

Figure 17–9 Aortic coarctation. From a suprasternal notch (SSN) window, continuous-wave Doppler of the coarctation shows an increased velocity in systole with persistent antegrade flow into diastole. Imaging of the coarctation often is suboptimal in adults.

and ascending aorta with loss of a clearly defined sinotubular junction (see Chapter 16). Aortic annular dilation results in aortic regurgitation and consequent LV volume overload. Aortic dissection occurs frequently and can occur even when aortic dilation is not severe. With an aortic root diameter of more than 50 mm in adults, the risk of spontaneous rupture is high, so many clinicians recommend periodic echocardiographic examination with prophylactic aortic root replacement with a valved aortic conduit when ascending aortic diameter exceeds this limit, or at even smaller diameters depending on patient size, the specific genetic defect, and family history.

Sinus of Valsalva Aneurysm

A congenital aneurysm of the aortic sinuses of Valsalva appears as a thin, dilated area that projects into adjacent cardiac structures, often with a fistulous communication depending on which sinus is involved. On echocardiographic imaging, a congenital aneurysm often has a "wind sock" appearance with a long, convoluted, mobile sac of tissue extending from the aortic sinus into adjacent cardiac structures (see Fig. 16–3). This appearance contrasts with the more symmetrical dilation seen in aneurysms due to endocarditis. An aneurysm of the noncoronary sinus projects into the RA, the left coronary cusp into the LA, and the right coronary cusp into the RV outflow tract. If a fistula is present, pulsed and color Doppler flow imaging demonstrate a left-to-right shunt with a flow disturbance in the receiving chamber. Continuous-wave (CW) Doppler shows a high-velocity systolic and diastolic flow signal.

Coronary Anomalies

Coronary Arteriovenous Fistula

A coronary arteriovenous fistula is a rare congenital anomaly that may present in young adults as a continuous murmur. Abnormal communication from a coronary artery to the coronary sinus or RA has been described. A coronary arteriovenous fistula is recognized echocardiographically as an abnormal area of dilation with diastolic or continuous flow plus a flow disturbance at the site of entry into the cardiac chamber (Fig. 17–10).

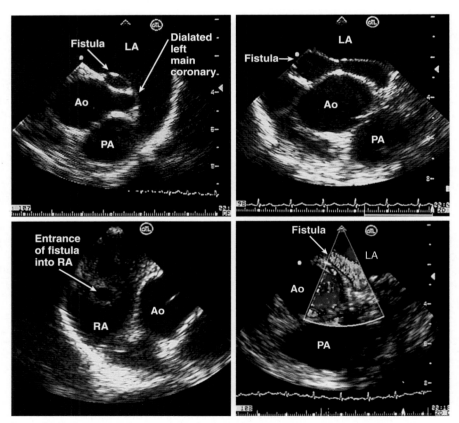

Figure 17–10 Coronary arteriovenous fistula from the left main coronary artery to the RA in a 20-year-old woman with a continuous murmur on auscultation. Transthoracic imaging showed an abnormal flow pattern in the RA. TEE imaging showed a dilated left main coronary artery (*top left*) with a tortuous channel (*top right*) leading to an entrance in the RA (*bottom left*). Color flow imaging shows disturbed systolic and diastolic flow in the fistula (*bottom right*).

Anomalous Origins of the Coronary Arteries

Other coronary artery abnormalities may be diagnosed on echocardiography, particularly when TTE or TEE images are of high quality, allowing identification of the proximal coronary arteries, such as the origin of the circumflex coronary artery from the right sinus of Valsalva, the origin of the right coronary artery from the left sinus of Valsalva, or the origin of the left main coronary from the right sinus of Valsalva. An anomalous coronary artery arising from the pulmonary artery only occasionally is diagnosed initially in adulthood because the resulting myocardial ischemia usually leads to significant clinical manifestations at a younger age.

Congenital Regurgitant Lesions

Ebstein Anomaly of the Tricuspid Valve

Ebstein anomaly is characterized by adherence of the basal segments of one (most often the septal) or more of the leaflets of the tricuspid valve to the RV endocardium, resulting in the appearance of apical displacement of the tricuspid valve attachment (Fig. 17–11). In Ebstein anomaly, the distance between the tricuspid and mitral annulus exceeds the normal 10-mm difference. In severe cases, the tricuspid valve may be displaced nearly to the RV apex. In addition, the tricuspid valve leaflets are thickened and malformed. Functionally, tricuspid regurgitation nearly always is present and may be severe. Typically, there is no antegrade obstruction to RV diastolic filling (Fig. 17–12).

As a result of the apical displacement of the tricuspid leaflet insertion, a portion of the anatomic RV physiologically serves as part of the RA. This "atrialized" ventricle adds to the appearance of RA enlargement, which is augmented by chronic atrial volume

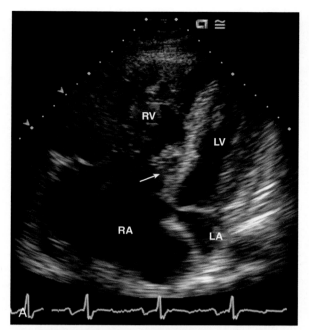

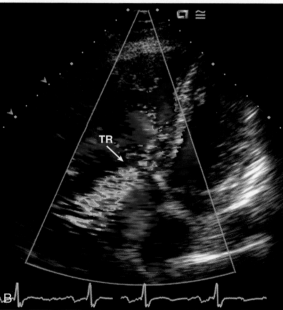

Figure 17–12 Apical four-chamber view (**A**) of an adult with Ebstein anomaly showing the apically displaced tricuspid valve (*arrow*), compared to the tricuspid annulus (*dashed line*), with RV and RA enlargement. Color flow Doppler (**B**) shows severe tricuspid regurgitation (TR).

Ebstein Anomaly

Figure 17–11 Schematic diagram of Ebstein anomaly showing apical displacement of the tricuspid valve and "atrialization" of the base of the RV. Tricuspid regurgitation (TR) with RV and RA enlargement typically is present.

overload from tricuspid regurgitation. Ebstein anomaly may be seen as an isolated anatomic defect or may be associated with an aberrant atrioventricular conduction bypass tract (Wolff-Parkinson-White syndrome), an ASD, or other congenital anomalies (e.g., ventricular inversion). Ebstein anomaly of the anatomic tricuspid valve in a patient with corrected transposition results in systemic atrioventricular valve regurgitation and chronic volume overload of the systemic ventricle.

Myxomatous Mitral Valve Disease

Like a bicuspid aortic valve, myxomatous mitral valve disease may be silent clinically until late in life, when progressive leaflet changes result in significant mitral regurgitation and symptom onset (see Chapter 12). The thickened, redundant mitral valve leaflets of myxomatous disease may result in slowly increasing severity of chronic mitral regurgitation with progressive volume overload of the LV and LA. Alternatively, chordal rupture can result in acute mitral regurgitation with abrupt symptom onset. Myxomatous involvement of tricuspid and, less often, aortic valves also may be present.

Atrial Septal Defects

Anatomy

There are three basic anatomic types of ASD (Fig. 17–13). The most common is a secundum defect, in which the central section of the atrial septum (the fossa ovalis) is absent due to failure of the secundum atrial septum to cover the foramen secundum during development.

A primum ASD is absence of the section of the interatrial septum adjacent to the central fibrous body. Developmentally, there is abnormal formation of the septum primum with failure of closure of the foramen primum, which often is associated with abnormalities of the atrioventricular valves, especially a cleft anterior mitral leaflet. The cleft in the anterior leaflet is seen in the parasternal short-axis view, while lateral-to-medial angulation in the long-axis image plane shows the differing patterns of motion of the medial and lateral leaflet segments (see Fig. 17–2) A cleft mitral valve may be competent if there is adequate systolic apposition of leaflet segments or may result in mitral regurgitation if closure is functionally inadequate. In a more severe developmental abnormality—called an atrioventricular canal or endocardial cushion defect—the entire central fibrous body is absent, resulting in a primum ASD, a VSD, and abnormalities of the atrioventricular valves.

The third type of ASD is the sinus venosus defect. This abnormal communication between RA and LA is developmentally related to abnormal fusion between the embryologic sinus venosus and the atrium—and thus is located near the junction of the atrium with either the superior or the inferior vena cava. Partial anomalous pulmonary venous return may be associated with a sinus venosus defect or may be seen as an isolated defect, which may not be diagnosed until adulthood. Anomalous pulmonary

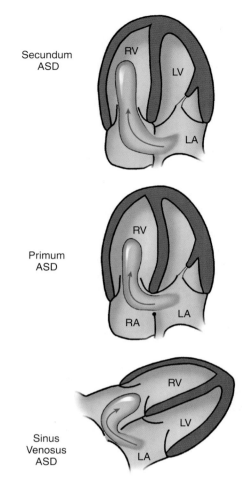

Figure 17–13 Schematic of primum, secundum, and sinus venosus atrial septal defects (ASDs). A secundum ASD is seen in the midsection of the atrial septum with prominent left-to-right flow on color imaging (*stippled area*). Paradoxical septal motion and RV and RA enlargement are present when the shunt is significant. A primum ASD is located near the atrioventricular connection and may be associated with abnormalities of the atrioventricular valves. A sinus venosus ASD is located at the base. Imaging of a sinus venosus defect may be difficult on transthoracic views but sometimes can be demonstrated from a subcostal approach.

veins can drain directly into the RA or into the superior or inferior vena cava.

Imaging

Ultrasound imaging of an ASD is most reliable from a subcostal approach so that the ultrasound beam is perpendicular to the plane of the interatrial septum. From apical or parasternal windows, apparent loss of signal from the atrial septum may be due to a parallel alignment between the ultrasound beam and the structures of interest (i.e., no ultrasound is reflected back to the transducer).

Secundum ASDs are seen in the central portion of the atrial septum (Fig. 17–14), and primum defects (Figs. 17–15 and 17–16) are seen adjacent to the annuli

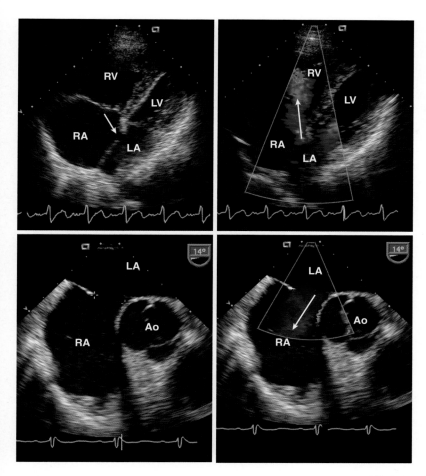

Figure 17–14 A secundum atrial septal defect is seen on transthoracic imaging (*top*) in a fore-shortened apical four-chamber view (*arrow*) in association with marked RV and RA enlargement due to the left-to-right shunt seen on color flow imaging (*top right*). TEE imaging allows more precise localization and measurement of the septal defect (*bottom*). Left-to-right flow across the defect is low velocity, since the pressure difference is small, so a uniform color signal is seen.

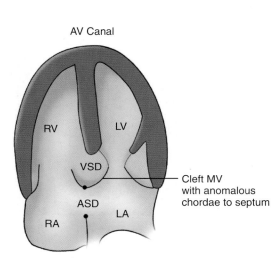

Figure 17–15 Schematic of an atrioventricular (AV) canal defect in a four-chamber view.

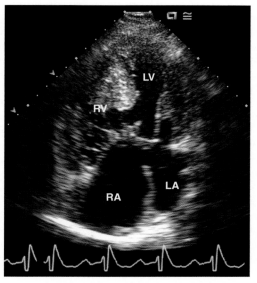

Figure 17–16 Ostium primum atrial septal defect (ASD) with an accompanying ventricular septal defect (VSD)—also called an atrioventricular canal—in a young woman with Down syndrome. This apical four-chamber view in systole shows the ASD, VSD, and common atrioventricular valve. RV and LV pressures are equal in systole, and pressure in all four chambers is equal in diastole. These findings are consistent with Eisenmenger's physiology unless severe pulmonic stenosis is present.

of the atrioventricular valves. Imaging of a sinus venosus defect may not be possible on a TTE study. However, because the defect is located in the superior and posterior aspects of the interatrial septum, a subcostal approach can visualize the defect in some patients. TTE from a subcostal approach has a sensitivity of 89% for detection of a secundum ASD and 100% for a primum defect, but only 44% for a sinus venosus defect. Sinus venosus defects are well demonstrated from the TEE approach (Figs. 17–17 to 17–19).

If an ASD is associated with a significant left-to-right shunt, RA enlargement, RV enlargement, and paradoxical septal motion consistent with right-sided volume overload (Figs. 17–20 and 17–21) are uniformly present. In fact, evidence for right-sided heart volume overload often is the first abnormality noted during the echocardiographic examination. When evidence for right-sided heart volume overload is present in the absence of a visualized ASD or other definable cause for volume overload (e.g., tricuspid regurgitation), TEE imaging should be performed to evaluate for the possibility of a sinus venosus defect or partial anomalous pulmonary venous return.

Doppler Examination

Color flow imaging often allows reliable identification of the ASD flow based on the spatial distribution of the flow disturbance from the LA to RA. However, multiple tomographic image planes are needed for correct identification of the origin of the flow signal. In some cases, the diastolic/systolic low-velocity flow signal across the ASD can be difficult to distinguish from other venous flow signals in the RA. Care must be taken to avoid mistaking superior vena cava flow into the RA, which often streams along the interatrial septum, for ASD flow. This appearance can be particularly misleading in high-volume flow states, such as pregnancy. Occasionally, a tricuspid regurgitant jet directed along the interatrial septum results in a confusing flow pattern, as well.

The subcostal window is optimal for color imaging of flow across the ASD, since the direction of flow is parallel to the ultrasound beam. Color flow imaging from other windows (including parasternal and apical) also is helpful, because it is the location and timing of the flow disturbance—rather than the absolute velocity of flow—that are diagnostic of the defect in the atrial septum. Color flow imaging shows a broad flow stream from LA to RA in both diastole and systole with a more prominent diastolic component. With large shunts, the flow across the atrial septum extends across the open tricuspid valve into the RV in diastole. Proximal flow acceleration on the LA side of the septum usually is evident.

TEE imaging is helpful for further definition of the site and size of an ASD if TTE images are suboptimal and for device sizing before percutaneous closure. In

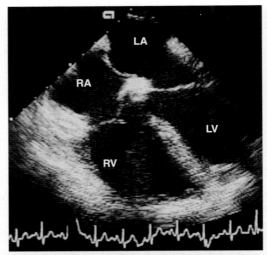

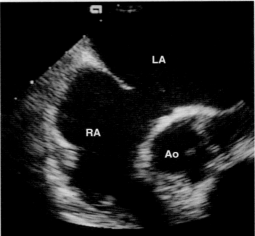

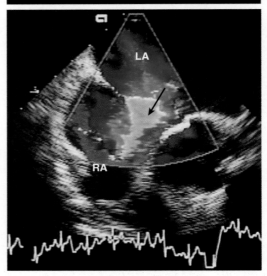

Figure 17–17 Transesophageal demonstration of an atrial septal defect in a 53-year-old woman. In a standard four-chamber view the septum appears intact (*top*). However, with slight anterior angulation, a defect is seen adjacent to the aortic root (*middle*) with color flow showing left-to-right flow across the defect (*bottom*).

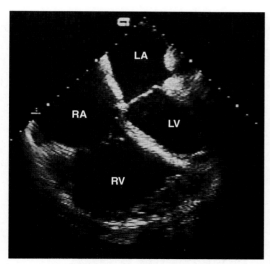

Figure 17–18 Sinus venosus atrial septal defect in a 74-year-old man. Although the TEE four-chamber view shows marked volume overload of the right side of the heart, the atrial septum appears intact in this view.

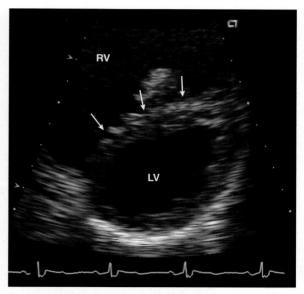

Figure 17–20 RV enlargement due to a secundum atrial septal defect. This parasternal short-axis view in diastole shows the flattened septal curvature (*arrows*), consistent with RV volume overload.

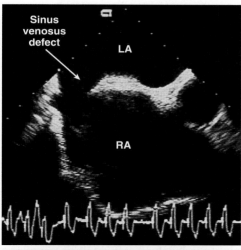

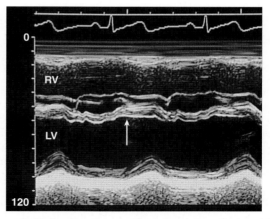

Figure 17–21 Paradoxical septal motion (note anterior motion in systole) and RV enlargement on M-mode in a 21-year-old woman with an ASD.

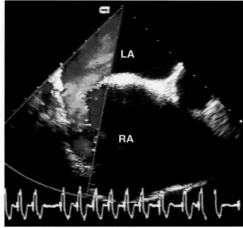

Figure 17–19 In the same patient as in Figure 17–18, the region of the atrial septum just inferior to the superior vena cava is absent (*top*), and color flow demonstrates left-to-right flow across this defect (*bottom*).

addition, TEE imaging usually is needed when a sinus venosus defect or partial anomalous pulmonary venous return is suspected. Using a biplane or multiplane approach, 2D and color flow imaging will identify the abnormal defect and flow communication in the superior aspect of the posterior portion of the interatrial septum. Small secundum defects also are most likely to be detected from a TEE approach. The severity of left-to-right shunting across the ASD can be measured as described previously (Fig. 17–22).

Contrast Echocardiography

In a patient with a primum or secundum ASD, peripheral venous injection of echo contrast material

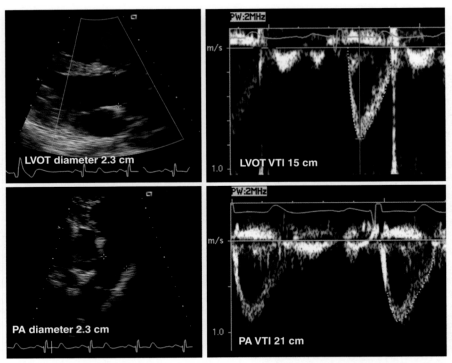

Figure 17–22 Calculation of the shunt ratio in a patient with an atrial septal defect. Systemic flow (Q_s) is calculated from the LV outflow tract diameter (2.2 cm) and Doppler velocity time integral (VTI) (15 cm) (*top*), while pulmonary blood flow is calculated from the pulmonary artery diameter (2.3 cm) and Doppler VTI (21 cm) (*bottom*). In this example, Q_p is 87 and Q_s is 57 mL, so that Q_p/Q_s is only 1.5, a value of borderline significance.

shows passage of microbubbles across the interatrial septum, even when the shunt is predominantly left to right in direction. The explanation for this observation is that RA pressure transiently and briefly exceeds LA pressure, allowing passage of a small volume of blood from right to left. This small volume can be identified when contrast echoes from the RA appear in the LA. Dense contrast in the RA also allows demonstration of a "negative" contrast jet across the ASD; that is, the blood flow from the LA into the RA will appear as an area with no echo contrast.

Contrast echo studies are rarely needed for diagnosis of an ASD when typical 2D echo, Doppler, and color Doppler findings are present. The principle of using echo contrast to identify very small degrees of right-to-left shunting can be used to detect a patent foramen ovale as a potential etiology for a systemic embolic event (see Chapter 15).

After Atrial Septal Defect Repair

With a prior ASD repair or closure, there may be mild residual RV and RA dilatation. More than mild persistent dilation should prompt a search for a residual defect or a leak around the patch repair or closure device.

Ventricular Septal Defects

Anatomy

There are four anatomically different types of VSDs (Fig. 17–23). The most common type is a perimembranous VSD located in the region of the membranous septum immediately inferomedial to the aortic valve and lateral to the septal leaflet of the tricuspid valve. Small membranous VSDs may close spontaneously during childhood by approximation of the tricuspid valve septal leaflet across the defect. A completely closed defect may be undetectable in adulthood, or a residual anatomic abnormality—a ventricular septal aneurysm—may be visualized at the closure site without evidence of blood flow from the LV to the RV. Incomplete closure leads to a persistent, albeit smaller, VSD, which may be difficult to distinguish from septal aneurysm on 2D imaging. However, color flow and CW Doppler show typical evidence for an abnormal flow communication between the LV and RV even when the defect is small.

Muscular VSDs occur at any location in the muscular portion of the septum and may be multiple. When the defect is small, imaging may not be possible with a tomographic imaging technique (such as echocardiography) even when multiple image planes

Membranous VSD

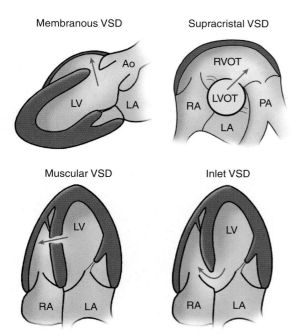

Supracristal VSD

Muscular VSD

Inlet VSD

Figure 17–23 Schematic of types of ventricular septal defects (VSDs). A membranous VSD is seen in a medially angulated parasternal long-axis view, immediately adjacent to the aortic valve. A supracristal VSD is seen well in a short-axis view just below the aortic valve with flow from the LV outflow tract into the outflow region of the RV. A muscular VSD can be located anywhere in the muscular portion of the ventricular septum and may be multiple. An inlet VSD is seen in the apical four-chamber view and may be associated with an atrioventricular canal defect.

are examined. Again, Doppler data are diagnostic in this situation.

Inlet VSDs are the result of failure of complete formation of the central fibrous body. This defect is located inferior to the aortic valve plane, adjacent to the mitral and tricuspid valve annuli. Inlet defects often are associated with other anomalies of the central fibrous body such as a primum ASD, atrioventricular valve abnormalities, or a complete atrioventricular canal defect.

Supracristal VSDs are located in the RV outflow portion of the septum (above the crista ventricularis), lateral and just inferior to the aortic valve. These defects are rarely initially diagnosed in adulthood.

Imaging

As noted, while large defects may be visualized easily with 2D echocardiography, small defects may be very difficult to demonstrate. Peri-membranous VSDs are imaged best in a parasternal long-axis view angulated slightly medially (see Figure 17–3). In the short-axis view just below the aortic valve level, the VSD is seen in a 10-o'clock position inferior to the right coronary cusp of the aortic valve and adjacent to the septal leaflet of the tricuspid valve. In this view, a supracristal VSD is located at the 2-o'clock position, inferior to the left coronary leaflet of the aortic valve and adjacent to the pulmonic valve. A supracristal VSD is imaged in the long-axis plane by lateral angulation of the transducer from the standard long-axis view. Muscular VSDs may be seen in sequential basal-to-apical short-axis views of the LV or in the apical four-chamber view. Inlet VSDs are best imaged in the apical four-chamber view or from the parasternal window in a short-axis view at the mitral valve level.

Most VSDs seen in adults are associated with a very small flow volume so that chamber sizes and ventricular function are normal. When there is a significant volume of left-to-right flow across a VSD, dilation of the LV and LA occur due to volume overload of these chambers. RV size usually is normal, since the systolic flow across the defect is ejected directly into the PA and LV systolic function typically is preserved because the shunt flow is ejected into the low-impedance pulmonary vascular bed. With large shunts, pulmonary vascular hypertension supervenes, resulting in Eisenmenger's physiology with RV hypertrophy and dilation (Fig. 17–24).

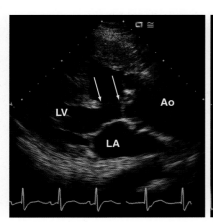
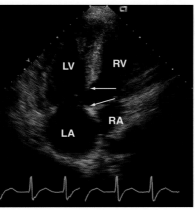

Figure 17–24 Large ventricular septal defect (*between arrows*) in a 26-year-old woman with Eisenmenger's physiology seen in a parasternal long-axis view (*left*) and apical four-chamber view (*right*). Severe RV hypertrophy is present. Doppler examination will show low-velocity bidirectional flow across the defect due to equalization of RV and LV pressures.

Doppler Findings

Color Doppler flow imaging shows a flow disturbance on the right side of the ventricular septum (with a left-to-right shunt). The presence and location of this flow disturbance are diagnostic even in the absence of a demonstrable defect on 2D imaging. The flow disturbance is detectable in the defect itself with proximal acceleration on the left side of the septum, immediately adjacent to the defect. Doppler ultrasound has a sensitivity of 90% and a specificity of 98% for detection of a VSD.

CW Doppler ultrasound shows a high-velocity left-to-right signal, with the shape of the velocity curve similar to that of mitral regurgitation, as determined by the instantaneous LV-to-RV pressure differences. In diastole, left-to-right shunting persists at a lower velocity (proportional to the diastolic LV-to-RV pressure differences) with the shape of the time-velocity curve similar to that of mitral stenosis. Brief reversal of flow may be, but is not always, present during isovolumic relaxation and contraction phases. Both the diastolic flow and brief reversals during the isovolumic periods are low velocity and thus may not be appreciated except at low high-pass filter settings on the Doppler spectral recording. Because this reversal of flow may not occur, intravenous injection of echo contrast material is less sensitive for detection of an intracardiac shunt at the ventricular level than at the atrial level.

Calculation of a pulmonic-to-systemic shunt ratio rarely is needed in adults with VSDs because either (1) the defect is small with a small volume of left-to-right shunt, or (2) a large defect with a significant shunt in childhood now has resulted in Eisenmenger's physiology with equalization of RV and LV pressures. If calculation of a shunt ratio is needed, systemic flow can be calculated in the aorta, and pulmonary flow can be calculated either in the PA (if not disturbed by the septal defect flow) or across the mitral valve (pulmonary venous return).

Patent Ductus Arteriosus

A patent ductus arteriosus often is difficult to image in adults because of limited acoustic access. However, the chronic volume overload of the LA and LV is manifested as dilation of these chambers. Left-to-right flow through the ductus can be detected with either conventional pulsed or color Doppler flow imaging using both parasternal short-axis and RV outflow views of the PA (Figs. 17–25 and 17–26). Diastolic ductal flow in the PA, typically seen along the lateral wall of this vessel, has a sensitivity of

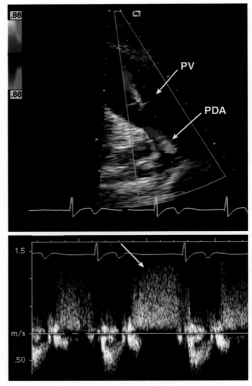

Figure 17–26 Patent ductus arteriosus (PDA) in a 22-year-old patient referred for an asymptomatic murmur. The parasternal RV outflow view shows the pulmonary artery with a color jet of pulmonic regurgitation at the pulmonary valve (PV) level and a second color jet in diastole in the PA. Pulsed Doppler of the patent ductus flow shows characteristic diastolic flow reversal (*arrow*) extending into early systole. The pulmonic regurgitant signal was shorter with a lower velocity.

Figure 17–25 Schematic of a patent ductus arteriosus. Flow (*arrow*) from the descending aorta into the pulmonary artery (PA) often streams along the lateral wall of the PA on color flow imaging. Pulsed or continuous-wave Doppler shows holodiastolic flow reversal in the PA. Systolic flow typically is abnormal as well, since aortic pressure exceeds pulmonary artery pressure throughout the cardiac cycle (giving rise to a continuous murmur on auscultation).

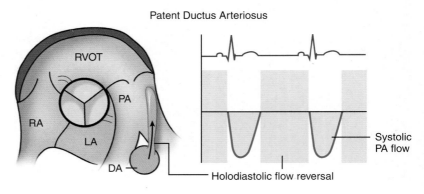

Patent Ductus Arteriosus

96% and specificity of 100% for diagnosis of a patent ductus arteriosus. Recording of flow in the descending aorta, from a suprasternal notch approach, shows holodiastolic flow reversal due to antegrade flow into the ductus in diastole. This finding must be distinguished from diastolic flow reversal due to aortic regurgitation, because the two conditions may coexist in adult patients.

Corrected Transposition of the Great Arteries

Congenitally corrected transposition of the great arteries (L-TGA) is sometimes called "ventricular inversion," because the anatomic RV serves as the systemic ventricle, and the anatomic LV serves as the pulmonic ventricle. Thus, physiologically the pathway of pulmonic and systemic blood flow is normal in uncomplicated corrected transposition (Fig. 17–27) Systemic venous blood returns to the RA, crosses the mitral valve into an anatomic LV, and then is ejected into the PA. Pulmonary venous return to the LA crosses the tricuspid valve into an anatomic RV and then is ejected into the aorta. In the absence of associated defects, the diagnosis may be made "incidentally" in adulthood (Fig. 17–28). However, associated defects are common, including VSDs, pulmonic stenosis, complete heart block, and Ebstein anomaly of the "inverted" tricuspid valve. Dilation, and eventual systolic dysfunction, of the systemic ventricle is common, although it is unclear whether this is due to the anatomy of the RV being less suited to performing as the systemic ventricle, to inadequate coronary blood flow via the right coronary artery, or to associated systemic atrioventricular valve regurgitation.

On echocardiographic examination, corrected transposition is recognized by identifying the anatomic ventricles in a side-by-side orientation and demonstrating the pathway of blood flow. Associated defects have 2D echo and Doppler findings as described for each abnormality. In addition, the position of the great vessels is abnormal, with the two semilunar valves lying in the same image plane (best seen in parasternal short-axis views) and with the great vessels parallel to each other (best seen in parasternal long-axis views). Typically, the aortic annulus is anterior and to the left of the pulmonic valve (hence the "L" in L-TGA). Corrected transposition also is associated with dextroversion (apex points toward the right), which makes the echocardiographic examination technically more difficult because the cardiac structures lie directly behind the sternum, limiting acoustic access.

"Incidental" Congenital Anomalies

A few congenital anomalies have no known adverse clinical effects but are important in that, if not recognized, they can be mistaken for pathologic conditions

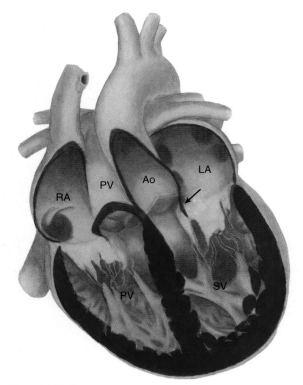

Figure 17–27 Illustration of congenitally corrected transposition (L-TGA). The systemic venous blood returns to the RA, passes across the mitral valve into an anatomic LV (the pulmonary ventricle [PV]), and is ejected into the pulmonary artery (PA). Pulmonary venous return into the LA is directed across the tricuspid valve into an anatomic RV (the systemic ventricle [SV]) and from there into the aorta (Ao). Common associated abnormalities are an Ebstein-type malformation of the tricuspid valve resulting in systemic atrioventricular valve regurgitation, pulmonic stenosis, a VSD, and complete heart block. The Ao is anterior and toward the patient's left side, and the Ao and PA are parallel to each other. *(From Gurvitz M: General echocardiographic approach to th adult with suspected congenital heart disease. In Otto CM [ed]: The Practice of Clinical Echocardiography, 3rd ed. Philadelphia: Elsevier/Saunders 2007.)*

and prompt other (possibly harmful) diagnostic tests. A persistent left superior vena cava is seen in a small percentage (0.3% to 0.5%) of otherwise normal individuals and in a higher percentage (3% to 10%) of patients with other congenital heart abnormalities. Since this vein drains into the coronary sinus, dilation of the coronary sinus is seen on parasternal long- and short-axis views and on an apical four-chamber view angulated posteriorly (see Fig. 15–5). This latter view nicely illustrates the entry of the dilated coronary sinus into the RA. The diagnosis can be confirmed (if questions remain) by injection of echo contrast material into the left arm, which will first opacify the coronary sinus and then the RA. Injection of echo contrast material into the right arm will opacify only the RA. The dilated coronary sinus can protrude into

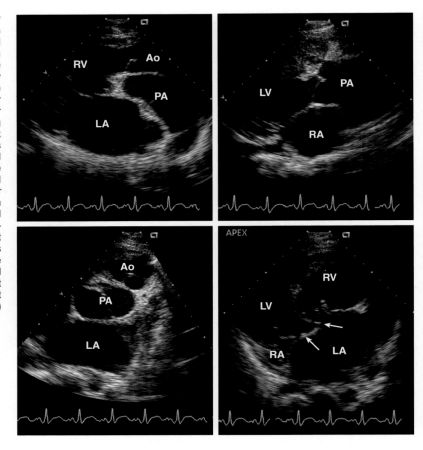

Figure 17-28 In a patient with congenitally corrected transposition of the great arteries (L-TGA), two long-axis images are obtained from a parasternal position with the aorta and pulmonary artery (PA) in a side-by-side orientation. The systemic RV and anteriorly located Ao are seen (*upper left*) with the muscular separation between the atrioventricular valve and semilunar valve evident. This anterior great vessel was identified as the Ao by following it superiorly to the arch and head and neck vessels. With slight lateral angulation, a long-axis view of the pulmonary LV and posteriorly located (and dilated) PA is seen (*upper right*). Note the fibrous continuity between the atrioventricular and semilunar valves. In the short-axis view (*lower left*) the aortic and pulmonic valves are both seen in cross-section with the aortic valve located anterior to the pulmonic valve. The apical four-chamber view in the standard display format demonstrates the anatomic RV on the patient's left, which serves as the systemic ventricle. Note apical displacement of the tricuspid valve septal leaflet as compared with the mitral leaflet insertion (*arrows*). This patient has significant regurgitation of the systemic (anatomic tricuspid) atrioventricular valve resulting in LA enlargement.

the LA, particularly on the parasternal long-axis view, sometimes being mistaken for an LA mass.

Idiopathic dilation of the PA is another uncommon benign abnormality. The diagnosis is made when the PA is enlarged, but there is no evidence of pulmonic stenosis (which might result in post-stenotic dilation) or other congenital abnormalities.

A Chiari network is a prominent inferior vena cava valve with fibrous extensions to the crista terminalis and/or coronary sinus valve seen in 2% of patients undergoing TEE. These fibrous connections are fenestrated and lax, forming a "network" which shows rapid chaotic motion during the cardiac cycle. On 2D imaging, the appearance of small, echogenic targets moving rapidly in the RA suggests this diagnosis. Although the Chiari network itself is benign, there is a high likelihood of an associated atrial septal aneurysm or patent foramen ovale.

Other Congenital Cardiac Diseases Presenting in Adults

In addition to conditions considered under the category of congenital heart disease, other cardiac diseases in adults are congenital (or genetic) in origin but usually present in adulthood. For example, hypertrophic

cardiomyopathy and Marfan syndrome are inherited disorders (see Chapters 9 and 16). Other types of cardiomyopathy may show a familial pattern, suggesting a genetic component. As our knowledge of molecular cardiology expands, other "acquired" diseases may be found to be genetic in origin.

ADULT CONGENITAL HEART DISEASE WITH PRIOR SURGICAL PROCEDURES

Classification of Types of Procedures

Numerous palliative and corrective surgical treatments for congenital heart disease have been developed since the first closure of a patent ductus arteriosus in 1938. These procedures can be grouped in several categories, as indicated in Table 17-2 and as listed here.

- ❏ Relief of stenosis
- ❏ Closures
- ❏ Shunts
- ❏ Pulmonary banding
- ❏ Atrial switch
- ❏ Arterial switch
- ❏ Conduits

TABLE 17–2   Common Operations for Congenital Heart Disease Seen in Surviving Adults

Type	Procedure	Defects Treated	Description	Years
Shunts	Blalock-Taussig	Reduced pulmonary blood flow (TOF, TGA, pulmonary atresia, tricuspid atresia)	Classic: Anastomosis of subclavian artery to PA (with or without modification)	1945–1990s
			Interposition tube graft (subclavian remains intact)	1945–present
	Potts	Alternate to Blalock	Descending aorta to left PA	1946–mid-1960s
	Waterston	Alternate to Blalock	Ascending aorta to right PA	1962–1980s
	Glenn	Tricuspid atresia, pulmonic atresia	SVC to divided right PA only	1959–1980s
			Bidirectional Glenn = SVC to right PA without isolation from left PA	1985–1990s
Atrial mixing	Surgical atrial septostomy	TGA (early palliation), mitral atresia, complex congenital heart disease	Also called Blalock-Hanlon procedure	1950–early 1980s
	Balloon atrial septostomy	TGA, tricuspid atresia	Percutaneous atrial septostomy, also called Rashkind balloon procedure	1966–present
Closures	Atrial septal defect (ASD) closure	ASD with significant shunt	Primary or patch closure	1954–present
			Percutaneous closure	1990–present
	Ventricular septal defect (VSD) closure	Isolated VSD or with other anomalies (TOF)	Primary or patch closure	1954–present
	Patent ductus arteriosus (PDA) ligation	Patent ductus arteriosus	Ligation ± division of PDA	1938–present
			Transcatheter technique	1981–present
	Endocardial cushion defect repair	Endocardial cushion defect (also called atrioventricular canal defect)	Closure of ASD and VSD, repair of atrioventricular valve abnormalities (e.g., cleft mitral leaflet)	1955–present
PA banding	Surgical reduction in flow area of PA	Large left-to-right shunt lesions	PA band to decrease PA flow and pressure	1952–present
Atrial baffles	Mustard	TGA (replaced by arterial switch procedures at many centers)	Dacron or pericardial baffle directs systemic venous return to PA via anatomic LV, pulmonary venous return to aorta via anatomic RV	1964–1990s
	Senning	TGA (replaced by arterial switch procedures at many centers). May be used as part of "double switch" procedure for L-TGA	RA free wall and interatrial septal tissue used for interatrial baffle similar to a Mustard repair.	1959–1964, 1980–present
Relief of stenosis	Aortic coarctation repair	Aortic coarctation	Various procedures including end-to-end anastomosis, patch enlargement, Gore-Tex graft; balloon dilation for recoarctation	1944–present
				Balloon dilation 1983–present
	Pulmonic valvotomy	TOF, pulmonic stenosis	Brock trans-RV approach	1948–1960s
			Direct surgical repair	1960s–present
			Balloon dilation	1982–present
	Aortic valvotomy	Congenital aortic stenosis	Direct surgical valvotomy or percutaneous balloon dilation	1954–present

Continued

TABLE 17–2—Cont'd

Type	Procedure	Defects Treated	Description	Years
Relief of stenosis— cont'd	Mitral repair	Congenital mitral stenosis	Surgical commissurotomy— initially a "closed" procedure without cardiopulmonary bypass	1949–1990s (closed) 1960s–present (open)
	Konno procedure	LV outflow obstruction not amenable to valvotomy and LVOT too small for an adequate size prosthetic valve	LVOT enlargement by creation of a VSD that is then patched, plus aortic valve replacement	1976–present
Complex repairs	Arterial switch	TGA	Switch of aortic root and PA trunk, coronaries transposed to neoaorta (also called Jatene procedure)	1988–present
	Fontan procedure	Tricuspid atresia, double-inlet ventricle with pulmonic stenosis.	Direct connection of systemic venous return to PA with no intervening right ventricle via (1) right atrial to PA anastomosis, (2) intracardiac conduit or (3) lateral tunnel. See Figure 17–34.	1971–present
	Rastelli procedure	TGA + VSD + subvalvular pulmonic stenosis, truncus arteriosus, double-outlet RV	Valved conduit from RV to transected PA. LV to aorta via VSD and intraventricular patch	1968–present
	Double switch procedure	L-TGA	Interatrial baffle (Mustard or Senning) plus arterial switch	2000–present
	TOF repair	TOF	VSD patch closure, relief of pulmonic stenosis, often with transannular patch	1954–present

ASD, atrial septal defect; L-TGA, congenitally corrected transposition of the great arteries; LVOT, left ventricular outflow tract; PA, pulmonary artery; PDA, patent ductus arteriosus; SVC, superior vena cava; TGA, transposition of the great arteries; TOF, tetralogy of Fallot; VSD, ventricular septal defect.

The approximate years during which each procedure was performed are shown to indicate which are likely to be encountered in a patient of a given age and to provide a historical explanation of why a patient may have had a particular procedure. Current surgical and interventional approaches provide a more complete anatomic and physiologic correction than earlier procedures. However, many patients with older surgical procedures continue to be seen as they grow to adulthood.

Procedures to relieve congenital stenotic lesions include aortic coarctation repair; pulmonic, aortic, or mitral valvotomy either with direct surgical inspection or with a percutaneous balloon; and the Konno procedure to relieve LV outflow obstruction. A residual gradient may be present after these procedures, and valvular regurgitation may be induced.

Procedures to close congenital intracardiac shunts— ASDs, VSDs, patent ductus arteriosus—are conceptually straightforward and may be performed by suturing the edges of the defect (primary closure), by using a surgical pericardial or synthetic patch or by a percutaneous closure device. The most common long-term complication of a shunt closure is a residual shunt.

In conditions with low pulmonary blood flow, such as tetralogy of Fallot, transposition of the great arteries, pulmonary atresia, or tricuspid atresia, an intracardiac shunt can be created to increase pulmonary blood flow. Shunts may redirect flow from a systemic artery to the pulmonary artery (Blalock-Taussig, Potts, Waterston), from a systemic vein to the pulmonary bed (Glenn), or at the atrial level (Blalock-Hanlon or balloon atrial septostomy). In some cases these shunts are removed ("taken down") at the time of subsequent corrective surgery. Complications of surgical shunts include:

❒ Inadequate pulmonary blood flow due to kinking or closure of the shunt
❒ Excessive pulmonary blood flow resulting in pulmonary hypertension
❒ Thrombus formation

Pulmonary banding is a palliative procedure that creates functional pulmonary stenosis to reduce pulmonary blood flow and "protect" the pulmonary vasculature from irreversible pulmonary hypertension. Banding is performed in patients with a large left-to-right shunt when definitive repair is not possible or must be delayed. If the degree of banding is not adequate, pulmonary hypertension still may ensue. Distal migration of the band can result in unequal right versus left pulmonary artery obstruction.

Other intracardiac repairs include the Fontan procedure, which directs systemic venous return to the pulmonary artery without an intervening RV in patients with an absent right heart (e.g., tricuspid atresia) and other more complex repairs as indicated in Table 17–2. When patients with previous surgical procedures for congenital heart disease present for echocardiographic evaluation, more detailed references on congenital heart disease can be helpful in planning, performing, and interpreting the echocardiographic examination.

Tetralogy of Fallot

The three primary characteristics of tetralogy of Fallot (Figs. 17–29 and 17–30) are:

- A membranous VSD
- A large aorta positioned across the VSD ("overriding")
- An RV outflow obstruction that may be sub-, supra-, or valvular in location

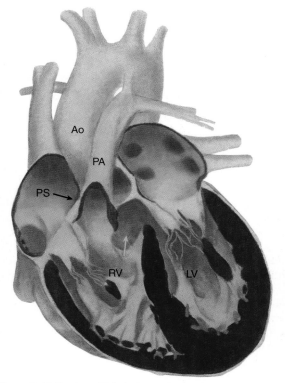

Figure 17–29 Tetralogy of Fallot is characterized by a large ventricular septal defect (*cyan arrow*) with an enlarged Ao that spans (or overrides) the defect, pulmonic stenosis (PS, which may be subpulmonic or valvular), and compensatory RV hypertrophy. *(From King ME: Echocardiographic evaluation of the adult with unoperated congenital heart disease. In Otto CM [ed]: The Practice of Clinical Echocardiography, 3rd ed. Philadelphia: Elsevier/Saunders, 2007.)*

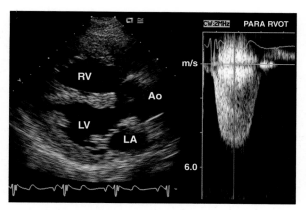

Figure 17–30 A 23-year-old man with an unrepaired tetralogy of Fallot. The overriding Ao and ventricular septal defect are seen in the parasternal long-axis view (*left*). The continuous-wave Doppler signal across the stenotic pulmonic valve has a maximum velocity of 5 m/s, consistent with severe pulmonic stenosis and low pulmonary pressures (*right*).

The fourth feature of this tetralogy is RV hypertrophy secondary to outflow obstruction. Adults with an untreated tetralogy of Fallot are rarely seen due to the high mortality of this condition without surgical intervention. In adults with a repaired tetralogy of Fallot, the VSD patch is evident, the aortic root is enlarged, and some degree of residual RV outflow obstruction may be present. However, the major long-term issue in adults with surgically treated tetralogy of Fallot is late pulmonic regurgitation (Fig. 17–31). With severe pulmonic regurgitation, color Doppler may be unimpressive because diastolic reverse

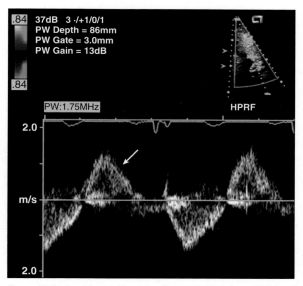

Figure 17–31 In a 34-year-old woman with a repaired tetralogy of Fallot and progressive RV enlargement, the continuous-wave Doppler signal across the pulmonic valve shows laminar forward and reverse low-velocity flow consistent with severe pulmonic regurgitation. Because the flow velocity is low, this finding may be missed on real-time viewing of the images, emphasizing the importance of frame-by-frame review when this diagnosis is suspected.

flow is laminar and low velocity. The pulsed or CW Doppler signal is diagnostic with diastolic reversal of flow equal in signal strength to antegrade flow with the signal reaching the zero baseline before end-diastole, due to equalization of pulmonic and RV diastolic pressures. Evaluation of RV size and systolic function on serial studies is particularly important, which may be supplemented by quantitative cardiac magnetic resonance (CMR) measurement of RV volumes and ejection fraction.

Complete Transposition of the Great Arteries

Adults with an atrial switch for complete transposition procedure are still often seen given the more recent introduction of the arterial switch procedure (Fig. 17–32). Atrial switch (Mustard or Senning) procedures for complete transposition are designed to redirect systemic venous return to the PA (via the anatomic mitral valve and LV) and pulmonary venous return to the aorta (via the anatomic tricuspid valve and RV). The 3D anatomy of these baffles is

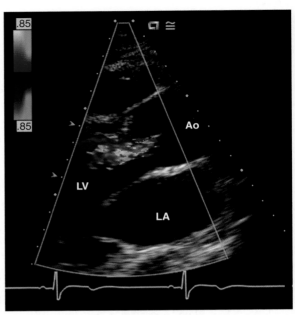

Figure 17–33 Parasternal long-axis view of the aortic valve (originally the pulmonic valve) in a 24-year-old man with complete transposition of the great arteries and a great vessel switch procedure as a child. Moderate aortic regurgitation now is present, and the aortic root is dilated.

complex and may be difficult to demonstrate on a TTE study due to poor ultrasound penetration at that depth. A TEE approach improves image quality, but an experienced examiner and multiple tomographic planes are needed to fully assess the interatrial baffle. Late complications of this procedure include baffle obstruction, baffle leaks, systolic dysfunction of the systemic (anatomic right) ventricle, and arrhythmias.

The arterial switch procedure now has largely replaced the interatrial baffle repair for complete transposition. The aorta and PA are transected and reconnected to the correct ventricular chambers, resulting in a physiologic normal flow pattern. Complications of this procedure are related to reimplantation of the coronary arteries and supravalvular great vessel obstruction at the anastomotic sites. In the long term, dilation of the "aortic sinuses" with aortic regurgitation (the anatomic pulmonary root and valve) also may be seen (Fig. 17–33). The transposed position of the aorta and PA may be demonstrated on echocardiography, and with other imaging approaches in patients with complete transposition, even after an atrial or arterial switch procedure.

Fontan Physiology

The Fontan procedure connects systemic venous return to the PA without an intervening RV. This connection may be from the RA to PA or, more commonly, from the inferior vena cava directly to the PA (lateral tunnel or extracardiac), with the superior

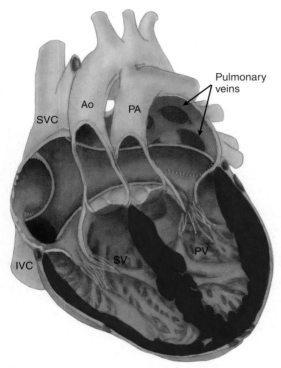

Figure 17–32 Illustration of interatrial baffle repair for transposition of the great arteries that directs systemic venous return to the pulmonary (anatomic LV) ventricle (PV) (and then to the pulmonary artery) and pulmonary venous return to the systemic (anatomic RV) ventricle (SV) (and then Ao). Adequate visualization of the interatrial baffle usually requires TEE imaging in adults. *(From Child J: Echocardiographic evaluation of the adult with postoperative congenital heart disease. In Otto CM [ed]: The Practice of Clinical Echocardiography, 3rd ed. Philadelphia: Elsevier/Saunders, 2007.)*

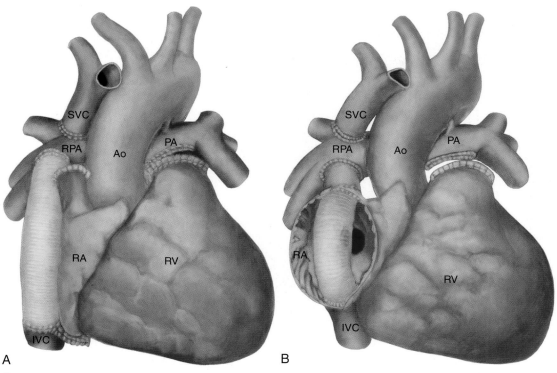

Figure 17–34 Fontan conduit directing systemic venous return to the pulmonary artery (PA) using (**A**) an extracardiac tube from the inferior vena cava (IVC) plus a superior vena cava (SVC) anastomosis to the right pulmonary artery (RPA) in a patient with tricuspid atresia or (**B**) an internal lateral tunnel from the IVC to the reconnected SVC. The early Fontan repair connected the RA directly to the PA. Patients with an RA-to-PA connection often have severe RA enlargement at long-term follow-up. *(From Child J: Echocardiographic evaluation of the adult with postoperative congenital heart disease. In Otto CM [ed]: The Practice of Clinical Echocardiography, 3rd ed. Philadelphia: Elsevier/Saunders, 2007.)*

vena cava connected to the PA (a bidirectional Glenn connection) (Fig. 17–34). Evaluation of patients with a Fontan procedure is complicated by the numerous variations of the surgical approach in the method of connecting systemic venous return to the pulmonary vasculature. TEE imaging often is required for adequate visualization (Fig. 17–35). Late complications of the Fontan procedure include baffle obstruction, interatrial shunts, and thrombus formation.

LIMITATIONS OF ECHOCARDIOGRAPHY/ALTERNATE APPROACHES

Measurement of Right Ventricular Volumes and Ejection Fraction

Accurate quantitative measures of RV size and function often are needed for clinical decision making in adults with congenital heart disease; for example, in repaired tetralogy of Fallot patients with pulmonic regurgitation. Echocardiography allows categorization of RV size as normal versus mild, moderate, or severe dilation and allows a similar qualitative estimate of systolic function. CMR now allows accurate

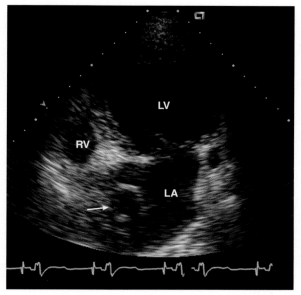

Figure 17–35 Apical "four-chamber" view in a patient with tricuspid atresia and a Fontan conduit, seen as a circulation structure (*arrow*) adjacent to the LA. Often TEE is needed for better visualization of the Fontan conduit.

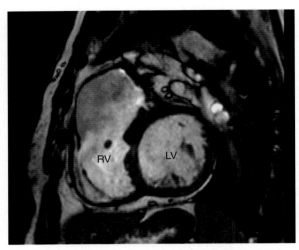

Figure 17–36 CMR images showing severe dilation of the RV in a patient with severe pulmonic regurgitation after childhood repair of tetralogy of Fallot. Quantitative RV volumes and ejection fraction can be measured by tracing the end-diastolic and end-systolic borders on a series of parallel slices that encompass the RV chamber.

measurement of RV size and volume and often is used in conjunction with periodic echocardiography in patient management (Fig. 17–36).

Calculations of Shunt Ratios

Accurate calculation of shunt ratios by Doppler echocardiography depends on accurate stroke volume determinations at two intracardiac sites. Each of these stroke volume determinations can be affected by several factors, as discussed in Chapter 6. Specifically, both the mean spatial flow velocity and the area of flow must be measured correctly. Flow at each site is assumed to be laminar with a flat flow velocity profile. Furthermore, accuracy depends on a parallel intercept angle between the direction of blood flow and the ultrasound beam. The flow area typically is assumed to be circular and is calculated from a 2D echo diameter measurement. Small errors in diameter measurement (which is squared in calculating a circular area) translate into large errors in stroke volume determinations. In adult patients, imaging of the diameter of the PA often is difficult and thus is the major source of error in Doppler-derived shunt ratios.

Alternate methods for calculation of pulmonary to systemic shunt ratios include (1) cardiac catheterization with measurement of intracardiac oxygen saturations and total body oxygen consumption, and (2) first-pass radionuclide estimation from the early recirculation pattern of the time-activity curve.

Imaging

2D TTE imaging in adult patients with congenital heart disease may be limited by poor acoustic access (Table 17–3). Even when image quality is acceptable, evaluation of posterior structures may be limited by lateral resolution at the depth of interest. This can be a problem, particularly in the evaluation of posterior conduits, interatrial baffle repair procedures, sinus venous ASDs, or anomalous pulmonary venous return. TEE imaging offers improved image quality, especially of posterior structures, and is a useful adjunct to TTE imaging in this patient population (Fig. 17–37).

Evaluation of extracardiac anatomy also is difficult. This limits evaluation of the PA branches, systemic arterial or venous shunts to the PA, and abnormalities of the ascending aorta and aortic arch. Other tomographic imaging techniques are especially helpful in assessing the position of the cardiac structures in the chest and in evaluating mediastinal abnormalities not accessible by ultrasound. Both chest computed tomography (CT) and cardiac magnetic resonance imaging (CMR) can be used, with the advantage of a wide field of view for both techniques. With CMR the data can be reformatted, in an orientation based on the long axis of the LV, into standard long- and short-axis views, facilitating identification of abnormal structures.

Other limitations of echocardiography are due to the use of a tomographic approach. For example, coronary anatomy cannot be assessed adequately with tomographic techniques. Angiography, with injection of dye into the coronary arteries, followed by cine- or digital radiographic recording is needed. Another example of potential shortcomings of echocardiography is that multiple VSDs may be missed unless careful evaluation in numerous tomographic planes is performed. A silhouette technique, such as ventriculography from an angle where the septum forms one of the borders of the ventricular chamber, has a higher reliability for this diagnosis. Limitations of angiography include the risks of contrast dye injection and its cost and invasive nature. Recent improvements in 3D echocardiographic displays may soon provide a clinically useful approach to evaluation of complex congenital heart disease.

Intracardiac Hemodynamics

While the definitive method for assessment of intracardiac hemodynamics remains cardiac catheterization with direct pressure measurement, much indirect information on intracardiac hemodynamics can be derived from the CW Doppler signal. Pulmonary artery pressures can be approximated by evaluation of pulmonic regurgitation and/or the tricuspid regurgitant jet. Maximum and mean pressure gradients across stenotic valves can be measured accurately with Doppler techniques. Inferences about the chronicity of regurgitation and the presence or absence of v-waves can be made from the shape of the regurgitant velocity curve. Estimates of LV end-diastolic pressure may be possible based on aortic regurgitant velocity at end-diastole, the pattern of LV diastolic filling, or pulmonary venous

TABLE 17–3 Alternate Diagnostic Imaging Procedures in Congenital Heart Disease

Diagnostic Test	Strengths	Weaknesses
Echocardiography (transthoracic, including Doppler)	Detailed 2D anatomy allowing identification of anatomic chambers, valves, and great vessels; blood flow pathway; structural abnormalities Assessment of stenotic and regurgitant lesions by Doppler Detection of intracardiac shunts Assessment of ventricular size and systolic function $Q_p:Q_s$ calculations Estimate of PA pressure Noninvasive, no discomfort	Poor acoustic access limits image quality in some individuals. Definition of posterior structures is suboptimal. $Q_p:Q_s$ calculation depends on accurate diameter measurements. No direct measures of intracardiac pressures Limited quantitation of RV size and function
Transesophageal echocardiography	Excellent image quality, especially of posterior structures Detailed Doppler evaluation of pulmonary veins, interatrial septum atrioventricular valves is possible.	Anterior cardiac structures now in far field of ultrasound image Apex may not be visualized. Oblique image planes limit quantitative measurements of chamber size. Some risk of procedure, plus discomfort to patient
Computed tomography	Detailed anatomic images gated to cardiac cycle Excellent for aortic anatomy and dimension, coronary artery anatomy, extra-cardiac abnormalities and exact position of cardiac structures in the chest	Intravenous contrast injection Radiation exposure Few physiologic data
Cardiac magnetic resonance (CMR) imaging	Detailed anatomic images gated to cardiac cycle Excellent for posterior structures, extracardiac vascular abnormalities, and position related to chest wall Blood has intrinsic "contrast" using different imaging sequences. Images can be realigned to cardiac major and minor axes. Cine-CMR images allow assessment of ventricular function and quantitation of RV size and function. Valve stenosis and regurgitation can be measured.	Expensive, not portable Pacer or defibrillator precludes CMR imaging Some patients are claustrophobic.
Cardiac catheterization	Direct measurement of intracardiac pressures Detection and quantitation of intracardiac shunts Assessment of ventricular size and systolic function Coronary anatomy. Calculation of pulmonary vascular resistance	Invasive (risks and discomfort) Expensive Requires contrast injection for visualization of structures

EF, ejection fraction; PA, pulmonary artery; $Q_p:Q_s$, pulmonary-to-systemic shunt ratio.

flow patterns. However, invasive pressure measurements still are often needed for appropriate clinical decision making in adults with congenital heart disease. In particular, evaluation of pulmonary vascular resistance, which requires invasive data, is an essential factor in patient management.

Integrating the Diagnostic Approach

Whichever diagnostic imaging procedure is performed first in an individual patient—be it echocardiography, catheterization, or CMR imaging—the next step should be to consider the data acquired in terms of both the anatomic and physiologic diagnoses and the certainty that these diagnoses are correct. Then, the remaining important clinical questions should be formulated and the most appropriate study to answer those questions performed next. When this approach is used, the echocardiogram may be the initial test to assess cardiac anatomy and physiology or may be performed only to answer a specific clinical question.

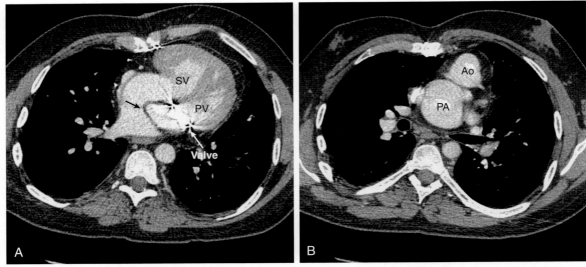

Figure 17–37 A, Computed tomographic imaging with contrast in a patient with complete TGA shows the interatrial baffle repair (*black arrow*) directing pulmonary venous return to the systemic ventricle (SV). This patient also has a mechanical pulmonary atrioventricular valve replacement. **B,** At the level of the great arteries, the aorta (Ao) is anterior and slightly leftward to the pulmonary artery (PA). PV, pulmonary ventricle.

SUGGESTED READING

1. Gurvitz M: General echocardiographic approach to the adult with suspected congenital heart disease. In Otto CM (ed): The Practice of Clinical Echocardiography, 3rd ed. Philadelphia: Elsevier/Saunders, 2007, pp 1021–1041.
   A detailed discussion of the echocardiographic approach to segmental analysis of the heart and a review of the echocardiographic features of frequently encountered complex congenital cardiac defects.

2. King ME: Echocardiographic evaluation of the adult with unoperated congenital heart disease. In Otto CM (ed): The Practice of Clinical Echocardiography, 3rd ed. Philadelphia: Elsevier/Saunders, 2007, pp 1042–1080.
   Advanced discussion of the echocardiographic evaluation of adults with congenital valvular abnormalities, obstructive outflow lesions, septal defects and shunt lesions, coronary fistulas, and complex congenital heart disease.

3. Child JS: Echocardiographic evaluation of the adult with postoperative congenital heart disease. In Otto CM (ed): The Practice of Clinical Echocardiography, 3rd ed. Philadelphia: Elsevier/Saunders, 2007, pp 1081–1107.

   Review of echocardiographic findings in adults with previous surgical procedures for congenital heart disease with an emphasis on expected findings and common complications. Topics include general postoperative issues, palliative procedures, corrective procedures for simple lesions (e.g., septal defects), and repair of complex malformations.

4. Li W, Henein M, Gatzoulis MG: Echocardiography in Adult Congenital Heart Disease. London: Springer, 2007.
   This 185-page book reviews the pathology, physiology, and echocardiographic findings in adult congenital heart disease.

5. Perloff JD, Child JS, Aboulhosn J: Congenital Heart Disease in Adults. Philadelphia: WB Saunders, 2008.
   This comprehensive 504-page textbook covers all aspects of adult congenital heart disease including diagnosis, pathophysiology, natural history, and medical and surgical management.

6. Popelova J, Oechslin E, Kaemmere H et al: Congenital Heart Disease in Adults. London: Informa Healthcare, 2008.
   This 192-page textbook provides numerous echocardiographic images in adults with congenital heart disease and drawings illustrating the anatomic findings.

7. Allen HD, Driscoll DJ, Shaddy RE et al (eds): Moss and Adams, Heart Disease

   in Infants, Children and Adolescents (Including the Fetus and Young Adult), 7th ed. Philadelphia: Lippincott Williams & Wilkins, 2007.
   Comprehensive (1680 pages) detailed textbook of pediatric cardiology. Useful reference for descriptions of congenital abnormalities, clinical presentation and management, and surgical procedures.

8. Sommer RJ, Hijazi ZM, Rhodes JF Jr: Pathophysiology of congenital heart disease in the adult. Part I: Shunt lesions. Circulation 117:1090–1094, 2008.
   Review of the anatomy, pathophysiology, natural history, and indications for intervention for ASDs, patent foramen ovale, VSDs, and patent ductus arteriosus. In addition, pulmonary arteriovenous malformations and coronary fistulas are discussed. 84 references.

9. Rhodes JF, Hijazi ZM, Sommer RF: Pathophysiology of congenital heart disease in the adult. Part II: Simple obstructive lesions. Circulation 117:1228–1237, 2008.
   Review of the pathophysiology, natural history, and indications for intervention for valvular, subvalvular, and supravalvular pulmonary stenosis, branch PA stenosis, subaortic stenosis, congenital aortic valve stenosis, supravalvular aortic stenosis, and aortic coarctation. Figures show examples of angiographic and hemodynamic findings. 89 references.

10. Sommer RJ, Hijazi ZM, Rhodes JF: Pathophysiology of congenital heart disease in the adult. Part III: Complex congenital heart disease. Circulation 117:1340–1350, 2008.

Discussion of the pathophysiology, clinical presentation, natural history, and indications for intervention in adults with unoperated complex congenital disease including Ebstein anomaly of the tricuspid valve, corrected transposition (L-TGA), and unrepaired tetralogy of Fallot. Patients with prior surgery are also discussed including atrial or arterial switch procedures for complete transposition of the great arteries, surgical correction for tetralogy of Fallot, and patients with a Fontan circulation. Schematic diagrams illustrate the anatomy.

11. Attenhofer Jost CH, Connolly HM, Dearani JA, et al: Ebstein's anomaly. Circulation 115:277–285, 2007.

Excellent illustrations of the anatomy of Ebstein anomaly with examples of pathology, echocardiographic imaging, and approaches to surgical repair.

12. Warnes CA: Transposition of the great arteries. Circulation 114:2699–2709, 2006.

Detailed discussion of the anatomy and surgical repair for complete TGA (or D-TGA) and congenitally corrected TGA (or L-TGA).

13. Skinner J, Hornung T, Rumball E: Transposition of the great arteries: from fetus to adult. Heart 94:1227–1235, 2008.

Long-term complications after great vessel switch surgery for TGA include coronary ischemia due to anatomic issues with the reimplanted coronary ostium or to inadequate coronary flow reserve, dilation of the neo-aortic root, and progressive aortic regurgitation.

14. Aboulhosn J, Child JS: Left ventricular outflow obstruction: Subaortic stenosis, bicuspid aortic valve, supravalvar aortic stenosis, and coarctation of the aorta. Circulation 114:2412–2422, 2006.

In addition to obstruction at the aortic valve level, young adults may present with obstruction at the subaortic or supravalvular level. A bicuspid aortic valve is present in 20% to 40% of patients with an aortic coarctation.

15. Paranon S, Acar P: Ebstein's anomaly of the tricuspid valve: from fetus to adult: Congenital heart disease. Heart 94:237–243, 2008.

Detailed review of the anatomy, clinical features, diagnostic imaging, and clinical outcomes with Ebstein anomaly. Management of arrhythmias and surgical options are discussed. 20 annotated references.

16. Bashore TM: Adult congenital heart disease: right ventricular outflow tract lesions. Circulation 115:1933–1947, 2007.

Review of congenital lesions that result in RV outflow obstruction including pulmonary valve stenosis, tetralogy of Fallot, double-chambered RV, double-outlet RV, and truncus arteriosus. For each lesion the anatomy is described and illustrated, in addition to a discussion of clinical presentation, diagnostic imaging, and options for intervention. 140 references.

17. Khairy P, Fernandes SM, Mayer JE Jr, et al: Long-term survival, modes of death, and predictors of mortality in patients with Fontan surgery. Circulation 117:85–92, 2008.

Long-term follow-up (median 12.2 years) of 261 patients with prior Fontan surgery found that perioperative mortality declined over time and that those who survived surgery had a 20-year actuarial survival of about 83%. Late deaths were due to thromboembolic events, heart failure, or sudden death.

18. Gersony WM: Fontan operation after 3 decades: What we have learned. Circulation 117:13–15, 2008.

Concise editorial that outlines the long-term outcome in patients with a Fontan correction and current areas of controversy including the type of repair, timing of intervention, role of fenestration, protein-losing enteropathy, arrhythmias, and long-term anticoagulation.

19. Huehnergarth KV, Gurvitz M, Stout KK, Otto CM: Repaired tetralogy of Fallot in the adult: Monitoring and management. Heart 94:1663–1669, 2008.

This article summarizes the anatomic features, clinical presentation, and imaging approach to tetralogy of Fallot. A practical approach to patient evaluation, follow-up, and management is proposed.

20. Schwerzmann M, Samman AM, Salehian O, et al: Comparison of echocardiographic and cardiac magnetic resonance imaging for assessing right ventricular function in adults with repaired tetralogy of Fallot. Am J Cardiol 99:1593–1597, 2007.

The accuracy of the myocardial performance index (MPI) for evaluation of RV systolic function was compared to CMR measurement of ejection fraction in 57 adults with repaired tetralogy of Fallot. MPI was calculated from spectral Doppler measurement of the duration of tricuspid regurgitation (TR) and the pulmonary valve (PV) ejection time:

$$RV\ MPI = (TR_{duration} - PV_{ejection\ time})/PV_{ejection\ time}$$

An RV MPI $\geq$ 0.40 had a sensitivity of 81% and a specificity of 85% for detection of an RV ejection fraction < 35%. A MPI < 0.25 indicated normal RV systolic function (ejection fraction $\geq$ 50%) with a specificity of 89% but a sensitivity of only 70%.

21. Niemann PS, Pinho L, Balbach T, et al: Anatomically oriented right ventricular volume measurements with dynamic three-dimensional echocardiography validated by 3-Tesla magnetic resonance imaging. J Am Coll Cardiol 50:1668–1676, 2007.

RV volumes calculated from 3D echocardiographic images acquired using a matrix array transducer correlated well (r = 0.99) with CMR imaging volumes. The measurement variability for ejection fraction was 4% for ultrasound and 5% for CMR. This may provide a useful clinical approach in the adult with RV volume overload due to congenital heart disease.

22. Pettersen MD, Du W, Skeens ME, et al: Regression equations for calculation of z scores of cardiac structures in a large cohort of healthy infants, children, and adolescents: An echocardiographic study. J Am Soc Echocardiogr 21:922–934, 2008.

Measurements of 21 structures in 782 patients (age 1 day to 18 years) were used to develop regression equations for cardiac structure normalized to body surface area. Both graphical displays and regression equations are provided for LV and RV dimensions, wall thickness, aortic size (at multiple sites), PA, LA, and atrioventricular valve annulus dimensions. These equations allow calculation of Z-scores for echocardiographic measurements in children and adolescents.

23. Crean A: Cardiovascular MR and CT in congenital heart disease. Heart 93:1637–1647, 2008.

A concise review, with excellent illustrations, of the utility of cardiac CT and CMR in evaluation of congenital heart disease. This information is useful to the echocardiographer in recommending additional studies, depending on the findings of the echocardiographic examination. CMR is particularly useful for quantitation of RV volumes and ejection fraction, detection of myocardial scar, and evaluation of PA anatomy. Both CT and CMR can visualize anomalous coronary arteries and are useful for examination of the full length of the aorta.

24. Bharucha T, Roman KS, Anderson RH, et al: Impact of multiplanar review of three-dimensional echocardiographic data on management of congenital heart disease. Ann Thorac Surg 86:875–881, 2008.

Three-dimensional echocardiographic imaging with multiplanar review in 300 patients with congenital heart disease provided additional information, compared to 2D imaging, which changed management or altered the diagnosis in 11% of cases. The authors recommend multiplane 3D images for evaluation of patients with congenital heart disease.

18 Intraoperative Transesophageal Echocardiography

T ransesophageal echocardiography (TEE) is a key element in the management of patients undergoing cardiac procedures in the operating room, cardiac catheterization laboratory, and hybrid procedure suites. Intraoperative TEE typically is performed by appropriately trained cardiovascular anesthesiologists or cardiologists. The principles of diagnostic TEE and intraoperative TEE are identical in terms of image plane orientation, anatomic findings, and Doppler flow patterns (see Chapter 3). In addition, standard methods for evaluation of ventricular systolic and diastolic function, valve dysfunction, congenital heart disease, and so on, as described in previous chapters, are also utilized for intraoperative TEE.

Typically, baseline TEE data are recorded after induction of anesthesia but before cardiopulmonary bypass. TEE data are again recorded after the surgical intervention and weaning from cardiopulmonary bypass. As with diagnostic TEE, intraoperative TEE provides images of great clarity and diagnostic value. However, intraoperative TEE differs from a standard diagnostic TEE in several respects:

❏ Time constraints may require a focused examination.

❏ Altered loading conditions may affect evaluation of valve and ventricular dysfunction.
❏ Baseline and post-intervention evaluations must have matched loading conditions.
❏ Urgent decision making based on imaging information may be necessary.
❏ Any limitations of the TEE information must be promptly recognized.
❏ Clear communication between the echocardiographer and surgeon is essential.

This chapter provides an introduction to the basic principles and major clinical applications of intraoperative TEE. Echocardiographers who practice intraoperative TEE should review training guidelines and refer to the additional books and articles included in the Suggested Reading at the end of this chapter (Table 18–1).

BASIC PRINCIPLES

Indications

The indications for intraoperative TEE range from basic monitoring of cardiovascular function to eval-

TABLE 18–1   Recommendations for Training in Basic and Advanced Perioperative Echocardiography*

Qualifications	Basic	Advanced	Maintenance of Competence
TEE studies interpreted and reported (supervised)	150	300	50 exams/yr (25 personally performed)
TEE studies performed (supervised)	50	150	15 hr category I CME every 3 yr
Program director	Advanced perioperative training	Advanced training plus 150 additional exams	Participation in a CQI program
Program (perioperative exam volume and diversity)	Wide variety	Full spectrum	
Documentation of training	NBE certification OR Verification by training director		

*This table shows the minimum number of procedures recommended to achieve and maintain competency. Summarized from Mathew JP, Glas K, Troianos CA, et al; Council for Intraoperative Echocardiography of the American Society of Echocardiography: ASE/SCA recommendations and guidelines for continuous quality improvement in perioperative echocardiography. Anesth Analg 103:1416–1425, 2006. The specific cognitive and technical skills needed for competency are listed in the reference.
CME, continuing medical education in echocardiography; NBE, National Board of Echocardiography.

uation of function after complex intracardiac surgical repairs (Table 18–2). In addition to traditional surgical approaches in the operating room with full cardiopulmonary bypass, intraoperative (or intraprocedural) TEE now also is utilized with alternate surgical and percutaneous techniques. The role of TEE has become more important as imaging replaces direct visualization of cardiac structure and function. Specific clinical indications are discussed in more detail below.

Preoperative Diagnosis

For elective surgical procedures, the diagnosis and surgical plan should be determined before the operative date (Fig. 18–1). Often a diagnostic TEE is performed as part of surgical planning to ensure an optimal surgical approach in addition to other diagnostic imaging studies, such as coronary angiography, cardiac magnetic resonance, or computed tomographic imaging. This allows time to review and discuss the diagnostic data, resolve any apparent discrepancies, and obtain additional data, as needed. In addition, the surgical options can be reviewed and discussed with the patient.

Preoperative assessment is particularly important for valvular and congenital heart disease both for technical and physiologic reasons. From a technical point of view, valve stenosis is best evaluated by transthoracic (TTE) imaging, which allows multiple interrogation angles to ensure that the maximum jet velocity is recorded. On TEE, the constraints in transducer position often result in underestimation

of stenosis severity. From a physiologic point of view, the altered loading conditions during anesthesia may result in underestimation of regurgitant severity, for example, if afterload is reduced.

Even when the preoperative diagnostic evaluation is complete, a baseline intraoperative TEE is important to:

- Confirm the diagnosis
- Provide additional information on valve repairability
- Serve as a baseline comparison for the postprocedure study
- Check for other abnormalities
- Monitor left ventricular (LV) function

When unexpected findings are present on the baseline intraoperative TEE in elective cases, management is individualized based on the specific findings and the urgency of the procedure. Usually, the surgical procedure can be modified as needed, for example, closure of an incidental patent foramen ovale (PFO) at the time of mitral valve repair. However, major unexpected findings may require consultation with the patient's primary cardiologist or rescheduling of the procedure.

In emergency cases, the intraoperative TEE recorded before cardiopulmonary bypass may be the primary diagnostic study. For example, with an acute aortic dissection, promptly transferring the patient to the operating room and obtaining TEE images quickly after induction of anesthesia may be optimal. In these situations, the echocardiographer should ensure that the diagnosis is correct, evaluate

TABLE 18–2 Indications for Intraoperative Transesophageal Echocardiography

Monitoring ventricular function
    Before and after CPB in high-risk patients
    During noncardiac surgery in high-risk patients

Evaluation of surgical procedure
    Mitral regurgitation
        Mechanism of regurgitation
        Severity of regurgitation
        Functional assessment after mitral valve repair
        Complications after mitral valve repair
    Complex valve procedures
        Aortic valve resuspension and aortic root repair
        Coronary artery reimplantation
    Endocarditis
        Valve involvement and dysfunction
        Assessment after repair or valve replacement
    Prosthetic valves
        Evaluation after valve implantation
        Detection of complications
    Hypertrophic cardiomyopathy
        Evaluation before and after myectomy
    Aortic disease
        Aortic dissection
        Aortic atheroma
    Congenital heart disease—before and after
        surgical repair

Placement of intracardiac devices
    Cannula placement
    Ventricular assist devices

Pericardial disease, including loculated effusion

General surgical complications
    Intracardiac air

CBP, cardiopulmonary bypass.

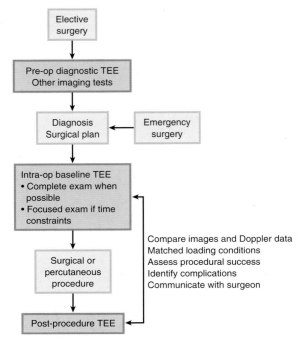

Figure 18–1 Flow chart illustrating integration of intraoperative TEE into clinical decision making.

for complications, and promptly communicate this information to the surgeon.

Hemodynamics

Assessment of cardiac hemodynamics and ventricular function in the operating room is affected by:

- ❏ Positive pressure mechanical ventilation
- ❏ Volume status
- ❏ Myocardial "stunning" secondary to aortic cross-clamping
- ❏ Effects of cardiopulmonary bypass
- ❏ Pharmacologic therapy

Typically, general anesthesia is provided by inhalational agents with supplemental opioids and muscle relaxants, all of which may alter preload and afterload. Many agents impair myocardial contractility and/or decrease systemic vascular resistance. During weaning from cardiopulmonary bypass, vasodilators or vasopressors may be used to maintain a normal systemic vascular resistance, and inotropic agents may be used if ventricular systolic function is impaired. Positive pressure ventilation at baseline and after cardiopulmonary bypass may reduce systemic venous return because of the increase in intrathoracic pressure, and this effect may be most pronounced when ventricular filling volumes are low. The combination of changes in preload, afterload, and contractility may result in variation in the severity of valve regurgitation (Fig. 18–2). Antegrade velocities and pressures gradients also will vary with volume flow rates.

TEE images and Doppler data optimally are recorded at loading conditions similar to the patient's baseline state and with matched loading conditions on the baseline and post–cardiopulmonary bypass studies. Basic parameters, such as heart rate and blood pressure, should be recorded on the echocardiographic images to ensure comparable loading conditions, with measures of systemic vascular resistance, filling pressures, and cardiac output also noted, when possible. After weaning from cardiopulmonary bypass, preload on the postbypass study can be optimized with volume infusion, often using TEE images of LV size as a measure of LV filling status, and afterload can be adjusted using pharmacologic agents as needed, to match the baseline study.

Surgical Manipulation and Instrumentation

During an open cardiac surgical procedure, the effects of surgical manipulation are directly observable on the TEE images (Fig. 18–3). For example, if the left atrial (LA) appendage was inverted during a

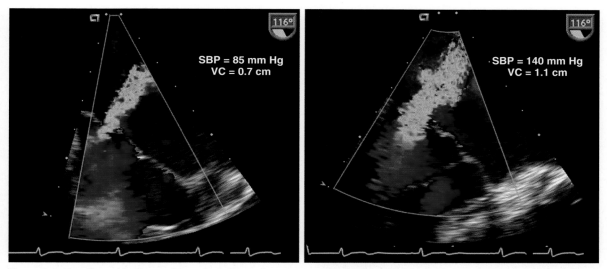

Figure 18–2 The effects of loading conditions on mitral regurgitant severity as assessed by color Doppler flow imaging are illustrated with a vena contracta (VC) width of 0.7 cm when the systolic blood pressure (SBP) is 85 mm Hg and compared to VC width of 1.1 cm at a SBP of 140 mm Hg on images taken a few minutes apart with no other intervention. *(Courtesy of Donald C. Oxorn, MD.)*

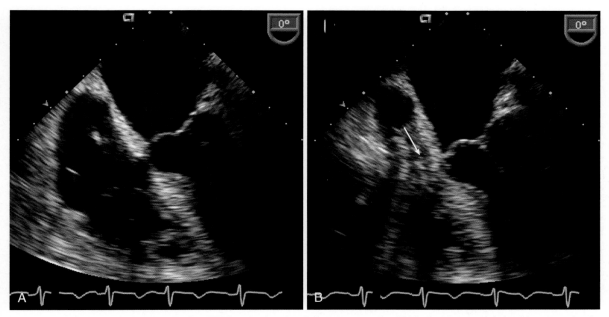

Figure 18–3 Comparison of the normal baseline TEE four-chamber view (*left*) to the same view (*right*) when the surgeon's hand is compressing the right heart (*arrow*). *(Courtesy of Donald C. Oxorn, MD.)*

mitral valve repair procedure, the inverted appendage may appear as a "mass" in the LA that disappears when the appendage resumes its normal shape. Cannulas for cardiopulmonary bypass may be visualized to confirm correct positioning but also may result in shadowing and reverberations that limit evaluation of cardiac function. Infusion of cardioplegia results in a contrast effect that may be visualized as increased echogenicity of the perfused myocardium. Intracardiac air related to the open surgical procedure has a characteristic bright appearance,

which can be used to ensure there is no intracardiac air at the end of the procedure (Fig. 18–4). Electronic interference from electrocautery creates an artifact on TEE images and disrupts the color Doppler signal.

Time Constraints

A complete systematic TEE examination is recommended during intraoperative evaluation whenever possible. However, when clinical urgency limits the time available for imaging, the data needed are

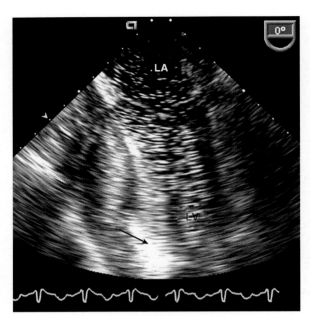

Figure 18–4 Intracardiac air appears as multiple bright mobile echo densities in the cardiac chambers in this TEE four-chamber view. A collection of intracardiac air (*arrow*) appears as a very bright mass in the RV. *(Courtesy of Donald C. Oxorn, MD.)*

prioritized and the most important images and Doppler data are recorded first, taking care to ensure that adequate data are recorded for any clinical decision making. Most patients have had a complete diagnostic study before entering the operating room, so that the baseline intraoperative TEE focuses on the views needed for comparison to the postprocedure images.

Quantitative approaches that are simple and fast are preferred over more complex methods, when possible. For example, valve regurgitation may be quantitated by measurement of vena contracta width, rather than optimizing the proximal isovelocity signal or comparing volume flow rates across the regurgitant and a normal valve. LV ejection fraction most often is visually estimated, rather than tracing end-diastolic and end-systolic borders for a biplane ejection fraction calculation. However, the echocardiographer also needs to be cognizant of any limitations in the data and communicate those issues to the surgeon. If the echocardiographic data are essential for decision making, adequate time for imaging without electronic artifacts needs to be provided.

ECHOCARDIOGRAPHIC APPROACH

Views

Transducer position and image planes are identical for a diagnostic and intraoperative TEE. The primary goal of an intraoperative TEE is to address the specific clinical issue in that patient, so that a focused examination is appropriate in many situations. However, a complete examination requires only a few minutes and is recommended whenever possible. The American Society of Echocardiography and Society of Cardiovascular Anesthesiologists recommend a standard series of 20 views (Fig. 18–5). Each view is recorded as a 2-second cine loop, so that all these images can be recorded within 10 minutes by an experienced operator, even assuming an average of 30 seconds to obtain each view. Additional time is needed for evaluation of abnormal findings, color and Doppler spectral recordings, and discussions between the anesthesiologist, surgeon, and cardiologist.

In addition to imaging data, a screening Doppler study is recommended in most patients. A basic intraoperative TEE includes color Doppler evaluation for regurgitation of aortic, mitral, and tricuspid valves in at least two orthogonal views. Evaluation of the pulmonic valve is more difficult and is only needed in specific situations, such as congenital pulmonic valve disease, post–cardiac transplantation, or with right ventricular (RV) assist device placement. Additional Doppler data recordings are tailored to the specific clinical indication. For example, when significant regurgitation is present, additional color Doppler data, such as vena contracta, are recorded. Color Doppler also allows detection of intracardiac shunts, including a PFO. Continuous-wave (CW) Doppler recordings may be helpful for evaluation of valve stenosis and regurgitation and for estimation of pulmonary pressures, if a pulmonary artery catheter has not been placed. Pulsed Doppler recordings can be used to evaluate LA filling via the pulmonary veins, LV diastolic filling, and atrial appendage function.

Sequence

There are several possible sequences of image acquisition, all of which are appropriate as long as the needed diagnostic images are obtained. Some echocardiographers prefer to obtain all the views from each transducer position:

- ❐ Mid-esophageal
- ❐ Transgastric
- ❐ Upper esophageal

This approach minimizes the time needed for acquisition and is easy to remember.

In this sequence (see Fig. 18–5), starting in a mid-esophageal four-chamber view with depth adjusted to show the entire LV, the image plane is rotated toward the two-chamber and then long-axis view (Fig. 18–6). The "mitral commissural" view describes a two-chamber plane in which both the medial and lateral commissures are seen and may be identical to the standard two-chamber view at about 60° rotation.

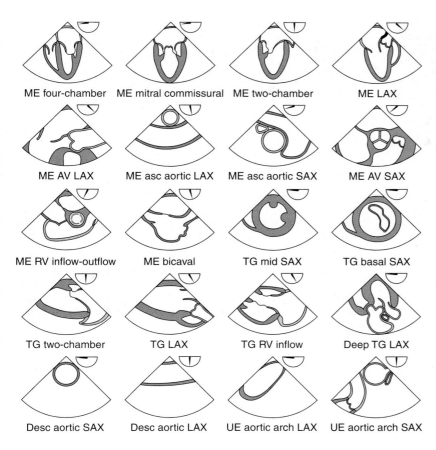

ME four-chamber   ME mitral commissural   ME two-chamber   ME LAX

ME AV LAX   ME asc aortic LAX   ME asc aortic SAX   ME AV SAX

ME RV inflow-outflow   ME bicaval   TG mid SAX   TG basal SAX

TG two-chamber   TG LAX   TG RV inflow   Deep TG LAX

Desc aortic SAX   Desc aortic LAX   UE aortic arch LAX   UE aortic arch SAX

Figure 18–5 The 20 transesophageal views recommended for a complete intraoperative examination by the American Society of Echocardiography and Society of Cardiovascular Anesthesiology. See text for details. asc, ascending; AV, aortic valve; LAX, long axis; ME, mid-esophageal; SAX, short axis; UE, upper esophageal. *(Modifed from Shanewise JS, Cheung AT, Aronson S, et al: ASE/SCA guidelines for performing a comprehensive intraoperative multiplane transesophageal echocardiography examination: recommendations of the American Society of Echocardiography Council for Intraoperative Echocardiography and the Society of Cardiovascular Anesthesiologists Task Force for Certification in Perioperative Transesophageal Echocardiography. Anesth Analg 89:870–884, 1999.)*

An additional "two-chamber" view at about 90° rotation provides visualization of additional segments of the mitral valve and the LA appendage. These views also allow sequential evaluation of regional wall motion in the four-chamber view (inferior septum and lateral wall), two-chamber view (inferior wall and anterior wall), and the long-axis view (posterior wall and anterior septum).

From the long-axis view, depth is decreased to focus on the aortic and mitral valves. Then the transducer is moved superiorly in the esophagus to visualize the ascending aorta, first in long axis, followed by rotation of the image plane to a short-axis view of the ascending aorta, with the pulmonary artery seen in long axis. The probe is advanced to a short-axis view of the aortic valve and then the tricuspid and pulmonic valves. Turning the probe to the right with further rotation of the image plane yields the bicaval view of the right atrium (RA; Fig. 18–7).

From the transgastric position, standard views include the short-axis views at the mid-LV and mitral valve levels, followed by rotation of the image plane to about 90° to show the two-chamber view. The probe is then turned rightward for a long-axis view that includes the aorta, and an RV inflow view. From the deep transgastric position, an anteriorly

angulated four-chamber view can be obtained in some patients. The descending thoracic aorta is examined in sequential short-axis views from the level of the diaphragm to the arch, as the probe is slowly withdrawn in the esophagus. These short-axis views are supplemented with long-axis views at 90° rotation, when abnormalities are seen. The arch is seen from an upper esophageal position by turning the image plane rightwards with a short-axis view obtained by rotation of the image plane.

Another approach is to evaluate each structure of interest in at least two orthogonal views, combining imaging, color, and spectral Doppler evaluation of each structure. With this approach, a complete examination includes:

- All four cardiac chambers (LV, RV, LA, RA)
- All four valves (aortic, mitral, tricuspid, pulmonic)
- Both great arteries (aorta, pulmonary artery)
- Systemic and pulmonary venous return (inferior vena cava, superior vena cava, four pulmonary veins)
- Atrial septum and LA appendage

This approach is useful with a focused examination, starting with the primary structures of interest and continuing on to evaluation of other structures

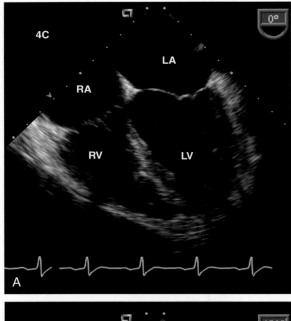

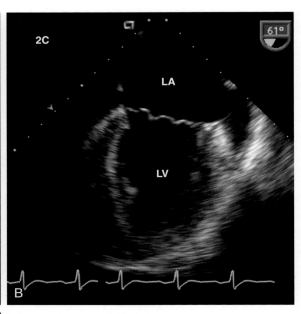

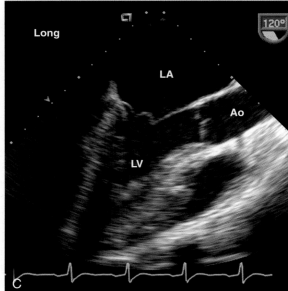

Figure 18–6 Mid-esophageal views of the LV in (**A**) four-chamber (4C) view showing the inferior septum and lateral wall, (**B**) two-chamber (2C) view showing the inferior and anterior walls, and (**C**) long-axis view showing the posterior wall and anterior septum. Transducer frequency and depth have been adjusted to include the entire LV and optimize endocardial definition; however, apical foreshortening still is likely, since it often is difficult to obtain an image plane that includes the LV apex.

at time allows. Even when a different sequence of imaging is used, the anatomic approach also provides a quick checklist to ensure that every structure has been evaluated before the examination is completed.

Reporting and Image Storage

Intraoperative TEE results are communicated directly to the surgeon at the time of data acquisition to facilitate prompt decision making. Intraoperative TEE results should be available throughout the surgical procedure, verbally or in written format. In addition, a permanent written or electronic report should be included in the medical record that includes indications, a description of the procedure, and diagnostic findings. The report should indicate if a comprehensive examination (most of the 20 recommended views) was recorded or if it was a focused or limited examination to address a specific clinical issue. Intraoperative TEE images should be stored with other echocardiographic images at each medical center, preferably in a digital format, for later review and for comparison with subsequent studies.

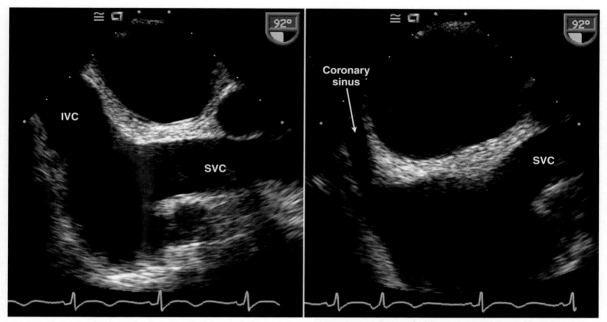

Figure 18–7 The bicaval view of the superior vena cava (SVC) and inferior vena cava (IVC) entering the RA is seen at about 90° rotation from a mid-TEE probe position. Turning the probe (and image plane) leftward shows the entrance of the coronary sinus into the RA. *(Courtesy of Donald C. Oxorn, MD.)*

LIMITATIONS/TECHNICAL CONSIDERATIONS

Image Plane Orientation

As with any echocardiographic study, intraoperative TEE images should be aligned in standard image planes corresponding to long-axis, short-axis, four-chamber, and two-chamber views, with scanning between standard image planes to ensure a comprehensive study. For example, the long-axis view includes a long-axis view of the aorta, aortic valve, and mitral valve, and shows the LV apex in long axis. Internal anatomic landmarks are used to define correct image alignment; the rotation angles provided in tables only serve as a guide to the typical angle needed for a given view; the actual rotation angle varies from patient to patient. In addition, individual variability in the anatomic relationship of the esophagus and heart results in variability in image plane orientation so that correct alignment of views is not always possible.

Doppler Interrogation Angle

A parallel alignment between the Doppler beam and blood flow of interest is not always possible on TEE imaging. The probe position is constrained by the anatomic relationship between the esophagus and heart, so that even with careful adjustment of transducer position

and rotation of the image plane, the interrogation angle may still be nonparallel, with potential underestimation of flow velocities. Intercept angle has limited impact on the diagnostic value of color Doppler, because the color Doppler flow image corresponds to the spatial pattern of the flow disturbance, even though exact velocities cannot be accurately measured. For spectral Doppler recordings, a near-parallel alignment is easily obtained by TEE for LV inflow across the mitral valve and for LA appendage and pulmonary veins flow (Fig. 18–8). From a high esophageal position, flow in the pulmonary artery also can be recorded at a near-parallel intercept angle. However, alignment of the Doppler beam with LV outflow tract and transaortic flow is problematic. On mid-esophageal views, parallel alignment is not possible. Sometimes better alignment can be obtained from a transgastric long-axis view or a deep transgastric anteriorly angulated four-chamber view. However, underestimation of velocity is likely and should be considered, particularly in TEE evaluation of aortic stenosis severity.

Technical Issues in the Operating Room

During an intraoperative or intraprocedural TEE, the echocardiographer needs to be alert to interference or technical artifacts. Cannula, catheters, and other devices may cause acoustic shadows or reverberations, obscuring the structure or flow of interest (Fig. 18–9).

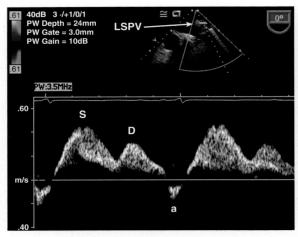

Figure 18–8 A pulsed Doppler sample volume is positioned about 1 cm into the left superior pulmonary vein (LSPV) to record normal systolic (S) and diastolic (D) pulmonary venous inflow into the LA, and a slight reversal of flow with atrial contraction (a) in a patient in sinus rhythm.

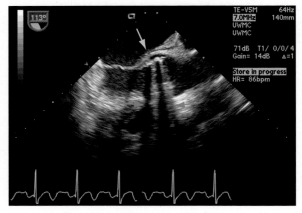

Figure 18–9 The long-axis TEE view in a patient with endocarditis of a mechanical aortic valve prosthesis shows shadows and reverberations originating from the posterior aspect of the prosthetic valve (*yellow arrow*) extending in alternating bands (*between blue arrows*) of dark (shadows) and white (reverberations) to obscure more distal structures, including the anterior aspect of the valve and the LV outflow tract.

Electronic interference from electrocautery or other procedures precludes diagnostic images or Doppler data (Fig. 18–10). If reverberations and shadowing cannot be avoided by repositioning the probe, alternate approaches such as epicardial scanning with a sterile transducer may need to be considered. Electronic devices should be paused when possible to allow recording of echocardiographic data without interference artifacts.

Optimization of Instrument Settings

Intraoperative TEE is facilitated by pre-setting the instrument settings to optimize image recording with minimal additional adjustment of parameters during

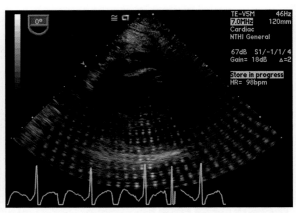

Figure 18–10 In a transgastric short-axis view, electronic artifact from the surgical cautery system not only creates a geometric artifact pattern but also obscures the two-dimensional image. Doppler flow data are not reliable when electronic artifact is present.

the examination. Images are recorded using 1- or 2-beat cine-loop image acquisition triggered to the QRS signal or setting a fixed recording time (if the electrocardiographic signal is not adequate for consistent triggering). Other instrument settings include starting with a standard transducer frequency, depth, gain, processing, and sector width settings.

However, each of these parameters may be need to be adjusted for optimal image recording during the TEE study. A higher transducer frequency (7 MHz) should be used to optimize resolution of near structures, such as the LA appendage, whereas lower frequencies (5 or 3.5 MHz) may be needed for optimal penetration to visualize the LV apex in the four-chamber view or on transgastric views. Depth should be adjusted to show the structure of interest; for example, starting with a depth of 15–16 cm in the four-chamber view for ventricular function and then decreasing depth to just beyond the mitral valve for examination of valve function (Fig. 18–11). Zoom mode provides improved image resolution and frame rate when examining the atrial appendage, or the aortic or mitral valve. Gain should be adjusted as needed based on image quality.

With color Doppler imaging, the color sector is adjusted so that depth just includes the flows of interest, which allows a higher frame rate due to the shorter pulse repetition frequency at a greater depth. However, the color sector should always extend to the top of the image because frame rate is not improved by excluding this section of the image. Usually color flow data are recorded initially with a relatively wide sector width to ensure that the spatial extent of the flow disturbance is visualized, with the sector width then narrowed to allow a higher frame rate. For vena contracta or proximal isovelocity surface area calculations, the color scale baseline and Nyquist limit also are adjusted to provide clear definition of the jet width and proximal acceleration zone (Fig. 18–12).

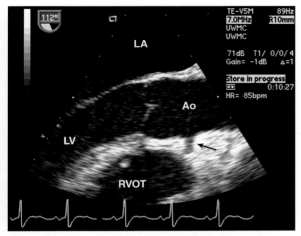

Figure 18–11 The aortic valve and aortic sinuses are evaluated in a long-axis view using a shallow depth and zoom mode with a high transducer frequency to optimize image resolution. The origin of the right coronary artery (RCA) is seen. RVOT, RV outflow tract.

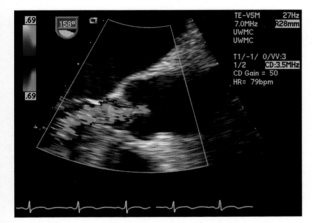

Figure 18–12 Measurement of vena contracta width is most accurate using zoom mode to enlarge the area of interest. The image plane and color parameters are adjusted to show the proximal flow acceleration, the narrow vena contracta (*arrow*), and distal jet expansion. Using a color scale without variance also may be helpful. In this example vena contracta width is 3 mm.

Spectral Doppler is recorded using the same principles as for any Doppler recording. Gray-scale gain and low-pass ("wall") filters are adjusted to optimize the flow signal, the velocity scale is adjusted so the flow signal fits within but nearly fills the velocity range, the zero baseline may be adjusted up or down depending on the flow of interest, and data are recorded with the time scale at 50 to 100 mm/s.

CLINICAL UTILITY

Clinical applications of intraoperative and intraprocedural TEE continue to evolve as new surgical and percutaneous approaches are developed. Some of

the current established indications are briefly discussed here as examples of the clinical utility of this approach. Echocardiographers performing TEE during surgical or percutaneous procedures should obtain additional training and consult additional reference sources as appropriate.

Monitoring Ventricular Function

Intraoperative TEE is useful in high-risk patients undergoing cardiac or noncardiac surgical procedures. Images of the LV provide continuous monitoring of:

- ❒ Ventricular preload (LV volume)
- ❒ Overall LV systolic function
- ❒ Regional LV function
- ❒ RV function

In general, the size of the ventricular chamber is a direct reflection of filling volume and can be used to optimize preload. Typically, ventricular size is evaluated qualitatively during the procedure, although a quick measurement of end-diastolic and end-systolic dimension provides a useful scale factor at baseline. In most patients, increases in filling volumes and pressures correlate with increases in ventricular volumes. Conversely, ventricular size may be small, despite adequate filling pressures, in patients with restrictive cardiomyopathy, pericardial constraint, severe right heart dysfunction, or in high contractility states.

Overall systolic function is usually estimated visually in the transgastric short-axis view. The area change in ventricular size provides a quick and accurate visual correlate of ejection fraction (see Chapter 6). Although quantitative ejection fractions, measured from four- and two-chamber views, are well validated, this approach is rarely used given the rapid time course of hemodynamic changes in the operating room. Similarly, although Doppler cardiac output measurements in the aorta or pulmonary artery can be reliably made, time factors make these approaches unrealistic. In addition, cardiac output typically is continuously monitored by right heart catheter techniques. Newer approaches for evaluation of ventricular function in the operating room such as tissue Doppler or speckle tracking are under evaluation.

The transgastric short-axis view is also useful for monitoring regional ventricular function, since it includes myocardium supplied by all three major coronary arteries (Fig. 18–13). An acute change in regional ventricular function suggests coronary ischemia, although changes in regional wall motion are not always due to epicardial coronary disease. Other causes of regional dysfunction include hypovolemia, conduction defects, and myocardial stunning after cardiopulmonary bypass. TEE monitoring of ventricular function during interventions to reverse ischemia allow

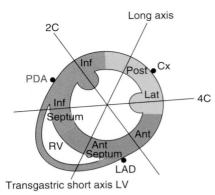

Figure 18-13 Schematic transgastric short-axis view showing the relationship between regional wall motion and coronary anatomy. The intersecting lines show which myocardial segments are seen in the mid-esophageal four-chamber (4C), two-chamber (2C), and long-axis views. Typically, the inferior (inf) septum and inferior wall are perfused by the posterior descending coronary artery (PDA; the anterior (ant) septum and anterior wall by the left anterior descending (LAD) coronary artery; and the lateral and posterior walls by branches of the circumflex (Cx) coronary artery.

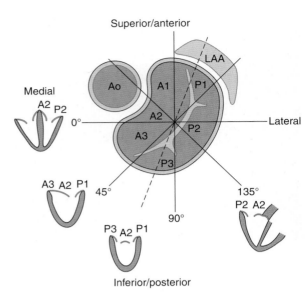

Figure 18-14 Reference view demonstrating the relationship of the transesophageal echocardiographic rotational imaging planes to the mitral valve with the probe positioned in the standard mid-esophageal position. (A1, A2, A3 = anterior leaflet sections; P1, P2, P3 = posterior leaflet sections.) *(From Foster GP, Isselbacher EM, Rose GA, et al: Accurate localization of mitral regurgitant defects using multiplane transesophageal echocardiography. Ann Thorac Surg 65:1025–1031, 1998.)*

assessment of the effects of therapy. Evaluation of RV systolic function is important because dysfunction may occur due to inadequate cardioplegia or air embolism, which preferentially affects the right coronary artery when separating from cardiopulmonary bypass. Coronary ischemia in the distribution of a coronary bypass graft may also be due to mechanical occlusion or a kink in a vein graft or spasm of an internal mammary graft.

Valvular Heart Disease

Mitral Valve Repair

In patients undergoing elective mitral valve repair, the baseline intraoperative TEE provides additional detailed information on mitral valve anatomy and the mechanism and severity of regurgitation. Annular size also may be measured in four-chamber and long-axis views.

Even when a comprehensive preoperative examination has been done, the echocardiographer in the operating room needs to be familiar with, and record, images demonstrating the baseline pathology for comparison with the post-repair study. Standard terminology for mitral valve anatomy facilitates communication between the echocardiographer and surgeon (Fig. 18–14). The anterior and posterior leaflets meet at the medial and lateral valve commissures, with the posterior leaflet extending around more of the annulus than the anterior leaflet. The posterior mitral leaflet typically has three distinct scallops, which were labeled from the perspective of a surgeon looking at the valve from the LA side. Thus, posterior leaflet scallops are numbered from lateral (P1) to medial

(P3), with central (P2) in the middle, with corresponding terms for the anterior leaflet.

Using rotational scanning from a mid-esophageal transducer position, both the four-chamber and long-axis views show the central (A2 and P2) scallops of both leaflets. As the image plane is rotated from 0° to 45°, first A3 and P1 are seen and then, with further rotation, both P3 and P1 are seen in the "bicommissural view," typically at a rotation angle of 60° to 90° (Fig. 18–15). In this view both the medial and lateral commissures are seen, with the P3 and P1

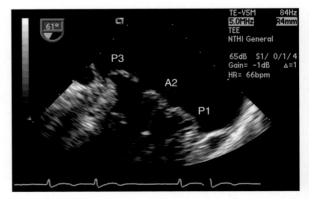

Figure 18-15 TEE two-chamber or bicommissural view in zoom mode in systole in a patient with myxomatous mitral valve disease and bileaflet prolapse. The medial (P3) and lateral (P1) segments of the posterior leaflet and the central (A2) segment of the anterior leaflet are seen.

posterior leaflet scallops at their attachments to the annulus. The central (A2) anterior leaflet scallop fills the center section of the annulus, moving in and out of the image during the cardiac cycle.

Another approach to visualization of the mitral leaflet scallops is to start in the four-chamber view and then either tilt the image plane superiorly or to slightly withdraw the probe, to show the more anterior/lateral scallops (A1 and P1), followed by tilting posteriorly or advancing the probe to show the posterior/medial segments (A3 and P3) (Fig. 18–16). From the two-chamber or bicommissural plane, turning the image plane toward the patient's right side shows all three scallops of the anterior leaflet and turning leftward shows all three scallops of the posterior leaflet. Transgastric short-axis views at the mitral valve level also are helpful.

Mitral valve anatomy in patients undergoing surgical repair for mitral regurgitation is well visualized by three-dimensional (3D) echocardiography (Fig. 18–17). The position of the TEE transducer posterior to the mitral valve, with the ultrasound imaging beam relatively perpendicular to the surface of the closed valve, results in excellent image quality and the ability to include the entire valve in the image field. As 3D imaging becomes widely available in formats that allow real-time or rapid image reconstruction, 3D imaging of the mitral valve likely will become the standard approach to evaluation in the operating room.

The mechanism of regurgitation in patients undergoing mitral valve repair may be primary leaflet disease, most often myxomatous disease, with fewer cases of rheumatic valve disease. With primary leaflet disease, anatomy is described for each leaflet segment

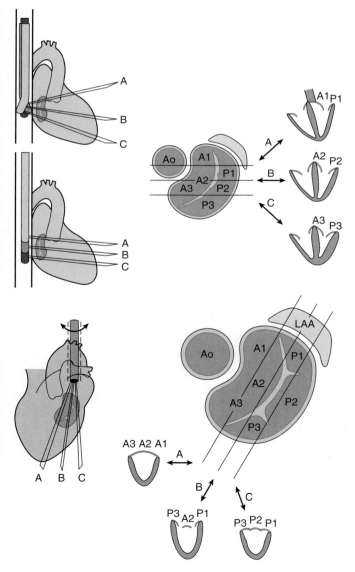

Figure 18–16 A, Effect of flexion or withdrawal and retroflexion or advancement of the transesophageal probe tip on the imaging plane in relation to the mitral valve at a transducer rotational angle of 0°. **B,** Effect of clockwise and counterclockwise turning of the probe on the imaging plane in relation to the mitral valve with the transducer rotational angle adjusted to the major axis of the mitral orifice (typically 45°–90°). (A1, A2, A3, anterior leaflet sections; LAA, LA appendage; P1, P2, P3, posterior leaflet sections.) *(From Foster GP, Isselbacher EM, Rose GA, et al: Accurate localization of mitral regurgitant defects using multiplane transesophageal echocardiography. Ann Thorac Surg 65:1025–1031, 1998.)*

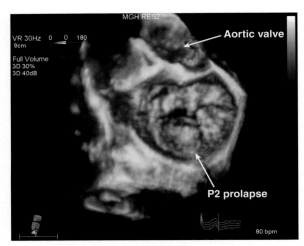

Figure 18–17 Three-dimensional transesophageal view of the mitral valve, viewed from the perspective of the LA, in a patient with prolapse of the P2 segment of the posterior leaflet. *(Image courtesy of Judy W. Hung, MD, Boston, MA.)*

in terms of thickness, redundancy, and motion, and any areas of calcification or chordal fusion and shortening are described. Prolapse describes motion of the leaflet into the LA in systole with a curved shape in systole due to intact chordal attachments (Fig. 18–18A). A flail segment indicates chordal rupture with the tip of the disrupted segment directed toward the LA in systole. Secondary mitral regurgitation often is due to ischemic disease. With secondary mitral regurgitation, leaflet motion typically is restricted with a tethering effect due to LV dilation and regional wall motion resulting in inadequate systolic leaflet coaptation. Restricted leaflet motion also may be seen with rheumatic valve disease or with dilated cardiomyopathy.

Color Doppler imaging is helpful for determining the mechanism of mitral regurgitation. The origin of the regurgitant jet as it crosses the valve indicates the area of inadequate coaptation. The direction of the regurgitant jet in the atrium tends to be anterior with posterior leaflet dysfunction, posterior with anterior leaflet dysfunction, and central with functional regurgitation (Fig. 18–18B). Complex or multiple jets may be seen when there is more than one mechanism of regurgitation.

Regurgitant severity is best evaluated before the patient is anesthetized in the operating room, due to the potential effects of altered loading conditions. However, baseline measures of regurgitant severity are needed for comparison to the post-repair images. Jet size and shape are not reliable indicators of regurgitant severity, because they are affected by many other factors, including driving pressure, chamber size, and compliance and cardiac rhythm. The recommended basic measurements of mitral regurgitant severity in the operating room are:

❑ Vena contracta width
❑ CW Doppler signal intensity relative to antegrade flow
❑ Pulmonary vein systolic flow reversal

A simple reliable measure of regurgitant severity is vena contracta width, taking care to measure the narrowest diameter between the proximal jet acceleration on the ventricular size of the valve and the area of jet expansion in the LA. Accuracy is enhanced using zoom images, a fast frame rate, and careful image alignment (see Chapter 12). The CW Doppler signal density compared to antegrade flow also provides a quick qualitative measure of regurgitant severity (Fig. 18–19). Pulmonary vein systolic flow reversal indicates severe regurgitation in patients in sinus

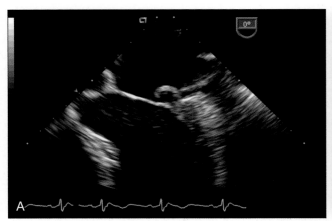

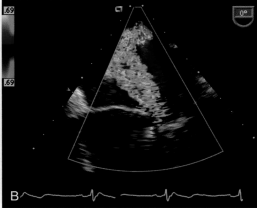

Figure 18–18 A, TEE four-chamber view in a patient with posterior mitral valve prolapse. The posterior leaflet is displaced into the LA (*arrow*), but the tip curves to point toward the LV apex. With a partial flail segment, the tip would point toward the roof of the LA. **B,** Color Doppler flow imaging in the same view shows an anteriorly directed jet, consistent with posterior leaflet prolapse being the primary mechanism of valve dysfunction.

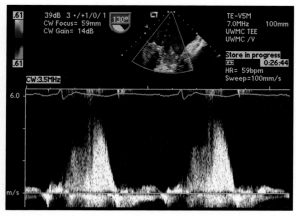

Figure 18–19 Continuous-wave Doppler recording of mitral regurgitation shows flow toward the transducer in systole with a high velocity (about 5 m/s) consistent with the LV-to-LA systolic pressure difference. The late-systolic signal is more dense than early systole due to predominantly late-systolic regurgitation resulting from mitral valve prolapse.

rhythm, although interrogation of all four pulmonary veins is needed with eccentric jets. In non-sinus rhythms, the pulmonary vein flow pattern is altered due to the rhythm and is not an accurate reflection of regurgitant severity. If further quantitation is needed, the proximal isovelocity surface area approach can be applied in the operating room. Measurement of volume flow rate across two valves is rarely utilized due to intercept angle limitations and time constraints.

After the surgical valve repair and weaning from cardiopulmonary bypass, imaging and Doppler studies of the mitral valve are repeated. Loading conditions should be adjusted to match conditions at the time of the baseline study, as much as possible, and the same image planes and Doppler flows should be recorded with the same instrument settings. The most common mitral valve repair is quadrangular resection of a posterior leaflet scallop (usually P2) with reapproximation and suturing of the resected edges and placement of an annuloplasty ring. The exact repair varies from patient to patient; more complex repairs include modifications to the anterior leaflets, use of artificial chords, and chordal transfer or shortening. Knowledge of the exact repair is needed for the post-pump TEE evaluation to ensure expected postoperative changes are distinguished from abnormal findings. The use of intraoperative TEE is associated with a higher rate of successful mitral valve repair, at both academic and community medical centers.

Complications of mitral valve repair detectable by TEE include:

❐ Persistent mitral regurgitation
❐ Systolic anterior mitral leaflet motion
❐ Mitral stenosis
❐ Ventricular systolic dysfunction
❐ Injury of the circumflex artery
❐ Tricuspid regurgitation

With a successful mitral valve repair, there is no or minimal residual mitral regurgitation. More than trivial mitral regurgitation, after optimization of loading conditions, may prompt consideration of an additional repair or valve replacement. Excessive reduction in mitral annular size may be associated with systolic anterior motion of the mitral leaflet with resultant LV outflow obstruction and mitral regurgitation, although this complication is infrequent with current surgical techniques. Functional mitral stenosis can occur with some repairs and is easily detected by recording the antegrade mitral flow velocity after valve repair. Ventricular dysfunction may be transient due to cardioplegia; persistent dysfunction suggests preoperative dysfunction that is more evident with a competent mitral valve or a complication of the procedure, such as coronary artery air embolism. Tricuspid regurgitation often accompanies mitral valve disease and should be evaluated both at baseline and on the post-repair study.

Valve Stenosis

Whenever possible, aortic stenosis should be fully evaluated before the patient is in the operating room (see Chapter 11). TEE calculation of continuity equation valve area is possible in some cases if LV outflow and aortic flow velocities can be recorded from transgastric long-axis planes. Unfortunately, this approach may significantly underestimate stenosis severity because of the inability to align the Doppler beam parallel to flow from a TEE approach resulting in inaccurate velocity data. TEE short-axis views of the valve are accurate for determination of valve anatomy, and planimetry of valve area may be possible in many cases (Fig. 18–20). In other cases, the complex 3D geometry of the orifice and distortion of

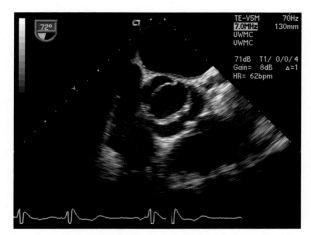

Figure 18–20 Transesophageal short-axis view of the aortic valve confirms a bicuspid valve with the leaflets open in systole. There is a raphe in the anterior leaflet due to congenital fusion of the right and left coronary cusps.

valve anatomy are challenging; ensuring measurement at the minimal orifice is facilitated with 3D imaging. Reverberations and shadowing by valve calcification may affect accuracy of planimetry with either two- or three-dimensional approaches.

Some specific circumstances when intraoperative TEE evaluation is especially helpful include the following:

❏ Detection of bicuspid valve
❏ Degree of valve calcification
❏ Aortic sinus and ascending aorta dilation

For example, in the patient undergoing coronary bypass grafting, aortic valve replacement is appropriate with moderate or severe asymptomatic stenosis. In equivocal cases the finding of a bicuspid aortic valve or extensive valve calcification on TEE may tip the balance toward valve replacement. Conversely, a trileaflet valve with minimal calcification and only mild-moderate aortic stenosis may not need intervention. Bicuspid aortic valve disease often is accompanied by aortic dilation. Intraoperative TEE may provide improved images and measurements of the aortic sinuses and ascending aorta. The surgical approach may be modified to include aortic root replacement if significant aortic dilation is present that was not recognized preoperatively. With percutaneous or hybrid approaches to aortic valve replacement, intraprocedural TEE is used to monitor the procedure, ensure correct placement of the valve, and provide immediate assessment of valve function.

Mitral stenosis procedures are most often performed percutaneously, and intracardiac or TEE assessment of stenosis and regurgitation severities is used routinely for these procedures. In a patient with rheumatic mitral stenosis undergoing surgical valve repair, TEE can be used to measure transmitral gradients and pressure half-times, because the Doppler beam is easily aligned with flow from the mid-esophageal four-chamber view. Mean pressure gradients may be more useful than pressure half-time valve areas in the acute setting, due to concurrent rapid changes in LA and LV volumes and compliance. Regurgitation severity is evaluated as with any mitral valve procedure.

Endocarditis

Intraoperative TEE is essential in patients undergoing valve surgery for endocarditis (see Chapter 14) The TEE study should include assessment of:

❏ Presence and location of vegetations
❏ Mechanism of valve dysfunction
❏ Severity of regurgitation
❏ Paravalvular abscess
❏ Other complications—fistulas, pseudoaneurysms

Given the complex patterns of valve destruction with endocarditis, careful review of the images with the surgeon is essential for planning the operative repair. Even with a complete presurgical evaluation, additional changes may occur between the time of that study and the surgical procedure, so the echocardiographer should perform a complete study. The baseline intraoperative study also provides a comparison to the postprocedure images.

Prosthetic Valve Dysfunction

After implantation of a prosthetic valve, TEE evaluation is helpful to confirm normal function. In addition to the normal patterns of mild regurgitation for prosthetic valves, a small amount of paravalvular regurgitation is not unusual immediately after implantation (Fig. 18–21). However, a significant paravalvular leak suggests suture dehiscence and may require immediate intervention. Occasionally, mechanical-valve disk motion will be impaired by excessive retained mitral leaflet tissue or other anatomic factors. The antegrade velocity and pressures gradient across a prosthetic valve are compared to published normal values for that valve type and size. Often, velocities and pressure gradients are higher than expected in the early postoperative setting due to increased adrenergic tone and a high-output state. In this situation, distinguishing prosthetic valve stenosis or patient-prosthesis mismatch from normal valve function is challenging (see Chapter 13).

Aortic Disease

Aortic Dissection

Intraoperative TEE is accurate for diagnosis of the presence and extent of an aortic dissection. Often these patients are promptly transferred to the operating room after a computed tomography scan showing an ascending aortic dissection, with no prior TEE imaging. The intraoperative study confirms the presence and origin of the dissection flap and provides assessment of aortic valve function (Fig. 18–22). It is particularly important to determine if the dissection involves the ascending aorta (type A), requiring surgical intervention, or only affects the descending aorta (type B), often managed medically.

A complete examination of the aorta includes mid-esophageal views of the sinuses and ascending aorta in both short- and long-axis views, ensuring the aorta is examined from the annulus level as far superiorly as possible with slow withdrawal of the probe (see Chapter 16). Aortic diameters are measured at end-diastole, from the inner edge to inner edge of the black/white interface, at the annulus, sinuses, sinotubular junction, and mid-ascending aorta. The descending thoracic aorta is imaged from the transgastric position to a very high esophageal position with slow withdrawal of the probe in the esophagus. Sequential short-axis views ensure that the entire endocardial surface

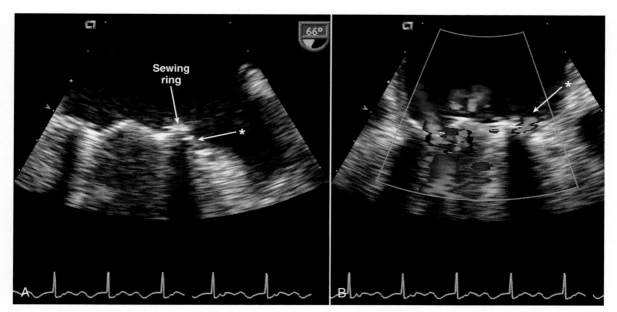

Figure 18–21 Immediately after implantation of a bileaflet mechanical mitral valve replacement, two-dimensional images (**A**) show the sewing ring and sutures (*arrow*), and color Doppler shows a slight amount of regurgitation (**B**) lateral to the sewing ring at this site. This regurgitation disappeared before the patient left the operating room, after reversal of anticoagulation. *(Courtesy of Donald C. Oxorn, MD.)*

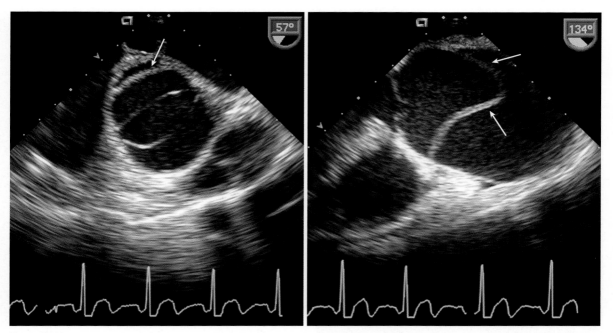

Figure 18–22 Aortic dissection in a patient with a bicuspid aortic valve. The dissection flap extends to leaflet level in the short-axis view (*left*) and is seen traversing the ascending aorta in the long–axis view (*right*). In real time the dissection flap had a motion pattern independent of the aortic wall. *(Courtesy of Donald C. Oxorn, MD.)*

is visualized. Supplemented long-axis views at each level are appropriate, especially when abnormal findings are present, but abnormalities medial or lateral to the long-axis plane may be missed with this approach. Descending aortic diameter is measured in the distal, mid-, and proximal descending aorta. The

aortic arch is seen from a high TEE position with the image plane turned and tilted to show the length of the arch. In each view, depth and gain setting are adjusted to optimize visualization of a dissection flap, intramural hematoma, or atheroma. Color Doppler is helpful in showing flow patterns in the true and false lumens when a dissection is present. The spectral Doppler pattern, recorded in a long-axis view of the descending aorta, shows holodiastolic flow reversal when severe aortic regurgitation is present.

Other key findings are (1) regional wall motion abnormalities due to involvement of the right coronary artery or (2) pericardial effusion, due to impending aortic rupture. After the repair, a dissection flap typically persists in the descending aorta, and the post-repair TEE images serve as a baseline for future follow-up studies. If the aortic valve has been resuspended, post-repair imaging of leaflet opening and Doppler evaluation for regurgitation are essential.

Aortic Atheroma

Cardiac surgery usually involves cannulation or manipulation of the aorta that is associated with adverse neurologic events due to embolization of aortic atheroma. Detection of protruding, mobile, or large (>3 mm) atheroma is a marker of increased risk. Atheroma can be detected by TEE, although epiaortic scanning provides higher accuracy due to more complete imaging of the entire endothelial surface of the ascending aorta (Fig. 18–23). The recommended minimum epiaortic examination consists of three short-axis views of the ascending aorta (proximal, mid-, and distal) and two long-axis views (proximal and distal). The location of any plaques should be described, with measurement of plaque thickness and notation of any mobile components.

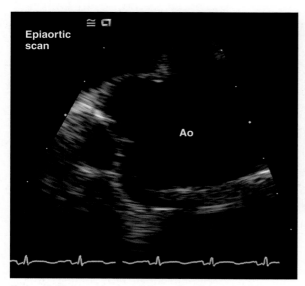

Figure 18–23 Long-axis view of the aortic valve, aortic sinuses, and proximal ascending Ao on an epiaortic scan with the transducer in a sterile sleeve placed directly on the anterior surface of the heart during the cardiac surgical procedure. There are no significant atheromas seen on this view.

Aortic Valve Resuspension and Coronary Reimplantation

When a graft replacement of the ascending aorta is performed for an acute aortic dissection, the aortic valve may be "resuspended" by the three commissures at the proximal graft anastomosis site. In these patients, post-pump TEE evaluation of aortic valve anatomy and Doppler flows is important to ensure valve competency. In patients with connective tissue disorders, such as Marfan syndrome, the proximal graft anastomosis site is at the aortic annulus, with replacement of the sinuses, as well as ascending aorta, and reimplantation of the coronary ostia into the graft with a small "button" of native aortic tissue. The native aortic valve may be resuspended in the tube graft, or a combined prosthetic valve and conduit may be used. Post-pump TEE evaluation in these patients includes visualization of the coronary ostium, if possible, to ensure patency and lack of kinking, as well as evaluation of valve function.

Cardiomyopathies

Hypertrophic Cardiomyopathy

Intraoperative TEE is used to guide the extent of myectomy in patients with LV outflow obstruction due to hypertrophic cardiomyopathy to assess:

❒ Severity and location of septal hypertrophy
❒ Immediate hemodynamic results
❒ Complications of the procedure

Careful evaluation of the degree and location of hypertrophy in terms of distance from the aortic valve and by myocardial segment, allows tailoring of the depth, width, and length of the myotomy-myectomy (see Chapter 9). Imaging is performed from both mid-esophageal and transgastric transducer positions, using multiple image planes to fully assess septal anatomy. Color Doppler localizes the level of obstruction at the site of flow acceleration in the LV outflow tract and is useful for detection and evaluation of associated mitral regurgitation. The LV outflow gradient may be recorded with CW Doppler from a deep transgastric view or the transgastric long-axis view, although underestimation is likely due to a nonparallel intercept angle.

After the procedure, TEE allows assessment of residual outflow obstruction and detection of complications, such as a ventricular septal defect. Often LV outflow obstruction due to systolic anterior motion of the mitral valve is accompanied by significant mitral regurgitation, which resolves when normal mitral leaflet motion is restored. Postoperative TEE results in additional surgical procedures in about 4% of cases. Intraprocedural TEE or TTE imaging also is used to monitor percutaneous catheter septal ablation procedures.

Ventricular Assist Devices

When placement of a ventricular assist device is considered, intraoperative TEE can ensure that there are no preexisting conditions that may affect pump function. For example, significant aortic regurgitation would result in inability to unload the LV. Another example is a PFO, which may result in right-to-left shunting when left-sided pressures are reduced, leading to arterial oxygen desaturation or paradoxical embolism. The presence of aortic atheroma may influence placement of the aortic inflow cannula. LV or LA clot also should be excluded.

In addition, intraoperative TEE can assist with placement of ventricular assist devices by assessment of:

- ❏ Placement of inflow and outflow cannula
- ❏ Ventricular volumes and systolic function
- ❏ Doppler inflow and outflow velocities
- ❏ De-airing of the pump before activation

LV assist devices include extracorporeal devices that use cannulas and an external pump to direct blood from the LV apex into the aorta. The pump may provide pulsatile flow or axial (continuous) flow. Some devices can be placed percutaneously, directing blood from the LA (via a trans-septal cannula) into the aorta. There also are intracorporeal devices that fit inside the heart. Because these devices are currently in development, there are frequent changes in technology so the echocardiographer needs information on each specific device, including use of cannulas, optimal device or cannula placement, and expected flow patterns (Fig. 18–24). Complications of ventricular assist devices include intracardiac thrombus formation, obstruction of inflow or outflow cannula due to positioning or thrombus formation,

regurgitation of the pump valves, and inadequate flow volumes. Nonpulsatile devices are challenging to evaluate by TEE, but ventricular size may be one factor in adjusting flow rates for these devices. With continuous-flow devices, excessive LV drainage may result in collapse of the ventricular chamber leading to obstruction of the inflow cannula and a drop in flow rates.

Heart Transplantation

After heart transplantation, intraoperative TEE is used to evaluate the anastomoses to the aorta and pulmonary artery. The RA and LA anastomoses also are evaluated to ensure there is no obstruction to systemic or pulmonary venous return and to serve as a baseline for atrial anatomy on subsequent diagnostic studies. With lung transplantation, all four pulmonary veins are imaged with recording of Doppler flow to ensure normal flow patterns. Evaluation of RV size and systolic function is particularly important after either heart or lung transplantation.

Congenital Heart Disease

Intraoperative TEE is essential in the surgical and percutaneous management of patients with congenital heart disease (see Chapter 17). Postprocedure evaluation ensures complete closure of ventricular and atrial septal defects, functional status of repaired or replacement valves, and patency of conduits. Except for simple defects, such as closure of an isolated atrial septal defect, intraoperative TEE for congenital heart disease should be performed by echocardiographers with additional training and experience in pediatric or adult congenital heart disease.

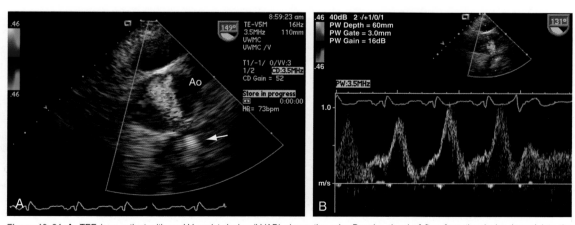

Figure 18–24 A, TEE in a patient with an LV assist device (LVAD) shows the color Doppler signal of flow from the device (*arrow*) into the ascending aorta (Ao). **B,** Pulsed Doppler interrogation of this flow shows predominant systolic flow about 1 m/s in velocity, with persistent antegrade flow in diastole. The inlet cannula (not shown here) was positioned in the LV apex.

ALTERNATE APPROACHES

TEE has many advantages compared to other imaging techniques in the operating room setting. The imaging probe is out of the surgical field, images can be continuously acquired without interrupting the procedure or subjecting the patient or staff to ionizing radiation, and the relatively small ultrasound system fits into the space with other monitoring equipment. In addition, the intraoperative TEE is now a standard monitoring approach used by the cardiovascular anesthesiologist so that additional personnel are not needed, and the data are acquired by the same physician who is managing hemodynamics and pharmacologic therapy.

When TEE image quality is limited by shadowing, reverberations, or distance of structures from the transducer, epicardial imaging with a sterile transducer is an option. This approach is useful for evaluation of aortic atheroma and often is useful in patients with hypertrophic cardiomyopathy. In theory, an epicardial transducer position might allow better angulation for measuring aortic stenosis jet velocity; in practice, transducer positioning is still limited by the thoracotomy, an apical transducer position is rarely possible, and time constraints largely preclude this approach.

Direct measurement of hemodynamics may be considered when this information is needed for decision making and TEE data may be inaccurate. Right heart pressures are routinely measured in the operation room, but LV, LA, and aortic pressures also can be measured by having the surgeon place an appropriate catheter in each chamber. As with any hemodynamic measurements, accurate data requires attention to catheter and transducer positioning, damping, frequency response, and timing in the cardiac cycle.

SUGGESTED READING

General

1. Oxorn DC, Otto CM: Atlas of Intraoperative Echocardiography: Surgical and Radiologic Correlations. Philadelphia: Elsevier/Saunders, 2007.

   This combination DVD and printed atlas uses a case-based format to show cine and still-frame echocardiographic and Doppler images with correlation with the clinical presentation and outcome, radiologic studies, and surgical findings. Suggested readings are provided for each case. Over 145 cases are included spanning the full range of intraoperative TEE studies including coronary disease, mitral and aortic valve disease, endocarditis, prosthetic valves, right-sided valve disease, adult congenital heart disease, hypertrophic cardiomyopathy, pericardial disease, disease of the great vessels, and cardiac masses.

2. Sidebotham D, Merry A, Legget M: Practical Perioperative Transesophageal Echocardiography. Philadelphia: Butterworth-Heinemann, 2003.

   A useful concise book summarizing the use of intraoperative echocardiography. A nice handbook for quick reference by cardiologists and anesthesiologists. Includes a CD with video clips of intraoperative studies.

3. Oxorn DC: Intraoperative echocardiography. Heart 94: 1236–1243, 2008.

   A brief review that provides an overview of intraoperative TEE for the general cardiologist including a list of evidence-based indications and illustrations of typical findings. There are 32 key references with annotations.

Monitoring Ventricular Function and Noncardiac Surgery

4. Oxorn DC: Monitoring ventricular function in the operating room: impact on clinical outcomes. In Otto CM (ed): The Practice of Clinical Echocardiography, 3rd ed. Philadelphia: Elsevier/ Saunders, 2007, p 31–61.

   Review of the use of TEE by a cardiac anesthesiologist for monitoring ventricular function in the operating room. This chapter also has detailed sections on special situations including separation from cardiopulmonary bypass, off-pump coronary bypass surgery, positioning of intravascular devices, and transplant surgery. 139 references.

5. Denault AY, Couture P, McKenty S, et al: Perioperative use of transesophageal echocardiography by anesthesiologists: impact in noncardiac surgery and in the intensive care unit. Can J Anaesth 49: 287–293, 2002.

   In 214 patients undergoing TEE by anesthesiologists in the noncardiac operating room or recovery room (74%), or in the intensive care unit (26%), TEE findings resulted in a change in therapy in 60% of those with a definite indication for TEE. Most often these were changes in medical therapy. Findings leading to a new or modified surgical procedure included cardiac tamponade in eight patients, aortic dissection in two patients, and RV dysfunction in two patients. In a table summarizing 22 previous studies, TEE during noncardiac surgery changed clinical management in between 11% and 80% of patients, depending on the study group, and resulted in changes in surgical management in 3% to 24% of patients overall.

6. Memtsoudis SG, Rosenberger P, Loffler M, et al: The usefulness of transesophageal echocardiography during intraoperative cardiac arrest in noncardiac surgery. Anesth Analg 102: 1653–1657, 2006.

   In 22 patients with unexpected intraoperative hemodynamic collapse during noncardiac surgery, intraoperative TEE provided an etiologic diagnosis in 19 (84%), including thromboembolic events in 9, acute myocardial ischemia in 6, hypovolemia in 2, and pericardial tamponade in 2 patients. In 12 of these patients (55%), the TEE diagnosis led to additional surgical procedures.

7. Norrild K, Pedersen TF, Sloth E: Transesophageal tissue Doppler echocardiography for evaluation of myocardial function during aortic valve replacement. J Cardiothorac Vasc Anesth 21: 367–370, 2007.

   This pilot study showed that accurate tissue Doppler velocity data can be acquired by intraoperative TEE at baseline and after cardiopulmonary bypass. However, strain and strain rate measurements were often unreliable during and after cardiopulmonary bypass.

Mitral Valve Repair

8. Stewart WJ, Griffin BF: Intraoperative echocardiography in mitral valve repair. In Otto CM (ed): The Practice of Clinical Echocardiography, 3rd ed.

Philadelphia: Elsevier/Saunders, 2007, p 459–480.

This chapter provides details on intraoperative echocardiography for decision making and assessing the results of mitral valve repair procedures. The pre-pump and post-pump findings and clinical significance are reviewed and complications of mitral valve repair are illustrated. 102 references.

9. Shah P: Intraoperative echocardiography for mitral valve disease. In Otto CM, Bonow R: Valvular Heart Disease, A Braunwald Companion. 3rd ed. Philadelphia: Elsevier/Saunders, 2009, Chapter 20.

This chapter includes a comprehensive discussion of the indications, approach, and findings of intraoperative TEE for mitral valve repair. Clear explanations of terminology for leaflet anatomy and motion with examples of TEE views used to examine the valve. Other topics include quantitation of regurgitant severity and impact of TEE findings on surgical management and long-term clinical outcome. More than 20 illustrations.

10. Foster GP, Isselbacher EM, Rose GA, et al: Accurate localization of mitral regurgitant defects using multiplane transesophageal echocardiography. Ann Thorac Surg 65: 1025–1031, 1998.

Clear description and diagrams of the TEE approach to evaluation of the segmental anatomy of the mitral valve. Source of Figures 18–14 and 18–16 are redrawn from this article.

11. Fedak PW, McCarthy PM, Bonow RO: Evolving concepts and technologies in mitral valve repair. Circulation 117: 963–974, 2008.

Excellent review article discussing the most common mitral valve pathologies leading to valve surgery—myxomatous, functional, and ischemic—followed by descriptions and illustrations of current and emerging approaches to mitral valve repair. 120 references.

Hypertrophic Cardiomyopathy

12. Ommen SR, Park SH, Click RL, et al: Impact of intraoperative transesophageal echocardiography in the surgical management of hypertrophic cardiomyopathy. Am J Cardiol 90: 1022–1024, 2002.

The findings with intraoperative monitoring of surgical myectomy in 256 consecutive patients are reported. In addition to monitoring the procedure, baseline evaluation is important for detection of other structural abnormalities. After the procedure, unexpected severe mitral regurgitation was seen in 8 patients and a ventricular septal defect was found in 2 patients.

13. Woo A, Wigle ED, Rakowski H: Echocardiography in the evaluation and management of patients with hypertrophic cardiomyopathy. In Otto CM (ed): The Practice of Clinical Echocardiography, 3rd ed. Philadelphia: Elsevier/Saunders, 2007, p 459–480.

This chapter on all aspects of echocardiography in patients with hypertrophic cardiomyopathy includes a section on intraoperative echocardiography and on outcomes following myectomy. There are several figures on intraoperative evaluation and more than 20 references in this section.

Ventricular Assist Devices

14. Chumnanvej S, Wood MJ, MacGillivray TE, et al: Perioperative echocardiographic examination for ventricular assist device implantation. Anesth Analg 105: 583–601, 2007.

A well-written and detailed review of ventricular assist device function, echocardiography before implantation, evaluation of assist device function, and detection of device complications. Includes excellent illustrations and over 150 references.

15. Wu AH: End-stage heart failure: ventricular assist devices and the post-transplant patient. In Otto CM (ed): The Practice of Clinical Echocardiography, 3rd ed. Philadelphia: Elsevier/Saunders, 2007, p 735–752.

About half of this chapter details echocardiographic evaluation of ventricular assist devices. The types of devices and changes in cardiac structure after device implantation are also summarized. Approaches to diagnosing assist device malfunction and assessing myocardial recovery are reviewed.

16. Sukernik MR, Bennett-Guerrero E: The incidental finding of a patent foramen ovale during cardiac surgery: Should it always be repaired? A core review. Anesth Analg 105: 602–610, 2007.

A PFO is a common finding on intraoperative TEE given the normal prevalence of 20% to 30% in the general population. PFO closure is considered when there is a high risk of hypoxemia and after placement of a left ventricular assist device or when closure can be performed easily, for example at the time of mitral valve surgery. If PFO closure is deferred at the time of surgery but then needed later, percutaneous closure is an option.

Guidelines

17. Shanewise JS, Cheung AT, Aronson S, et al: ASE/SCA guidelines for performing a comprehensive intraoperative multiplane transesophageal echocardiography examination: Recommendations of the American Society of Echocardiography Council for Intraoperative Echocardiography and the Society of Cardiovascular Anesthesiologists Task Force for Certification in Perioperative Transesophageal Echocardiography. Anesth Analg 89: 870–884, 1999.

The article defines the standard intraoperative TEE examination as summarized in Figure 18–5. The probe positions and rotation angle for image acquisition are detailed, and technical aspects of data acquisition are addressed.

18. Cahalan MK, Stewart W, Pearlman A, et al; American Society of Echo-cardiography and Society for Cardio-vascular Anesthesiologists Task Force. Guidelines for Training in Per-ioperative Echocardiography. J Am Soc Echocardiogr 15: 647–652, 2002.

Training guidelines for anesthesiologists using echocardiography are proposed with a distinction between Basic Training (use of echocardiography for monitoring and screening) and Advanced Training (use of echocardiography for diagnosis and quantitation of cardiac disease).

19. Mathew JP, Glas K, Troianos CA, et al; Council for Intraoperative Echocardiography of the American Society of Echocardiography: ASE/SCA recommendations and guidelines for continuous quality improvement in perioperative echocardiography. Anesth Analg 103: 1416–1425, 2006.

These guidelines provide detailed tables of the cognitive and technical skills needed to perform basic and advanced intraoperative TEE. Training guidelines and recommendations for maintenance of competence are summarized. In addition to training guidelines, specific recommendations for continuous quality improvement are provided, including equipment standards, periodic review, continuing medical education, utilization review, and continuous quality improvement documentation.

20. Glas KE, Swaminathan M, Reeves ST, et al; Council for Intraoperative Echocardiography of the American Society of Echocardiography; Society of Cardiovascular Anesthesiologists; Society of Thoracic Surgeons. Guidelines for the performance of a comprehensive intraoperative epiaortic ultrasonographic examination:*

Recommendations of the American Society of Echocardiography and the Society of Cardiovascular Anesthesiologists; endorsed by the Society of Thoracic Surgeons. Anesth Analg 106:1376–1384, 2008.

Epiaortic scanning is more sensitive than TEE for detection of ascending aortic atheroma and is recommended in patients undergoing open-heart surgery who are at increased risk of embolic stroke. A comprehensive study includes three short-axis views of the ascending aorta (proximal, mid-, and distal) and two long-axis views (proximal and distal). The location of any plaques should be described, with measurement of plaque thickness and notation of any mobile components. There is an increased risk of adverse neurologic outcomes with plaques >3 mm thick or with mobile components, which should be discussed with the surgeon before manipulation of the aorta.

The Echo Exam: Quick Reference Guide

Basic Principles

Optimization of Echocardiographic Images		
Instrument Control	**Data Optimization**	**Clinical Issues**
Transducer	• Different transducer types and transmission frequencies are needed for specific clinical applications. • Transmission frequency is adjusted for tissue penetration in each patient and for ultrasound modality (Doppler vs imaging).	• A higher transducer frequency provides improved resolution but less penetration. • A larger aperture provides a more focused beam.
Power output	• Power output reflects the amount of ultrasound energy transmitted to the tissue. • Higher power output results in greater tissue penetration.	• Potential bioeffects must be considered. • Exam time and mechanical and thermal indexes should be monitored.
Imaging mode	• 2D imaging is the clinical standard for most indications. • M-mode provides high time resolution along a single scan line. • 3D imaging provides appreciation of spatial relationships.	• Optimal measurement of cardiac chambers and vessels may require a combination of imaging modes.
Transducer position	• Acoustic windows allow ultrasound tissue penetration without intervening lung or bone tissue. • Transthoracic acoustic windows include parasternal, apical subcostal, and suprasternal. • TEE acoustic windows include high esophageal and transgastric.	• Optimal patient positioning is essential for acoustic access to the heart. • Imaging resolution is optimal when the ultrasound beam is reflected perpendicular to the tissue interface. • Doppler signals are optimal when the ultrasound beam is aligned parallel to flow.
Depth	• Depth is adjusted to show the structure of interest. • Pulse repetition frequency (PRF) depends on maximum image depth.	• PRF is higher at shallow depths, which contributes to improved image resolution. • Axial resolution is the same along the entire length of the ultrasound beam. • Lateral and elevations resolution depends on the 3D shape of the ultrasound beam at each depth.
Sector width	• Standard sector width is 60° but a narrower sector allows a higher scan-line density and faster frame rate.	• Sector width should be adjusted as needed to optimize the image. • Too narrow a sector may miss important anatomic or Doppler findings.
Gain	• Overall gain affects the display of the reflected ultrasound signals.	• Excessive gain obscures border identification. • Inadequate gain results failure to display reflections from tissue interfaces.
TGC	• Time gain compensation (TGC) adjusts gain differentially along the length of the ultrasound beam to compensate for the effects of attenuation.	• An appropriate TGC curve results in an image with similar brightness proximally and distally in the sector image.
Gray scale/ dynamic range	• Ultrasound amplitude is displayed using a decibel scale in shades of gray.	• The range of displayed amplitudes is adjusted to optimize the image using the dynamic range or compression controls.

Continued

Optimization of Echocardiographic Images—Cont'd

Instrument Control	Data Optimization	Clinical Issues
Harmonic imaging	• Harmonic frequencies are proportional to the strength of the fundamental frequency but increase with depth of propagation.	• Harmonic imaging improves endocardial definition and decreases near-field and side-lobe artifacts. • Flat structures, such as valves, appear thicker with harmonic than with fundamental imaging. • Axial resolution is reduced.
Focal depth	• Transducer design parameters that affect focal depth include array pattern, aperture size, and acoustic focusing.	• The ultrasound beam is most focused at the junction between the near zone and far field of the beam pattern. • Transducer design allows a longer focal zone. In some cases, focal zone can be adjusted during the examination.
Zoom mode	• The ultrasound image can be restricted to a smaller depth range and narrow section. The maximum depth still determines PRF, but scan-line density and frame rate can be optimized in the region of interest.	• Zoom mode is used to examine areas of interest identified on standard views.
ECG	• The ECG signal is essential for triggering digital cine loop acquisition.	• A noisy signal or low-amplitude QRS results in incorrect triggering or inadvertent recording of an incomplete cardiac cycle.

Optimization of Doppler Recordings

Modality	Data Optimization	Common Artifacts
Pulsed	• 2D guided with "frozen" image • Parallel to flow • Small sample volume • Velocity scale at Nyquist limit • Adjust baseline for aliasing • Use low-wall filters • Adjust gain and dynamic range	• Nonparallel angle with underestimation of velocity • Signal aliasing; Nyquist limit = ½ PRF • Signal strength/noise
Continuous wave (CW)	• Dedicated non-imaging transducer • Parallel to flow • Adjust velocity scale so flow fits and fills the displayed range • Use high-wall filters • Adjust gain and dynamic range	• Nonparallel angle with underestimation of velocity • Range ambiguity • Beam width • Transit-time effect
Color flow	• Use minimal depth and sector width for flow of interest (best frame rate) • Adjust gain just below random noise • Color scale at Nyquist limit • Decrease 2D gain to optimize Doppler signal	• Shadowing • Ghosting • Electronic interference

Transthoracic Echocardiography: Core Elements

A Complete Transthoracic Echo Exam Consists of Core Elements + Additional Components			
Modality	**Window**	**View/Signal**	**Basic Measurements**
Clinical data		Indication for echo Key history and physical findings Previous cardiac imaging data	Blood pressure at time of echo exam
2D imaging	Parasternal	Long-axis Short-axis aortic valve Short-axis mitral valve Short-axis LV (papillary muscle level) RV-inflow	LV ED and ES dimensions LV ED wall thickness Aortic ED sinus dimension LA dimension
	Apical	Four-chamber Anteriorly angulated four-chamber Two-chamber Long-axis	Visual estimate or biplane EF
	Subcostal	Four-chamber IVC with respiration Proximal abdominal aorta	
	Suprasternal	Aortic arch	
Pulsed Doppler	Parasternal	PA-flow	PA velocity
	Apical	LV-inflow	*E*-velocity *A*-velocity
		LV-outflow	LV outflow velocity
Color flow	Parasternal	Long-axis: aortic and mitral valves Short-axis: aortic and pulmonic valves RV-inflow: tricuspid valve	Color flow to identify regurgitation of all four valves. If more than mild, measure vena contracta.
	Apical	Four-chamber: mitral and tricuspid valves Long-axis: aortic and mitral valves	
CW Doppler	Parasternal	Tricuspid valve Pulmonic valve	TR-jet velocity
	Apical	Aortic valve Mitral valve Tricuspid valve	Aortic velocity TR jet (pulmonary pressures)

A, atrial; *E*, early-diastolic; EF, ejection fraction; ES, end-systolic; IVC, inferior vena cava; LV, left ventricle; PA, pulmonary artery; RV, right ventricle; TR, tricuspid regurgitant.

Transthoracic Echo: Additional Components

Transthoracic Echocardiography: Additional Components

Abnormality on Core Elements	Additional Echo Exam Components (Chapter)
Reason for Echo	**Additional Components to Address Specific Clinical Question***
Left Ventricle	
Decreased EF	See Systolic Function (6)
Abnormal LV filling velocities	See Diastolic Function (7)
Regional wall motion abnormality	See Ischemic Cardiac Disease (8)
Increased wall thickness	See Hypertrophic Cardiomyopathy, Restrictive Cardiomyopathy, and Hypertensive Cardiac Disease (9)
Valves	
Imaging evidence for stenosis or an increased antegrade transvalvular velocity	See Valvular Stenosis (11)
Regurgitation greater than mild on color flow imaging or CW Doppler	See Valvular Regurgitation (12)
Prosthetic valve	See Prosthetic Valves (13)
Valve mass or suspected endocarditis	See Endocarditis and Cardiac Masses (14,15)
Right Heart	
Enlarged RV	See Pulmonary Heart Disease and Congenital Heart Disease (9,17)
Elevated TR-jet velocity	See Pulmonary Pressures (6)
Pericardium	
Pericardial effusion	See Pericardial Effusion (10)
Pericardial thickening	See Pericardial Constriction (10)
Great Vessels	
Enlarged aorta	See Aortic Disease (16)

*The echo exam should always include additional components to address the clinical indication. For example, if the indication is "heart failure," additional components to evaluate systolic and diastolic function are needed even if the Core Elements do not show obvious abnormalities. If the indication is "cardiac source of embolus," the Additional Components for that diagnosis are needed.

Principles of Doppler Quantitation

Method	Assumptions/Characteristics	Examples of Clinical Applications
Volume flow $SV = CSA \times VTI$	• Laminar flow • Flat flow profile • Cross-sectional area (CSA) and velocity time integral (VTI) measured at same site	• Cardiac output • Continuity equation for valve area • Regurgitant volume calculations • Intracardiac shunts, pulmonary-to-systemic flow ratio
Velocity-pressure relationship $\Delta P = 4v^2$	• Flow-limiting orifice • CW Doppler signal recorded parallel to flow	• Stenotic valve gradients • Calculation of pulmonary pressures • LV dP/dt
Spatial flow patterns	• Proximal flow convergence region • Narrow flow stream in orifice (vena contracta) • Downstream flow disturbance	• Detection of valve regurgitation and intracardiac shunts • Level of obstruction • Quantitation of regurgitant severity

Basic Transesophageal Exam

Basic Transesophageal Exam			
Probe Position	**Rotation Angle**	**Views**	**Focus**
High esophageal *Set depth to include LV apex.*	0° 60° 120°	Four-chamber Two-chamber Long-axis	• LV size, global and regional function • RV size and systolic function • LA and RA size
High esophageal ↓*Depth to optimize valves*	120° 120° → 0°	Long-axis Two-chamber Four-chamber	• Mitral valve
	120° 30°–50°	Long-axis Short-axis	• Aortic valve • Aorta
	0° 60° 90°	↓Depth	• LA appendage (resolution mode, 7 MHz) • Pulmonary veins
	0° → 90°	Rotational scan	• Atrial septum
	0° 90°	Four-chamber Bicaval view	• RV • RA • Superior and inferior vena cava
	0° 60° 90°	Four-chamber Short-axis RV-outflow	• Tricuspid valve • Pulmonic valve and pulmonary artery
Transgastric (TG)	0°	Short-axis	• LV wall motion, wall thickness, chamber dimensions • RV size and function
	90°	Long-axis	• LV and mitral valve • Turn medially to image RV and tricuspid valve
TG apical	0°	Four-chamber	• Useful for antegrade aortic flow but may still be nonparallel intercept angle
TG to high esophageal	0°	Short-axis descending aorta	• Image aorta from the diaphragm to aortic arch

Advanced Echocardiographic Modalities

Advanced Echocardiographic Modalities

Modality	Instrumentation	Clinical Utility	Special Training
3D Echo	Volumetric or 2D image acquisition Various display formats	• Rapid acquisition for LV regional function • Mitral valve anatomy • Atrial septal defects (ASDs)	• Image acquisition and analysis
Tissue Doppler strain rate and strain	Tissue Doppler and 2D imaging are used to measure strain rate: $SR = (V_2 - V_1)/D$	• Strain rate is a measure of ventricular contractility. • Strain rate is integrated to determine strain, a measure of regional myocardial function.	• Data acquisition and analysis • Clinical interpretation of data
Myocardial speckle tracking	Strain is measured directly from the motion of myocardial speckles as: $[(L - L_o)/L_o] \times 100\%$	• Myocardial speckle tracking is angle independent. • Analysis can be performed after image acquisition.	• Data acquisition and analysis • Clinical interpretation of data
Myocardial dyssynchrony	Multiple 2D, pulsed Doppler, and tissue Doppler methods	• The degree of dyssynchrony may predict the response to dual-chamber pacer therapy.	• Data acquisition and analysis • Clinical interpretation of data
Contrast echo	Microbubbles for right or left heart contrast	• Detection of patent foramen ovale • LV endocardial definition	• IV administration of contrast agents • Knowledge of potential risks
Intracardiac echo	5–10 MHz catheter-like intracardiac probe	• Interventional procedures (ASD closure) • Electrophysiology procedures	• Invasive cardiology training and experience
Intravascular ultrasound	30–50 MHz intracoronary catheter	• Degree of coronary narrowing and plaque morphology	• Interventional cardiology training
Hand-held ultrasound	Small, inexpensive ultrasound instruments	• Besides evaluation by physician for pericardial effusion, LV global and regional function	• At least Level 1 echo training

Diagram of the level of echocardiography training and the level of training in other skills for each of the echocardiographic modalities. All physicians perform physical examinations. Although hand-held echocardiography extends the physical examination, at least basic training and experience are needed for accurate clinical use. TTE is followed in level of training by TEE. The practice of stress echocardiography, contrast echocardiography, and 3D echocardiography requires other skills in addition to echocardiography, for example, the safe performance of a stress study. Intravascular ultrasound typically requires advanced skills as an interventional cardiologist but only basic ultrasound training. ICE requires advanced invasive cardiology skills, preferably in combination with Level 2 training in Echocardiography given the complexity of the imaging data available with this modality.

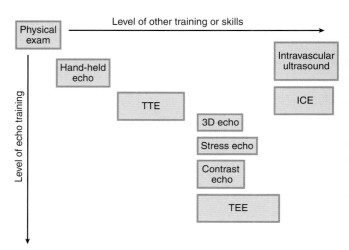

Indications for Echocardiography

Clinical Diagnosis	Key Echo Findings	Limitations of Echo	Alternate Approaches
Valvular Heart Disease			
Valve stenosis	Etiology of stenosis, valve anatomy Transvalvular ΔP, valve area Chamber enlargement and hypertrophy LV and RV systolic function Associated valvular regurgitation	Possible underestimation of stenosis severity Possible coexisting coronary artery disease	Cardiac cath CMR
Valve regurgitation	Mechanism and etiology of regurgitation Severity of regurgitation Chamber enlargement LV and RV systolic function PA pressure estimate	TEE may be needed to evaluate MR severity and valve anatomy (esp. before mitral valve repair).	Cardiac cath CMR
Prosthetic valve function	Evidence for stenosis Detection of regurgitation Chamber enlargement Ventricular function PA pressure estimate	Imaging prosthetic valves is limited by shadowing and reverberations. TEE is needed for suspected prosthetic MR due to "masking" of the LA on TTE.	Cardiac cath Fluoroscopy
Endocarditis	Detection of vegetations (TTE sensitivity 70% to 85%) Presence and degree of valve dysfunction Chamber enlargement and function Detection of abscess Possible prognostic implications	TEE more sensitive for detection of vegetations (>90%) A definite diagnosis of endocarditis also depends on bacteriologic criteria. TEE more sensitive for abscess detection	Blood cultures and clinical findings also are diagnostic criteria for endocarditis.
Coronary Artery Disease			
Acute myocardial infarction	Segmental wall motion abnormality reflects "myocardium at risk." Global LV function (EF) Complications: Acute MR vs VSD Pericarditis LV thrombus, aneurysm RV infarct	Coronary artery anatomy itself not directly visualized	Coronary angio (cath or CT) Radionuclide or PET perfusion imaging

Continued

475

Clinical Diagnosis	Key Echo Findings	Limitations of Echo	Alternate Approaches
Angina	Global and segmental LV systolic function Exclude other causes of angina (e.g., AS, HOCM)	Resting wall motion may be normal despite significant coronary artery disease. Stress echo needed to induce ischemia and wall motion abnormality.	Coronary angio (cath or CT) Radionuclide or PET perfusion imaging ECG exercise stress test
Pre- and post-revascularization	Assess wall thickening and endocardial motion at baseline. Improvement in segmental function post-procedure	Dobutamine stress and/or contrast echo needed to detect viable but nonfunctioning myocardium	CMR Coronary angio (cath or CT) Radionuclide or PET perfusion imaging Contrast echo
End-stage ischemic disease	Overall LV systolic function (EF) PA pressure Associated MR LV thrombus RV systolic function		Coronary angio (cath or CT) Radionuclide or PET perfusion imaging CMR for myocardial viability
Cardiomyopathy			
Dilated	Chamber dilation (all four) LV and RV systolic function (qualitative and EF) Coexisting mitral valve regurgitation PA systolic pressure LV thrombus	Indirect measures of LV EDP Accurate EF may be difficult if image quality poor.	Radionuclide EF LV and RV angio
Restrictive	LV wall thickness LV systolic function LV diastolic function PA systolic pressure	Must be distinguished from constrictive pericarditis.	Cardiac cath with direct, simultaneous RV and LV pressure measurement after volume loading
Hypertrophic	Pattern and extent of LV hypertrophy Dynamic LVOT obstruction (imaging and Doppler) Coexisting MR Diastolic LV dysfunction		
Hypertension	LV wall thickness and chamber dimensions LV mass LV systolic function Aortic root dilation Aortic regurgitation		

	Findings	Comments	Alternative Techniques
Pericardial Disease			
	Pericardial thickening 2D signs of tamponade physiology Detection, size, and location of effusion Doppler signs of tamponade physiology	Diagnosis of tamponade is a hemodynamic and clinical diagnosis. Constrictive pericarditis is a difficult diagnosis. Not all patients with pericarditis have an effusion.	Intracardiac pressure measurements for tamponade or constriction CMR or CT to detect pericardial thickening
Aortic Disease			
Aortic dilation	Etiology of aortic dilation Accurate aortic diameter measurements Anatomy of sinuses of Valsalva (esp. Marfan syndrome) Associated aortic regurgitation		CT, CMR, aortography
Aortic dissection	2D images of ascending aorta (PLAX, PSAX), aortic arch (SSN), descending thoracic (A2C), and proximal abdominal (SC) aorta Imaging of dissection "flap" Associated aortic regurgitation Ventricular function	TEE more sensitive (97%) and specific (100%) Cannot assess distal vascular beds.	Aortography CT CMR TEE
Cardiac Masses			
LV thrombus	High sensitivity and specificity for diagnosis of LV thrombus Suspect with apical wall motion abnormality or diffuse LV systolic dysfunction	Technical artifacts can be misleading. 5-MHz or higher frequency transducer and angulated apical views needed	LV thrombus may not be recognized on radionuclide or contrast angio.
LA thrombus	Low sensitivity for detection of LA thrombus, although specificity is high Suspect with LA enlargement, mitral valve disease	TEE is needed to detect LA thrombus reliability.	TEE
Cardiac tumors	Size, location, and physiologic consequences of tumor mass	Extracardiac involvement not well seen Cannot distinguish benign from malignant, or tumor from thrombus	TEE CT CMR Intracardiac echo

Continued

Indications for Echocardiography—Cont'd

Clinical Diagnosis	Key Echo Findings	Limitations of Echo	Alternate Approaches
Pulmonary Hypertension			
	Estimate of PA pressure Evidence of left-sided heart disease to account for increased PA pressures RV size and systolic function (cor pulmonale) Associated tricuspid regurgitation	Indirect PA pressure measurement Unable to determine pulmonary vascular resistance accurately	Cardiac cath
Congenital Heart Disease			
	Detection and assessment of anatomic abnormalities Quantitation of physiologic abnormalities Chamber enlargement Ventricular function	No direct intracardiac pressure measurements Complicated anatomy may be difficult to evaluate if image quality is poor (TEE helpful).	CMR with 3D reconstruction Cardiac cath TEE 3D echo

2D, two-dimensional; A2C, apical two-chamber; Angio, angiography; AS, aortic stenosis; Cath, catheterization; CMR, cardiac magnetic resonance imaging; CT, computed tomography; EF, ejection fraction; HOCM, hypertrophic obstructive cardiomyopathy; LA, left atrial; LV, left ventricular; LVEDP, left ventricular end-diastolic pressure; LVOT, left ventricular outflow tract; MHz, megahertz; MR, mitral regurgitation; ΔP, pressure gradient; PA, pulmonary artery; PET, positron emission tomography; PLAX, parasternal long-axis; PSAX, parasternal short-axis; RV, right ventricular; SC, subcostal; SSN, suprasternal notch; TEE, transesophageal echocardiography; TR, tricuspid regurgitation; TTE, transthoracic echocardiography; VSD, ventricular septal defect.

Ventricular Systolic Function

The Echo Exam: Ventricular Systolic Function

	TTE	TEE
Indications	A standard echo exam includes measures of LV and RV size and global and regional systolic function	Nondiagnostic TTE Intraoperative and procedural TEE monitoring Whenever TEE is performed for other indications
LV size and wall thickness	Linear 2D or M-mode LV internal dimensions and wall thickness LV volumes calculated from apical biplane method	Linear dimensions can be measured on transgastric short-axis views. LV volumes can be calculated by the biplane method.
LV EF	Biplane method using four-chamber and two-chamber views, taking care to image from tip of LV apex	Biplane method using TEE four-chamber and two-chamber views, taking care to include LV apex by angulation of the image plane.
LV regional wall motion	Apical four-chamber, apical two-chamber, and long-axis views plus parasternal long- and short-axis views.	TEE four-chamber, two-chamber and long-axis views plus transgastric short-axis view. Apical wall motion may be difficult to assess.
Doppler cardiac output	LVOT and transmitral flows from apical approach. PA flow from parasternal views.	Transmitral flow in four-chamber view. PA flow from high TEE view. LVOT flow sometimes obtained from transgastric long-axis view, but intercept angle may be nonparallel.
LV dP/dt	CW Doppler MR jet	CW Doppler MR jet
RV size and systolic function	Apical and subcostal four-chamber views plus parasternal long- and short-axis views	TEE four-chamber view plus transgastric short-axis and RV-inflow views
PA pressure estimates	TR jet recorded from parasternal and apical views with dedicated CW Doppler transducer	TR jet may be recorded on TEE four-chamber or short-axis views, but underestimation may occur due to a nonparallel intercept angle.

LVOT, left ventricular outflow tract; MR, mitral regurgitation; TR, tricuspid regurgitation.

Technical Details

Parameter	Modality	View	Recording	Measurements
Ejection fraction	2D	A4C and A2C	Adjust depth, optimize endocardial definition, harmonic imaging, contrast if needed.	Careful tracing of endocardial borders at ED and ES in both views
dP/dt	CW Doppler	MR jet, usually from apex	Patient positioning and transducer angulation to obtain highest velocity MR jet, decrease velocity scale, increase sweep speed	Time interval between 1 m/s and 3 m/s on Doppler MR velocity curve
PA pressures	CW Doppler	Parasternal and apical	Patient positioning and transducer angulation to obtain highest velocity TR jet	Estimate of RA pressure from size and appearance of IVC
Cardiac output	2D and pulsed Doppler	Parasternal LVOT diameter	Ultrasound beam perpendicular to LVOT with depth decreased and gain adjusted to see mid-systolic diameter	LVOT diameter from inner edge to inner edge in mid-systole, adjacent and parallel to aortic valve.
		Apical LVOT VTI	LVOT velocity from anteriorly angulated A4C view with sample volume just on LV side of aortic valve	Trace modal velocity of LVOT spectral Doppler envelope.

A2C, apical two-chamber view; A4C, apical four-chamber view; CW, continuous-wave; ED, end-diastole; ES, end-systole; IVC, inferior vena cava; LVOT, left ventricular outflow tract; MR, mitral regurgitation; VTI, velocity-time integral.

Example

A 68-year-old man with a recent inferior MI now is hypotensive. Echocardiography shows:

LV wall thickness (diastole)	8 mm
LV end-diastolic dimension	50 mm
LV end-systolic dimension	33 mm
Apical biplane	
End-diastolic volume (EDV)	106 mL
End-systolic volume (ESV)	62 mL
Time interval between 1 and 3 m/s on MR jet	34 ms
LV segmental wall motion	Akinesis of basal and mid-LV segments of inferior and inferior-lateral walls
RV size	Moderately increased
RV systolic function	Severely decreased
TR-jet velocity (V_{TR})	2.7 m/s
Inferior vena cava	
Diameter	2.0 cm
Inspiratory change	<50%
LVOT diameter ($LVOT_D$)	2.3 cm
LVOT velocity-time integral (VTI_{LVOT})	11 cm
Heart rate	88 beats/min

Interpretation

The LV is normal to small in size, based on diastolic dimensions and volumes, with a mildly reduced ejection fraction (EF) and regional wall motion abnormalities consistent with a recent inferior myocardial infarction. EF is calculated from the apical biplane volumes as:

$$EF = (EDV - ESV)/EDV \times 100\%$$
$$= (106 \text{ mL} - 62 \text{ mL})/106 \text{ mL} \times 100\%$$
$$= 42\%$$

Qualitative evaluation of EF is used only when image quality is too poor for tracing endocardial borders. LV dP/dt is calculated from the time interval between 1 and 3 m/s on the MR-jet signal (dt) as:

$$dP/dt = \left[4(V_2)^2 - 4(V_1)^2\right]/dt$$
$$= [4(3)^2 - 4(1)^2/dt = [36 - 4 \text{ mm Hg}]/.036 \text{ s}$$
$$= 941 \text{ mm Hg/s}$$

which is mildly reduced (normal > 1000 mm Hg/s).

RV size and systolic function are graded qualitatively. The findings of a moderately dilated RV with severe systolic dysfunction in this patient are consistent with RV infarction accompanying the inferior LV infarction, as the coronary artery that supplies the LV inferior wall also often supplies the RV free wall.

RA pressure is moderately elevated (estimate 10-15 mm Hg) as shown by the <50% respiratory change in the diameter of a dilated inferior vena cava (see Table 6-7).

Pulmonary arterial systolic pressure (PAP) is calculated from the TR-jet velocity (V_{TR}) and estimate of RA pressure as:

$$PAP = 4(V_{TR})^2 + RAP = 4(2.7)^2 + 10 = 29 + 10$$
$$= 39 \text{ mm Hg}$$

This is consistent with mild pulmonary hypertension.

Cardiac output is calculated using the LVOT diameter to calculate the circular cross-sectional area (CSA) of flow:

$$CSA_{LVOT} = \pi(LVOT_D/2)^2 = 3.14(2.3/2)^2 = 4.2 \text{ cm}^2$$

Stroke volume (SV) across the aortic valve ($cm^3 = mL$), then is:

$$SV_{LVOT} = (CSA_{LVOT} \times VTI_{LVOT})$$
$$= 4.2 \text{ cm}^2 \times 11 \text{ cm} = 46 \text{ cm}^2$$

CO is:

$$CO = SV \times HR = 46 \text{ mL} \times 88 \text{ beats/min}$$
$$= 4020 \text{ mL/min or } 4.02 \text{ L/min}$$

Cardiac index (CI) is:

$$CI = CO/BSA = 4.02 \text{ L/min}/1.8 \text{ m}^2$$
$$= 2.23 \text{ L/min/m}^2$$

The low CI (normal >2.5 L/min/m^2) is due to the RV infarction resulting in reduced LV preload in combination with mild LV systolic function.

As an internal check of the consistency of the echo data, SV and CO can also be calculated from the 2D apical biplane volume data:

$$SV = EDV - ESV = 106 \text{ mL} - 62 \text{ mL} = 44 \text{ mL}$$
$$CO = SV \times HR = 44 \text{ mL} \times 88 \text{ beats/min}$$
$$= 3872 \text{ mL/min or } 3.87 \text{ L/min}$$

The differences between SVs and COs calculated by the two methods (Doppler and 2D) are consistent with normal measurement error. If significant mitral regurgitation were present, transaortic Doppler SV would be less than the 2D apical biplane SV (see Chapter 12).

Diastolic Dysfunction

Quantitation of Diastolic Function

Parameter	Modality	TTE View	TEE View	Recording	Measurements
LV inflow at leaflet tips	Pulsed Doppler	Apical four-chamber view (A4C) with 2- to 3-mm sample volume positioned at mitral leaflet tips	High TEE 4-chamber view with sample volume at leaflet tips	Parallel to flow Normal expiration Low wall filters	E = early diastolic filling velocity (m/s) A = filling velocity after atrial contraction (m/s) E/A ratio DT = deceleration time (ms)
LV inflow at annulus	Pulsed Doppler	A4C with 2-mm sample volume at mitral annulus	High TEE 4-chamber view with sample volume at mitral annulus	Parallel to flow, normal expiration, low wall filters	A_{dur} = duration of atrial filling velocity in ms
Myocardial tissue Doppler	Pulsed Doppler	A4C with 2- to 3-mm sample volume placed within basal segment of septal wall	High TEE 4-chamber view with 2- to 3-mm sample volume placed within basal segment of septal wall	Very low gain settings Low wall filters	E' = early diastolic tissue Doppler velocity (m/s) A' = diastolic tissue Doppler velocity after atrial contraction (m/s) E/E' = ratio of LV inflow E velocity to tissue Doppler E' velocity
IVRT	Pulsed Doppler	Anteriorly angulated A4C with 3- to 5-mm sample volume midway between aortic and mitral valves	High TEE 4-chamber view angulated toward aortic valve with a 3- to 5-mm sample volume midway between aortic and mitral valves	Clear aortic closing click and clear onset of transmitral flow, low wall filters	IVRT = isovolumic relaxation time (ms)
Pulmonary vein (PV)	Pulsed Doppler (color to guide location)	Right superior PV in A4C view using color flow to visualize flow	Left superior PV from high TEE view (all 4 veins can be used)	2-mm sample volume 1–2 cm into pulmonary vein	PV_S = peak systolic velocity PV_D = peak diastolic velocity PV_a = peak atrial reversal velocity a_{dur} = PV atrial reversal duration (ms)

Diastolic Dysfunction

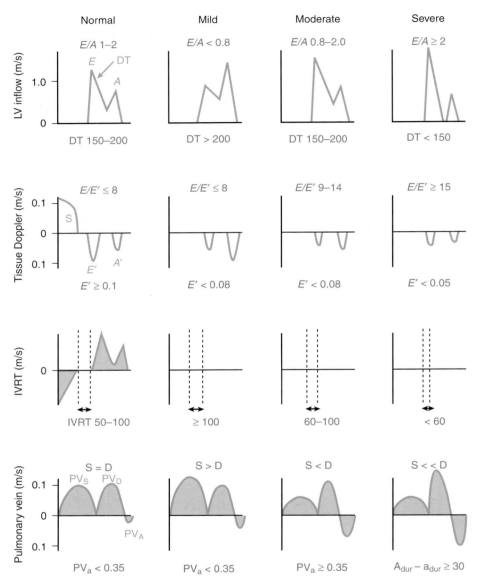

Diagram comparing typical Doppler findings in patients with normal, mild, moderate, and severe diastolic dysfunction. The top row shows LV inflow with early (E) and atrial (A) phases of diastolic filling, the second row shows tissue Doppler recorded at the septal side of the mitral annulus with the myocardial early (E') and atrial (A') velocities and the expected ratio of E/E', the third row shows the isovolumic relaxation time (IVRT), and the bottom row shows the pulmonary vein (PV) inflow pattern with systolic (S) and diastolic (D) antegrade flow and the pulmonary vein atrial (PV_a) reversal of flow.

Classification of Diastolic Dysfunction

Pathophysiology	Normal	Mild ↓ Relaxation	Moderate ↓ Relaxation and ↑ LV EDP	Severe* ↓ Compliance and ↑↑ LV EDP
E/A ratio	1–2	<0.8	0.8–2.0‡	≥2.0
DT (ms)	150–200	>200	150–200	<140
E' velocity (cm/s)	≥10	<8	<8	<5
E/E' ratio	≤8	<8	9–14	≥15
IVRT (ms)	50–100	≥100	60–100	≤60
PV S/D	≅1	S>D	S<D	S ≪ D
PV_a (m/s)	<0.35	<0.35†	≥0.35	≥0.35
$a_{dur} - A_{dur}$ (ms)	<20	<20†	≥30	≥30 ms

DT, deceleration time.

*An additional grade of irreversible severe dysfunction is characterized by the absence of a decrease in E velocity with the strain phase of the Valsalva maneuver.

†PV_a duration and velocity may be increased if filling pressures are elevated.

‡E/A with Valsalva is <1.0.

Modified from Canadian Consensus Guidelines (Rakowki et al: J Am Soc Echocardiogr 9:736–760, 1996; Yamada et al: J Am Soc Echocardiogr 15:1238–1244, 2002; Redfield, JAMA 289:194–202, 2003; Lester et al: J Am Coll Cardiol 51:679–689, 2008.

Example

A 62-year-old man with amyloidosis has an echocardiogram that shows a symmetric increase in wall thickness with an EF of 52%. The following parameters of diastolic function are recorded.

E velocity	1.0 m/s
A velocity	0.6 m/s
DT	160 ms
A_{dur}	130 ms
E'	0.07 m/s
E'/A' ratio	<1
IVRT	40 ms
PV_S/PV_D	<1
PV_a	0.4 m/s
a_{dur}	155 ms

The E/A ratio is >1, but the E'/A' ratio is <1, indicating a pattern of pseudo-normalization suggestive of moderate diastolic dysfunction with decreased compliance. Moderate diastolic dysfunction is confirmed by the short isovolumic relaxation time (IVRT) and relatively short deceleration time (DT).

There also is evidence of elevated filling pressures with an equivocal E/E' ratio of 14, but a $PV_a >$ 0.35 m/s and with the duration of PV atrial flow minus the duration of atrial flow at the mitral annulus >20 ms.

Ischemic Cardiac Disease

Myocardial Ischemia

Stress Echo Modalities

Treadmill exercise
Supine bicycle
Dobutamine

Digital Cine-Loop Views

Short-axis midcavity
Apical four-chamber
Apical two-chamber
Apical (or parasternal) long-axis

Interpretation

Exercise duration
Heart rate and blood pressure
Symptoms
Wall motion at rest and with stress
Ejection fraction at rest and with stress

Utility

Diagnosis of coronary artery disease
Severity of disease
  Number of vessels involved,
  Extent of myocardium at risk
Overall LV systolic function
Diastolic LV function
Clinical prognosis

End-Stage Ischemic Disease

LV Systolic Dysfunction

Decreased ejection fraction
Decreased *dP/dt*
Regional pattern may be seen

RV Systolic Dysfunction

May be present if RV infarction or if pulmonary
  pressures elevated

Mitral Regurgitation

Diverse mechanisms of ischemic MR
  LV dilation and systolic dysfunction
  Regional wall motion abnormality
  PM dysfunction or rupture
Quantitate severity (see Chapter 12)

LV Aneurysm

Diastolic contour abnormality with dyskinesis
Thrombus formation

Differentiation of Left Ventricular Systolic Dysfunction Due to End-Stage Ischemic Disease from Dilated Cardiomyopathy or Chronic Valvular Disease

Findings	End-Stage Ischemic Disease	Dilated Cardiomyopathy	Chronic Valvular Disease
LV ejection fraction	Moderate to severely depressed	Moderate to severely depressed	Moderate to severely depressed
Segmental wall motion abnormalities	May be present	Absent	Absent
RV systolic function	Normal	Decreased	Variable
Pulmonary pressure	Elevated	Elevated	Elevated
Mitral regurgitation	Moderate	Moderate	Moderate to severe
Aortic regurgitation	Not significant	Not significant	Moderate to severe

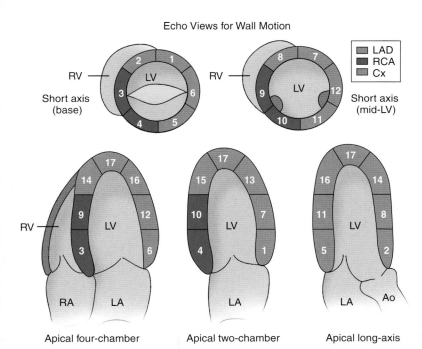

Echo Views for Wall Motion

Echocardiographic views for wall motion evaluation. In the short-axis view, at the base and midventricular levels, the LV is divided into the anterior (1,7), anterior-septal (2, 8), inferior septal (3, 9), inferior (4, 10), inferolateral (5, 11), and anterolateral (6, 12) segments. In the apical region there are four segments: anterior (13), septal (14), inferior (15), and lateral (16), plus the tip of the apex (17). The territory of the LAD artery is indicated in green, the RCA in red, and the left Cx coronary artery in yellow.

Stress Echocardiography

Parameter	Modality	View	Recording	Interpretation
Resting regional wall motion	2D	PSAX mid-cavity level A4C A2C Apical long-axis	Depth that includes only LV, optimize endocardial definition, use contrast if needed	Select optimal image from series of digital cine-loops
Stress regional wall motion	2D	PSAX mid-cavity level A4C A2C Apical long-axis	Same depth as baseline, optimize endocardial definition, use contrast if needed	Compare optimal baseline and stress images in same views
Clinical and hemodynamic data		Symptoms Heart rate and rhythm Blood pressure	Continuous during exam, report values at each stage of stress	Maximal workload affects accuracy of echo results for detection of ischemia
LV systolic function	2D and Doppler	EF dP/dt	Biplane apical EP CW Doppler MR jet	

A2C, apical two-chamber; A4C, apical four-chamber; EF, ejection fraction; PSAX, parasternal short-axis.

Acute Myocardial Infarction

Detection of wall motion abnormalities
Evaluation of recurrent chest pain
Assessment of the response to reperfusion
Complications of acute myocardial infarction
    LV systolic dysfunction
    LV thrombus
    Aneurysm formation
    Acute mitral regurgitation
    Ventricular septal defect
    LV rupture (pseudoaneurysm)
    Pericardial effusion

Cardiomyopathies, Hypertensive and Pulmonary Heart Disease

Echo Differential Diagnosis of Heart Failure

Ischemic disease
Valvular disease
Hypertensive heart disease
Cardiomyopathy
   Dilated
   Hypertrophic
   Restrictive
   Other
Pericardial disease
   Constriction
   Tamponade
Pulmonary heart disease

Cardiomyopathies: Typical Features

	Dilated	Hypertrophic	Restrictive	Athlete's Heart
LV systolic function	Moderately–severely ↓	Normal	Normal	Normal
LV diastolic function	May be abnormal	Abnormal	Abnormal	Normal
LV hypertrophy	↑ LV mass due to LV dilation with normal wall thickness	Asymmetric LV hypertrophy	Concentric LV hypertrophy	Normal wall thickness
Chamber dilation	All four chambers	LA and RA dilation if MR is present	LA and RA dilation	LV dilation
Outflow tract obstruction	Absent	Dynamic LV outflow tract obstruction may be present.	Absent	Absent
LV end-diastolic pressure	Elevated	Elevated	Elevated	Normal
Pulmonary pressure	Elevated	Elevated	Elevated	Normal

MR, mitral regurgitation.

Differentiation of Cause of Increased Wall Thickness

	Hypertensive Heart Disease	Hypertrophic Cardiomyopathy	Restrictive Cardiomyopathy
LV hypertrophy	Present	Present	Present
Pattern of hypertrophy	Concentric	Asymmetric	Concentric
Clinical history of hypertension	Present	Absent	Absent
Outflow obstruction	Midventricular cavity obliteration	Dynamic subaortic obstruction	Absent
RV hypertrophy	Absent	May be present	Present
Pulmonary hypertension	Mild	Mild	Moderate
LV systolic function	Normal initially but may be reduced late in disease course	Normal	Normal initially but may be reduced late in disease course
LV diastolic function	Abnormal	Abnormal	Abnormal

Echo Approach to the Cardiomyopathies

Modality	Echo Views and Flows	Measurements
Imaging	LV size and systolic function	LV EDV, LV ESV Apical biplane EF
	Degree and pattern of LV hypertrophy	LV mass
	Evidence for dynamic outflow tract obstruction	SAM of the mitral valve
	RV size and systolic function	Aortic valve mid-systolic closure
	LA size	
Doppler echo	Associated valvular regurgitation	Measure vena contracta, quantitate if more than mild
	LV diastolic function	Standard diastolic function evaluation with classification of severity and estimate of LV EDP
	LV systolic function	dP/dt from MR jet Calculation of CO
	Pulmonary pressures	TR jet and IVC for PA systolic pressure Evaluate PR jet for PA diastolic pressure Estimate pulmonary resistance
	Color, pulsed, and CW Doppler to quantitate outflow obstruction	Maximum outflow tract gradient

EDP, end-diastolic pressure; EDV, end-diastolic volume; EF, ejection fraction; ESV, end-systolic volume; IVC, inferior vena cava; MR, mitral regurgitation; PA, pulmonary artery; PR, pulmonic regurgitation; SAM, systolic anterior motion; TR, tricuspid regurgitation.

Pericardial Disease

Pericardial Effusion

Views
  Parasternal
  Apical
  Subcostal
Distinguish from pleural fluid
Size
  Small (<0.5 cm)
  Moderate (0.5–2.0 cm)
  Large (>2.0 cm)
Diffuse versus loculated
Evaluate for tamponade physiology if moderate
  or large
TEE if needed, especially in post-op pts

Pericardial Tamponade

Clinical Findings

Low cardiac output
Elevated venous pressures
Pulsus paradoxus
Hypotension

2D Echo

Moderate to large effusion
RA systolic collapse (duration greater than ⅓ of
  systole)
RV diastolic collapse
Reciprocal respiratory changes in RV and LV volumes
Inferior vena cava plethora

Doppler

Respiratory variation in RV and LV diastolic filling
Increased RV filling on first beat after inspiration
Decreased LV filling on first beat after inspiration

Constrictive Pericarditis

M-mode/2D

Pericardial thickening
Normal LV size and systolic function
LA enlargement
Flattened diastolic wall motion
Abrupt posterior motion of the ventricular septum
  in early diastole
Dilated inferior vena cava and hepatic veins

Doppler

Prominent y descent on hepatic vein
  or superior vena cava flow pattern
LV inflow shows prominent E velocity
  with a rapid early-diastolic deceleration slope
  and a small or
  absent A velocity
Increase in LV IVRT by >20%
  on first beat after inspiration
Respiratory variations in RV/LV diastolic filling
  (difference >25%) with
  inspiratory ↑RV ↓LV filling
Tissue Doppler ↑E′
Pulmonary venous flow shows
  prominent a-wave and
  blunting of systolic phase

LV Pseudoaneurysm

Abrupt transition from normal myocardium to
  aneurysm
Acute angle between myocardium and aneurysm
Narrow neck
Ratio of neck diameter to aneurysm diameter <0.5
May be lined with thrombus

Aortic Stenosis

Aortic Stenosis: Echo Approach

Valve anatomy	Calcific Bicuspid (2 leaflets in systole) Rheumatic
Stenosis severity	Jet velocity (V_{max}) Mean pressure gradient (ΔP_{mean}) LVOT/AS velocity ratio Aortic valve area
Coexisting AR	Qualitative evaluation of severity
LV response	LV hypertrophy LV dimensions or volumes LV ejection fraction
Other findings	Pulmonary pressures Mitral regurgitation

AR, aortic regurgitation.

Example

An 82-year-old woman presents with dyspnea on exertion and is noted to have a 3/6 systolic murmur at the base, radiating to the carotids with a single S2 and a diminished carotid upstrokes.

Echocardiography shows a calcified aortic valve with:

Aortic jet velocity (V_{max})	4.2 m/s
Velocity-time integral (VTI_{AS})	68 cm
Mean gradient	45 mm Hg
LV outflow tract diameter ($LVOT_D$)	2.1 cm
LV outflow tract velocity (V_{LVOT})	0.9 m/s
Velocity-time integral (VTI_{LVOT})	14 cm

The *maximum jet velocity* of 4.2 m/s indicates severe stenosis, which is confirmed by calculation of maximum and mean pressure gradients.

Maximum pressure gradient is calculated from maximum aortic jet velocity (V_{max}) as:

$$\Delta P_{max} = 4(V_{max})^2 = 4(4.2)^2 = 71 \text{ mm Hg}$$

Mean pressure gradient is calculated by tracing the outer edge of the continuous wave Doppler velocity curve, with the echo instrument calculating and then averaging instantaneous pressure gradients over the systolic ejection period. The simplified method for estimation of mean gradient is:

$$\Delta P = 2.4(V_{max})^2 = 2.4(4.2)^2 = 42 \text{ mm Hg}$$

In order to correct for transvalvular volume flow rate, the velocity ratio and valve area are calculated:

Velocity ratio is:

$$V_{LVOT}/V_{max} = 0.9/4.2 = 0.21$$

(dimensionless index)

Aortic valve area is:

$$AVA = (CSA_{LVOT} \times VTI_{LVOT})/VTI_{AS\text{-}jet}$$

where cross sectional area (CSA) of the LVOT is:

$$CSA_{LVOT} = \pi(LVOT_D/2)^2 = 3.14(2.1/2)^2 = 3.46 \text{ cm}^2$$

Thus:

$$AVA = (3.46 \text{ cm}^2 \times 14 \text{ cm})/68 \text{ cm} = 0.71 \text{ cm}^2$$

Simplified formula for valve area is:

$$AVA = (CSA_{LVOT} \times V_{LVOT})/V_{max}$$

Thus:

$$AVA = (3.46 \text{ cm}^2 \times 0.9 \text{ cm/s})/4.2 \text{ cm/s} = 0.74 \text{ cm}^2$$

This mean gradient (>40 mm Hg), velocity ratio (<0.25), and valve area (<1.0 cm²) are all consistent with severe stenosis.

Classification of Aortic Stenosis Severity

	Mild	Severe
Jet velocity (m/s)	<3.0	>4.0
Mean gradient (mm Hg)	<20	>40
Velocity ratio	>0.50	<0.25
Valve area (cm²)	>1.5	<1.0

Quantitation of Aortic Stenosis Severity

Components	Modality	View	Recording	Measurements
LVOT diameter ($LVOT_D$)	2D	Parasternal long-axis	Adjust depth, optimize endocardial definition, zoom mode	Inner edge to inner edge of LVOT, parallel and adjacent to aortic valve, mid-systole
LVOT flow V_{LVOT} VTI_{LVOT}	Pulsed Doppler	Apical four-chamber (anteriorly angulated)	Sample volume 2–3 mm, envelope of flow with defined peak, start with sample volume at valve and move apically	Trace modal velocity of spectral velocity curve
AS jet V_{max} VTI_{AS-jet}	CW Doppler	Apical, SSN, other	Examination from multiple windows, careful positioning, and transducer angulation to obtain highest velocity signal	Measure maximum velocities at edge of intense velocity signal $\Delta P_{max} = 4(V_{max})^2$
Continuity equation aortic valve area (AVA)			$AVA(cm^2) = [\pi(LVOT_D/2)^2 \times VTI_{LVOT}]/VTI_{AS-jet}$	
Simplified continuity equation			$AVA(cm^2) = [\pi(LVOT_D/2)^2 \times V_{LVOT}]/V_{AS-jet}$	
Velocity ratio			Velocity ratio $= V_{LVOT}/V_{AS-jet}$	

AS, aortic stenosis; CW, continuous-wave; LVOT, left ventricular outflow tract; SSN, suprasternal notch; V_{LVOT}, LVOT velocity; V_{max}, maximum velocity; VTI, velocity-time integral.

Mitral Stenosis

Mitral Stenosis: Echo Approach

Valve anatomy	Valve thickness and mobility Calcification Commissural fusion Subvalvular involvement
Stenosis severity	2D valve area Mean pressure gradient Pressure half-time valve area
LA	Size TEE for thrombus pre-valvuloplasty
Coexisting MR	Qualitative evaluation of severity
Pulmonary vasculature	Pulmonary systolic pressure RV size and function
Other findings	Aortic valve involvement LV size and systolic function

2D, two-dimensional; MR, mitral regurgitation; TEE, transthoracic echocardiogram.

Example

A 26-year-old pregnant woman presents with dyspnea and is noted to have a diastolic murmur at the apex. Echocardiography shows rheumatic mitral stenosis with:

MVA_{2D}	$0.8\ cm^2$
Mean ΔP	5 mm Hg
$T^{1/2}$	260 ms
MV morphology score:	
Leaflet thickness	2
Mobility	1
Calcification	1
Subvalvular	2
TOTAL	6
Tricuspid regurgitant jet velocity	3.1 m/s
Estimated RA pressure	10 mm Hg
Mitral regurgitation	Mild

Mean pressure gradient is calculated by tracing the outer edge of the continuous-wave Doppler velocity curve, with the echo instrument calculating and then averaging instantaneous pressure gradients over the systolic ejection period.

Doppler mitral valve area ($MVA_{Doppler}$) is calculated as:

$$MVA_{Doppler} = 220/T^{1/2} = 220/260 = 0.85\,cm^2$$

The 2D mitral-valve area and the pressure half time valve area show reasonable agreement, and both are consistent with severe mitral stenosis.

Pulmonary artery pressure (PAP) is:

$$PAP = 4(V_{TR})^2 + RAP = 4(3.1)^2 + 10 \text{ mm Hg}$$
$$= 48 \text{ mm Hg}$$

Pulmonary pressure is moderately elevated consistent with a secondary response to severe mitral stenosis.

The mitral morphology score is low and only mild mitral regurgitation is present, indicating a high likelihood of immediate and long-term success with balloon mitral valvuloplasty. TEE is needed just before mitral valvuloplasty to evaluate for LA thrombus.

Classification of Mitral Stenosis Severity

	Mild	Severe
Mean gradient (mm Hg)	<5	>15
Pulmonary pressure (mm Hg)	<30	>60
Valve area (cm^2)	>1.5	<1.0

Quantitation of Mitral Stenosis Severity

Parameter	Modality	View	Recording	Measurements
2D valve area	2D	Parasternal short-axis	Scan from apex to base to identify minimal valve area.	Planimetry of inner edge of dark/light interface
Mean ΔP	HPRF Doppler	Apical four-chamber or long-axis	Align Doppler beam parallel to stenotic, jet. Adjust angle to obtain smooth envelope with a clear peak and linear deceleration slope.	Trace maximum velocity of spectral velocity curve.
Pressure half-time	HPRF Doppler	Apical four-chamber or long-axis	Same as mean gradient. Adjust scale so velocity curve fills the screen. HPRF Doppler often has less noise than CW Doppler signal.	Place line from maximum velocity along mid-diastolic linear slope. MVA = 220/T½

2D, two-dimensional; CW, continuous-wave; HPRF, high pulse repetition frequency; MVA, mitral valve area.

Aortic Regurgitation

Aortic Regurgitation: Echo Approach	
Etiology	Valve abnormality Dilated aorta
Severity of regurgitation	Vena contracta width Descending aorta holosystolic flow reversal CW Doppler deceleration slope Calculation of RSV, RF, and ROA
Coexisting aortic stenosis	Aortic jet velocity
LV response	LV dimensions or volumes LV ejection fraction *dP/dt*
Other findings	Dilation of sinuses or ascending aorta Aortic coarctation (with bicuspid valve)

CW, continuous-wave; RF, regurgitant fraction; ROA, regurgitant orifice area; RSV, regurgitant stroke volume.

Example

A 37-year-old man presents with an asymptomatic diastolic murmur. Echocardiography shows a bicuspid aortic valve with more than mild aortic regurgitation (AR) with:

Vena contracta width	5 mm
Descending aorta	Holodiastolic flow reversal in descending thoracic, but not proximal abdominal, aorta
CW Doppler	AR signal less dense than antegrade flow $\text{VTI}_{AR} = 150$ cm
LVOT diameter (LVOT_D)	2.8 cm
VTI_{LVOT}	24 cm
Mitral annulus (MA) diameter	3.1 cm
VTI_{MA}	12 cm

The *vena contracta width* indicates more than mild AR, but this could be moderate or severe.

Holodiastolic flow reversal in the proximal abdominal aorta would be consistent with severe AR. Flow reversal in the descending thoracic aorta indicates at least moderate AR but is less specific for severe AR.

CW Doppler signal density indicates at least moderate AR and a deceleration slope >3 m/s^2 but <5 m/s^2 is also consistent with moderate or severe aortic regurgitation.

Next, regurgitant stroke volume (RSV), regurgitant fraction (RF), and regurgitant orifice area (ROA) are calculated.

Using the left ventricular outflow tract (LVOT) and mitral annulus (MA) diameters, the circular cross-sectional areas of flow are calculated:

$$\text{CSA}_{LVOT} = \pi(\text{LVOT}_D/2)^2 = 3.14(2.7/2)^2 = 6.2\,\text{cm}^2$$
$$\text{CSA}_{MA} = \pi(\text{MA}_D/2)^2 = 3.14(3.1/2)^2 = 7.5\,\text{cm}^2$$

Stroke volume (SV) across each valve (cm^3 = mL), then is:

$$\begin{aligned}\text{SV}_{LVOT} &= (\text{CSA}_{LVOT} \times \text{VTI}_{LVOT})\\ &= 6.2\,\text{cm}^2 \times 24\,\text{cm}\\ &= 149\,\text{cm}^3\\ \text{SV}_{MA} &= (\text{CSA}_{MA} \times \text{VTI}_{MA})\\ &= 7.5\,\text{cm}^2 \times 12\,\text{cm} = 91\,\text{cm}^3\end{aligned}$$

Regurgitant stroke volume (RSV) is calculated from total stroke volume (TSV) across the aortic valve and forward stroke volume (FSV) across the mitral valve, as:

$$\text{RSV} = \text{TSV} - \text{FSV} = 149\,\text{mL} - 91\,\text{mL} = 58\,\text{mL}$$

Regurgitant fraction (RF) is:

$$\text{RF} = \text{RSV/TSV} \times 100\% = 58\,\text{mL}/149\,\text{mL} \times 100\%$$
$$= 39\%$$

Regurgitant orifice area (ROA) is:

$$\text{ROA} = \text{RSV}/\text{VTI}_{AR} = 58\,\text{cm}^3/204\,\text{cm} = 0.28\,\text{cm}^2$$

The RSV, RF, and ROA all are consistent with moderate (but nearly severe) AR.

Quantitation of Aortic Regurgitation Severity

Parameter	Modality	View	Recording	Measurements and Calculations
Vena contracta width	Color flow imaging	Parasternal long-axis	Angulate, decrease depth, narrow sector, zoom	Narrowest segment of regurgitant jet between proximal flow convergence and distal jet expansion
Descending aortic diastolic flow reversal	Pulsed Doppler	Subcostal and SSN	Sample volume 2–3 mm, decrease wall filters, adjust scale.	Evidence for holodiastolic flow reversal
CW Doppler signal (intensity, slope, VTI)	CW Doppler	Apical	Careful positioning, and transducer angulation to obtain clear signal	Compare signal intensity of retrograde to antegrade flow, measure slope along edge of dense signal.
Volume flow at 2 sites (RSV, RF, ROA)	2D and pulsed Doppler	Parasternal (2D) and apical	LVOT diameter and VTI Mitral annulus diameter and VTI	$TSV = SV_{LVOT} = (CSA_{LVOT} \times VTI_{LVOT})$ $FSV = SV_{MA} = (CSA_{MA} \times VTI_{MA})$ $RSV = TSV - FSV$ $ROA = RSV/VTI_{AR}$

2D, two-dimensional; CSA, cross-sectional area; CW, continuous-wave; FSV, forward stroke volume; RF, regurgitant fraction; ROA, regurgitant orifice area; RSV, regurgitant stroke volume; SSN, suprasternal notch; TSV, total stroke volume; VTI, velocity-time integral.

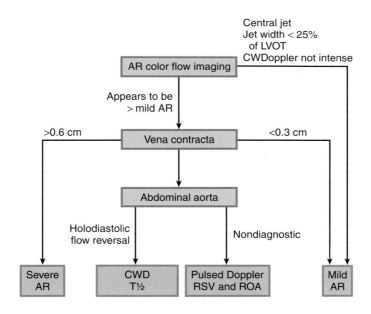

Mitral Regurgitation

Mitral Regurgitation: Echo Approach	
Etiology	Primary valve disease Secondary (functional)

Severity of regurgitation	Vena contracta width
	Jet direction (central, eccentric)
	CW Doppler signal
	Calculation of RSV, RF, and ROA
	Central jet: PISA method
	Eccentric jet
	  Volume flow at two sites
	  Pulmonary vein flow reversal

LV response	LV dimensions or volumes LV ejection fraction dP/dt
Pulmonary vasculature	Pulmonary systolic pressure RV size and systolic function
Other findings	LA size

CW, continuous-wave; RF, regurgitant fraction; ROA, regurgitant orifice area; RSV, regurgitant stroke volume, PISA, proximal isovelocity surface area.

Example

A 52-year-old man with a dilated cardiomyopathy presents with worsening heart failure symptoms.

Echocardiography shows a dilated LV with an EF of 32% and a central jet of mitral regurgitation (MR) with:

Vena contracta width	8 mm
CW Doppler	MR signal as dense as antegrade flow with no evidence for a v-wave $dP/dt = 840$ mm Hg/s Maximum MR velocity $= 4.6$ m/s $VTI_{MR} = 130$ cm
PISA radius	1.2 cm
Aliasing velocity	30 cm/s
Right superior pulmonary vein	Systolic flow reversal

The *vena contracta width* indicates severe mitral regurgitation (MR).

CW Doppler signal density indicates moderate-to-severe MR, and the absence of a v-wave suggests a chronic disease process. The dP/dt is <1000 mm Hg/s, consistent with decreased LV contractility.

Color flow indicates a central jet, so the proximal isovelocity surface area (PISA) method can be used to quantitate regurgitant severity.

The PISA is calculated from the radius measurement as:

$$PISA = 2\pi r^2 = 2\pi(1.0 \text{ cm})^2 = 6.3 \text{ cm}^2$$

The maximum *instantaneous regurgitant flow rate* (R_{FR}) is calculated from PISA and the aliasing velocity ($V_{aliasing}$) as:

$$R_{FR} = PISA \times V_{aliasing} = 6.3 \text{ cm}^2 \times 30 \text{ cm/s}$$
$$= 189 \text{ cm}^3/\text{s}$$

Maximum regurgitant orifice area (ROA) (instantaneous) then is calculated from the R_{FR} and MR jet velocity (where 4.6 m/s $= 460$ cm/s):

$$ROA_{max} = R_{FR}/V_{MR} = (189 \text{ cm}^3/\text{s})/460 \text{ cm/s}$$
$$= 0.41 \text{ cm}^2$$

This ROA is consistent with severe MR.

Regurgitant stroke volume (RSV) over the systolic flow period can be estimated as:

$$RSV = ROA \times VTI_{MR} = 0.41 \text{ cm}^2 \times 130 \text{ cm}$$
$$= 53 \text{ cm}^3 \text{ or mL}$$

This RSV is consistent with moderate MR.

If the jet is eccentric, quantitation should be performed using transaortic (forward) stroke volume and transmitral (total) stroke volume calculations, as illustrated for aortic regurgitation.

Quantitation of Mitral Regurgitation Severity

Parameter	Modality	View(s)	Recording	Measurements and Calculations
Vena contracta width	Color flow imaging	Parasternal long-axis	Angulate, decrease depth, narrow sector, zoom.	Narrowest segment of regurgitant jet between proximal flow convergence and distal jet expansion
Color flow imaging	Color flow imaging	Parasternal and apical	Narrow sector, decrease depth	Central vs eccentric, anterior vs posteriorly directed
CW Doppler signal	CW Doppler	Apical	Careful positioning and transducer angulation to obtain clear signal	Compare signal intensity of retrograde to antegrade flow.
PISA	Color flow imaging	A4C or A long-axis	Decrease depth, narrow sector, zoom mode. Adjust aliasing velocity so PISA is hemispherical, measure from aliasing boundary to orifice.	$PISA = 2\pi r^2$ $R_{FR} = PISA \times V_{aliasing}$ $ROA_{max} = R_{FR}/V_{MR}$ $RSV = ROA \times VTI_{MR}$
Volume flow at 2 sites	2D and pulsed Doppler	Parasternal and apical	LVOT diameter and VTI. Mitral annulus (MA) diameter and VTI	$TSV = SV_{MA} = (CSA_{MA} \times VTI_{MA})$ $FSV = SV_{LVOT} = (CSA_{LVOT} \times VTI_{LVOT})$ $RSV = TSV - FSV$ $ROA = RSV/VTI_{MR}$
2D LV total and Doppler LVOT FSV	2D and pulsed Doppler	Parasternal and apical	LVOT diameter and VTI. Apical biplane LV volumes	$TSV = EDV - ESV$ (on 2D LV volumes) $FSV = SV_{LVOT} = (CSA_{LVOT} \times VTI_{LVOT})$ $RSV = TSV - FSV$ $ROA = RSV/VTI_{MR}$
Pulmonary vein flow	Pulsed Doppler	A4C on TTE but TEE often needed	Pulmonary venous flow in all four veins	Qualitative, systolic flow reversal

A4C; apical four-chamber view; CW, continuous-wave; CSA, cross-sectional area; EDV, end diostolic volume; ESV, end systolic volume; FSV, forward stroke volume; LVOT, left ventricular outflow tract; PISA, proximal isovelocity surface area; R_{FR}, regurgitant instantaneous flow rate; ROA, regurgitant orifice area; RSV, regurgitant stroke volume; TSV, total stroke volume; VTI, velocity-time integral.

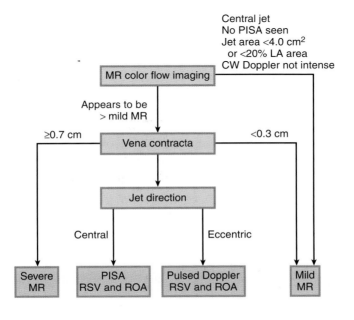

495

Prosthetic Valves

Transthoracic Examination

Imaging	Valve leaflet thickness and motion
	LV size, wall thickness, and systolic function
Doppler	Antegrade prosthetic valve velocity
	Evaluate for stenosis
	Search carefully for regurgitation
	Pulmonary artery pressures

Transesophageal Examination

Imaging	Valve leaflet thickness and motion
	Examine atrial side of mitral prostheses
	LV size, wall thickness, and systolic function
Doppler	Antegrade prosthetic valve velocity
	Evaluate for stenosis.
	Search carefully for regurgitation
	Pulmonary artery pressures

Transthoracic Doppler Evaluation of Prosthetic Valves

Components	Modality	View	Recording	Measurements
Antegrade flow velocity	Pulsed or CW Doppler	Apical	Antegrade transmitral or transaortic velocity	Peak velocity (compare to normal values for valve type and size)
Measures of valve stenosis	Pulsed and CW Doppler	Apical	Careful positioning to obtain highest velocity signal	Mean gradient Aortic valves: ratio of LVOT to aortic velocity Mitral valve: pressure half-time
Valve regurgitation	Color imaging and CW Doppler	Parasternal, apical, SSN	Jet origin, direction and size on color Doppler CW Doppler of each valve Pulmonary vein flow Descending aorta flow	Vena contracta width Intensity of CW Doppler signal Pulmonary vein systolic flow reversal (MR) Descending aorta flow reversal (AR)
Pulmonary pressures	CW Doppler	RV inflow and apical	TR jet velocity IVC size and variation	Calculate PA systolic pressure as $4v^2$ of TR jet plus estimated RA pressure.

AR, aortic regurgitation; CW, continuous-wave; IVC, inferior vena cava; LVOT, left ventricular outflow tract; MR, mitral regurgitation; PA, pulmonary artery; SSN, suprasternal notch; TR, tricuspid regurgitation.

Echocardiographic Signs of Prosthetic Valve Dysfunction

Increased antegrade velocity across the valve
Decreased valve area (continuity equation or $T_{1/2}$)
Increased regurgitation on color flow
Increased intensity of CW Doppler signal
Progressive chamber dilation
Persistent LV hypertrophy
Recurrent pulmonary hypertension

Example

A 62-year-old man with a mechanical mitral valve replacement 2 years ago for myxomatous mitral valve disease presents with increasing heart failure symptoms and a systolic murmur. He is in chronic atrial fibrillation.

Transthoracic echocardiography shows:

LA anterior-posterior dimension	5.7 cm
LV dimensions (systole/diastole)	6.2/3.8 cm
Ejection fraction	56%
Transmitral E velocity	1.8 m/s
Mitral pressure half-time	100 ms
TR jet velocity	3.2 m/s
IVC size and variation	Normal

Color flow imaging shows ghosting and reverberations in the LA region, but no definite regurgitant jet can be identified. CW Doppler shows a mitral regurgitant (MR) signal that is incomplete in duration and not as dense as antegrade flow.

This transthoracic study is difficult to interpret without a previous study for comparison. The LA and LV dilation and the borderline ejection fraction may be residual from before the valve surgery or

TEE Evaluation of Prosthetic Valves

Components	Modality	View	Recording	Limitations
Valve imaging	2D echo	High esophageal	Mitral valve in high esophageal four-chamber view Aortic valve in high esophageal long- and short-axis views	Aortic valve prosthesis may shadow anterior segments of the aortic valve. With both aortic and mitral prostheses, the aortic shadow may obscure the mitral prosthesis.
Antegrade flow velocity	Pulsed or CW Doppler	High esophageal or transgastric apical	Antegrade transmitral or transaortic velocity	Alignment of Doppler beam with transaortic valve flow may be problematic; compare with TTE data.
Measures of valve stenosis	Pulsed and CW Doppler	High esophageal or transgastric apical	Careful positioning to obtain highest velocity signal	Mean gradient Aortic valves: ratio of LVOT to aortic velocity (alignment may be suboptimal) Mitral valve: pressure half-time
Valve regurgitation	Color imaging and CW Doppler	High esophageal with rotational scan	Document origin of jet and proximal flow acceleration, and jet size and direction.	Measure vena contracta, record pulmonary venous flow pattern, search carefully for eccentric jets.
Pulmonary pressures	CW Doppler	RV inflow and apical	TR jet velocity IVC size and variation	Calculate PAP as $4v^2$ of TR jet plus estimated right atrial pressure. May be difficult to align Doppler beam parallel to TR jet, correlate with TTE data.

2D, two-dimensional; CW, continuous-wave; IVC, inferior vena cava; LVOT, LV outflow tract; TR, tricuspid regurgitation; TTE, transthoracic echocardiography.

could represent progressive changes after valve replacement. Pulmonary artery pressure (PAP) is moderately elevated at:

$$PAP = 4(V_{TR})^2 + RAP = 4(3.2)^2 + 10 = 41 + 10$$
$$= 51 \text{ mm Hg}$$

Again, pulmonary hypertension may be residual or recurrent after valve surgery, but the presence of pulmonary hypertension suggests the possibility of significant prosthetic MR. Although a clear regurgitant jet is not demonstrated due to shadowing and reverberations from the valve prosthesis, the high antegrade flow velocity with a short pressure half time and detection of regurgitation with CW Doppler indicate that further evaluation is needed.

TEE demonstrates a paravalvular MR jet with a proximal acceleration region seen at the lateral aspect of the annulus, a vena contracta width of 7 mm, and an eccentric jet directed along the posterior-lateral LA wall. The left pulmonary veins show definite systolic flow reversal; the right pulmonary veins show blunting of the normal systolic flow pattern. These findings are consistent with severe paraprosthetic regurgitation.

On TEE imaging the LV was not well visualized due to shadowing and reverberations from the mitral prosthesis; although transgastric short-axis views were obtained, ejection fraction could not be calculated. The maximum TR jet obtained on TEE was 2.9 m/s. Because a higher jet was obtained on TTE imaging, the TEE jet most likely underestimates pulmonary pressures.

In summary, this patient has severe paraprosthetic MR with LA and LV dilation, moderate pulmonary hypertension and a borderline ejection fraction. As is typical with prosthetic valves, the combination of TTE and TEE imaging was needed for diagnosis.

Endocarditis

Duke Criteria (Short Version)

Definite endocarditis =	2 major or 1 major + 3 minor or 5 minor criteria
Major criteria =	Bacteremia with a typical organism Echo evidence of endocarditis
Minor criteria =	Predisposing condition Fever Vascular phenomenon Immunologic phenomenon Other microbiologic evidence

Echocardiographic Approach

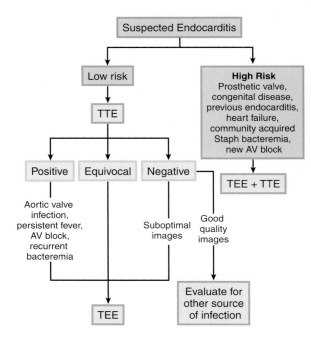

Diagnostic Echo Findings in Endocarditis

	Definition	Exam Points	Diagnostic Value	Limitations
Valvular vegetations	Mass attached to leaflet with independent motion	Use multiple acoustic windows and image planes. Angle between standard views. Use a high-frequency transducer and zoom mode.	Vegetations have high specificity for diagnosis of endocarditis. TEE is more sensitive than TTE for detection of vegetations.	Noninfective masses, healed vegetations, and artifacts may be mistaken for a vegetation.
Leaflet destruction	New or worsening valve regurgitation	Use standard Doppler approaches for detection and quantitation of valve dysfunction.	Valve dysfunction in association with a vegetation is diagnostic for endocarditis.	Other causes of valve dysfunction must be considered. With prosthetic MV, TEE is essential for evaluation of valve function when endocarditis is suspected.
Abscess	Infected area adjacent to valve, usually in the aortic or mitral annulus	Use multiple acoustic windows and image planes. Angle between standard views. Use zoom mode.	TEE is much more sensitive than TTE for detection of paravalvular abscess.	Cardiac abscesses may be echo-lucent or echo-dense.
Aneurysm or pseudoaneurysm	Localized dilation of a valve leaflet, aortic sinus or aortic-mitral intervalvular fibrosa (aneurysm) or a contained rupture (pseudoaneurysm).	Look for an abnormal contour of valve leaflets, aortic sinuses, or a space between the base on the anterior mitral leaflet and aortic root. Examine the para-aortic region for excess echodensity. Use color Doppler to examine flow in these regions.	Echo findings of aneurysm or pseudoaneurysm are accurate and can be used for clinical decision making.	TEE often is needed for accurate diagnosis.
Fistula	Abnormal communication between cardiac chambers or great vessels	An aortic paravalvular abscess can rupture into the LV, LA or RA, or RVOT.	Color Doppler detection of abnormal flow combined with pulsed and CW Doppler to define flow hemodynamics is diagnostic for a fistula.	The full extent of tissue destruction is difficult to assess with imaging approaches.
Prosthetic valve dehiscence	Detachment (partial) of the prosthetic valve from the annular tissue	Look for excess motion ("rocking") of the prosthetic valve (>20°).	Valve dehiscence usually is accompanied by severe paravalvular regurgitation.	Valve "rocking" is diagnostic but rarely seen.

CW, continuous-wave; MV, mitral valve; RVOT, right ventricular outflow tract; TEE, transesophageal echocardiography; TTE transthoracic echocardiography.

Example

A 28-year-old man with a known bicuspid aortic valve (BAV) presents with a 2-week history of fevers and fatigue. Physical examination shows a blood pressure of 120/40 mm Hg and a harsh diastolic murmur at the left sternal border. Blood cultures (3 sets) are positive for *Streptococcus viridans*. With a predisposing factor, fevers, and positive blood cultures with a typical organism, the pre-test likelihood of endocarditis is very high (>90%).

TTE imaging shows a BAV with a mass on the ventricular side of the leaflets with independent motion. LV size and systolic function are normal. Color flow Doppler shows aortic regurgitation (AR) with an eccentric jet and a vena contracta width of 7 mm, CW Doppler shows a dense signal with a deceleration slope of 120 ms, and there is holodiastolic flow reversal in the proximal abdominal aorta.

The TTE findings are diagnostic for endocarditis, so that this patient now has 2 major Duke criteria and a diagnosis of *definite endocarditis*. With his BAV, there may have been some degree of underlying AR. However, the normal LV size and the steep deceleration slope of the CW AR jet are consistent with superimposed *acute* AR. AR is *severe* as evidenced by a wide vena contracta and holodiastolic flow reversal in the aorta.

The following day, a prolonged PR interval (first-degree AV block) is noted on the ECG, and TEE imaging is performed. The TEE shows an echolucent area in the aortic annulus region consistent with abscess, and the patient is referred for prompt surgical intervention.

Cardiac Masses and Source of Embolus

Structures That May Be Mistaken for an Abnormal Cardiac Mass	
Left atrium	Dilated coronary sinus (persistent left superior vena cava) Raphe between left superior pulmonary vein and leftatrial appendage Atrial suture line after cardiac transplant Beam-width artifact from calcified aortic valve, aortic valve prosthesis, or other echogenic target adjacent to the atrium Interatrial aneurysm
Right atrium	Crista terminalis Chiari network (eustachian valve remnants) Lipomatous hypertrophy of the interatrial septum Trabeculation of RA appendage Atrial suture line after cardiac transplant Pacer wire, Swan-Ganz catheter, or central venous line
Left ventricle	Papillary muscles LV web (aberrant chordae) Prominent apical trabeculations Prominent mitral annular calcification
Right ventricle	Moderator band Papillary muscles Swan-Ganz catheter or pacer wire
Aortic valve	Nodules of Arantius Lambl's excrescences Base of valve leaflet seen *en face* in diastole
Mitral valve	Redundant chordae Myxomatous mitral valve tissue
Pulmonary artery	Left atrial appendage (just caudal to pulmonary artery)
Pericardium	Epicardial adipose tissue (especially anteriorly) Fibrinous debris in a chronic organized pericardial effusion

Distinguishing Characteristics of Intracardiac Masses

Characteristic	Thrombus	Tumor	Vegetation
Location	LA (especially when enlarged or associated with MV disease) LV (in setting of reduced systolic function or segmental wall abnormalities)	LA (myxoma) Myocardium Pericardium Valves	Usually valvular Occasionally on ventricular wall or Chiari network
Appearance	Usually discrete and somewhat spherical in shape or laminated against LV apex or LA wall	Various: may be circumscribed or may be irregular	Irregular shape, attached to the proximal (upstream) side of the valve with motion independent from the valve
Associated findings	Underlying etiology usually evident LV systolic dysfunction or segmental wall motion abnormalities (exception: eosinophilic heart disease) MV disease with LA enlargement	Intracardiac obstruction depending on site of tumor Clinically: fevers, systemic signs of endocarditis, positive blood cultures	Valvular regurgitation usually present

MV, mitral valve.

Disease of the Great Vessels

Aortic Dissection

Dissection flap
   In aortic lumen
   Independent motion
   True and false lumen
   Entry sites
   Thrombosis of false lumen
Intramural hematoma
Indirect findings
   Aortic dilation
   Aortic regurgitation
   Coronary ostial involvement
   Pericardial effusion

Sinus of Valsalva Aneurysm

Congenital
   Complex shape
   Protrusion into RVOT
   Fenestrations
Acquired
   Infection or inflammation
   Symmetric shape
   Communication with aorta
   Potential for rupture

Complications of Thoracic Aortic Dissection

Aortic valve regurgitation
   Due to aortic root dilation
   Due to leaflet flail
Coronary artery occlusion
   Ventricular fibrillation
   Acute myocardial infarction
Distal vessel obstruction or occlusion
   Carotid (stroke)
   Subclavian (upper limb ischemia)
Aortic rupture
   Into the pericardium
   Pericardial effusion
   Pericardial tamponade
Into the mediastinum
Into the pleural space
   Pleural effusion
   Exsanguination

Aortic Atheroma

Complex ($\geq$4 mm or mobile)
Associated with
   Coronary artery disease
   Cerebroembolic events

Examination of the Aorta

Aortic Segment	Modality	View	Recording	Limitations
Aortic root	TTE	PLAX	Images of sinuses of Valsalva, aortic annulus, and STJ	Shadowing of posterior aortic root
	TEE	High esophageal long-axis	Standard long-axis plane by rotating to about 120–130°	
Ascending	TTE	PLAX	Move transducer superiorly to image STJ and ascending Ao.	Only limited segments visualized, variable between patients.
	TTE Doppler	Apical	LVOT and ascending Ao flow recorded with pulsed or CW Doppler from an anteriorly angulated four-chamber view	Velocity underestimation if the angle between the Doppler beam and flow is not parallel.
	TEE	High esophageal long-axis	From long-axis view, move transducer superiorly to image ascending Ao	The distal ascending Ao may not be visualized.
Arch	TTE	Suprasternal	Long- and short-axis views of aortic arch	Descending aorta appears to taper as it leaves the image plane.
	TEE	High esophageal	From the short-axis view of the initial segment of the descending thoracic Ao, turn the probe toward the patient's right side and angulate inferiorly.	View not obtained in all patients. The aortic segment at the junction of the ascending Ao and arch may not be visualized.
Descending thoracic	TTE	Parasternal and modified apical views	Rotate from long-axis view to image thoracic Ao in long axis posterior to LV. From apical two-chamber view, use lateral angulation and counterclockwise rotation to image Ao.	Depth of thoracic Ao on TTE limits image quality. TEE usually needed for diagnosis.
	TTE Doppler	Suprasternal	Descending aorta flow recorded with pulsed Doppler from SSN view	Low wall filters needed to evaluate for holodiastolic flow reversal
	TEE	Short-axis aorta	Sequential short-axis views of the aorta from the level of the diaphragm to the arch with the image plane turned posteriorly and the transducer slowly withdrawn in the esophagus	Long-axis views allow further evaluation of abnormal findings
Proximal abdominal	TTE	Subcostal	Long axis of proximal abdominal Ao	Only the proximal segment is visualized.
	TTE Doppler	Transgastric	Proximal abdominal Ao flow recorded with pulsed Doppler	Low wall filters needed to evaluate for holodiastolic flow reversal
	TEE	Transgastric	From the transgastric position, portions of the abdominal Ao may be seen posteriorly.	Does not allow evaluation of entire abdominal Ao.

Ao; aorta; PLAX, parasternal long-axis; SSN, suprasternal notch view; STJ, sinotubular junction; TEE, transesophageal echocardiography; TTE, transthoracic echocardiography.

Adult Congenital Heart Disease

Categories of Congenital Heart Disease

Congenital Stenotic Lesions

Subvalvular
Valvular
Supravalvular
Peripheral great vessels (aortic coarctation)

Congenital Regurgitant Lesions

Myomatous valve disease
Ebstein's anomaly

Abnormal Intracardiac Communications

Atrial septal defect
Ventricular septal defect
Patent ductus arteriosus

Abnormal Chamber and Great Vessel Connections

Transposition of the great arteries
Congenitally corrected transposition (L-TGA)
Tetralogy of Fallot
Tricuspid atresia
Truncus arteriosus

Approach to the Echocardiographic Examination in Adults with Congenital Heart Disease

Before the Examination

Review the clinical history
Obtain details of any prior surgical procedures
Review results of prior diagnostic tests
Formulate specific questions

Sequence of Examination

Identify cardiac chambers, great vessels, and their connections
Identify associated defects, and evaluate the physiology of each lesion
Regurgitation and/or stenosis (quantitate as per Chapters 11 and 12)
Shunts (calculate $Q_p:Q_s$)
Pulmonary hypertension (calculate pulmonary pressure)
Ventricular dysfunction (measure ejection fraction if anatomy allows)

After the Examination

Integrate echo and Doppler findings with clinical data
Summarize findings
Identify which clinical questions remain unanswered, suggest appropriate subsequent diagnostic tests

Clues to the Identification of Cardiac Structures in Adults with Congenital Heart Disease

Structure	Anatomic Feature	Echo Approach
Right atrium	Inferior vena cava enters right atrium	Start with subcostal approach to identify RA
Right ventricle	Prominent trabeculation Moderator band Infundibulum Tricuspid valve Apical location of annulus	Apical four-chamber view to compare annular insertions of two ventricles, parasternal for valve anatomy and infundibulum
Pulmonary artery	Bifurcates	Parasternal long-axis view or apical four-chamber view angulated very anteriorly
Left atrium	Pulmonary veins usually enter left atrium	TEE imaging for pulmonary vein anatomy
Left ventricle	Mitral valve Basal location of annulus Fibrous continuity between anterior mitral leaflet and semilunar valve	Apical four-chamber view and parasternal long- and short-axis views.
Aorta	Gives rise to aortic arch and arterial branches.	Start with parasternal long-axis view and move transducer superiorly to follow vessel to its branches.

Examples

1. A 24-year-old with a history of a cardiac murmur has an echocardiogram which shows:

RV outflow velocity	1.6 m/s
Pulmonary artery (PA) velocity	3.1 m/s
Tricuspid regurgitant (TR) jet	3.4 m/s
Estimated RA pressure	5 mm Hg (small IVC with normal respiratory variation)

Because the RV outflow velocity is elevated, the maximum pulmonic valve gradient should be calculated using the proximal velocity in the Bernoulli equation:

$$\Delta P = 4(V_{jet}^2 - V_{prox}^2)$$
$$\Delta P = 4[(3.1)^2 - (1.6)^2] = 4[9.6 - 2.6] = 28 \text{ mm Hg}$$

If the proximal velocity is not included, the gradient would be overestimated at 38 mm Hg.

Estimated PA systolic pressure (PAP) is calculated by subtracting the pulmonic valve gradient from the estimated RV pressure because pulmonic stenosis is present:

$$PAP = (\Delta P_{RV-RA} + P_{RA}) - \Delta P_{RV-PA}$$
$$PAP = (4V_{TR}^2 + P_{RA}) - \Delta P_{RV-PA} = [4(3.4)^2 + 5] - 28$$
$$= 23 \text{ mm Hg}$$

Thus, PA systolic pressure is normal even though the TR jet correctly indicates a RV systolic pressure of 51 mm Hg.

2. A 26-year-old woman undergoes echocardiography for symptoms of decreased exercise tolerance. She is found to have an enlarged RA and RV with paradoxic septal motion and the following Doppler data:

RV outflow velocity	1.8 m/s
Velocity-time integral (VTI_RVOT)	32 cm
Diameter	2.6 cm
LV outflow velocity	1.1 m/s
Velocity-time integral (VTI_LVOT)	16 cm
Diameter	2.4 cm

The right heart enlargement suggests an atrial septal defect may be present. The shunt ratio is calculated from the ratio of pulmonary flow (Q_p), measured in the RV outflow tract and systemic flow (Q_s), measured in the LV outflow tract. At each site, cross-sectional area (CSA) is calculated as the area of a circle:

$$CSA_{RVOT} = \pi(D/2)^2 = 3.14(2.6/2)^2 = 5.3 \text{ cm}^2$$
$$CSA_{LVOT} = \pi(D/2)^2 = 3.14(2.4/2)^2 = 4.5 \text{ cm}^2$$

Flow (stroke volume) at each site then is calculated:

$$Q_p = CSA_{RVOT} \times VTI_{RVOT} = 5.3 \text{ cm}^2 \times 32 \text{ cm}$$
$$= 170 \text{ cm}^3$$

$$Q_s = CSA_{LVOT} \times VTI_{LVOT} = 4.5 \text{ cm}^2 \times 16 \text{ cm}$$
$$= 72 \text{ cm}^3$$

so that $Q_p/Q_s = 170/72 = 2.4$

These calculations are consistent with a significant shunt that most likely will require closure to prevent progressive right heart dysfunction.

Intraoperative Transesophageal Echocardiography

Basic Principles of Intraoperative Transesophageal Echocardiography

- Establish diagnosis preoperatively when possible
- The goals of the baseline TEE are to:
  - Confirm the diagnosis
  - Provide additional information on repairability
  - Serve as comparison to post-procedure study
  - Assess LV and RV function
  - Check for other abnormalities
- Perform a complete study unless there are clinical or time constraints
- Record post-procedure images at similar loading conditions to baseline
- Communicate and discuss findings at time of study
- Report TEE findings in medical record and store TEE images

Recommended Image Acquisition for Intraoperative TEE

Window	Image Plane	Rotation Angle (approx)	Structure Visualized
Mid esophagus	Four-chamber	0°	LV, RV, LA, RA, MV, TV
	Bicommissural	45°–60°	LV, LA, MV
	Two-chamber	60°–90°	LV, LA, LAA, MV
	Long-axis	120°–140°	LV, LA, MV, AV, Ao
	Long-axis, decreased depth	120°–140°	AV and sinuses, MV
	Long-axis, higher in esophagus	120°–140°	Asc. Ao
	Short-axis Asc. Ao	0°–30°	Asc. Ao, PA
	Short-axis AV	30°–60°	AV
	RV inflow-outflow	60°–90°	RA, TV, RVOT, PV
	Bicaval	80°–110°	SVC, RA, IVC
Transgastric	Short-axis LV	0°–20°	LV, RV
	Short-axis MV	0°–20°	MV
	Two-chamber	80°–100°	LV, MV, LA
	Long-axis	80°–100°	LV, MV, AV
	RV-inflow	80°–100°	RA, TV, RV
Deep transgastric	Four-chamber (with aorta)	0°–20° with anteflexion	LV, LA, Ao, RV
Descending aorta	Short-axis	0°	Desc. Ao
	Long-axis	90°–110°	Desc. Ao
Aortic arch	Long-axis	0°	Arch, L. brachio vein
	Short-axis	90°	Arch, PA

Arch, aortic arch; Asc Ao, ascending aorta; AV, aortic valve; Brachio, brachiocephalic; L, left; IVC, inferior vena cava; LAA, left atrial appendage; MV, mitral valve; PA, pulmonary artery; PV, pulmonary valve; SVC, superior vena cava; TV, tricuspid valve.
Modified from Shanewise JS, Cheung AT, Aronson S, et al: ASE/SCA guidelines for performing a comprehensive intraoperative multiplane transesophageal echocardiography examination: Recommendations of the American Society of Echocardiography Council for Intraoperative Echocardiography and the Society of Cardiovascular Anesthesiologists Task Force for Certification in Perioperative Transesophageal Echocardiography. Anesth Analg 89:870–884, 1999.

INDEX

Note: Numbers followed by f indicates figures and t indicates tables.